Muscle and Tendon Injuries

Gian Luigi Canata • Pieter d'Hooghe
Kenneth J. Hunt
Editors

Muscle and Tendon Injuries

Evaluation and Management

Springer

Editors
Gian Luigi Canata
Koelliker Hospital
Centre of Sports Traumatology
Torino
Italy

Pieter d'Hooghe
Department of Orthopaedic Surgery
Aspetar Hospital Aspire Zone
Doha
Qatar

Kenneth J. Hunt
Department of Orthopedics
University of Colorado Hospital
Aurora, Colorado
USA

ISBN 978-3-662-54183-8 ISBN 978-3-662-54184-5 (eBook)
DOI 10.1007/978-3-662-54184-5

Library of Congress Control Number: 2017941284

Printed on acid-free paper

This Springer imprint is published by Springer Nature
The registered company is Springer-Verlag GmbH Germany
The registered company address is: Heidelberger Platz 3, 14197 Berlin, Germany

Foreword

Dear ISAKOS member,

The Leg Ankle and Foot (LAF) has been recently created. Under the impulsion of the chairs Pieter d'Hooghe, Gian Luigi Canata, and Kenneth Hunt, recognized authors all around the world have worked together in order to provide the best current knowledge about muscle and tendon.

Several chapters are dedicated to basic science. These chapters are crucial to understand the management of lesions. They also allow to define future directions. In this booklet about muscles and tendons, surgical management is challenged by conservative management. Several studies with a high level of evidence had been published comparing these two approaches; it may help the sport medical doctor and surgeon and also the physiotherapist in their research and their clinical practice.

The collection of the ISAKOS booklets is chaired and coordinated by Joao Espregueira Mendes for a few years. These booklets are becoming one of the flags of the education program of ISAKOS.

Thanks to the authors who spent their time to summarize the state of the art in muscle and tendon anatomy, biology, biomechanics, and pathology, and congratulations to the LAF.

A great booklet useful for our young and experienced ISAKOS members!

ISAKOS President — Philippe Neyret

Preface

Muscle and tendon injuries are extremely common in sports activities and in work-induced physical loading: prevention, diagnosis and treatment of these pathologies are demanded to all those involved in sports medicine, orthopaedic surgery and rehabilitation.

This book is an updated presentation of the main aspects of muscle and tendon disorders.

It is practically impossible to write a scientific book without the help of co-workers. ISAKOS has been the nest where ideas can become reality, and the ISAKOS excellencies have done a great job. The LAF Committee has been the starter of this project, and the co-editors Pieter d'Hooghe, LAF Committee Chair, and Ken Hunt, Deputy Chair, must be commended for their extraordinary support and their friendship. The latest available information have been offered by world-renowned experts in the field to all those who wish to better treat patients with muscle and tendon problems. On behalf of all editors. we thank the authors who contributed to the excellence of this book giving their time and exceptional effort with enthusiasm, meeting the demands of deadlines and revisions.

Torino, Italy — Gian Luigi Canata

Acknowledgements

We wish to express our gratitude to ISAKOS who made this project possible, to the ISAKOS LAF Committee and the Education Committee for the great support, to Springer for their excellent editorial job, to Catena Cottone who coordinated with great care the various authors and to all the authors of this book for their invaluable cooperation.

Torino, Italy — Gian Luigi Canata
Doha, Qatar — Pieter d'Hooghe
Aurora, CO, USA — Kenneth J. Hunt

Contents

Functional Morphology of Muscles and Tendons

1

James N. Fisher, Alessia Di Giancamillo, Eliana Roveda, Angela Montaruli, and Giuseppe M. Peretti

Contents

J.N. Fisher
IRCCS Istituto Ortopedico Galeazzi,
Via R. Galeazzi, 4, 20161, Milano, Italy

A. Di Giancamillo
Department of Health, Animal Sciences and Food Safety, University of Milan, Milan, Italy

E. Roveda • A. Montaruli
Department of Biomedical Sciences for Health, University of Milan, Milan, Italy

G.M. Peretti (✉)
IRCCS Istituto Ortopedico Galeazzi,
Via R. Galeazzi, 4, 20161, Milano, Italy

Department of Biomedical Sciences for Health, University of Milan, Milan, Italy
e-mail: giuseppe.peretti@unimi.it

1.1 Muscle

Muscle is one of the four principal tissue types; it produces movement by pulling on the dense connective tissue which forms the tendons and periosteum.

In the human body there are four different types of muscle:

1. *Smooth muscle*, also known as *involuntary*, or *nonstriated* muscle, is responsible for the generation of the *tunica muscularis*, or muscle coat, of the internal organs and blood vessels and makes up the stroma of several visceral organs. The contraction of smooth muscle cells is involuntary, as opposed to the contraction of striated muscle; it is slower and requires less energy but can be maintained for longer periods of time. The sarcoplasm (cytoplasm of muscle cells) of smooth muscle cells is rich in myofibrils, which are not arranged in sarcomeres as in striated muscle types.
2. *Cardiac muscle*, also called *myocardium*, makes up the walls of the heart and is responsible for the pumping of blood. Cardiac muscle contraction is involuntary, unlike skeletal muscle, although it is characterised by striations similar to those in skeletal muscle which are due to the organised distribution of myofibrils within the cell sarcomere.
3. *Skeletal muscle*, also known as *striated* or *voluntary* muscle, is connected to the skeleton

G.L. Canata et al. (eds.), *Muscle and Tendon Injuries*, DOI 10.1007/978-3-662-54184-5_1

and is responsible for generating movement. Contraction is under voluntary control, and as a result the skeletal muscle is highly innervated by motoneurons: every muscle fibre is contacted by a motoneuron at the neuromuscular junction, which transmits the signal to contract.

1.1.1 Anatomy of Skeletal Muscle Tissue

Skeletal muscle represents about 40% of adult bodyweight and is characterised by elongated cylindrical cells of varying length and diameter, called *muscle fibres*. They are arranged parallel to one another, surrounded by a thin membrane of connective tissue that is richly innervated and vascularised. Technically, each muscle cell is a *polynuclear syncytium*, a cytoplasmic mass with multiple nuclei which form during embryonic and foetal development from the fusion of several mesodermal mononuclear fusiform progenitor cells, myoblasts.

Figure 1.1 shows the organisation of the muscle and its constitutive elements which are made up of fascicles, which are in turn composed of a number of muscle fibres. The individual fascicles are enveloped and separated by connective tissue that supports and protects the muscle. The connective tissue is rich in nerves and blood vessels that supply oxygen and nutrients and allow for the elimination of catabolic waste products, particularly lactic acid. Since muscle tissue undergoes contraction and extension, the vessels and nerves in muscle are looped back on themselves in a wave-like pattern. The epimysium surrounds the fascicles that form the whole muscle tissue; the perimysium wraps around single fascicle, grouping the bundles of muscle fibres; finally, the endomysium encloses each individual muscle fibre. The role of these connective tissues is to favour the transmission of mechanical force and at the same time protect the muscle fibres during contraction. The collagen fibres that make up these connective tissues overlap and, at the ends of the muscle, come together to form the tendons.

Muscle cells range in size from 10 to100 μm in diameter and from 1 mm to 20 cm in length. The sarcoplasm is rich in mitochondria needed to provide ATP and hosts a highly developed sarcoplasmic reticulum (SR; smooth endoplasmic reticulum of myocytes) which contains an elevated concentration of calcium ions (Ca^{++}) which is necessary for muscle contraction. The multiple nuclei are located peripherally adjacent to the sarcolemma, the plasma membrane that surrounds the muscle fibre and regulates the movement of chemical substances in and out of the cell. The sarcoplasmic reticulum is composed of tubules and cisternae which wrap around the myofibril. The tubules run

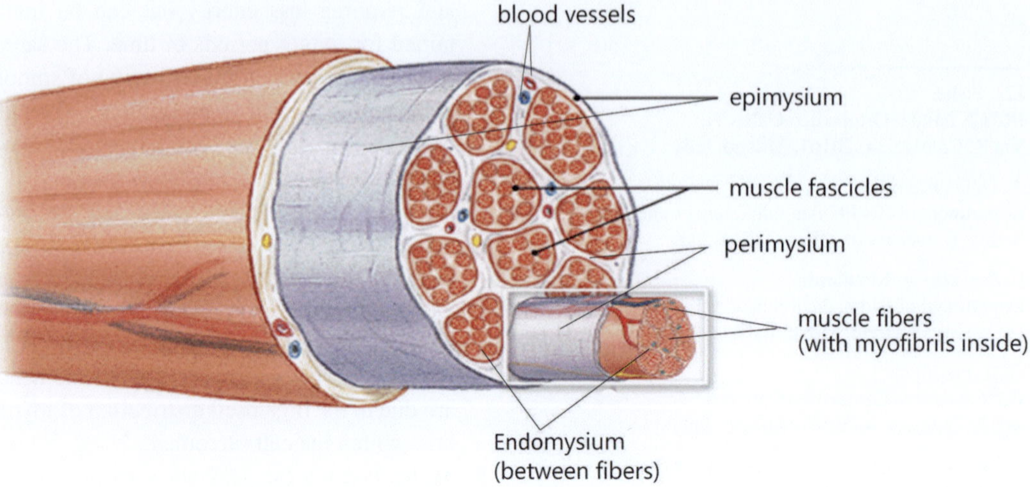

Fig. 1.1 Organisational levels and connective tissue sheaths in skeletal muscle. Courtesy of CIC Edizioni Internazionali—From "Il tendine e il muscolo" (Eds.: Giuseppe M. Peretti, Gian Luigi Canata), CIC Edizioni Internazionali, Rome 2014

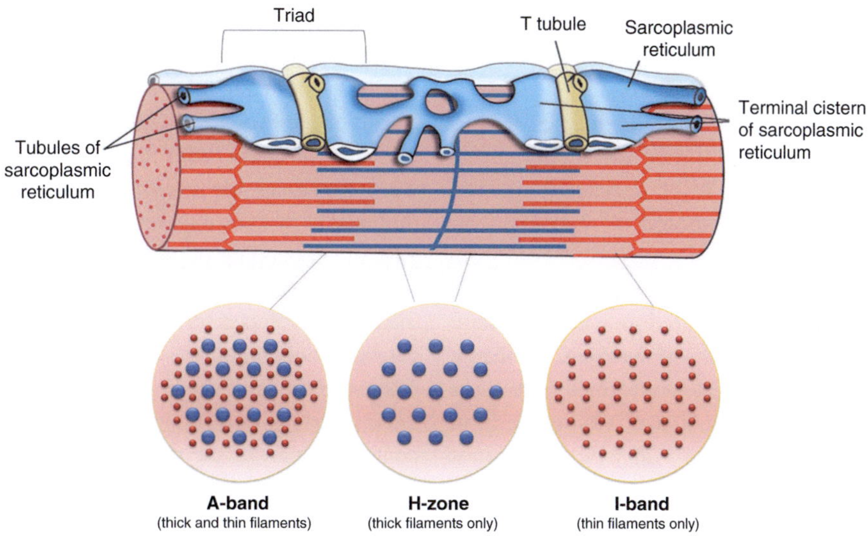

Fig. 1.2 **Sarcoplasmic** reticulum and T-tubules in the skeletal muscle fibres. The figure shows a cross-sectional view of a location within the sarcomere. Courtesy of CIC Edizioni Internazionali—From "Il tendine e il muscolo" (Eds.: Giuseppe M. Peretti, Gian Luigi Canata), CIC Edizioni Internazionali, Rome 2014

parallel to the myofibril and anastomose with one another within the H-zone, while between the A- and I-bands, they open into terminal cisternae which run perpendicularly to the axis of the muscle fibre (Fig. 1.2). The terminal cisternae are connected by transverse tubules (or T-tubules). The sarcoplasm also contains numerous myofibrils, composed of bundles of multiple myofilaments, which in turn are composed of specialised contractile proteins. Both myofilaments and myofibrils are distributed parallel to one another and to the longitudinal axis of the muscle fibre.

The contractile proteins within the myofibrils are distributed in a partially overlapping manner which gives the myofibrils the distinct banding pattern (striation) of dense and less dense areas seen in striated muscle. The contractile proteins that form the myofilaments are myosin, a filamentous protein with a globular head domain that forms the dense bands (*A*, anisotropic when viewed with polarised light), and actin which constitutes the thin filaments and, together with troponin and tropomyosin, makes up the less dense (*I*, isotropic) bands (Fig. 1.3). The Z-disc, a thin dark band, corresponds to either end of the sarcomere, while the M-line, a dark band in the centre of the lighter H-zone, marks the centre of the sarcomere where the thick filaments are stabilised by cross-linking (Agarkova and Perriard 2005). The thin

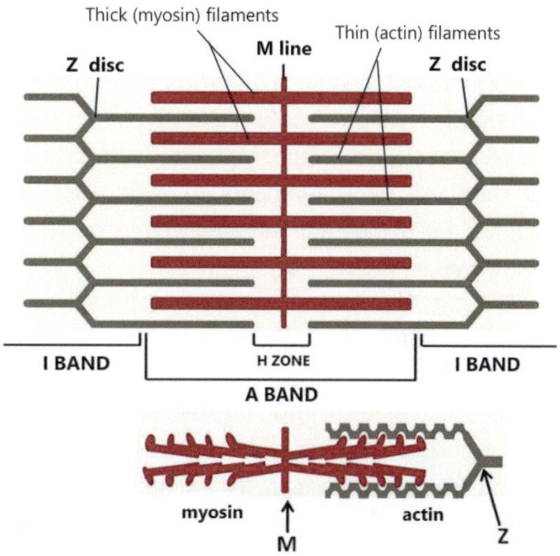

Fig. 1.3 Microscopic anatomy of the skeletal muscle fibre: basic structure of the sarcomere. Courtesy of CIC Edizioni Internazionali—From "Il tendine e il muscolo" (Eds.: Giuseppe M. Peretti, Gian Luigi Canata), CIC Edizioni Internazionali, Rome 2014

filaments (actin) are present in the A-band as well as myosin; however, the H-zone is occupied solely by myosin. Thus, the dark appearance of the A-band is due to the overlap of thin and thick filaments. Within the A-band each filament of myosin is surrounded by six actin filaments (Fig. 1.2). The sarcomere represents the functional unit of the muscle cell as it is the sliding movement of the overlapping actin and myosin strands that cause the contraction of the myofibril and thus muscle contraction (Huxley 2004).

The contractile proteins are therefore filamentous molecules that constitute the myofilaments present in the sarcomere of muscle fibres. The thick filaments are composed of myosin molecules; the globular head moieties project out from the filament and make contact with actin. The thin filaments are composed predominantly of actin and make transverse connections to one another at the Z-disc. Actin filaments are formed from three molecules of globular actin and assume the form of a polarised helical chain, with a plus and minus end, and a number of additional accessory proteins including tropomyosin and troponin. Tropomyosin forms two filaments that insert into the groove of actin and binds three molecules of troponin. When cellular Ca^{++} levels are low, the interaction of tropomyosin and troponin blocks interaction with myosin. Upon release from the SR, calcium ions bind troponin C and cause a conformational change in the troponin/tropomyosin complex which uncovers the myosin binding site on the actin molecule. Myosin binding causes the thin and thick filaments to slide past one another, due to the motor activity of myosin which is powered by the hydrolysis of ATP.

The calcium ions are rapidly removed from the sarcoplasm by a large number of ATP-dependent Ca^{++} pumps; tropomyosin, in the absence of calcium ions, returns to its original conformation blocking the actin active site, and the muscle returns to its resting length.

1.1.2 Classification of Skeletal Muscles

Skeletal muscles are located under the integumentary system, covered by a sheet of connective tissue which, in some points, may be attached to the periosteum that covers the bone surface. Their function is to produce movement, by pulling on the skeletal frame of the body, to maintain posture and to protect the underlying structures, particularly in areas lacking skeletal protection. In addition, muscular contraction causes thermogenesis and acts as a vascular pump.

The physical form differs greatly between different muscles, and some are flat and thin, while others are short and thick or long and spindly. The length of the muscle, excluding the tendon component, correlates with the contractile length, while the contractile force depends on the mass of the muscle in question, which may be used only partially depending on the level of force desired. The contractile mass is termed *muscle belly*; it is the most developed form of skeletal striated muscle and is both highly vascularised and innervated. The extremities of the muscle belly develop into either tendons or aponeuroses which attach the contractile part of the muscle to bones or, in the case of the facial muscles, to the skin.

Single muscle fibres may be orientated in one of two ways; parallel or oblique to the direction of muscle action. On this basis, the muscle can be classified as muscles in which the fascicle arrangement is *parallel* or muscles in which the fascicle arrangement is *oblique* to the body midline (Fig. 1.4). In the former case (Fig. 1.4a–c), the fibres run directly parallel to the long axis of the muscle, and the tendons are arranged in the same orientation as the muscle. Contraction of the muscle occurs in the same direction as the fibres are oriented, increasing the amplitude of the movement. Muscle of this type may assume various shapes, such as the *straplike* muscles (Fig. 1.4a) and *fusiform* muscles, with an expanded central *belly* and more thinned extremities where the muscle gives way to tendon (Fig. 1.4b) as well as muscles with *circular* pattern of fascicles, usually called *sphincters*, in which fibres are arranged in concentric rings (Fig. 1.4d). In triangular muscles, the fibres fan out over a wide area (Fig. 1.4e), converging on a thick central tendon. The triangular arrangement of the fibre allows the muscle to function in various planes of movement depending on the subset of fibres utilised; the trapezoid and pectoral muscles exemplify this type of muscle.

In the muscles in which the fascicle arrangement is oblique, the muscle fibres are shorter and attach obliquely to the tendon with respect to the direction of muscle action. These muscles are referred to as *pennate* muscles, due to the muscle structure which resembles the fibres of a feather (Fig. 1.4f–g). This arrangement maximises the

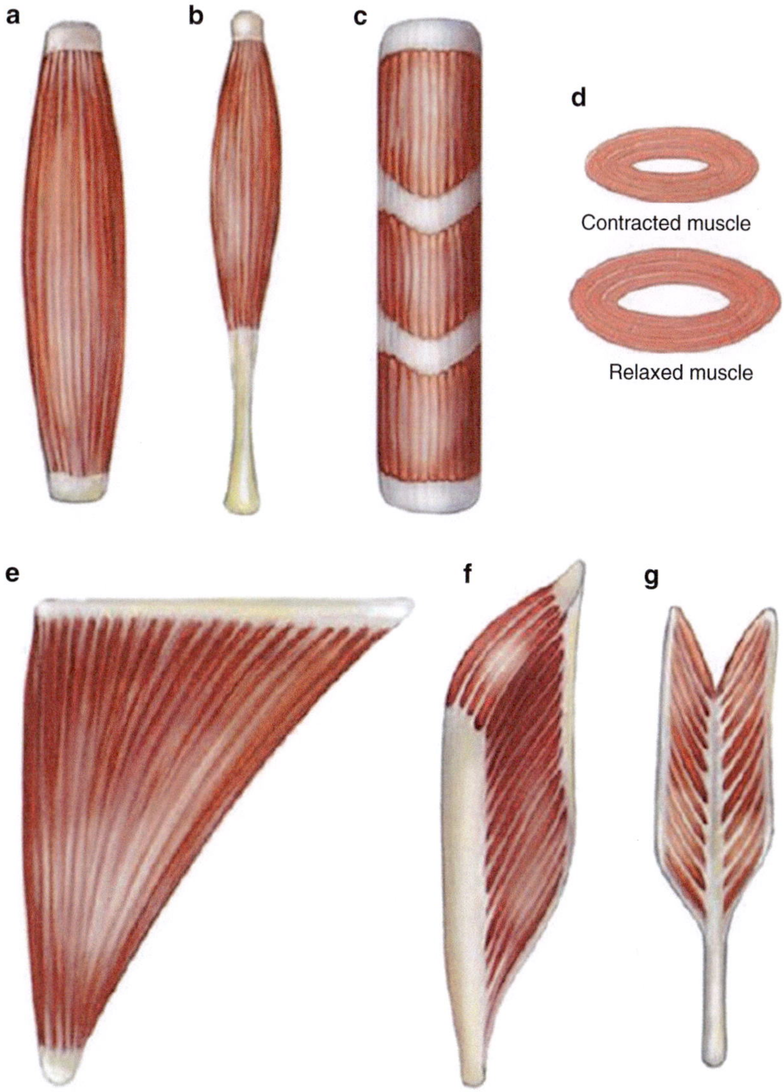

Fig. 1.4 Patterns of fascicle arrangement in muscles. In (**a**–**c**) the fibres are parallel to the long axis of the muscle. In (**d**) the fibres are arranged in concentric rings. In **e**, the origin of the muscle is broad, and the fibres converge towards a thick central tendon. In (**f**) and (**g**) muscle fibres are short and attach obliquely to a tendon. Courtesy of CIC Edizioni Internazionali—From "Il tendine e il muscolo" (Eds.: Giuseppe M. Peretti, Gian Luigi Canata), CIC Edizioni Internazionali, Rome 2014

number of fibres incorporated in a given area, and because a greater number of fibres result in a greater cross-sectional area, the force produced by these muscles will be greater. In reality, the force produced by a muscle is influenced by several morphological factors, including the cross-sectional area and the fascia angle (the angle formed by the longitudinal axis of the muscle and the tendon).

1.1.3 Number of Points of Origin

A muscle group may be composed of several independent muscles, called "muscle heads". These are named according to the number of muscles involved; examples include the biceps ("two heads"), triceps ("three heads") and quadriceps ("four heads") which are composed, respectively, of 2, 3 and 4 muscles with different origins that converge on a common tendon.

1.1.4 Mode of Action

On the base of functional criteria, muscles may be classified as flexors or extensors, abductors or adductors, pronators or supinators and internal or external rotators, depending on the movement generated by contraction. The names of many forearm and leg muscles begin with *extensor* or *flexor*, indicating how they move the hand, foot and digits. To transmit their action, a muscle must bridge a point of articulation and attach to two bones.

On the basis of the insertion point of the muscle to the skeleton, and how many articulations are involved, a muscle may be classified as mono-, bi- or polyarticular. Monoarticular muscles bridge one joint and join two bones; thus, movement is confined to one joint, e.g. the coracobrachialis muscle. Biarticular muscles span two joints; often these muscles have two or more tendons at one extremity and one tendon at the other end; one tendon is monoarticular, while the other is biarticular. Polyarticular muscles span more than two joints, with tendon insertions on several bone sites; these include very long muscles, usually located along the spinal column, that make contact with each vertebra.

1.1.5 Classification of Skeletal Muscle Fibres

The body is capable of a wide range of movements, from simple maintenance of posture to the capacity to engage in activities such as the high jump to running the marathon. The skeletal muscle is able to generate a finely tuneable output; the power generated represents the product of the force produced by the shortening of the muscle fibres multiplied by the velocity at which the muscles contract. The velocity of contraction is, to a large degree, determined by the expression of different isoforms of the myosin heavy chain (MHC), which have greatly differing ATPase activity. Type I, or slow fibres, contain MHC-1B; intermediate fibres, type IIa, contain MHC-IIA; and the fast fibres contain MHC-IIx. MHC-1B, in slow fibres, are seven to nine times slower than type IIx fibres which contain MHC-IIx. Therefore the power can be altered by regulating either of the two input variables: force and velocity; both of these variables depend on the properties of the muscle fibres, the characteristics of the motor units and by their recruitment.

Skeletal muscle fibres have different characteristics depending on their different molecular, metabolic, structural and contractile properties which permit their classification into three groups.

1. Type I fibres (also known as red fibres or slow oxidative (SO) fibres). These are small fibres, containing a high concentration of myoglobin, a red-pigmented molecule similar to haemoglobin which similarly stores oxygen. Thus, even at rest, the fibres contain a reserve of oxygen which is made available the instant of contraction. Tissues composed of these fibres are rich in capillaries, ensuring the supply of blood to the muscle. The sarcoplasm of type I fibres contains few myofibrils but many mitochondria. Type I fibrils are also known as slow fibres due to their slow speed of contraction. The large number of mitochondria produces more ATP than myosin can hydrolyse combined with the large reserve of myoglobin help to avoid fatigue. Therefore, this type of muscle fibre is prevalent in postural muscles, which must remain contracted for long periods of time.
2. Type II fibres, or white fibres, are fast-twitch glycolytic (FTG) fibres. Fibres of this group are much more voluminous that type I fibres due to the presence of increased numbers of myofibrils and which consequently produce more force. They contain fewer mitochondria and less myoglobin than type I fibres and contain fewer capillaries. Type II fibres are also known as fast fibres, as they contract at a greater velocity than type I, due to a faster form of myosin, as well as a system of T-tubules and a SR that is more efficient at releasing calcium ions. The cost of faster contraction is more rapid exhaustion of ATP, so type II fibres are more susceptible to fatigue with respect to type I. With fewer mitochondria, type II fibres rely on the cleavage of glycogen to produce ATP. Since anaerobic respiration is far less efficient at producing ATP, these muscles cannot maintain prolonged contraction. However, since these

fibres contract and relax rapidly, they are well suited to activities that require short bursts of intense power, such as sprinting.

3. Intermediate fibres are fast-twitch oxidative-glycolytic (FTOG) fibres. Recently discovered, these fibres are structurally, architecturally and biochemically a mix of the previous two types in that they consist of rapid contracting fibres that are resistant to fatigue. Histologically they are similar to fast fibres but contain a greater number of mitochondria and capillaries, and as a result they are more resistant to fatigue with respect to type II fibres while generating more force more rapidly than type I fibres. These fibres have been found in muscles which perform both rapid, high power tasks, such as jumping, but also work to maintain posture (e.g. in the leg).

The proportion of the diverse groups of fibres depends on the type of activities for which an individual uses their muscles, for example, athletes that practise endurance sports tend to have prevalently slow fibres. Training represents a stimulus for the recruitment of fibres or rather the motor units, which are activated in a precise order, depending on the intensity of the exercise. The type I fibres are recruited first during light exercise, before the intermediate type and finally the white fibres, which are most susceptible to fatigue (Table 1.1).

Unlike in animals where one may speak of *white meat* (such as chicken breast) or *red meat* (such as chicken leg), the skeletal muscles in humans are mixed, that is, all types of fibres are present albeit in different proportions, due to the varied functional demands placed on them. This diverse functionality that a given muscle may be used to satisfy different needs (maintenance of posture, very precise movements, repeated submaximal movements, contractions at maximum power) derives from precise organisation that requires the involvement of different types of muscle fibres and sophisticated nervous system control. The combination of fibre types within an individual's muscles is the result of genetic factors as well as an element of conditioning due to training and usage. Thus, slow fibres are utilised

Table 1.1 Characteristics of the muscle fibres found in skeletal muscle and their innervation

Fibre	Characteristics	Motor unit	Nerve axon diameter	Conduction velocity	Order of activation	Order of deactivation
Type I, slow oxidation	Small cells, high in myoglobin and mitochondria. Found in postural and low-power, high resistance muscles	FR	Thin	Slow	1	3
Intermediate, FTOG fibres	Recently described, fast contracting cells with intermediate resistance to fatigue	S	Intermediate	Intermediate	2	2
Type II, FTG, white fibres	Voluminous cells with lots of myofibrils but few mitochondria. Rapid and powerful contraction but susceptible to fatigue	FF	Large	Fast	3	1

FTG Fast-twitch glycolytic, *FTOG* fast-twitch oxidative-glycolytic, *FR* fast-resistant, *FF* fast-fatigable, *S* slow predominantly for postural control and for slow repeated contractions, while fast fibres give better performance in rapid, powerful and short duration contractions.

1.1.6 Motor Units and Their Recruitment

The motoneurons responsible for muscular contractions are found in the anterior horn of the grey matter in the spinal column. The motoneurons that innervate a single muscle constitute a *pool* of motoneurons. As all the muscle cells innervated by a single motoneuron contract simultaneously in response to an action potential, this group of myocytes are referred to as a *motor unit*. The motor unit represents the functional unit of movement; the ratio between the myocytes and the motoneurons that control them is referred to as the *innervation ratio* and can vary largely from a single motoneuron controlling hundreds of muscle fibres to very few fibres. Usually the innervation ratio is proportional to the volume of muscle; small muscles tend to be involved in tasks that require precision and fine control, whereas large muscles tend to be used for tasks involving greater power. The smaller the number of fibres within a given motor unit, the greater the possibility that exists for precise control over the muscle tension, increasing or decreasing the number of motor units involved; this concept is called *summation*.

The fibres that constitute a motor unit are distributed throughout the muscle rather than co-localising; the effect of this is to distribute the exerted force throughout the muscle, even if the number of fibres is relatively low. Additionally, the different motor units within a given muscle will contract asynchronously to produce a more constant force, which also helps reduce fatigue. As the muscle fibres within any motor unit have similar morphological and functional characteristics, they can be divided into three groups:

1. Fast-fatigable (FF). These are formed from FTG-type fatigable fast fibres, which produce rapid, powerful contractions but are susceptible to fatigue.
2. Fast-resistant (FR). These fast FTG-type fibres are capable of both rapid and sustained contractions and which are relatively resistant to fatigue.
3. Slow (S). Formed from SO fibres, these fibres produce relatively low levels of power and contract relatively slowly but are capable of maintaining their maximum level of power output for prolonged periods.

The class of motor unit and the type of motoneuron which are related in those muscle fibres which are more susceptible to fatigue are innervated by motoneurons which are larger than those that innervate slower motor units. In addition, as the nerve conduction velocity of axons with larger diameter is faster than in thinner axons, there is a correlation between the conduction velocity and contraction velocity.

Depending on the necessary force required, the pyramidal neurons of the cerebral cortex recruit increasing numbers of motor units, therefore increasing number of muscle fibres, according to the *size principle* which states that motoneurons are activated on the basis of cell size (Henneman et al. 1965). Muscular contraction is stimulated by the activation of motor units innervated initially by smaller (and thus, slower) motoneurons, followed by faster non-fatigable motor units, and finally motor units containing fast, fatigable muscle fibres which are activated by the largest motoneurons. The order of motor unit deactivation is reversed, i.e. the motoneurons which are activated first and deactivated last (Henneman 1957).

1.1.7 Vascularisation and Innervation

Striated muscle is highly vascularised, each muscle receiving blood from diverse arteries. The arteries enter the muscle at a point that is less subject to movement during contraction and rapidly branches to form a network of capillaries that run parallel to the muscle fibres and join via transverse anastomoses.

The muscles are permeated by an irregular network of motoneurons and sensory neurons, concentrated in certain areas. The nerves communicate with the muscle cells via neuromuscular junctions that are usually located about halfway along the muscle cell at a specialised area of the sarcolemma, the motor endplate.

There are two types of specialised sensory receptors, the Golgi tendon organ and the muscle spindles, which provide proprioception, control muscle movement and regulate muscle tone. The Golgi tendon organs are located at the musculotendon junction and are stimulated by the contraction of collagen fibres within the tendon during muscular contraction.

1.1.8 Muscle Plasticity

Skeletal muscle tissue undergoes significant changes over the course of a lifetime. This is associated with the manner in which it is utilised or to particular types of training, as well as the process of ageing. Despite the fact that the muscle fibres tend to maintain their morpho-functional characteristics, change from one type of muscle fibre to another is possible as the result of certain stimuli. Fast fibres, when subjected to prolonged stimuli, similar to those which activate slow fibres, can change their phenotype towards aerobic respiration, developing greater resistance to fatigue and a slower contractile velocity. During this change, the muscle cell volume does not change, but the number of fibres increases (hyperplasia). If the new "slow" stimulus is removed, the cells resume their original phenotype. Strength training, on the other hand, does increase the volume of the muscle, due to hypertrophy of the white fibres and an increase in contractile proteins without changing the biochemical profile of the cell.

1.2 Tendons

Tendons are fibrous connective tissue located between the muscles and bone whose role is to transmit force generated by skeletal muscle in a manner which maintains posture and joint movement.

1.2.1 Tendon Structure

Macroscopically, tendons present as mother of pearl in colour, with a viscous-elastic consistency with high mechanic resistance; in fact, being more rigid than muscles, tendons have a greater tensile strength and therefore can support greater loads while deforming less, which means that force generated by the muscles is transmitted without the dissipation of energy due to stretching (Redaelli and Montevecchi 2007). Form is dictated by function and vice versa; muscles responsible for precision movements, such as those in the fingers, end in long and slender tendons, while muscles that do a lot of work, such as the flexors and extensors of the thigh, have thick robust tendons.

The tendon is wrapped in a membrane or synovial sheath, which facilitates tendon movement, avoids friction and maintains the position of the tendon during muscular contraction. Furthermore tendons which have fibres with one predominant orientation, such as the Achilles tendon, are covered with an external sheath called the *paratenon* which consists of peritendineal sheets of loose fibrillar tissue which are predominantly formed of collagen types I–III and elastic fibres. The number of these sheets varies as a function of the type of tendon and anatomical location. The function of the paratenon is then to reduce tendon friction during movement (Strocchi et al. 1985). Immediately below the paratenon lies the *epitenon*, a thin sheath composed of dense connective tissue, and together the paratenon and epitenon make up the *peritenon* (Fig. 1.5). Internally adjacent to the epitenon lies the *endotenon*, a thin connective tissue membrane which functions to encompass and group collagen fibrils into bundles of varying dimensions and to organise the distribution of nervous system and vascular structures within the tendon. Alternatively, tendons that are subject to greater degrees of bending during movement, such as the flexor tendons of the fingers, are enclosed within a richly vascularised synovial sheath. The presence of synovial liquid between the external wall of the tendon and the

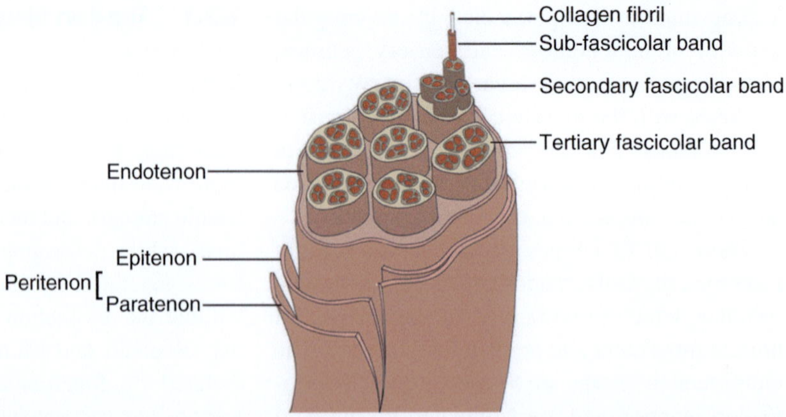

Fig. 1.5 Cross-sectional anatomy of the tendon. The figure illustrates the various substructures of the tendon. Courtesy of CIC Edizioni Internazionali—From "Il tendine e il muscolo" (Eds.: Giuseppe M. Peretti, Gian Luigi Canata), CIC Edizioni Internazionali, Rome 2014

internal wall of the sheath ensures minimal friction between the tendon and the bone.

The area where the tendons insert into the bone is called the osteotendinous junction (enthesis) and comprises four zones: the tendon, fibrocartilage, mineralised fibrocartilage and bone. The areas where the tendon meets the muscle is called the myotendinous junction; here the collagen fibrils make contacts with muscle cells forming *folds* which increase the contact surface area between muscle and tendon hence reducing the applied stress during muscular contraction (Charvet 2012).

Structurally the tendon is formed by numerous collagen bands covered externally by the peritenon. Internally we see tertiary, secondary and sub-fascicular bands as well as single collagen fibres, wrapped by and separated from others by the endotenon. The basic building blocks of the tendon are collagen fibres themselves composed of many collagen fibrils which have a diameter of 20–150 nm depending on the functional role of the tendon (Dyer and Enna 1976).

The majority of fibres are aligned with the main axis of the tendon, which makes the tendon very load resistant; this property is associated with the average diameter of the collagen fibres (Parry et al. 1978). Within the tendons, aggregates of collagen fibrils form fibres, which themselves form the bands of varying dimensions that are together called tendons. More precisely, a group of collagen fibrils form a primary band, or sub-band, and many of these primary bands surrounded by the endotenon form a secondary band or *fascicle*. A group of secondary bands form a tertiary band and many tertiary bands together constitute the tendon, enclosed within the endotenon.

Table 1.2 Biochemical makeup of the tendon

Component	Percentage (%)
Cells	3–6
Collagen I	25–31
Collagen III	2
Collagen IV	<1
Elastin	1
Proteoglycans	1–4
Water	60–65

Courtesy of CIC Edizioni Internazionali—From "Il tendine e il muscolo" (Eds.: Giuseppe M. Peretti, Gian Luigi Canata), CIC Edizioni Internazionali, Rome 2014

1.2.2 Biochemical Composition of the Tendon

From a biochemical perspective, the tendon is a complex structure comprising collagen fibres immersed in a proteoglycan matrix. The acellular portion of the tendon is composed of a water-rich matrix (60–65% water) made up of proteoglycans and glycosaminoglycans, elastin and collagen fibrils (Table 1.2) (Silver et al. 1992).

1.2.2.1 Collagen

Tendons have a modular structure, being formed by *fascicles*, which can reach up to 100 μm in diameter and which contain fibres whose cross-sectional area comprises between 1 and 300 μm. The fibres are made up of collagen fibrils, which vary from 20 to 280 nm in diameter and 0.3–2 mm in length and are made of multiple collagen molecules arranged in parallel. The collagen fibrils are then the smallest structural unit within the tendon. The majority of the collagen found in the tendon is type I (see Table 1.2), but type III is also present (Wang 2006). Type I collagen is found in two forms, as a homotrimer (5%) but predominantly as a heterotrimer (95%). Type I collagen has a triple-helical fibrillar structure made up of three left-handed polypeptide chains which are able to interact with one another to form a right-handed triple helix, the basic unit of the tendon matrix, tropocollagen. The cross-section of a microfibril is made up of five molecules of tropocollagen, and multiple microfibrils make up left-handed helical structure of collagen fibrils. Collagen type I is also found in numerous other tissues, including the skin, bone, ligaments, teeth as well as vascular and alveolar walls. The basic structure of collagen is composed of three amino acids: glycine (33%), proline (15%) and hydroxyproline (15%). Phenylalanine, leucine and glutamic acid can be substituted for proline, and arginine and leucine can take the place of hydroxyproline.

Over time, collagen undergoes non-enzymatic glycosylation whereby glucose and fructose react with lysine and arginine forming Schiff bases and Amadori products (Robins and Bailey 1972). This process, glycation, plays an important role in the senescence of connective tissue (Bailey 2005; Avery and Bailey 2005); the amount of glycosylated amino acids increases with time (Bailey 2005) and significantly alters the physical structure of collagen, increasing the mechanic resistance of the tendon (Avery and Bailey 2005).

1.2.2.2 Elastin

The dimension of elastin fibres varies from 0.3 to 2.0 μm; usually the individual fibres are widely distributed, forming an irregular net within the tissue. These fibres are synthesised by fibroblasts as a precursor called tropoelastin and polymerised extracellularly. Elastin fibre is organised with an amorphous and homogenous central core with a periphery of fibrillin, a glycoprotein with a width of approximately 110 angstrom. Elastin is synthesised by fibroblasts as a precursor form called tropoelastin and is polymerised extracellularly. Fibrillin is incorporated surrounding or within the elastin allowing the polymerisation of elastin. The elastin component of the tendon is higher in youth and decreases with senescence.

1.2.2.3 Proteoglycans

A three-dimensional net of proteoglycans (PG) exists between the collagen fibrils; PGs are composed of polysaccharides, i.e. polymers of simple sugars, prevalently in the form of glycosaminoglycans (GAGs) (Scott 1998, 2001). PGs slow the deformation of tissues and add to the viscoelastic component of the same tissues. In addition PGs have other functions inherent to the metabolism of the extracellular matrix, specifically large PGs such as aggrecan and versican function to occupy the intra-fibrillar space and prevent their collapse. Aggrecan is the second most abundant PG in tendons; it is a macromolecule which is alternately glycosylated and is concentrated in areas of the tendon that are subject to the greatest levels of compressive stress. It additionally acts as a lubricant allowing the fibrils to slide over one another (Yoon and Halper 2005). Aggrecan and versican bind hyaluronic acid (HA), and this association is fundamental for the integrity of the extracellular matrix.

Small PGs such as decorin function in the organisation and deposition of collagen fibrils. Decorin is the most expressed PG in tendons and is considered a crucial regulator of matrix assembly as it limits the diameter of the collagen fibrils and thus intervenes in the remodelling of the tendon in response to tension (McCormick 1999). Mechanical forces and pressure determine the expression of a range of PGs; it has been observed that decorin is synthesised during tension, while compression stimulated the synthesis of aggrecan (Robbins and Vogel 1994; Robbins et al. 1997).

1.2.3 Tendon Cells

The predominant cell type within the tendon is the fibroblast, which in the tendon is called the tenoblast-tenocyte and represents 90–95% of the cells present. Other cell types are also present in lesser quantities such as endothelial and nerve cells, lymphocytes, macrophages and mastocytes. Tenocytes are fusiform cells which align in columns along the direction of the collagen fibre; the tenocytes synthesise and organise the matrix, controlling the structure through the processes of degradation and remodelling.

In younger subjects, the cell-to-matrix ratio is very high, and tenocytes are distributed parallel to one another with variable forms and dimensions. During the initial stages of growth, the biosynthetic activity of the cell is very high, and this decreases in the later stages. With age, the morphology of the cell changes too; at the end of development, tenoblasts become elongated (up to 300 μm in length) and are called tenocytes. Tenocytes are responsible for the synthesis of tropocollagen molecules and also control fibrillogenesis and influence the orientation of the newly synthesised fibrils in the matrix. Tenocytes are able to sense mechanical deformation through physical and functional links to the matrix and stimulate an increased or decreased synthesis of the matrix (Galbraith and Sheetz 1998). The tenocyte cytoskeleton is linked to the matrix via adhesion molecules present in the cell membrane; the most important of these are composed of the integrin family. Integrins are transmembrane receptors that are composed of three domains:

1. Extracellular domain, which interacts with collagen structural PGs
2. Transmembrane domain
3. Cytoplasmic domain which interacts with cytoskeletal proteins

Integrins play a strategic role in signal transduction, transmitting mechanical signals from outside the cell to the interior and vice versa (Galbraith and Sheetz 1998), influencing protein synthesis and cell differentiation (Wang 2000, 2006), as well as cell decisions such as movement (Paul et al. 2016), growth and cell death (Gao et al. 2003; Vachon 2011).

1.2.4 Tendon Crimps

Tendons present with bands of fibre aligned along their main axis; these bands show a characteristic wave-like undulation, or tendon crimps, when observed under the microscope (Fig. 1.6) (Rowe 1985; Gathercole and Keller 1991; De Campos

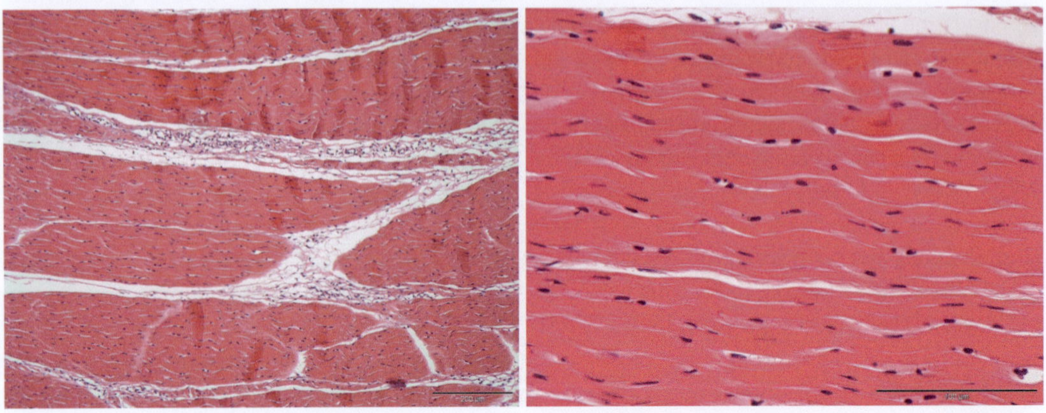

Fig. 1.6 Microscopic visualisation of tendon crimps. The characteristic undulating morphology of the tissue within the tendon is visible within this longitudinal section of the Achilles tendon. Staining: haematoxylin and eosin. Scale bar, *left* 200 μm, *right* 100 μm. Courtesy of CIC Edizioni Internazionali—From "Il tendine e il muscolo" (Eds.: Giuseppe M. Peretti, Gian Luigi Canata), CIC Edizioni Internazionali, Rome 2014

2003). In Fig. 1.6 the tendon can be seen to contain dense fibrous connective tissue in closely adjacent parallel bands separated by small quantities of intercellular material. These bands follow the "stress lines" to resist the forces of traction and the tensions generated during muscular movement.

1.2.5 Vascularisation

The tendons are vascularised by the perimysium, the periosteum and the paratenon; the flow of blood is slow (0.5 ml per 100 g tissue per minute) and is concentrated on the external surface of the tendon. For this reason the tendon is considered a poorly vascularised tissue and therefore is subject to prolonged regeneration times.

1.2.6 Innervation

The tendon is scarcely innervated, and the nerve branches form a course parallel to the main axis of the tendon with transversal and oblique anastomoses. In some cases, these branches terminate in contact with corpuscular receptors (Golgi, Pacini corpuscles, Ruffini corpuscles and Golgi-Mazzoni corpuscles) that are involved in proprioceptive sensitivity and myotatic reflexes (Perugia et al. 1981), while others terminate in free branched ends which are mostly found in the peritendinous sheets involved in nociception.

References

Agarkova I, Perriard JC (2005) The M-band: an elastic web that crosslinks thick filaments in the center of the sarcomere. Trends Cell Biol 15(9):477–485

Avery NC, Bailey AJ (2005) Enzymic and non-enzymic cross-linking mechanism in relation to turnover of collagen: relevance to aging and exercise. Scand J Med Sci Sports 15:231–240

Bailey AJ (2005) Molecular mechanisms of ageing in connective tissues. Mech Ageing Dev 122:735–755

Charvet B (2012) Muscles. Ligaments Tendons 2(2):53–63

De Campos VB (2003) Image analysis of tendon helical superstructure using interference and polarized light microscopy. Micron 34:423–432

Dyer RF, Enna CD (1976) Ultrastructural features of adult human tendon. Cell Tissue Res 168:247–259

Galbraith CG, Sheetz MP (1998) Forces on adhesive contacts affect cell function. Curr Opin Cell Biol 10:566–571

Gao C, Sun W, Christofidou-Solomidou M et al (2003) PECAM-1 functions as a specific and potent inhibitor of mitochondrial-dependent apoptosis. Blood 102(1):169–179

Gathercole LJ, Keller A (1991) Crimp morphology in the fibre-forming collagens. Matrix 11:214–234

Henneman E (1957) Relation between size of neurons and their susceptibility to discharge. Science 126:1345–1347

Henneman E, Somjen G, Carpenter DO (1965) Functional significance of cell size in spinal motoneurons. J Neurophysiol 28:560–580

Huxley HE (2004) Fifty years of muscle and the sliding filament hypothesis. Eur J Biochem 271(8):1403–1415

McCormick RJ (1999) Extracellular modifications to muscle collagen: implications for meat quality. Poult Sci 8:785–791

Parry DA, Barnes GRG, Craig AS (1978) A comparison of the size distribution of collagen fibrils in connective tissues as a function of age and a possible relation between fibril size distribution and mechanical properties. Proc R Soc Lond B Biol Sci 203:305–321

Paul CD, Shea J, Mahoney MR et al (2016) Interplay of the physical microenvironment, contact guidance, and intracellular signaling in cell decision making. FASEB J 30(6):2161–2170

Perugia L, Postacchini F, Ippolito E (1981) I tendini, biologia-patologia-clinica. Masson Italia Editori, Milano

Redaelli A, Montevecchi F (2007) Biomeccanica analisi multiscala di tessuti biologici. Patron Editore. 153–215

Robbins JR, Vogel KG (1994) Regional expression of mRNA for proteoglycans and collagen in tendon. Eur J Cell Biol 64:264–270

Robbins JR, Evanko SP, Vogel KG (1997) Mechanical loading and TGF-beta, regulate proteoglycan synthesis in tendon. Arch Biochem Biophys 342(2):203–211

Robins SP, Bailey AJ (1972) Age-related changes in collagen: the identification of reducible lysine-carbohydrate condensation products. Biochem Biophys Res Commun 48:76–84

Rowe RW (1985) The structure of rat tail tendon fascicles. Connect Tissue Res 14:21–30

Scott JE (1998) Proteoglycan-fibrillar collagen interactions. Biochem J 252(2):313–323

Scott JE (2001) Structure and function in extracellular matrices depend on interactions between anionic glycosaminoglycans. Pathol Biol 49(4):284–289

Silver D, Miller J, Harrison R, Prockop DJ (1992) Helical model of nucleation and propagation to account for the growth of type-I collagen fibrils from symmetrical pointed tips: a special example of self-assembly of rod-like monomers. Proc Natl Acad Sci USA 89(20):9860–9864

Strocchi R, Leonardi L, Guizzardi S et al (1985) Ultrastructural aspects of rat tail tendon sheaths. J Anat 140:57–67

Vachon PH (2011) Integrin signaling, cell survival, and anoikis: distinctions, differences, and differentiation. J Signal Transduct 2011:738137. doi:10.1155/2011/738137
Wang JH (2000) Substrate deformation determines actin cytoskeleton reorganization: a mathematical modeling and experimental study. J Theor Biol 202:33–41
Wang JH (2006) Mechanobiology of tendon. J Biomech 39(9):1563–1582
Yoon JH, Halper J (2005) Tendon proteoglycans: biochemistry and function. J Musculoskelet Neuronal Interact 5:22–34

Tendon Biomechanics

2

Zakary M. Beach, Daniel J. Gittings, and Louis J. Soslowsky

Contents

Z.M. Beach, B.S. • D.J. Gittings, M.D.
L.J. Soslowsky, Ph.D. (✉)
McKay Orthopaedic Research Laboratory,
Penn Center for Musculoskeletal Disorders,
University of Pennsylvania, 3450 Hamilton Walk,
425 Stemmler Hall, Philadelphia,
PA 19104-6180, USA
e-mail: soslowsk@upenn.edu

2.1 Introduction

Tendons are soft connective tissues that provide both joint stability and also act to transmit tensile loads between the muscle and bone. Furthermore, tendons may provide a mechanical advantage for force generated by the muscle by acting around a pulley or lengthening a lever arm. Additionally, viscoelastic material properties allow tendons to passively store and release energy during loading cycles. Similarly, tendons dissipate energy and prevent injury by maintaining joint alignment under high loads (O'Brien 1992; Dykyj and Jules 1991). Given the critical function of tendons, it is imperative to understand their structural and mechanical properties in order to optimize their function and healing response. Moreover, tendon injury and degeneration can be highly debilitating, and can result in substantial pain, disability, and health-care costs. Thus, the purpose of this chapter is to provide an overview of tendon biomechanics, including a description of tendon composition and structure, mechanical properties, mechanical testing, and factors that affect mechanics.

2.2 Composition and Structure

The basic composition and structure of tendons are paramount to their mechanical and functional properties. Like most connective tissues, tendons are composed primarily of water and collagen.

G.L. Canata et al. (eds.), *Muscle and Tendon Injuries*, DOI 10.1007/978-3-662-54184-5_2

Water comprises 50–60% of tendon weight. Collagen is approximately 75% of the dry weight, with 95% being type I collagen (Woo et al. 2008). Collagen molecule groups form fibrils that are embedded in an extracellular matrix (ECM) that consists of proteoglycans and other components. Proteoglycans consist of a core protein with chains of negatively charged glycosaminoglycans (GAGs). The combination of the structure of collagen fibrils and also the polarized nature of GAGs together contribute to the mechanical properties displayed by tendons.

Tendons are arranged in a hierarchical structure. The structure begins with a triple helix of collagen, then microfibrils, fibrils, fascicles, and ultimately the tendon itself (Fig. 2.1). Tenocytes synthesize the building blocks necessary for tendon structure. Tenocytes are spindle-shaped fibroblast-type cells that synthesize the collagen fibrils and ECM. The overall thickness and quality of the collagen fibrils are dictated by small leucine-rich proteoglycans (SLRPs) such as decorin and biglycan (Kalamajski and Oldberg 2009). The collagen fibrils also have a waveform structure known as crimp, which is present in all tendons. Furthermore, the ultrastructure of tendons shows "crimp" that can be viewed using a microscope (Fig. 2.2). Crimp is important to tendon mechanical properties, particularly in the early phase of loading.

2.3 Mechanics

Tendon's longitudinal and fibrillar structure results in anisotropic and nonlinear properties. Anisotropy refers to a material having directionally dependent properties. In the tendon, this results in mechanical properties that are up to 1000 times higher during tensile testing along the longitudinal versus transverse axes (Lake et al. 2010). In addition to anisotrophic properties, tendons also display nonlinear characteristics under an applied force, which results in an initial increase in stiffness as more force is applied. The nonlinear characteristics of the tendon result in two distinct regions in a load-elongation curve, termed the toe and linear regions (Fig. 2.3). The toe region of the load-elongation curve describes the behavior of tendons at low deformation, where the collagen fibril crimp is straightened. As deformation increases through the toe region into the linear region, crimp disappears and the collagen fascicle itself stretches (Dale et al. 1972; Diamant et al. 1972; Atkinson et al. 1999). As deformation continues to increase through the

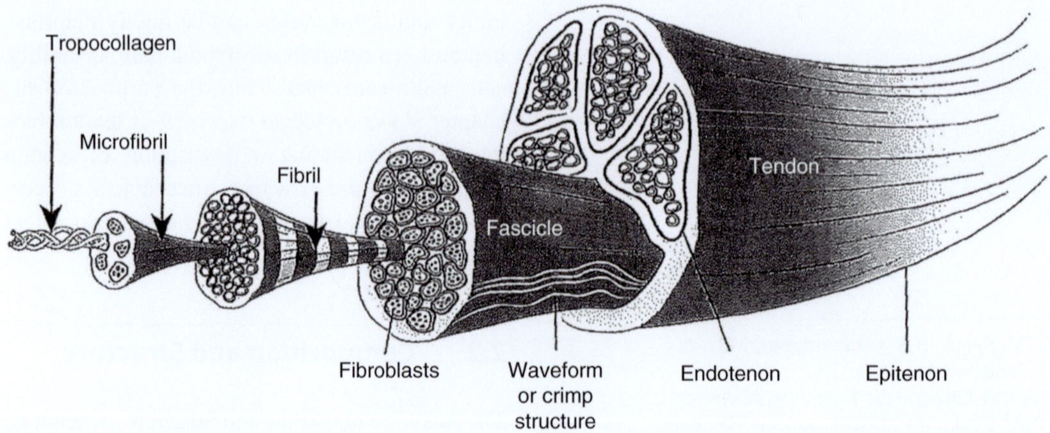

Fig. 2.1 Tendon hierarchical structure. Collagen molecules are assembled into progressively larger bundles, until the level of the tendon itself is reached. Reproduced with permission from Reuther KE, Gray CF, Soslowsky LJ: Form and Function of Tendon and Ligament, in O'Keefe RJ, Jacobs JJ, Chu CR, Einhorn TA (eds): *Orthopaedic Basic Science, 4th edition*. Rosemont, IL, American Academy of Orthopaedic Surgeons, 2013

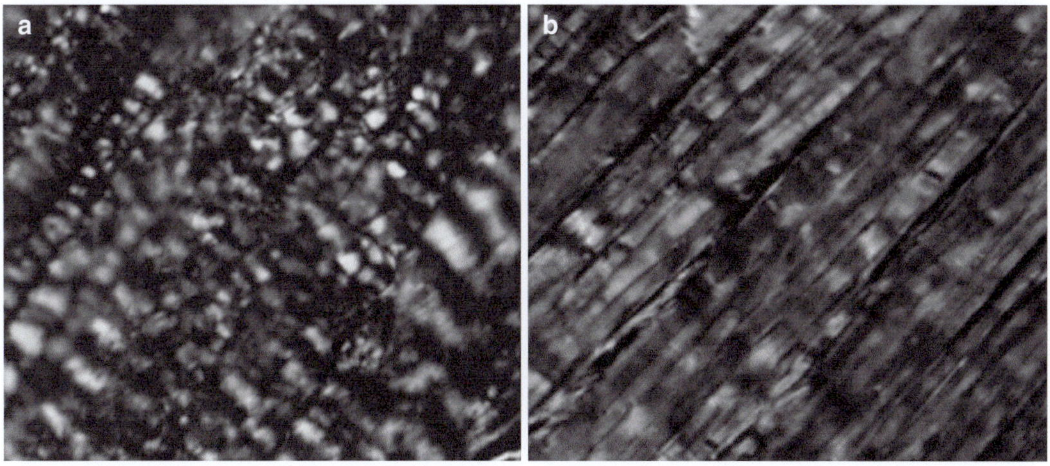

Fig. 2.2 Polarized light microscopy of crimp in a mouse supraspinatus tendon. (**a**) Collagen fibrils with crimp without an applied load. (**b**) Collagen fibrils uncrimped while under an applied tensile load. Reproduced with permission from Miller, KS, Connizo, BK, Feeney, F, Soslowsky, LJ: Characterizing local collagen fiber re-alignment and crimp behavior throughout mechanical testing in a mature mouse supraspinatus tendon model. *J Biomech* 2012; 45(12)

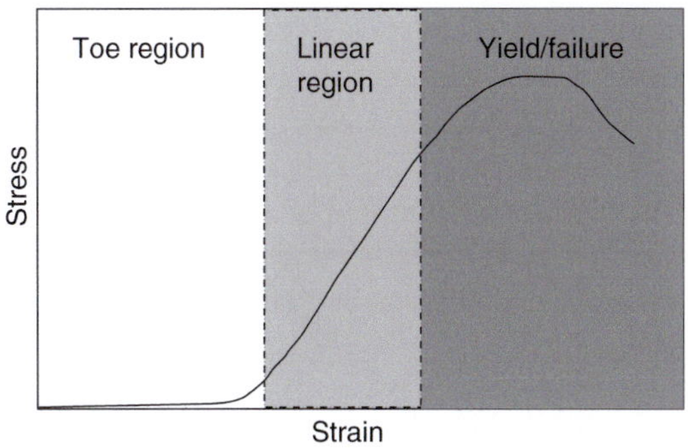

Fig. 2.3 Stress-strain curve demonstrating the toe and linear regions

linear region, the tendon accumulates irreversible damage and eventually ruptures. The anisotropic and nonlinear properties of tendons are further explained by other properties, such as viscoelasticity.

Viscoelasticity is the ability for materials to display both elastic and viscous behavior. One component of a viscoelastic material is viscosity, a measure of resistance to deformation. Although it has been traditionally used to characterize fluids, it can also describe other materials, such as rubber, glass, and biopolymers. Elasticity is the ability of a material to return to its original shape after forces that cause deformation are removed. The elasticity of a material can be described in the context of structural or material properties. Stiffness is a structural property that defines the extent to which a material resists deformation from an applied force. Stiffness is derived from the slope of the load-elongation curve (Fig. 2.4a). In contrast with structural properties, material properties are normalized properties, taking into account tissue size or shape. Material properties are calculated using stress and strain. Stress is the intensity of the load or force normalized by the cross-sectional area. Strain is a relative measure of deformation, a change in length divided by the original length. These parameters are used to calculate Young's modulus, a material property that describes elasticity and is defined as the slope of the stress-strain curve (Fig. 2.4b). Both load-elongation and stress-strain curves are generated through mechanical testing. Mechanical testing protocols can be adapted to measure different types of properties, including viscoelastic properties.

Dynamic mechanical analysis is one methodology used to assess tendon viscoelastic properties. This analysis is performed by applying an oscillatory stress and measuring the strain response. A phase lag is a delay between the applied stress and resulting strain response.

Phase lags may be measured to describe the viscous or elastic behavior of a material. In purely elastic materials, there is no phase lag; the strain response occurs simultaneously with the applied stress (Fig. 2.5a). In purely viscous materials, strain lags stress by 90° or one quarter cycle behind the stress applied (Fig. 2.5b). The phase lag for any material will always be between 0° and 90°, making purely elastic and purely viscous materials both the upper- and lower-bounds for phase lag, respectively. Additionally, viscoelasticity of tendons can also be characterized via hysteresis. Hysteresis represents the amount of energy dissipated as a result of internal friction during mechanical loading and unloading. Like all materials, tendon dissipates energy throughout loading and unloading cycles. Thus, hysteresis can be derived from the area between loading and unloading load-elongation curves during mechanical testing (Fig. 2.6).

The viscoelastic properties of tendon also lead to phenomena known as creep and stress relaxation. Creep is an increase in deformation of a material under a constantly applied load. Initially, elongation under a constant load occurs quickly, however, this response slows with time (Fig. 2.4c). Cyclic creep occurs during cyclic dynamic testing, where each consecutive load cycle generally causes an increase in the amount of deformation. In contrast with creep, stress relaxation holds strain constant. Stress relaxation in tendon is demonstrated when a measured load in a tendon decreases over time with a constant strain (Fig. 2.4d). This load initially decreases under a constant strain quickly, but the rate of change decreases over time as it approaches equilibrium. Cyclic stress relaxation also generally occurs when a tendon is exposed to cycling dynamic testing, requiring a decreased force to reach a constant strain over time.

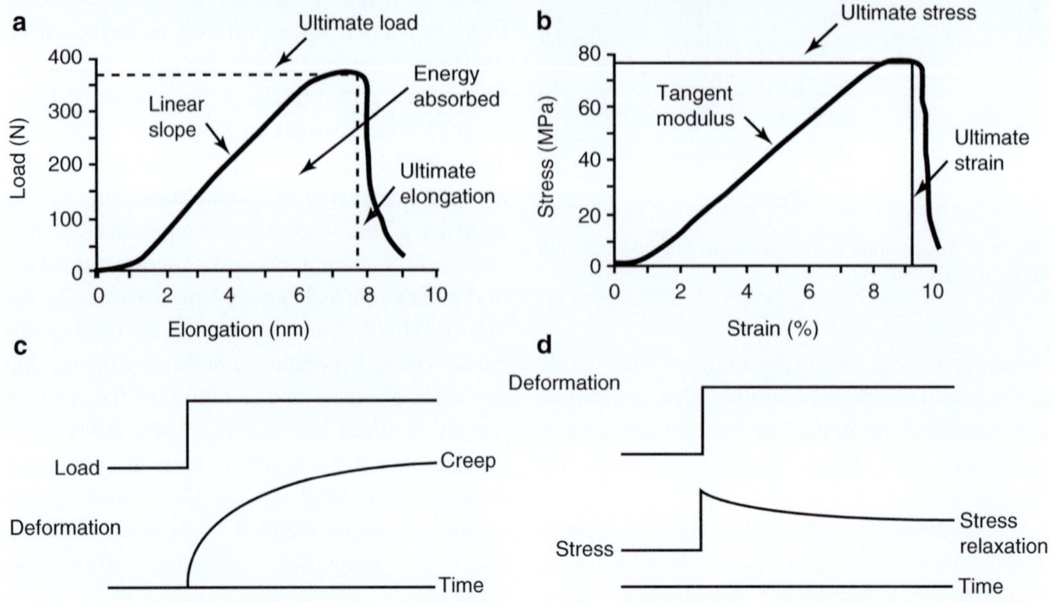

Fig. 2.4 (**a**) Tendon load-elongation curve. Various material properties can be derived from this curve. (**b**) Tendon stress-strain curve. This curve normalizes properties to each individual tendon's parameters, including length and area. Reproduced with permission from Woo SL, Debski RE, Withrow JD, Janushek MA: Biomechanics of knee ligaments. *Am J Sports Med* 1999; 27(4):533–543. (**c**) Creep test where load is held constant and amount of tendon deformation is measured. (**d**) Stress relaxation test where deformation is held constant and stress is measured. Both the creep test and stress relaxation test demonstrate viscoelastic behavior of tendon in response to load

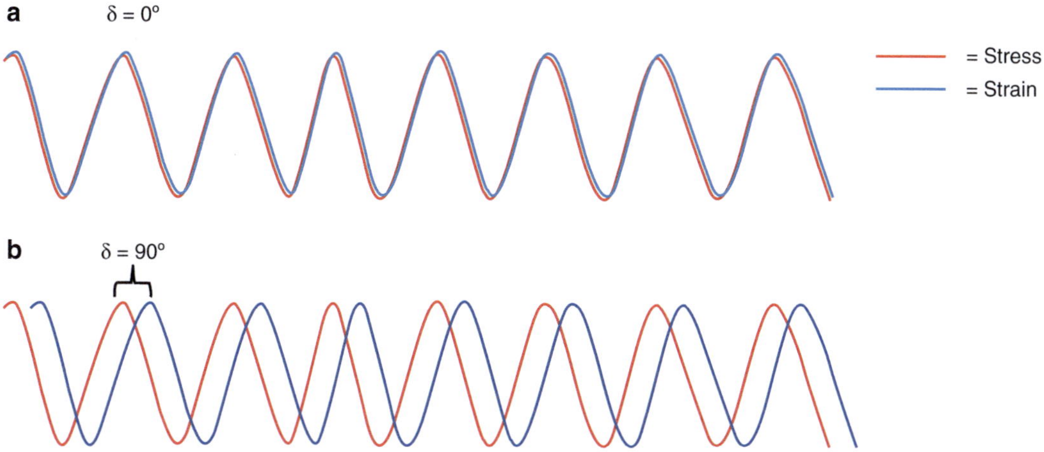

Fig. 2.5 Stress and strain response curves that represent a perfectly elastic material (**a**), with 0° phase lag between stress and strain, and a perfectly viscous material (**b**), with a 90° phase lag between stress and strain

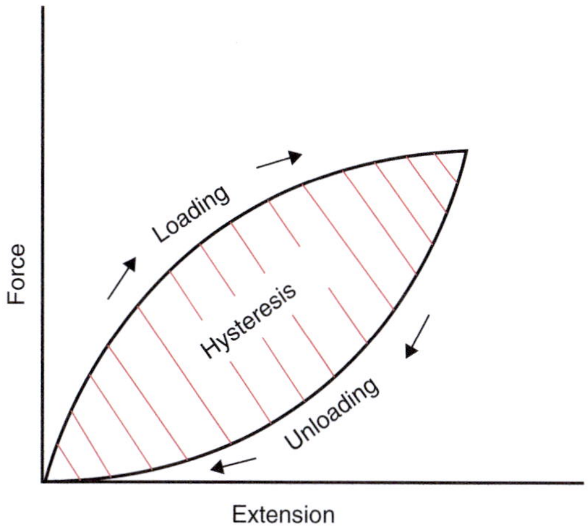

Fig. 2.6 A graph showing the loading and unloading curves of an idealized rubber band, with the area between the curves, highlighted by red lines, representing hysteresis

2.4 Mechanical Testing Methods

There are many parameters that affect the results of mechanical testing. In order to standardize measurements for comparison, cyclic preconditioning is commonly performed before mechanical testing. Preconditioning is performed at low loads to stretch the tendon without causing irreversible damage. After applying a preconditioning protocol, a steady state is reached where no further changes occur unless the protocol is altered (Fung 1993; Miller et al. 2012). After preconditioning, many mechanical testing methods such as ramp to failure, dynamic cyclic, and fatigue testing can be used to assess tendon mechanical properties.

Ramp to failure testing is the most common form of mechanical testing used to assess tendons. One purpose of this method is to find the maximum force and displacement a sample can endure before failure. It is typically performed by applying a constantly increasing displacement on the sample until failure. In addition, this test is also used to determine the stiffness and modulus of both the toe and linear regions and the transition point between these regions. It is not uncommon for ramp to failure testing to be performed in series with dynamic testing. This is because the low strains used in dynamic testing to measure creep and stress relaxation do not alter the tendon's integrity, making it is possible to combine these tests together (Fig. 2.7).

Many different parameters set during dynamic cyclic testing affect tendon response due to the viscoelastic nature of the tissue. The dynamic modulus derived from cyclic dynamic testing is defined as the stress amplitude divided by the strain amplitude. Thus, the dynamic modulus measurement is affected by testing parameters, based on the strains and frequencies that are selected. These moduli describe how tendons

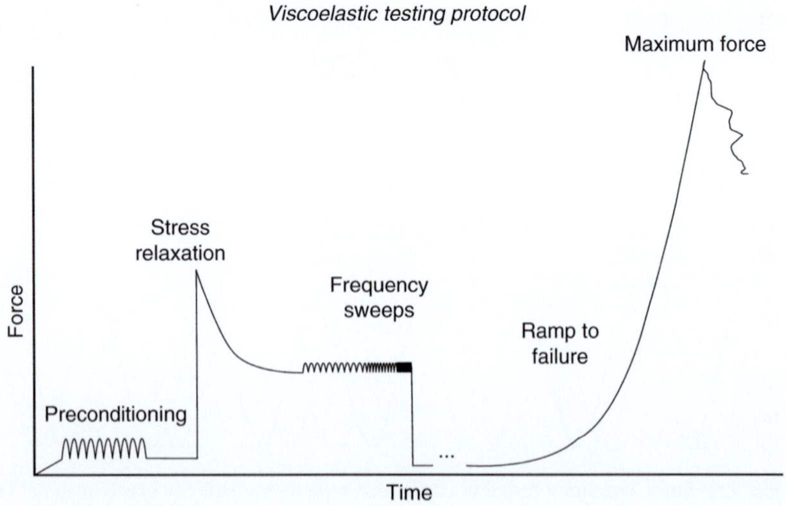

Fig. 2.7 An example of a tendon viscoelastic testing protocol. The test begins with preconditioning, followed by a stress relaxation and a series of frequency sweeps. Multiple stress relaxations can be performed at higher strains, followed by more frequency sweeps. The test ends with a ramp to failure test

behave depending on rate of loading and loading history. As previously discussed, creep and stress relaxation can also be used to characterize the viscoelastic behavior of tendons. Creep and stress relaxation are affected by the magnitude of force or strain, respectively. A more comprehensive method of evaluating creep and stress relaxation is to perform dynamic testing using various magnitudes of force. Examining these properties across a range of values provides a deeper insight into the viscoelastic characteristics of the sample.

Fatigue testing is another type of cyclic testing which consists of cycling within a defined range of force or displacement, and recording the number of cycles until failure. During this testing, tendons have three phases marked by changes in stiffness (Freedman et al. 2014). Initially, the tendon increases in stiffness, reaches a maximum, and finally descreases in stiffness, demonstrating a triphasic behavior pattern. This decrease in stiffness is attributed to an accumulation of sub-rupture damage, which results in increases in deformation and decreases in stiffness prior to failure. This testing is useful for characterization of tendons that undergo repetitive loads, such as the Achilles tendon and other tendons that function in locomotion (Fung et al. 2009, 2010; Wren et al. 2003).

2.5 Experimental Factors Influencing Tendon Mechanics

Several technical aspects must be considered when preparing for testing of tendon mechanical properties. The overall process typically includes sample isolation, storage, preparation, and testing. Tendons are prepared by isolating them for independent testing by removing bony or muscular attachments that may confound results. This process may be labor intensive, thus, it is not uncommon to store samples in a freezer before further preparation and testing. However, when storing these samples prior to testing, freeze-thaw cycles must be taken into consideration. While studies have reported no changes in mechanics with less than five freeze-thaw cycles (Suto et al. 2012), other studies have noted a decline in mechanics with each cycle and to use caution when exposing tendons to more than five cycles (Chen et al. 2011; Huang et al. 2011). The environment in which the tendon is tested also requires careful consideration. Specifically, hydration and temperature of the tendon must be controlled, as changed in either of these parameters will have profound effects on tendon behavior. For example, dehydration of tendon has been shown to cause a shortening of the collagen molecules, resulting in the generation of large stresses (Masic et al. 2015). Decreases in temperature make tendon behavior less viscous and more elastic (Huang et al. 2009). For these reasons, a water bath is typically used to immerse the tendon in order to control for hydration and temperature during testing.Before proceeding with testing, accurate measurement of tendon cross-sectional area is vital to ensure that material properties are properly reported. This is most robust when done through noncontact methods, such as laser-based systems, to reduce error (Favata 2006). Once cross-sectional area is measured, tendons are mounted in an anatomical orientation, where the fibers are loaded longitudinally, in order to model the in vivo scenario. Grips placed on the tendon ends properly are important to isolate the tendon and also prevent errors associated with slipping and stress concentrations. To reduce these errors, tendons are ideally tested with a high length versus width ratio. Furthermore, errors from grip slippage can be further reduced by using optical or other noncontact techniques to accurately calculate strain and measure finite levels of local deformation (e.g., finding the deformation at the insertion or midsubstance) (Peltz et al. 2009). During testing, the rate of loading also has an impact on data. For tendon, specifically, rate-dependent mechanical changes have been associated with altered uncrimping and volumetric contraction (Buckley et al. 2013).

2.6 Biological Factors Influencing Tendon Mechanics

Several non-modifiable and modifiable biologic factors significantly affect tendon mechanical properties. Non-modifiable factors include age, gender, and anatomic location. Advanced age is a risk factor for increased incidence of tendon injury (Abate et al. 2009; Langberg et al. 2001; Birch et al. 2016). Although there appears to be diminished mechanical properties with age, the mechanisms behind these phenomena are still under investigation. Additionally, gender has also been shown to be a risk factor for injury susceptibility and altered healing characteristics (Pardes et al. 2016; Fryhofer et al. 2016). Sex hormones regulate the collagen composition leading to altered mechanical properties (Hansen and Kjaer 2016). Anatomic location of the tendon within the body is another non-modifiable factor that affects tendon mechanical properties. Similar to what is seen ex vivo in the laboratory, variations of the loading environment such as load cycles and local temperature in various anatomic regions of the body affect the mechanical properties (Maganaris 2002). In contrast with non-modifiable factors, modifiable factors offer greater potential for optimizing therapeutic strategies for tendon pathology. Modifiable factors include comorbidities and activity level. Comorbidities such a diabetes, hypercholesterolemia, tobacco use, and renal disease have all been shown to adversely affect tendon mechanics (Connizzo et al. 2014; Beason et al. 2013; Ichinose et al. 2010; Taşoğlu et al. 2016; Artan and Basgoze 2015). Exercise also profoundly affects tendon mechanics, with increased activity increasing modulus compared to age-matched control tendons (Arnoczky et al. 2008). Furthermore, return to early activity after acute tendon injury has been shown to improve mechanical properties (Freedman et al. 2016).

Conclusion

Tendon composition, structure, mechanical properties, and testing methods provide insight into the fundamental mechanisms that govern tendon function. The collagen matrix composition and crimp structure promote viscoelastic mechanical properties of tendons. By testing these mechanical properties, the physiologic and pathologic behavior of tendons is better understood. Translation of tendon biomechanics to the bedside aids clinicians in improving the care of patients.

References

Abate M et al (2009) Pathogenesis of tendinopathies: inflammation or degeneration? Arthritis Res Ther 11:235

Arnoczky SP et al (2008) Loss of homeostatic strain alters mechanostat 'set point' of tendon cells in vitro. Clin Orthop Relat Res 466:1583–1591

Artan AS, Basgoze B (2015) Bilateral quadriceps tendon rupture in a hemodialysis patient. Clin Exp Nephrol 19:755–756

Atkinson TS, Ewers BJ, Haut RC (1999) The tensile and stress relaxation responses of human patellar tendon varies with specimen cross-sectional area. J Biomech 32:907–914

Beason DP et al (2013) Hypercholesterolemia increases supraspinatus tendon stiffness and elastic modulus across multiple species. J Shoulder Elb Surg 22:681–686

Birch HL, Peffers MJ, Clegg PD (2016) Influence of ageing on tendon homeostasis. Adv Exp Med Biol 920:247–260. doi:10.1007/978-3-319-33943-6_24

Buckley MR, Sarver JJ, Freedman BR, Soslowsky LJ (2013) The dynamics of collagen uncrimping and lateral contraction in tendon and the effect of ionic concentration. J Biomech 46:2242–2249

Chen L et al (2011) Effect of repeated freezing-thawing on the Achilles tendon of rabbits. Knee Surg Sports Traumatol Arthrosc 19:1028–1034

Connizzo BK, Bhatt PR, Liechty KW, Soslowsky LJ (2014) Diabetes alters mechanical properties and collagen fiber re-alignment in multiple mouse tendons. Ann Biomed Eng 42:1880–1888

Dale WC, Baer E, Keller A, Kohn RR (1972) On the ultrastructure of mammalian tendon. Experientia 28:1293–1295

Diamant J, Keller A, Baer E, Litt M, Arridge RG (1972) Collagen; ultrastructure and its relation to mechanical properties as a function of ageing. Proc R Soc Lond B Biol Sci 180:293–315

Dykyj D, Jules KT (1991) The clinical anatomy of tendons. J Am Podiatr Med Assoc 81:358–365

Favata M (2006) Scarless healing in the fetus: implications and strategies for postnatal tendon repair. University of Pennsylvania, Philadelphia

Freedman BR, Sarver JJ, Buckley MR, Voleti PB, Soslowsky LJ (2014) Biomechanical and structural response of healing Achilles tendon to fatigue loading following acute injury. J Biomech 47:2028–2034

Freedman B et al (2016) Nonsurgical treatment and early return to activity leads to improved Achilles tendon fatigue mechanics and functional outcomes during early healing in an animal model. J Orthop Res n/a--n/a. doi:10.1002/jor.23253

Fryhofer GW et al (2016) Postinjury biomechanics of Achilles tendon vary by sex and hormone status. J Appl Physiol 121:1106–1114

Fung Y-C (1993) Biomechanics: mechanical properties of living tissues. Springer, New York

Fung DT et al (2009) Subrupture tendon fatigue damage. J Orthop Res 27:264–273

Fung DT et al (2010) Early response to tendon fatigue damage accumulation in a novel in vivo model. J Biomech 43:274–279

Hansen M, Kjaer M (2016) Sex hormones and tendon. Adv Exp Med Biol 920:139–149. doi:10.1007/978-3-319-33943-6_13

Huang C-Y, Wang VM, Flatow EL, Mow VC (2009) Temperature-dependent viscoelastic properties of the human supraspinatus tendon. J Biomech 42:546–549

Huang H, Zhang J, Sun K, Zhang X, Tian S (2011) Effects of repetitive multiple freeze-thaw cycles on the biomechanical properties of human flexor digitorum superficialis and flexor pollicis longus tendons. Clin Biomech 26:419–423

Ichinose R et al (2010) Alteration of the material properties of the normal supraspinatus tendon by nicotine treatment in a rat model. Acta Orthop 81:634–638

Kalamajski S, Oldberg A (2009) Homologous sequence in lumican and fibromodulin leucine-rich repeat 5-7 competes for collagen binding. J Biol Chem 284:534–539

Lake SP, Miller KS, Elliott DM, Soslowsky LJ (2010) Tensile properties and fiber alignment of human supraspinatus tendon in the transverse direction demonstrate inhomogeneity, nonlinearity, and regional isotropy. J Biomech 43:727–732

Langberg H, Olesen J, Skovgaard D, Kjær M (2001) Age related blood flow around the Achilles tendon during exercise in humans. Eur J Appl Physiol 84:246–248

Maganaris CN (2002) Tensile properties of in vivo human tendinous tissue. J Biomech 35:1019–1027

Masic A et al (2015) Osmotic pressure induced tensile forces in tendon collagen. Nat Commun 6:5942

Miller KS, Edelstein L, Connizzo BK, Soslowsky LJ (2012) Effect of preconditioning and stress relaxation on local collagen fiber re-alignment: inhomogeneous properties of rat supraspinatus tendon. J Biomech Eng 134:31007

O'Brien M (1992) Functional anatomy and physiology of tendons. Clin Sports Med 11:505–520

Pardes AM et al (2016) Males have inferior Achilles tendon material properties compared to females in a rodent model. Ann Biomed Eng 44:2901–2910

Peltz CD, Perry SM, Getz CL, Soslowsky LJ (2009) Mechanical properties of the long-head of the biceps tendon are altered in the presence of rotator cuff tears in a rat model. J Orthop Res 27:416–420

Suto K et al (2012) Repeated freeze-thaw cycles reduce the survival rate of osteocytes in bone-tendon constructs without affecting the mechanical properties of tendons. Cell Tissue Bank 13:71–80

Taşoğlu Ö, Ekiz T, Yenigün D, Akyüz M, Özgirgin N (2016) Bilateral quadriceps and triceps tendon rupture in a hemodialysis patient. Hemodial Int 20:E19–E21

Woo SLY, Fisher MB, Feola AJ (2008) Contribution of biomechanics to management of ligament and tendon injuries. Mol Cell Biomech 5:49–68

Wren TAL, Lindsey DP, Beaupré GS, Carter DR (2003) Effects of creep and cyclic loading on the mechanical properties and failure of human Achilles tendons. Ann Biomed Eng 31:710–717

Pathophysiology of Tendinopathy

3

Michael Girdwood, Sean Docking, Ebonie Rio, and Jill Cook

Contents

Tendon injuries are common, especially in athletic populations, and result in pain and dysfunction in the tendon (called tendinopathy). Clinicians require a thorough understanding of normal structure and behaviour of tendons, as well as factors contributing to pathology to be able to successfully manage tendinopathy.

3.1 Structure and Histology

Tendons connect muscles to bones and help transmit force. They vary in size and length in different regions of the body, and they may be long, broad, flat, round or aponeurotic. Tendons lie around bony pulleys (peroneal tendons around the malleoli), enclose sesamoids (flexor hallucis longus) and may also be located in intramuscular situations, as well as connecting different muscle bellies to each other (intermediate tendon) (Benjamin et al. 2008).

Tendons are organised in a hierarchical pattern to form strong, fibrous structures. Tendon cells (tenocytes) manufacture all of the components of tendon in response to the environment (both load and chemical signalling). Tendons are primarily made up of collagen, which transmits tensile load

M. Girdwood (✉) • S. Docking • E. Rio
J. Cook
La Trobe Sport and Exercise Medicine Research Centre, Melbourne, VIC, Australia
e-mail: m.girdwood@latrobe.edu.au; s.docking@latrobe.edu.au; e.rio@latrobe.edu.au; j.cook@latrobe.edu.au

G.L. Canata et al. (eds.), *Muscle and Tendon Injuries*, DOI 10.1007/978-3-662-54184-5_3

through the long axis of the tendon. Collagen is the major component of the *extracellular matrix* (ECM). The ECM also contains *ground substance*, which includes water, proteoglycans (PGs), glycoproteins and glycosaminoglycans (GAGs).

The tendon as a whole is enveloped by the *peritendon*, made up of the *paratenon* (loose outer layer) and *epitenon* (thin inner layer) (Grant et al. 2013). This allows the tendon to glide against the surrounding tissue (Elliot 1965). Paratenon lined with synovial cells is called a *tenosynovium*, while one with a double-layer sheath without synovial cells is known as a *tenovagium*. Peritendinous structures are highly variable depending on location and function of each tendon. The long finger flexor and extensor tendons exhibit a highly organised and structured peritendon due to the amount of movement against surrounding tissues, while those in the hip and knee have a negligible peritendon. Peritendon cells are responsive to loading (Langberg et al. 1999, 2001) and appear more sensitive and reactive to stimuli than intratendinous cells (Rempel and Abrahamsson 2001). Their importance and exact role in maintaining tendon structure and contributing to pathology, however, are not fully known.

3.2 Tenocytes

Tenocytes are arranged sparsely and longitudinally between collagen fibrils (Benjamin et al. 2008). They communicate through cell processes and gap junctions (McNeilly et al. 1996; Kraushaar and Nirschl 1999; O'Brien 1997). These gap junctions transfer ions and small metabolites (Waggett et al. 2006). Adherens junctions are also found between cells forming cell-cell adhesions, mediating cell proliferation, polarisation and migration (Kjaer et al. 2009).

Tenocytes modify their shape, function and cellular regulation (Kjaer et al. 2009) in response to load such as tensile strain and compression, as well as in response to growth factors and hydrostatic pressure (Leadbetter 1992). The gap junctions between tenocytes are important in response to load, with a higher rate of turnover and increased formation of gap junctions following loading (Waggett et al. 2006; Wall and Banes 2005; Banes et al. 1999). This enables greater collagen synthesis (Kjaer et al. 2009). Adherens junctions also exhibit force-dependent behaviour (Nagafuchi 2001) and are likely involved in mechanotransduction (Schwartz and DeSimone 2008) and also in adaption to loading (Kjaer et al. 2009).

Along with cell-to-cell attachments, the cell has direct contact with the extracellular matrix. Focal adhesion complexes link the internal cytoskeleton with the surrounding ECM (Ingber 1997). These focal adhesion complexes consist of actin filaments of the cytoskeleton, actin-associated molecules intracellularly, and integrin molecules that have direct contact with the ECM. The internal cytoskeleton has been shown to be critical in the detection of mechanical stimuli, with disruption of the cytoskeleton resulting in the cell being unable to detect mechanical stimuli (Lavagnino and Arnoczky 2005; Gardner et al. 2012). As these focal adhesion complexes physically link the internal compartment of the cell to the ECM, it is likely to have a critical role in detecting mechanical stimuli and converting it into a biochemical response (Arnoczky et al. 2007).

3.3 Extracellular Matrix

Tendon ECM is predominantly made up of Type I collagen, though many other collagens also contribute to the fibrillar matrix (Riley 2005). Collagen is arranged in a hierarchical manner (Kastelic et al. 1978). Tenocytes assemble procollagen within the cell, before being cleaved into tropocollagen (Kjaer 2004; Robins 1988). The tropocollagen molecule is made up of three polypeptide chains, forming a triple-helical structure (Kadler et al. 1996). These are bound together by enzymes to form the smallest 'unit' of collagen, a collagen fibril. Collagen molecules overlap one another in an orderly fashion, to reinforce the fibril (O'Brien 1997; Robins 1988). Fibrils are arranged mostly longitudinally but some are transversely to reinforce and protect tendon against forces from a variety of directions (Robins 1988; Khan et al. 1999). Cross-links between molecules are an important part of force transmission (Depalle et al. 2015) and contribute to the mechanical properties of the tendon (Magnusson et al. 2010; Kjaer 2004). Molecular gliding occurs between fibrils to allow tendon elongation (Fratzl et al. 1998; Screen et al. 2004; Benjamin et al. 2008). Fibrils are grouped together to become fibres, which are then bound together into larger bundles and finally fascicles (Kastelic et al. 1978). Fascicles are visible on ultrasonographic examination. A tendon is made up of many fascicles, and this is thought to be a protective mechanism against failure of individual fibre bundles (Benjamin and Ralphs 1997).

The collagen matrix provides the tensile strength for force transmission in tendons. It allows for stiffness and strength when loaded but flexibility when bent or twisted (Amiel et al. 1984). However, it remains unknown whether microdamage to individual fibrils or changes to the non-collagenous components are responsible for alterations to tendon capacity (Magnusson et al. 2010).

Collagen fibres and fascicles (but not fibres) are surrounded by connective tissue, known as *endotendon (Screen et al. 2015)*. The endotendon allows for blood vessels, nerves and lymphatics to supply the tendon at a fascicle level (Grant et al. 2013; Elliott 1965). The endotendon also contains small amounts of Type III collagen (smaller diameter and looser more reticular bundles) (Williams et al. 1984).

3.3.1 Ground Substance

Ground substance is the non-collagenous components of the ECM, mainly made up of proteoglycans and glycoproteins. Proteoglycans are formed from an association between a protein core and glycosaminoglycan (GAG) side chain/s (Yoon and Halper 2005). PGs are hydrophilic (water attracting) and hence water makes up 60–80% of the weight of ground substance. Proteoglycans and water are thought to be responsible for lubricating and spacing collagen fibrils in tendons and play an important role in viscoelasticity (Screen et al. 2005; Kjaer 2004). They also appear to have a role in aligning and orientating collagen (Baldock et al. 2001).

Small proteoglycans (that have fewer GAG chains and therefore bind less water) are the most abundant in normal tendon and include decorin, biglycan and fibromodulin (Birch et al. 2013). Decorin appears to have a role in inhibiting the fusion of adjacent collagen fibrils, with high concentration in decorin resulting in a high proportion of small-diameter collagen fibrils. Larger proteoglycans (with more protein cores and GAG chains) such as aggrecan and versican are less common but integral to viscoelasticity of a tendon and resistance to compressive loading (Yoon and Halper 2005).

Glycoproteins are also found within the ECM. They are made up of protein and carbohydrates, such as tenascin-C, which is an anti-adhesive protein found to respond to mechanical loading and contribute to the elasticity of the tendon (Martin et al. 2003; Mehr et al. 2000). Elevated levels are found in tendons subject to compression and heavy mechanical loading (Jarvinen et al. 2003; Midwood and Orend 2009; Riley et al. 1996). The ECM also contains integrin-associated proteins, which form cell-to-ECM connections that are involved in controlling and signalling adaptive cell responses to loading (Chiquet et al. 2003). They may remain elevated for as long as four days after loading (Mehr et al. 2000).

3.4 Blood and Nerve Supply

Tendons are relatively avascular when compared with the muscle and skin (Benjamin and Ralphs 1997), with blood vessels making up only 1–2% of the area of the ECM (Kjaer 2004). Vascular supply to a tendon arises from three distinct zones: the musculotendinous junction, the bone-tendon junction, and surrounding more highly vascularised peritendon (Fenwick et al. 2002; Zantop et al. 2003; Ahmed et al. 1998; Schatzker and Branemark 1969). Vessels enter the tendon via the endotendon (Grant et al. 2013).

Blood supply is variable and affected by factors such as muscle contraction, stretching and shearing (Cook et al. 2005a; Khan et al. 1999;

Benjamin and Ralphs 1997). Blood flow is adequate throughout tendons (Astrom and Westlin 1994), and poor regional blood flow (such as in the Achilles mid-portion) does not contribute to pathology (Chen et al. 2009).

Tendons have an almost exclusively afferent nerve supply that is located mostly near the muscle-tendon junction to assist in mediating proprioception (Kirkendall and Garrett 1997; O'Brien 1997; O'Brien 1992). Most nerve fibres do not enter the tendon proper, and supply to the mid-tendon is minimal (Ackermann et al. 2005). Similarly to the vascular supply, the paratenon is richly innervated.

3.5 Structural Regions in Tendons

All tendons connect the muscle to bone via a region called the enthesis. The enthesis is the zone of transition between the tendon and bone, where collagen fibres become integrated into mineralised bony tissue. Different types of entheses (fibrous and fibrocartilaginous) have been described (Biermann 1957; Woo 1988; Hems and Tillman 2000) (Benjamin and Ralphs 1997; Apostolakos et al. 2014).

A fibrous enthesis occurs when a tendon inserts directly into the bone or periosteum and contains dense fibrous connective tissue (Benjamin and Ralphs 1997). They insert into the metaphysis or diaphysis, typically over a large surface area, and are seen on long bones, such as linea aspera on the femur (Benjamin et al. 2006; Apostolakos et al. 2014). They rarely cause pain or pathology.

Fibrocartilaginous entheses are seen at tendons inserting into the epiphysis or apophysis (Benjamin and Ralphs 1997; Apostolakos et al. 2014). They have four distinct zones to form continuity from uncalcified tendon to fully calcified the bone: the tendon, fibrocartilage, calcified fibrocartilage and then bone (Benjamin et al. 1986, 2006; Shaw and Benjamin 2007; Apostolakos et al. 2014). These represent a change in tissue flexibility (Hems and Tillman 2000). Other structures exist around fibrocartilaginous tendon insertions, such as bursae, fat pads and retinaculum, and have been collectively termed the *enthesis organ* (Benjamin and McGonagle 2001). The fat pad and bursae are innervated structures that help to maintain tendon function (distribute stress) (Kumai and Benjamin 2002) and also may provide proprioceptive information (Shaw and Benjamin 2007).

3.6 Response to Load

Tendons are responsive to load through a complex primarily cell-driven response. Tensile loading leads to matrix and cell deformation, which leads to ECM protein production and/or change in mechanical strength that improves tissue capacity and tolerance to subsequent load (Magnusson et al. 2010). Tendon loading changes both collagen degradation and production (Magnusson et al. 2010), with peak synthesis at around 24 h, and relative elevated production for up to 72 h (Langberg et al. 1999). Increased turnover likely maintains normal homeostasis (Heinemeier and Kjaer 2011; Rees et al. 2009). Different contraction types do not affect the synthesis or degradation of collagen, and differences between concentric, eccentric or isometric loading are related to the total tendon strain (Kjaer et al. 2009; Heinemeier et al. 2007). Other matrix proteins, including a number of proteoglycans (PGs), also exhibit increased turnover in response to exercise.

Compressive or shearing forces on tendons result in increased production of larger PG, such as aggrecan (Docking et al. 2013; Vogel et al. 2004; Giori et al. 1993). This expression is thought to be a homeostatic response to loading, similar to that of collagen production(Koob et al. 1992). Compressive forces may also increase fibrocartilaginous tissue near the compressed areas of a tendon insertion (Docking et al. 2013; Benjamin and Ralphs 1998).

On a molecular level, loading leads to an increase in growth factors and cytokines, such as insulin-like growth factor 1 (IGF-1), transforming growth factor β (TGF-β) and interleukin 6 (IL-6) (Nourissat et al. 2015; Magnusson et al.

2010; Kjaer et al. 2009). Many of these regulate collagen production via tendon cells (Andersen et al. 2011) and remain elevated for at least 36 h after loading (Langberg et al. 2002). Other responses include release of substance P and calcitonin gene-related peptide (CGRP) (Danielson et al. 2007). Substance P has been shown to be elevated after 1 week of loading in animal models (Backman et al. 2011a). In vitro research also suggests substance P released after loading is involved in upregulating proliferation of tenocytes and can regulate tendon homeostasis (Backman et al. 2011b; Zhou et al. 2015).

3.7 Function and Mechanics of Tendons

The properties of tendon are related to their shape and size that is in turn related to function (and forces placed on the tendon) (Roberts 2002). A larger tendon can withstand a higher load, while a longer tendon will be able to store more energy (Brughelli and Cronin 2008).

Mechanical properties of a tendon may be expressed as tensile stress or strain. Stress is calculated by dividing the total tensile load by the cross-sectional area at the point of loading (Brughelli and Cronin 2008). For example, the thinnest part of a tendon will be subjected to the most stress under a given load. Strain refers to the amount a tendon stretches while loaded compared with its unloaded length. The relationship between these two measures determines other mechanical properties such as Young's modulus.

Tendons are also subject to compressive forces, when in contact with the bone, retinacula or fascia (Almekinders et al. 2003). They also experience shearing forces that are a vector of compressive and tensile loads (Benjamin et al. 2008).

Functionally, one of the most important functions of a tendon is to store and release energy, acting like a spring. This allows for the use of elastic energy to create movement (Holt et al. 2014; Kirkendall and Garrett 1997; Alexander 2002; Amiel et al. 1984). An example of this is the Achilles tendon during running, which recovers energy stored with tendon lengthening to be released during propulsion (push off) (Alexander et al. 1982; Dimery et al. 1986).

3.8 Summary

Tendons are complex structures that connect muscles and bones. They have two main functions: to transmit force from the muscle to bone to create joint movement and to store and release energy like a spring. Around the body they are seen in a variety of different shapes and sizes, which often reflect their purpose and location. Tendons are composed of a highly organised extracellular matrix (ECM), produced and regulated by tenocytes. At its insertion onto the bone, tendon structure transitions to the bone at the enthesis. Tendons have an almost exclusively afferent nerve supply and low but sufficient vasculaturity. Tendons are highly load tolerant and adaptable to changing stresses. This is mediated by an interplay of a range of different factors such as chemical changes and loading types. Understanding this complex interaction is required to accurately assess and treat tendinopathy.

Understanding how tendons transition from normal to injured and painful tendons is important when considering treatment. A number of factors impact on the development of tendon pathology. Historically a wide variety of terminology has been used to describe tendon pathology, such as tendinitis or tendinosis (Khan et al. 1999) (Maffulli et al. 1998).

3.9 Structural Changes in Tendon Pathology

End-stage degenerative tendon pathology is clearly described, characterised by changes in cell activity, disorganisation of the collagen matrix and increased neovascularisation (Kannus 1997). Histopathological studies of tendon pathology demonstrate increased proteoglycan and glycosaminoglycan content and in turn more bound water (Samiric et al. 2009; Xu and Murrell

2008). There are more tenocytes that are more active and rounded (Magnusson et al. 2010). Elevated levels of messenger RNA (mRNA) are seen for collagen production, proteoglycans, vascular growth and stress-responsive proteins, suggesting a hypercellular environment (Magnusson et al. 2010). Lower amounts of Type I and greater amounts of Type III collagen are synthesised in pathological tendons (Maffulli et al. 2000; Eriksen et al. 2002; Riley et al. 1994); Type III collagen has lower tensile strength and forms less organised bundles, possibly due to fewer cross-links (Goncalves-Neto et al. 2002). Increased neovascular ingrowth is present in the tendon (Alfredson et al. 2003). Other changes include increased substance P production (Fearon et al. 2014) and more substance P-positive nerve fibres (Schubert et al. 2005).

Tendons with pathology are often thickened and have an increased cross-sectional area (Abate et al. 2009). Thickened tendons were previously thought to be maladaptive; however new research proposes that a tendon may thicken to maintain a sufficient amount of aligned fibrillar structure to compensate for the area of pathology (Docking and Cook 2016).

3.10 Pathoaetiology

The primary change in tendon pathology may be collagen, tendon cell or inflammation or some combination of these. Tearing, disruption and degeneration of collagen fibres were originally considered the cause of tendinopathy (Leadbetter 1992). Models of failed healing have also been put forward; injury to tendon structure leads to a failed healing response, and this in turn leads to a clinical manifestation of tendon pain (Fu et al. 2010). While this model seemingly accounts for cellular findings listed above as well as structural changes, it does not explain the disconnect seen between pain and structure.

The presence, relevance and impact of inflammation in tendon pathology have long been debated amongst experts. While clinical inflammation (swelling, redness) is often described in cases of tendon pathology (Scott et al. 2004), research in Achilles, patellar and extensor carpi radialis brevis tendons all showed no difference in levels of prostaglandin E2 when comparing pathological tendons with controls (Alfredson et al. 1999, 2000, 2001) (Pingel et al. 2012; Jarvinen et al. 1997). Upregulation of inflammatory cytokines (such as endothelial growth factors, tumour necrosis factors, COX-2, PGE-2 and interleukins) (Mousavizadeh et al. 2014; Zhang and Wang 2010; Wang et al. 2004) may occur as a consequence of mechanical loading of a normal tendon (Kjaer et al. 2013).

Research showing elevated inflammatory cells in tendon disorders are cited as evidence of inflammation as a cause of tendon pain (Dean et al. 2016; Millar et al. 2010); however the link between these features and pain remains unclear. An inflammatory response may be a factor in the development of tendinopathy (Rees et al. 2014; Abate et al. 2009); however inflammation alone as a cause of tendinopathy is not supported, and the clinical importance of these processes remains unclear.

Other findings point to increased inflammatory cytokines not at the site of tendinopathy itself but in peritendinous structures (Riley 2008; Kjaer et al. 2013). While this may be consistent with theories suggesting the peritendon as a source of pain (Stecco et al. 2014), it does not explain the development of pathology in the tendon itself.

3.10.1 Continuum Model of Tendinopathy

The continuum of tendon pathology presents different stages of tendinopathy: reactive tendinopathy, tendon dysrepair and degenerative tendinopathy (Cook and Purdam 2009; Cook et al. 2016). Reactive tendinopathy is seen after acute tensile and/or compressive overload, resulting in a noninflammatory cell-based response. This is often seen after abusive loading, unaccustomed activity (both in athletes and sedentary populations) (Scott et al. 2007) or even a direct blow to the tendon (Garau et al. 2008). From a histopathological perspective, reactive tendinopathy is characterised by a hypercellular environment with an increase in large proteoglycans synthesised, and thus more bound water is observed (Magnusson et al. 2010). Clinically this is seen as a thickened tendon—a response that can reduce the stress on tendon tissue in the short term. While this stage is sometimes described clinically as 'inflamed' due to the swollen appearance and acute pain, there is no significant upregulation of inflammatory cells as a driver of this stage (Scott et al. 2007). Importantly there is structural change in the collagen matrix, and if the overload is sufficiently reduced, tendon structure can return to normal.

Tendon dysrepair marks the development of fibrillar disorganisation on the back of increased proteoglycan production. This stage may be similar to what has previously been described as 'failed healing' (Fu et al. 2010).

Degenerative tendon pathology is defined by irreversible degenerative tendon pathology and associated neurovascular changes. Collagen matrix degradation occurs and can be visualised as hypoechoic areas on ultrasound. The degenerative portion does not transmit any load and is thought of as mechanically silent. Importantly, tendons that have degenerative areas also have regions of normal tendon tissue. Tendon thickening is proposed as an adaption to maintain sufficient aligned fibrillar structure for loading (Docking and Cook 2015).

Patients present for clinical management when in pain; however at other times pathology may be asymptomatic or 'dormant'. The continuum model suggests that within this model two presentations are seen clinically: (1) reactive tendinopathy as first-time presentation of pain and (2) reactive-on-degenerative presentation—reactive part of previously normal tendon surrounding 'dormant' degenerative component. Therefore, it is the reactive state of pathology that is proposed to be nociceptive and not the degenerative portion of the tendon. Pain-free tendons may still demonstrate significant structural pathology but insufficient nociceptive signalling (Rio et al. 2015).

3.11 Pain in Tendinopathy

Tendon pain has some unique characteristics compared to other musculoskeletal conditions. Pain in tendinopathy remains highly localised (regardless of length of time of symptoms), is provoked by loading in an 'on/off' fashion and is not usually seen at rest, suggesting a primary tendon-based nociceptive driver of pain. This also infers that inhibitory control at the spinal cord is maintained in contrast with many other persistent pain presentations where spreading of pain is observed with chronicity. This may be due to the relationship with loading that prevents potentiation. The extent of structural disorganisation observed on imaging does not correlate with clinical symptoms. Inflammation in tendinopathy also does not provide an explanation for the clinical presentation of tendon pain.

The key drivers of nociception are unclear (Littlewood et al. 2013a; Rio et al. 2015). Tendons have poor sensory innervation, with almost no afferent fibres deep in the tendon itself (Ackermann et al. 2005). Paracrine signalling from the tendon has been proposed as a cause of tendon pain (Danielson et al. 2006), by sensitising more peripherally located nociceptive nerves (Rio et al. 2015). The peritendon has also been proposed as a source of pain in tendinopathy (Stecco et al. 2014), and this may be due to sensitisation of the peripheral nerve or from tendon swelling in a reactive tendinopathy presentation (Cook et al. 2016).

Nerve fibres positive for substance P are also sensitive to a number of other substances such as acetylcholine (ACh), glutamate and catecholamines (Danielson et al. 2007; Alfredson et al. 2001), which may be upregulated by the tenocyte, suggesting cell-driven signalling as a potential mechanism for tendon pain (Danielson 2009). These substances also impact on cell homeostasis, collagen production and other functions of tenocytes, which may contribute to the structural changes in tendinopathy (Danielson 2009). Ion channels in cell membranes may also be important in tendon pain (Rio et al. 2015). They are implicated in cell signalling and mechanotransduction. A decreased pH as a result of accumulation of lactate (Alfredson et al. 2002) may lead to altered expression of acid-sensing ion channels. These ion channels may also explain for the 'warm-up' phenomenon seen in tendinopathy, as they exhibit evidence of saturation (Jones et al. 2004). Changes in acid-sensing ion channels have been shown to impede cell function in the bone, cartilage and intervertebral discs (Jahr et al. 2005; Rong et al. 2012; Uchiyama et al. 2007).

The impact of peripheral nervous system (PNS) and CNS sensitisation is widely accepted in a variety of musculoskeletal conditions; however its involvement in tendinopathy is less clear. Evidence shows that contralateral sensory changes exist in tendinopathy (Heales et al. 2014); however these are also seen in other acute conditions such as ankle sprains and may be reversed instantly with anaesthetic (Ramiro-Gonzalez et al. 2012). In addition, secondary hyperalgesia is not seen in lower limb tendinopathy, as tendon pain remains highly localised, without spontaneous or spreading of pain. While development of bilateral symptoms or tendinopathy on the contralateral side to initial presentation can occur (Paavola et al. 2000), this process is likely complex and may involve central mechanisms, with alterations in loading patterns, morphological differences or systemic drivers. Isometric exercises performed on one side in bilateral presentations decrease ipsilateral symptoms but no impact on contralateral pain, also supporting the significance of locally driven factors in tendon pain (Rio et al. 2015).

All pain is an output of the brain; thus, it is critical the clinician understands and can communicate key messages about tendinopathy. For example, the use of the term 'tear' relating to tendon imaging is likely unhelpful, evokes fear and therefore will probably promote unloading. In our management of tendinopathy, we must educate patients to understand their tendon and the importance of rehabilitation.

3.12 Regional Changes in Tendinopathy

Other structures may also be affected by tendinopathy and are important differential diagnoses. The peritendon may become irritated and painful by friction loads and is seen commonly in the wrist, hands and feet. Peritendinitis has an inflammatory component (Kannus 1997; Reynolds and Worrell 1991). Chronic peritendinitis can lead to changes in the structure of the peritendon, with more connective tissue adhesions, vascular ingrowth and an influx of a variety of cells (Jarvinen et al. 1997; Kvist et al. 1992).

A number of other structures exist around a tendon, including fat pad and bursae, and coexist with tendinopathy. Bursitis is usually associated with tendon pathology. Some tendons may be adjoined by fat pads, which are highly innervated and may be a source of pain. Fat pads show an inflammatory response in painful presentations (Ward et al. 2016).

3.13 Epidemiology of Tendinopathy

Tendinopathy is primarily the result of load that exceeds a tendon's capacity. Tendinopathy is prevalent in active and sporting populations, though sedentary individuals who have a low capacity are also prone to overload and may be further compromised by other systemic factors (Ackermann and Renstrom 2012; Maffulli et al. 2003; Hopkins et al. 2016; Cook et al. 1998). Elite athletes in particular are prone to developing tendinopathy given their high training loads (Ackermann and Renstrom 2012; Cook and Purdam 2003). Tendinopathy and their associated aetiology occur in many common sites (Table 3.1) but can occur in any tendon (e.g. flexor hallucis longus, tibialis posterior and distal biceps brachii tendon).

The prevalence of tendinopathy may be underestimated as the condition may be mild, and patients may not present for diagnosis and management. This is also seen in a sporting context, where an athlete may continue to train and play with tendinopathy; tendinopathy may not register as an injury as injury statistics are usually recorded when there is a sporting time loss. It is worth noting that the burden is greater than missed participation as the impact on performance is difficult to measure.

Because of the varied definitions, diagnostic criteria, tendon studied and population, estimates

Table 3.1 Tendinopathy sites

Tendon	Site of tendinopathy	Loading factors	Age/sex
Achilles	Achilles insertion or mid-portion	Distance running, change of direction (combined tensile and compressive load at the calcaneus)	Men—elite and recreational (Jarvinen et al. 2005)
Patellar	Inferior pole of patella	Jumping and landing, fast change of direction, e.g. volleyball	Younger athletes (Cassel et al. 2015) <30 years old
Proximal hamstring	Ischial attachment of hamstring	Training errors Sprinting +– bending, e.g. hockey (combined compressive and tensile load)	Any age in an active person (Goom et al. 2016)
Gluteal	Greater trochanter	Stairs and walking	Postmenopausal women (Grimaldi et al. 2015)
Adductor	Adductor tendon or insertion	Kicking	Male athletes (Weir et al. 2015) Kicking sports
Lateral elbow	Common extensor origin	Manual work or gripping tasks, racquet sports (Roquelaure et al. 2006; Descatha et al. 2013)	>40 years old (Bisset and Vicenzino 2015)
Rotator cuff	Sub-acromial	Overhead activity (Seitz et al. 2011)	Young overhead athletes (Sein et al. 2010) Older than 50 years (Bodin et al. 2012)

of prevalence vary between studies. The general population have a 2–5% prevalence of tendinopathy (across all body sites) (Hopkins et al. 2016), though subgroups such as patellar tendinopathy in volleyball players have rates of up to 40%. Incidence of rotator cuff tendinopathy is estimated as high as 5.5% (Littlewood et al. 2013), while incidence of lateral epicondylalgia is around 1–2% (Gabel 1999; Allander 1974).

Prevalence of tendinopathy in elite sport also is highly dependent on the nature of the sport and thus the loading factors present (Ackermann and Renstrom 2012). Studies in soccer have shown 2.4% prevalence of patellar tendinopathy across a season; median absence from play was only 5 days per injury (Hagglund et al. 2011). An 11% lifetime prevalence of Achilles tendinopathy has been shown in runners (Jarvinen et al. 2005).

Pathology can be identified on imaging, but it may be asymptomatic, highlighting the poor connection between pain and structure (Docking et al. 2015). The presence of tendon pathology in pain-free individuals has been estimated as high as 50% in some populations, such as Australian football (Docking et al. 2015). Pathology on imaging is a risk factor for developing future symptoms (McAuliffe et al. 2016), though the risk is inconsistent across different tendons. In patellar and Achilles tendinopathy, the presence of pathology on greyscale ultrasound increased the risk of developing tendinopathy approximately five times (McAuliffe et al. 2016). Despite these findings, a number of other risk factors are involved in the development of tendinopathy. The majority of those with asymptomatic pathology will not develop symptoms and will never present for medical management; hence, caution in interpreting the importance of imaging abnormalities is required.

3.14 Intrinsic Risk Factors

Intrinsic factors may be modifiable or unmodifiable and relate to a person's body composition, lifestyle and general health. It is critical to investigate these factors and address systemic contributors for successful management.

3.14.1 Genetics

Genetic factors are implicated in the pathogenesis of tendinopathy. Identical twin studies have implicated genetic factors in lateral epicondylalgia (Hakim et al. 2003). A number of different genes have been found to be upregulated and downregulated in tendinopathy; however their significance is yet to be determined (September et al. 2007; Jelinsky et al. 2011; Magra and Maffulli 2008). Two variants for COL5A1 gene and the tenascin-C (TNC) gene have been implicated in tendon pathology. COL5A1 encodes for a component of Type V collagen, which aligns and organises Type I collagen (Birk et al. 1990). A specific phenotype results in more tightly packed collagen bundles leading to both better energy storage and also greater vulnerability to tendinopathy. Variations in the COL5A1 gene are linked to an increased risk of Achilles tendinopathy (Chauhan et al. 2015; Mokone et al. 2006; September et al. 2009). Tenascin-C is an anti-adhesive protein, which is important in the regulation of load capacity after tendon loading and compression (Jarvinen et al. 2000). Variants of the TNC gene have also been linked with Achilles tendinopathy, with certain polymorphisms increasing the risk of developing symptoms sixfold (Mokone et al. 2005). Polymorphisms within the TNC or COL5A1 gene have been suggested to be linked to other injuries such as ACL tears (September et al. 2007); however so far results have been conflicting (Stepien-Slodkowska et al. 2015; Posthumus et al. 2010).

Other factors involved in tissue repair in tendons include transforming growth factor β1 (TGF-β1) and growth/differentiation factor 5 (GDF-5) (Hou et al. 2009; Rickert et al. 2005). A genetic association study however showed no difference in TGF-β1 expression between people with tendinopathy and controls. Genes coding for GDF-5 however were significantly associated with Achilles tendinopathy, showing a modest two times elevated risk (Posthumus et al. 2010).

3.14.2 Sex

The impact of sex on tendinopathy varies across the population, as well as affecting different tendons. Postmenopausal women exhibit higher rates of tendinopathy (Frizziero et al. 2014) and tendon rupture (Maffulli et al. 2007); however this may be confounded by other factors such as increased blood lipids. There was no impact of gender in Achilles or patellar tendinopathy in masters athletes (Longo et al. 2009, 2011). Peritendon disorders such as De Quervain's tenosynovitis are more common in women (Wolf et al. 2009), and this may be linked to altered inflammatory responses in women (Hart et al. 1998).

3.14.3 Age

Ageing is thought of as a risk factor for developing degenerative pathology; however ageing alone does not explain tendon pathology. Ageing affects the structure and histology of tendons, with increased stiffness, deformation and cross-sectional area, as well as decreased peak tendon stress and strain (Carroll et al. 2008; Tuite et al. 1997). However, when force is normalised, there is no difference seen between young and old tendons in terms of deformation, strain and stiffness, suggesting change in force-output capacity may be more responsible for the alterations seen during ageing (Carroll et al. 2008). Other studies have shown increase in collagen cross-linking, decrease in water content and collagen concentration (Narici et al. 2008; Couppe et al. 2009), as well as a decrease in blood supply (Tuite et al. 1997). Together it seems that load capacity decreases with age, particularly with reference to energy storage and release loading. Ageing is a risk factor for tendon rupture (Pedowitz and Kirwan 2013), and cumulative loading may also be a factor, as past athletes exhibit higher rates of tendinopathy and rupture (Kujala et al. 2005).

Young athletes exhibit high rates of tendon pathology. In children, tendon pathology may be seen on imaging (Simpson et al. 2016); however pain is commonly attributed to the apophysis (such as Osgood-Schlatters disease). Evidence is however emerging to suggest that tendon pathology may be present in children and adolescents distant to the apophysis (Sailly et al. 2013).

3.14.4 Medications

Fluoroquinolones, a class of antibiotic, have been closely associated with the development of tendinopathy and tendon rupture (Lewis and Cook 2014). The Achilles tendon is the site most commonly affected (Lang et al. 2016; Khaliq and Zhanel 2003). Men appear to be at greater risk, with a dose-dependent response seen (Khaliq and Zhanel 2003; Lewis and Cook 2014). Fluoroquinolones are thought to have their effect by decreasing cell numbers and increasing matrix breakdown. Fluoroquinolone-associated tendinopathy may be slower to respond to treatment (Lewis and Cook 2014).

Statin medications have also been implicated as a risk factor for developing tendinopathy, though evidence is conflicting (Teichtahl et al. 2016; Kirchgesner et al. 2014). A number of case reports show increased incidence of tendinopathy (Kirchgesner et al. 2014; Marie et al. 2008); however a recent systematic review showed no increased risk (Teichtahl et al. 2016). Conversely simvastatin may actually slightly decrease the risk of tendinopathy (Contractor et al. 2015).

Finally local and systemic use of glucocorticoids has been suggested to negatively affect tendon tissue (Dean et al. 2014; Blanco et al. 2005). Local glucocorticoid injection leads to decreased collagen production, impaired cell proliferation, increased matrix disorganisation and hence lower mechanical load tolerance of the tendon cells (Dean et al. 2014). Long-term clinical outcomes were worse following corticosteroid injection in lateral epicondylalgia (Coombes et al. 2016). An association between local injection and rupture has been proposed (Kirchgesner et al. 2014; Blanco et al. 2005); however little evidence supports this (Scott et al. 2015a).

3.14.5 General Health

Obesity is considered a risk factor for a variety of musculoskeletal conditions and has also been shown as a risk factor for developing tendinopathy (Scott et al. 2015b; Gaida et al. 2008, 2009a; Franceschi et al. 2014). Elevated body mass index has been shown in tendinopathy compared to control, though a variety of interactions may be responsible (Scott et al. 2013; Klein et al. 2013; Gaida et al. 2008, 2009a). Increased waist circumference was also linked with asymptomatic tendon pathology. There are differences between fat distributions in men and women; men with tendinopathy have more central adiposity, while women exhibit peripheral distribution of fat (Gaida et al. 2010). This is supported by findings in men showing waist girth over 83 cm was a risk factor for patellar tendinopathy in volleyball players but not in women (Malliaras et al. 2007).

Obesity has both mechanical and systemic effects (Scott et al. 2014). Elevated load on tendons due to excessive weight has been postulated to be behind the elevated risk of tendinopathy. From a systemic viewpoint, obesity increases blood lipids, which have also been shown elevated in Achilles tendinopathy (Gaida et al. 2009b).

Systemic diseases and illnesses associated with obesity can predispose to tendinopathy. People with Type II diabetes mellitus have a 3.6 times greater prevalence of tendinopathy than controls (Ranger et al. 2016). Increased tendon thickness is also reported in diabetes (de Oliveira et al. 2011a). The mechanism may be via hyperglycaemia that reduces proteoglycan content and increased levels of transforming growth factor $\beta1$ (TGF-$\beta1$) (Burner et al. 2012). Diabetes also leads to increased formation of advanced glycation end products (AGE), which can create more collagen cross-links (Snedeker and Gautieri 2014; Abate et al. 2013; Reddy 2003). Increased

AGE content is shown to decrease the viscoelastic properties of tendons, by decreased sliding between fibres (Li et al. 2013; Fessel et al. 2014). Increased cross-linking can increase load to failure (Snedeker and Gautieri 2014) and increase stiffness, while other studies showed greater tissue fragility (Fox et al. 2011; de Oliveira et al. 2011b).

Dyslipidaemia may predispose tendons to pain and pathology by altering tendon structure and increased levels of immune and pro-inflammatory cells (Scott et al. 2014). The dyslipidaemia seen in Achilles tendinopathy is similar to that seen in insulin resistance, and it has been proposed that tendinopathy may be a comorbidity of metabolic syndrome and cardiovascular disease (Gaida et al. 2009b). This may also explain why decreased physical activity is associated with development of tendinopathy (Descatha et al. 2013). Tendon pain then further reduces physical activity.

Hypercholesterolaemia also appears to be associated with tendinopathy (Tilley et al. 2015; Esenkaya and Unay 2011), particularly in familial cases (Abate et al. 2013; Beeharry et al. 2006). Increased blood lipids increase the accumulation of pro-inflammatory cells, mast cells and macrophages, as well as increased deposition of low-density lipoproteins (LDLs) in the tendon matrix (Tilley et al. 2015). Association with lower physical activity levels or other comorbidities may be driving this link (Tilley et al. 2015). A number of other illnesses have been linked with elevated risk for tendinopathy including hyperuricaemia (Abate et al. 2013), systemic lupus, rheumatoid arthritis (Fredberg 1997), psoriatic arthritis (Gutierrez et al. 2010) and hypertension (Holmes and Lin 2006).

3.14.6 Flexibility and Joint Stiffness

Reduced flexibility of muscles attaching to the at-risk tendon as well as antagonist muscle groups has been shown to increase the risk of developing tendinopathy. Both quadriceps and hamstring inflexibility have been shown as a risk factor for development of patellar tendinopathy (Witvrouw et al. 2001; Silva et al. 2016; Crossley et al. 2007; Cook et al. 2002). Too much or too little ankle dorsiflexion range is a risk factor for developing Achilles and patellar tendinopathy (Backman and Danielson 2011; Malliaras et al. 2006; Crossley et al. 2007; Kaufman et al. 1999; Rabin et al. 2014; Mahieu et al. 2006).

There is little evidence that foot posture and mechanics are associated with tendinopathy nor that altering them with orthotics is effective despite widespread clinical use (Munteanu et al. 2015). Static foot posture has not been shown as a risk factor for patellar tendinopathy (de Groot et al. 2012; Crossley et al. 2007). Increased ankle inversion moments during landing and jumping tasks have been associated with patellar tendinopathy (Richards et al. 2002). Excessive foot pronation is often suggested as a risk factor for Achilles tendinopathy (Munteanu and Barton 2011); however quality research beyond anecdotal evidence is lacking (Dowling et al. 2014).

3.14.7 Strength

Clinically, poor strength is often associated with tendinopathy, likely mediated by pain. Decreased eccentric strength has been found in the quadriceps in people with patellar tendinopathy (Gaida et al. 2004) and gastrocnemius in those with Achilles tendinopathy (Silbernagel et al. 2006; Haglund-Akerlind and Eriksson 1993). Functional deficits such as decreased vertical jump and hopping ability (Silbernagel et al. 2006) have also been shown.

However a strength deficit has not been shown prospectively, with no relationship shown between quadriceps and hamstring strength and the development of patellar tendinopathy (Witvrouw et al. 2001). Consideration of kinetic chain deficits is important, as reduced strength in other regions may predispose a tendon to overload, and should be assessed on an individual basis when managing tendinopathy (Malliaras et al. 2015; Kountouris and Cook 2007).

3.15 Extrinsic Risk Factors

Extrinsic risk factors vary for each tendon. Lower limb tendinopathies are seen in weight-bearing sports, while shoulder tendinopathies are seen in overhead sports such as swimming and volleyball. Activities with high energy storage demands pose the highest risk for developing tendinopathy. Common examples of tensile (energy storage) overload include jumping in basketball or volleyball players, uphill running in runners and change of direction and kicking in field sports.

3.15.1 Load

Excessive loading above a tendon's capacity is a cause of tendinopathy. Clinically, activities requiring energy storage loads (such as running for the Achilles tendon) are associated with onset of tendon pain. While previous terminology has referred to tendinopathy as 'repetitive strain injuries', sports with high-frequency cyclical load such as cycling and rowing with low-energy storage components do not have high rates of tendinopathy. The clinician must understand load and use it as part of their differential diagnosis and decision making; the cyclist and rower are vulnerable to paratendinitis due to the repetitive friction in these activities and require different management.

The amount of loading may be critical; female basketball players with patellar tendon pathology trained 2.14 h more each week on average than their pain-free colleagues (Gaida et al. 2004). The number of hours trained significantly correlated with supraspinatus tendinopathy in swimmers (Sein et al. 2010). Training volume, as well as increased game exposure, was also a risk factor for patellar tendinopathy in volleyball players (Visnes and Bahr 2013). These findings are similar to other sports-related injuries, such as in those seen in throwers in baseball (Olsen et al. 2006) and bowlers in cricket (Hulin et al. 2014).

While total load is important, change in loading and training errors are key factors in a number of musculoskeletal pathologies, including tendinopathy. Consideration of the acute versus chronic workloads may be a factor to decrease risk of injury (Gabbett 2016). An optimum amount of loading appears to be protective while excess or insufficient loading precipitating greater risk. Orchard et al. (2015) found that medium-term workload (3 months) was protective for the development of tendon injuries in cricket bowlers. Clinically, tendinopathy presentations are very often seen after changes in training loads (Ferretti 1986). This may be change of training cycle, onset of intensive competitions, and even change in equipment or footwear. It is often common to see increased cases of tendinopathy in the beginning of a season after resumption of training, and this may also relate to underloading in the off-season and a relative increase in load with resumption of training.

While the majority of research concerns tendon overload, offloading or unloading may predispose a tendon to pain and symptoms as it may lower the load capacity, placing an individual at risk of tendinopathy (Kannus et al. 1997). Sedentary individuals are also at risk of developing tendinopathy, when they perform abusive loading or unaccustomed activity (as it exceeds their load capacity). This has been proposed in rotator cuff tendinopathy, often seen in older less active patients (Lewis 2010). Underload may also be seen when an athlete resumes training after a long layoff (such as the off-season) or injury. The importance of load is reinforced by the fact that complete rest of a symptomatic tendon will not cure a patient's presentation and often leads to a worsening tendinopathy once load is resumed.

References

Abate M, Silbernagel KG, Siljeholm C, Di Iorio A, De Amicis D, Salini V et al (2009) Pathogenesis of tendinopathies: inflammation or degeneration? Arthritis Res Ther 11(3):235. doi:10.1186/ar2723

Abate M, Schiavone C, Salini V, Andia I (2013) Occurrence of tendon pathologies in metabolic disorders. Rheumatology (Oxford) 52(4):599–608. doi:10.1093/rheumatology/kes395

Ackermann PW, Renstrom P (2012) Tendinopathy in sport. Sports Health 4(3):193–201. doi:10.1177/1941738112440957

Ackermann PW, Bring DK-I, Renström P (2005) Tendon innervation and neuronal response after injury. In: Maffulli N, Renström P, Leadbetter WB (eds) Tendon injuries: basic science and clinical medicine. Springer, London, pp 287–297

Ahmed IM, Lagopoulos M, McConnell P, Soames RW, Sefton GK (1998) Blood supply of the Achilles tendon. J Orthop Res 16(5):591–596. doi:10.1002/jor.1100160511

Alexander RM (2002) Tendon elasticity and muscle function. Comp Biochem Physiol A Mol Integr Physiol 133(4):1001–1011

Alexander RM, Maloiy GMO, Ker RF, Jayes AS, Warui CN (1982) The role of tendon elasticity in the locomotion of the camel (Camelus-Dromedarius). J Zool 198(November):293–313

Alfredson H, Thorsen K, Lorentzon R (1999) In situ microdialysis in tendon tissue: high levels of glutamate, but not prostaglandin E2 in chronic Achilles tendon pain. Knee Surg Sports Traumatol Arthrosc 7(6):378–381. doi:10.1007/s001670050184

Alfredson H, Ljung BO, Thorsen K, Lorentzon R (2000) In vivo investigation of ECRB tendons with microdialysis technique—no signs of inflammation but high amounts of glutamate in tennis elbow. Acta Orthop Scand 71(5):475–479. doi:10.1080/000164700317381162

Alfredson H, Forsgren S, Thorsen K, Lorentzon R (2001) In vivo microdialysis and immunohistochemical analyses of tendon tissue demonstrated high amounts of free glutamate and glutamate NMDAR1 receptors, but no signs of inflammation, in Jumper's knee. J Orthop Res 19(5):881–886. doi:10.1016/S0736-0266(01)00016-X

Alfredson H, Bjur D, Thorsen K, Lorentzon R, Sandstrom P (2002) High intratendinous lactate levels in painful chronic Achilles tendinosis. An investigation using microdialysis technique. J Orthop Res 20(5):934–938. doi:10.1016/S0736-0266(02)00021-9

Alfredson H, Ohberg L, Forsgren S (2003) Is vasculo-neural ingrowth the cause of pain in chronic Achilles tendinosis? An investigation using ultrasonography and colour Doppler, immunohistochemistry, and diagnostic injections. Knee Surg Sports Traumatol Arthrosc 11(5):334–338. doi:10.1007/s00167-003-0391-6

Allander E (1974) Prevalence, incidence, and remission rates of some common rheumatic diseases or syndromes. Scand J Rheumatol 3(3):145–153

Amiel D, Frank C, Harwood F, Fronek J, Akeson W (1984) Tendons and ligaments: a morphological and biochemical comparison. J Orthop Res 1(3):257–265. doi:10.1002/jor.1100010305

Andersen MB, Pingel J, Kjaer M, Langberg H (2011) Interleukin-6: a growth factor stimulating collagen synthesis in human tendon. J Appl Physiol (1985) 110(6):1549–1554. doi:10.1152/japplphysiol.00037.2010

Apostolakos J, Durant TJ, Dwyer CR, Russell RP, Weinreb JH, Alaee F et al (2014) The enthesis: a review of the tendon-to-bone insertion. Muscles Ligaments Tendons J 4(3):333–342

Arnoczky SP, Lavagnino M, Egerbacher M (2007) The mechanobiological aetiopathogenesis of tendinopathy: is it the over-stimulation or the under-stimulation of tendon cells? Int J Exp Pathol 88(4):217–226. doi:10.1111/j.1365-2613.2007.00548.x

Astrom M, Westlin N (1994) Blood flow in the human Achilles tendon assessed by laser Doppler flowmetry. J Orthop Res 12(2):246–252. doi:10.1002/jor.1100120214

Backman LJ, Danielson P (2011) Low range of ankle dorsiflexion predisposes for patellar tendinopathy in junior elite basketball players: a 1-year prospective study. Am J Sports Med 39(12):2626–2633. doi:10.1177/0363546511420552

Backman LJ, Andersson G, Wennstig G, Forsgren S, Danielson P (2011a) Endogenous substance P production in the Achilles tendon increases with loading in an in vivo model of tendinopathy-peptidergic elevation preceding tendinosis-like tissue changes. J Musculoskelet Neuronal Interact 11(2):133–140

Backman LJ, Fong G, Andersson G, Scott A, Danielson P (2011b) Substance P is a mechanoresponsive, autocrine regulator of human tenocyte proliferation. PLoS One 6(11):e27209. doi:10.1371/journal.pone.0027209

Baldock C, Koster AJ, Ziese U, Rock MJ, Sherratt MJ, Kadler KE et al (2001) The supramolecular organization of fibrillin-rich microfibrils. J Cell Biol 152(5):1045–1056

Banes AJ, Weinhold P, Yang X, Tsuzaki M, Bynum D, Bottlang M, Brown T et al (1999) Gap junctions regulate responses of tendon cells ex vivo to mechanical loading. Clin Orthop Relat Res (367 Suppl):S356–S370

Beeharry D, Coupe B, Benbow EW, Morgan J, Kwok S, Charlton-Menys V et al (2006) Familial hypercholesterolaemia commonly presents with Achilles tenosynovitis. Ann Rheum Dis 65(3):312–315. doi:10.1136/ard.2005.040766

Benjamin M, McGonagle D (2001) The anatomical basis for disease localisation in seronegative spondyloarthropathy at entheses and related sites. J Anat 199(Pt 5):503–526

Benjamin M, Ralphs JR (1997) Tendons and ligaments—an overview. Histol Histopathol 12(4):1135–1144

Benjamin M, Ralphs JR (1998) Fibrocartilage in tendons and ligaments—an adaptation to compressive load. J Anat 193(Pt 4):481–494

Benjamin M, Evans EJ, Copp L (1986) The histology of tendon attachments to bone in man. J Anat 149:89–100

Benjamin M, Toumi H, Ralphs JR, Bydder G, Best TM, Milz S (2006) Where tendons and ligaments meet bone: attachment sites ('entheses') in relation to exercise and/or mechanical load. J Anat 208(4):471–490. doi:10.1111/j.1469-7580.2006.00540.x

Benjamin M, Kaiser E, Milz S (2008) Structure-function relationships in tendons: a review. J Anat 212(3):211–228. doi:10.1111/j.1469-7580.2008.00864.x
Biermann H (1957) Die Knochenbildung im Bereich periostaler-diaphysärer Sehnen- und Bandansätze. Z Zellforsch Mikrosk Anat 46(6):635–671. doi:10.1007/BF00339370
Birk DE, Fitch JM, Babiarz JP, Doane KJ, Linsenmayer TF (1990) Collagen fibrillogenesis in vitro: interaction of types I and V collagen regulates fibril diameter. J Cell Sci 95(Pt 4):649–657
Bisset LM, Vicenzino B (2015) Physiotherapy management of lateral epicondylalgia. J Physiother 61(4):174–181. doi:10.1016/j.jphys.2015.07.015
Blanco I, Krahenbuhl S, Schlienger RG (2005) Corticosteroid-associated tendinopathies: an analysis of the published literature and spontaneous pharmacovigilance data. Drug Saf 28(7):633–643. doi:10.2165/00002018-200528070-00005
Bodin J, Ha C, Petit Le Manac'h A, Serazin C, Descatha A, Leclerc A et al (2012) Risk factors for incidence of rotator cuff syndrome in a large working population. Scand J Work Environ Health 38(5):436–446. doi:10.5271/sjweh.3285
Brughelli M, Cronin J (2008) A review of research on the mechanical stiffness in running and jumping: methodology and implications. Scand J Med Sci Sports 18(4):417–426
Burner T, Gohr C, Mitton-Fitzgerald E, Rosenthal AK (2012) Hyperglycemia reduces proteoglycan levels in tendons. Connect Tissue Res 53(6):535–541. doi:10.3109/03008207.2012.710670
Carroll CC, Dickinson JM, Haus JM, Lee GA, Hollon CJ, Aagaard P et al (2008) Influence of aging on the in vivo properties of human patellar tendon. J Appl Physiol (1985) 105(6):1907–1915. doi:10.1152/japplphysiol.00059.2008
Cassel M, Baur H, Hirschmuller A, Carlsohn A, Frohlich K, Mayer F (2015) Prevalence of Achilles and patellar tendinopathy and their association to intratendinous changes in adolescent athletes. Scand J Med Sci Sports 25(3):e310–e318. doi:10.1111/sms.12318
Chauhan AA, Morrissey D, Jones PR, Angioi M, Kumar B, Langberg H et al (2015) Genetic risk factors for mid-portion Achilles tendinopathy: a systematic review. Bone & Joint Journal Orthopaedic Proceedings Supplement, 97-B(SUPP 11), 32
Chen TM, Rozen WM, Pan WR, Ashton MW, Richardson MD, Taylor GI (2009) The arterial anatomy of the Achilles tendon: anatomical study and clinical implications. Clin Anat 22(3):377–385. doi:10.1002/ca.20758
Chiquet M, Renedo AS, Huber F, Fluck M (2003) How do fibroblasts translate mechanical signals into changes in extracellular matrix production? Matrix Biol 22(1):73–80
Contractor T, Beri A, Gardiner JC, Tang X, Dwamena FC (2015) Is statin use associated with tendon rupture? A population-based retrospective cohort analysis. Am J Ther 22(5):377–381. doi:10.1097/MJT.0000000000000039
Cook JL, Purdam CR (2003) Rehabilitation of lower limb tendinopathies. Clin Sports Med 22(4):777–789
Cook JL, Purdam CR (2009) Is tendon pathology a continuum? A pathology model to explain the clinical presentation of load-induced tendinopathy. Br J Sports Med 43(6):409–416. doi:10.1136/bjsm.2008.051193
Cook JL, Purdam C (2012) Is compressive load a factor in the development of tendinopathy? Br J Sports Med 46(3):163–168. doi:10.1136/bjsports-2011-090414
Cook JL, Khan KM, Harcourt PR, Kiss ZS, Fehrmann MW, Griffiths L, Wark JD (1998) Patellar tendon ultrasonography in asymptomatic active athletes reveals hypoechoic regions: a study of 320 tendons. Victorian Institute of Sport Tendon Study Group. Clin J Sport Med 8(2):73–77
Cook JL, Khan KM, Purdam C (2002) Achilles tendinopathy. Man Ther 7(3):121–130
Cook JL, Kiss ZS, Ptasznik R, Malliaras P (2005a) Is vascularity more evident after exercise? Implications for tendon imaging. AJR Am J Roentgenol 185(5):1138–1140. doi:10.2214/AJR.04.1205
Couppe C, Hansen P, Kongsgaard M, Kovanen V, Suetta C, Aagaard P et al (2009) Mechanical properties and collagen cross-linking of the patellar tendon in old and young men. J Appl Physiol (1985) 107(3):880–886. doi:10.1152/japplphysiol.00291.2009
Crossley KM, Thancanamootoo K, Metcalf BR, Cook JL, Purdam CR, Warden SJ (2007) Clinical features of patellar tendinopathy and their implications for rehabilitation. J Orthop Res 25(9):1164–1175. doi:10.1002/jor.20415
Danielson P (2009) Reviving the "biochemical" hypothesis for tendinopathy: new findings suggest the involvement of locally produced signal substances. Br J Sports Med 43(4):265–268. doi:10.1136/bjsm.2008.054593
Danielson P, Alfredson H, Forsgren S (2006) Immunohistochemical and histochemical findings favoring the occurrence of autocrine/paracrine as well as nerve-related cholinergic effects in chronic painful patellar tendon tendinosis. Microsc Res Tech 69(10):808–819. doi:10.1002/jemt.20351
Danielson P, Alfredson H, Forsgren S (2007) Studies on the importance of sympathetic innervation, adrenergic receptors, and a possible local catecholamine production in the development of patellar tendinopathy (tendinosis) in man. Microsc Res Tech 70(4):310–324. doi:10.1002/jemt.20413
Dean BJ, Lostis E, Oakley T, Rombach I, Morrey ME, Carr AJ (2014) The risks and benefits of glucocorticoid treatment for tendinopathy: a systematic review of the effects of local glucocorticoid on tendon. Semin Arthritis Rheum 43(4):570–576. doi:10.1016/j.semarthrit.2013.08.006
Dean BJ, Gettings P, Dakin SG, Carr AJ (2016) Are inflammatory cells increased in painful human tendinopathy? A systematic review. Br J Sports Med 50(4):216–220. doi:10.1136/bjsports-2015-094754
Depalle B, Qin Z, Shefelbine SJ, Buehler MJ (2015) Influence of cross-link structure, density and mechanical properties in the mesoscale deformation mecha-

nisms of collagen fibrils. J Mech Behav Biomed Mater 52:1–13. doi:10.1016/j.jmbbm.2014.07.008

Descatha A, Dale AM, Jaegers L, Herquelot E, Evanoff B (2013) Self-reported physical exposure association with medial and lateral epicondylitis incidence in a large longitudinal study. Occup Environ Med 70(9):670–673. doi:10.1136/oemed-2012-101341

Dimery NJ, Alexander RM, Ker RF (1986) Elastic extension of leg tendons in the locomotion of horses (Equus-Caballus). J Zool 210:415–425

Docking SI, Cook J (2016) Pathological tendons maintain sufficient aligned fibrillar structure on ultrasound tissue characterization (UTC). Scand J Med Sci Sports 26(6):675–683. doi:10.1111/sms.12491

Docking S, Samiric T, Scase E, Purdam C, Cook J (2013) Relationship between compressive loading and ECM changes in tendons. Muscles Ligaments Tendons J 3(1):7–11. doi:10.11138/mltj/2013.3.1.007

Docking SI, Ooi CC, Connell D (2015) Tendinopathy: is imaging telling us the entire story? J Orthop Sports Phys Ther 45(11):842–852. doi:10.2519/jospt.2015.5880

Dowling GJ, Murley GS, Munteanu SE, Smith MM, Neal BS, Griffiths IB et al (2014) Dynamic foot function as a risk factor for lower limb overuse injury: a systematic review. J Foot Ankle Res 7(1):53. doi:10.1186/s13047-014-0053-6

Elliott DH (1965) Structure and function of mammalian tendon. Biol Rev Camb Philos Soc 40:392–421

Eriksen HA, Pajala A, Leppilahti J, Risteli J (2002) Increased content of type III collagen at the rupture site of human Achilles tendon. J Orthop Res 20(6):1352–1357. doi:10.1016/S0736-0266(02)00064-5

Esenkaya I, Unay K (2011) Tendon, tendon healing, hyperlipidemia and statins. Muscles Ligaments Tendons J 1(4):169–171

Fearon AM, Twin J, Dahlstrom JE, Cook JL, Cormick W, Smith PN, Scott A (2014) Increased substance P expression in the trochanteric bursa of patients with greater trochanteric pain syndrome. Rheumatol Int 34(10):1441–1448. doi:10.1007/s00296-014-2957-7

Fenwick SA, Hazleman BL, Riley GP (2002) The vasculature and its role in the damaged and healing tendon. Arthritis Res 4(4):252–260. doi:10.1186/ar416

Ferretti A (1986) Epidemiology of jumper's knee. Sports Med 3(4):289–295

Fessel G, Li Y, Diederich V, Guizar-Sicairos M, Schneider P, Sell DR et al (2014) Advanced glycation end-products reduce collagen molecular sliding to affect collagen fibril damage mechanisms but not stiffness. PLoS One 9(11):e110948. doi:10.1371/journal.pone.0110948

Fox AJ, Bedi A, Deng XH, Ying L, Harris PE, Warren RF, Rodeo SA (2011) Diabetes mellitus alters the mechanical properties of the native tendon in an experimental rat model. J Orthop Res 29(6):880–885. doi:10.1002/jor.21327

Franceschi F, Papalia R, Paciotti M, Franceschetti E, Di Martino A, Maffulli N, Denaro V (2014) Obesity as a risk factor for tendinopathy: a systematic review. Int J Endocrinol 2014:670262. doi:10.1155/2014/670262

Fratzl P, Misof K, Zizak I, Rapp G, Amenitsch H, Bernstorff S (1998) Fibrillar structure and mechanical properties of collagen. J Struct Biol 122(1–2):119–122. doi:10.1006/jsbi.1998.3966

Frizziero A, Vittadini F, Gasparre G, Masiero S (2014) Impact of oestrogen deficiency and aging on tendon: concise review. Muscles Ligaments Tendons J 4(3):324–328

Fu SC, Rolf C, Cheuk YC, Lui PP, Chan KM (2010) Deciphering the pathogenesis of tendinopathy: a three-stages process. Sports Med Arthrosc Rehabil Ther Technol 2:30. doi:10.1186/1758-2555-2-30

Gabbett TJ (2016) The training-injury prevention paradox: should athletes be training smarter and harder? Br J Sports Med 50(5):273–280. doi:10.1136/bjsports-2015-095788

Gabel GT (1999) Acute and chronic tendinopathies at the elbow. Curr Opin Rheumatol 11(2):138–143

Gaida JE, Cook JL, Bass SL, Austen S, Kiss ZS (2004) Are unilateral and bilateral patellar tendinopathy distinguished by differences in anthropometry, body composition, or muscle strength in elite female basketball players? Br J Sports Med 38(5):581–585. doi:10.1136/bjsm.2003.006015

Gaida JE, Cook JL, Bass SL (2008) Adiposity and tendinopathy. Disabil Rehabil 30(20–22):1555–1562. doi:10.1080/09638280701786864

Gaida JE, Alfredson L, Kiss ZS, Wilson AM, Alfredson H, Cook JL (2009a) Dyslipidemia in Achilles tendinopathy is characteristic of insulin resistance. Med Sci Sports Exerc 41(6):1194–1197. doi:10.1249/MSS.0b013e31819794c3

Gaida JE, Ashe MC, Bass SL, Cook JL (2009b) Is adiposity an under-recognized risk factor for tendinopathy? A systematic review. Arthritis Rheum 61(6):840–849. doi:10.1002/art.24518

Gaida JE, Alfredson H, Kiss ZS, Bass SL, Cook JL (2010) Asymptomatic Achilles tendon pathology is associated with a central fat distribution in men and a peripheral fat distribution in women: a cross sectional study of 298 individuals. BMC Musculoskelet Disord 11:41. doi:10.1186/1471-2474-11-41

Garau G, Rittweger J, Mallarias P, Longo UG, Maffulli N (2008) Traumatic patellar tendinopathy. Disabil Rehabil 30(20–22):1616–1620. doi:10.1080/09638280701786096

Gardner K, Lavagnino M, Egerbacher M, Arnoczky SP (2012) Re-establishment of cytoskeletal tensional homeostasis in lax tendons occurs through an actin-mediated cellular contraction of the extracellular matrix. J Orthop Res 30(11):1695–1701. doi:10.1002/jor.22131

Giori NJ, Beaupre GS, Carter DR (1993) Cellular shape and pressure may mediate mechanical control of tissue composition in tendons. J Orthop Res 11(4):581–591. doi:10.1002/jor.1100110413

Goncalves-Neto J, Witzel SS, Teodoro WR, Carvalho-Junior AE, Fernandes TD, Yoshinari HH (2002)

Changes in collagen matrix composition in human posterior tibial tendon dysfunction. Joint Bone Spine 69(2):189–194
Goom TS, Malliaras P, Reiman MP, Purdam CR (2016) Proximal hamstring tendinopathy: clinical aspects of assessment and management. J Orthop Sports Phys Ther 46(6):483–493. doi:10.2519/jospt.2016.5986
Grant TM, Thompson MS, Urban J, Yu J (2013) Elastic fibres are broadly distributed in tendon and highly localized around tenocytes. J Anat 222(6):573–579. doi:10.1111/joa.12048
Grimaldi A, Mellor R, Hodges P, Bennell K, Wajswelner H, Vicenzino B (2015) Gluteal tendinopathy: a review of mechanisms, assessment and management. Sports Med 45(8):1107–1119. doi:10.1007/s40279-015-0336-5
de Groot R, Malliaras P, Munteanu S, Payne C, Morrissey D, Maffulli N (2012) Foot posture and patellar tendon pain among adult volleyball players. Clin J Sport Med 22(2):157–159. doi:10.1097/JSM.0b013e31824714eb
Gutierrez M, Filippucci E, De Angelis R, Filosa G, Kane D, Grassi W (2010) A sonographic spectrum of psoriatic arthritis: "the five targets". Clin Rheumatol 29(2):133–142. doi:10.1007/s10067-009-1292-y
Hagglund M, Zwerver J, Ekstrand J (2011) Epidemiology of patellar tendinopathy in elite male soccer players. Am J Sports Med 39(9):1906–1911. doi:10.1177/0363546511408877
Haglund-Akerlind Y, Eriksson E (1993) Range of motion, muscle torque and training habits in runners with and without Achilles tendon problems. Knee Surg Sports Traumatol Arthrosc 1(3–4):195–199
Hakim AJ, Cherkas LF, Spector TD, MacGregor AJ (2003) Genetic associations between frozen shoulder and tennis elbow: a female twin study. Rheumatology (Oxford) 42(6):739–742. doi:10.1093/rheumatology/keg159
Hart DA, Archambault JM, Kydd A, Reno C, Frank CB, Herzog W (1998) Gender and neurogenic variables in tendon biology and repetitive motion disorders. Clin Orthop Relat Res 351:44–56
Heales LJ, Lim EC, Hodges PW, Vicenzino B (2014) Sensory and motor deficits exist on the non-injured side of patients with unilateral tendon pain and disability—implications for central nervous system involvement: a systematic review with meta-analysis. Br J Sports Med 48(19):1400–1406. doi:10.1136/bjsports-2013-092535
Heinemeier KM, Kjaer M (2011) In vivo investigation of tendon responses to mechanical loading. J Musculoskelet Neuronal Interact 11(2):115–123
Heinemeier KM, Olesen JL, Haddad F, Langberg H, Kjaer M, Baldwin KM, Schjerling P (2007) Expression of collagen and related growth factors in rat tendon and skeletal muscle in response to specific contraction types. J Physiol 582(Pt 3):1303–1316. doi:10.1113/jphysiol.2007.127639
Hems T, Tillman B (2000) Tendon entheses of the human masticatory muscles. Anat Embryol 202(3):201–208
Holmes GB, Lin J (2006) Etiologic factors associated with symptomatic achilles tendinopathy. Foot Ankle Int 27(11):952–959
Holt NC, Roberts TJ, Askew GN (2014) The energetic benefits of tendon springs in running: is the reduction of muscle work important? J Exp Biol 217(Pt 24):4365–4371. doi:10.1242/jeb.112813
Hopkins C, Fu S-C, Chua E, Hu X, Rolf C, Mattila VM et al (2016) Critical review on the socio-economic impact of tendinopathy. Asia-Pacific J Sports Med Arthrosc Rehabil Technol 4:9–20. doi:10.1016/j.asmart.2016.01.002
Hou Y, Mao Z, Wei X, Lin L, Chen L, Wang H et al (2009) The roles of TGF-beta1 gene transfer on collagen formation during Achilles tendon healing. Biochem Biophys Res Commun 383(2):235–239. doi:10.1016/j.bbrc.2009.03.159
Hulin BT, Gabbett TJ, Blanch P, Chapman P, Bailey D, Orchard JW (2014) Spikes in acute workload are associated with increased injury risk in elite cricket fast bowlers. Br J Sports Med 48(8):708–712. doi:10.1136/bjsports-2013-092524
Ingber DE (1997) Tensegrity: the architectural basis of cellular mechanotransduction. Annu Rev Physiol 59:575–599. doi:10.1146/annurev.physiol.59.1.575
Jahr H, van Driel M, van Osch GJ, Weinans H, van Leeuwen JP (2005) Identification of acid-sensing ion channels in bone. Biochem Biophys Res Commun 337(1):349–354. doi:10.1016/j.bbrc.2005.09.054
Jarvinen M, Jozsa L, Kannus P, Jarvinen TL, Kvist M, Leadbetter W (1997) Histopathological findings in chronic tendon disorders. Scand J Med Sci Sports 7(2):86–95
Jarvinen TA, Kannus P, Jarvinen TL, Jozsa L, Kalimo H, Jarvinen M (2000) Tenascin-C in the pathobiology and healing process of musculoskeletal tissue injury. Scand J Med Sci Sports 10(6):376–382
Jarvinen TA, Jozsa L, Kannus P, Jarvinen TL, Hurme T, Kvist M et al (2003) Mechanical loading regulates the expression of tenascin-C in the myotendinous junction and tendon but does not induce de novo synthesis in the skeletal muscle. J Cell Sci 116(Pt 5):857–866
Jarvinen TA, Kannus P, Maffulli N, Khan KM (2005) Achilles tendon disorders: etiology and epidemiology. Foot Ankle Clin 10(2):255–266. doi:10.1016/j.fcl.2005.01.013
Jelinsky SA, Rodeo SA, Li J, Gulotta LV, Archambault JM, Seeherman HJ (2011) Regulation of gene expression in human tendinopathy. BMC Musculoskelet Disord 12:86. doi:10.1186/1471-2474-12-86
Jones NG, Slater R, Cadiou H, McNaughton P, McMahon SB (2004) Acid-induced pain and its modulation in humans. J Neurosci 24(48):10974–10979. doi:10.1523/JNEUROSCI.2619-04.2004
Kadler KE, Holmes DF, Trotter JA, Chapman JA (1996) Collagen fibril formation. Biochem J 316(Pt 1):1–11
Kannus P (1997) Etiology and pathophysiology of chronic tendon disorders in sports. Scand J Med Sci Sports 7(2):78–85
Kannus P, Jozsa L, Natri A, Jarvinen M (1997) Effects of training, immobilization and remobilization on tendons. Scand J Med Sci Sports 7(2):67–71
Kastelic J, Galeski A, Baer E (1978) The multicomposite structure of tendon. Connect Tissue Res 6(1):11–23

Kaufman KR, Brodine SK, Shaffer RA, Johnson CW, Cullison TR (1999) The effect of foot structure and range of motion on musculoskeletal overuse injuries. Am J Sports Med 27(5):585–593

Khaliq Y, Zhanel GG (2003) Fluoroquinolone-associated tendinopathy: a critical review of the literature. Clin Infect Dis 36(11):1404–1410. doi:10.1086/375078

Khan KM, Cook JL, Bonar F, Harcourt P, Astrom M (1999) Histopathology of common tendinopathies. Update and implications for clinical management. Sports Med 27(6):393–408

Kirchgesner T, Larbi A, Omoumi P, Malghem J, Zamali N, Manelfe J et al (2014) Drug-induced tendinopathy: from physiology to clinical applications. Joint Bone Spine 81(6):485–492. doi:10.1016/j.jbspin.2014.03.022

Kirkendall DT, Garrett WE (1997) Function and biomechanics of tendons. Scand J Med Sci Sports 7(2):62–66

Kjaer M (2004) Role of extracellular matrix in adaptation of tendon and skeletal muscle to mechanical loading. Physiol Rev 84(2):649–698. doi:10.1152/physrev.00031.2003

Kjaer M, Langberg H, Heinemeier K, Bayer ML, Hansen M, Holm L et al (2009) From mechanical loading to collagen synthesis, structural changes and function in human tendon. Scand J Med Sci Sports 19(4):500–510. doi:10.1111/j.1600-0838.2009.00986.x

Kjaer M, Bayer ML, Eliasson P, Heinemeier KM (2013) What is the impact of inflammation on the critical interplay between mechanical signaling and biochemical changes in tendon matrix? J Appl Physiol (1985) 115(6):879–883. doi:10.1152/japplphysiol.00120.2013

Klein EE, Weil L Jr, Weil LS Sr, Fleischer AE (2013) Body mass index and achilles tendonitis: a 10-year retrospective analysis. Foot Ankle Spec 6(4):276–282. doi:10.1177/1938640013489343

Koob TJ, Clark PE, Hernandez DJ, Thurmond FA, Vogel KG (1992) Compression loading in vitro regulates proteoglycan synthesis by tendon fibrocartilage. Arch Biochem Biophys 298(1):303–312

Kountouris A, Cook J (2007) Rehabilitation of Achilles and patellar tendinopathies. Best Pract Res Clin Rheumatol 21(2):295–316. doi:10.1016/j.berh.2006.12.003

Kraushaar BS, Nirschl RP (1999) Tendinosis of the elbow (tennis elbow). Clinical features and findings of histological, immunohistochemical, and electron microscopy studies. J Bone Joint Surg Am 81(2):259–278

Kujala UM, Sarna S, Kaprio J (2005) Cumulative incidence of achilles tendon rupture and tendinopathy in male former elite athletes. Clin J Sport Med 15(3):133–135

Kumai T, Benjamin M (2002) Heel spur formation and the subcalcaneal enthesis of the plantar fascia. J Rheumatol 29(9):1957–1964

Kvist M, Jozsa L, Jarvinen M (1992) Vascular changes in the ruptured Achilles tendon and paratenon. Int Orthop 16(4):377–382

Lang TR, Cook J, Rio E, Gaida JE (2016) What tendon pathology is seen on imaging in people who have taken fluoroquinolones? A systematic review. Fundam Clin Pharmacol. doi:10.1111/fcp.12228

Langberg H, Skovgaard D, Petersen LJ, Bulow J, Kjaer M (1999) Type I collagen synthesis and degradation in peritendinous tissue after exercise determined by microdialysis in humans. J Physiol 521(Pt 1):299–306

Langberg H, Rosendal L, Kjaer M (2001) Training-induced changes in peritendinous type I collagen turnover determined by microdialysis in humans. J Physiol 534(Pt 1):297–302

Langberg H, Olesen JL, Gemmer C, Kjaer M (2002) Substantial elevation of interleukin-6 concentration in peritendinous tissue, in contrast to muscle, following prolonged exercise in humans. J Physiol 542(Pt 3):985–990

Lavagnino M, Arnoczky SP (2005) In vitro alterations in cytoskeletal tensional homeostasis control gene expression in tendon cells. J Orthop Res 23(5):1211–1218. doi:10.1016/j.orthres.2005.04.001

Leadbetter WB (1992) Cell-matrix response in tendon injury. Clin Sports Med 11(3):533–578

Lewis JS (2010) Rotator cuff tendinopathy: a model for the continuum of pathology and related management. Br J Sports Med 44(13):918–923. doi:10.1136/bjsm.2008.054817

Lewis T, Cook J (2014) Fluoroquinolones and tendinopathy: a guide for athletes and sports clinicians and a systematic review of the literature. J Athl Train 49(3):422–427. doi:10.4085/1062-6050-49.2.09

Li Y, Fessel G, Georgiadis M, Snedeker JG (2013) Advanced glycation end-products diminish tendon collagen fiber sliding. Matrix Biol 32(3–4):169–177. doi:10.1016/j.matbio.2013.01.003

Littlewood C, Malliaras P, Bateman M, Stace R, May S, Walters S (2013a) The central nervous system—an additional consideration in 'rotator cuff tendinopathy' and a potential basis for understanding response to loaded therapeutic exercise. Man Ther 18(6):468–472. doi:10.1016/j.math.2013.07.005

Littlewood C, May S, Walters S (2013b) Epidemiology of rotator cuff tendinopathy: a systematic review. Should Elb 5(4):256–265. doi:10.1111/sae.12028

Longo UG, Rittweger J, Garau G, Radonic B, Gutwasser C, Gilliver SF et al (2009) No influence of age, gender, weight, height, and impact profile in achilles tendinopathy in masters track and field athletes. Am J Sports Med 37(7):1400–1405. doi:10.1177/0363546509332250

Longo UG, Rittweger J, Garau G, Radonic B, Gutwasser C, Gilliver SF et al (2011) Patellar tendinopathy in master track and field athletes: influence of impact profile, weight, height, age and gender. Knee Surg Sports Traumatol Arthrosc 19(3):508–512. doi:10.1007/s00167-010-1314-y

Maffulli N, Khan KM, Puddu G (1998) Overuse tendon conditions: time to change a confusing terminology. Arthroscopy 14(8):840–843

Maffulli N, Ewen SW, Waterston SW, Reaper J, Barrass V (2000) Tenocytes from ruptured and tendinopathic achilles tendons produce greater quantities of type III collagen than tenocytes from normal achilles tendons. An in vitro model of human tendon healing. Am J Sports Med 28(4):499–505

Maffulli N, Wong J, Almekinders LC (2003) Types and epidemiology of tendinopathy. Clin Sports Med 22(4):675–692

Maffulli N, Ajis A, Longo UG, Denaro V (2007) Chronic rupture of tendo Achillis. Foot Ankle Clin 12(4):583–596 . doi:10.1016/j.fcl.2007.07.007vi

Magnusson SP, Langberg H, Kjaer M (2010) The pathogenesis of tendinopathy: balancing the response to loading. Nat Rev Rheumatol 6(5):262–268. doi:10.1038/nrrheum.2010.43

Magra M, Maffulli N (2008) Genetic aspects of tendinopathy. J Sci Med Sport 11(3):243–247. doi:10.1016/j.jsams.2007.04.007

Mahieu NN, Witvrouw E, Stevens V, Van Tiggelen D, Roget P (2006) Intrinsic risk factors for the development of achilles tendon overuse injury: a prospective study. Am J Sports Med 34(2):226–235. doi:10.1177/0363546505279918

Malliaras P, Cook JL, Kent P (2006) Reduced ankle dorsiflexion range may increase the risk of patellar tendon injury among volleyball players. J Sci Med Sport 9(4):304–309. doi:10.1016/j.jsams.2006.03.015

Malliaras P, Cook JL, Kent PM (2007) Anthropometric risk factors for patellar tendon injury among volleyball players. Br J Sports Med 41(4):259–263 . doi:10.1136/bjsm.2006.030049discussion 263

Marie I, Delafenetre H, Massy N, Thuillez C, Noblet C and the Network of the French Pharmacovigilance Centers (2008) Tendinous disorders attributed to statins: a study on ninety-six spontaneous reports in the period 1990–2005 and review of the literature. Arthritis Rheum 59(3):367–372. doi:10.1002/art.23309

Martin JA, Mehr D, Pardubsky PD, Buckwalter JA (2003) The role of tenascin-C in adaptation of tendons to compressive loading. Biorheology 40(1–3):321–329

McAuliffe S, McCreesh K, Culloty F, Purtill H, O'Sullivan K (2016) Can ultrasound imaging predict the development of Achilles and patellar tendinopathy? A systematic review and meta-analysis. Br J Sports Med. doi:10.1136/bjsports-2016-096288

McNeilly CM, Banes AJ, Benjamin M, Ralphs JR (1996) Tendon cells in vivo form a three dimensional network of cell processes linked by gap junctions. J Anat 189(Pt 3):593–600

Mehr D, Pardubsky PD, Martin JA, Buckwalter JA (2000) Tenascin-C in tendon regions subjected to compression. J Orthop Res 18(4):537–545. doi:10.1002/jor.1100180405

Midwood KS, Orend G (2009) The role of tenascin-C in tissue injury and tumorigenesis. J Cell Commun Signal 3(3–4):287–310. doi:10.1007/s12079-009-0075-1

Millar NL, Hueber AJ, Reilly JH, Xu Y, Fazzi UG, Murrell GA, McInnes IB (2010) Inflammation is present in early human tendinopathy. Am J Sports Med 38(10):2085–2091. doi:10.1177/0363546510372613

Miller BF, Hansen M, Olesen JL, Schwarz P, Babraj JA, Smith K et al (2007) Tendon collagen synthesis at rest and after exercise in women. J Appl Physiol (1985) 102(2):541–546. doi:10.1152/japplphysiol.00797.2006

Mokone GG, Gajjar M, September AV, Schwellnus MP, Greenberg J, Noakes TD, Collins M (2005) The guanine-thymine dinucleotide repeat polymorphism within the tenascin-C gene is associated with achilles tendon injuries. Am J Sports Med 33(7):1016–1021. doi:10.1177/0363546504271986

Mokone GG, Schwellnus MP, Noakes TD, Collins M (2006) The COL5A1 gene and Achilles tendon pathology. Scand J Med Sci Sports 16(1):19–26. doi:10.1111/j.1600-0838.2005.00439.x

Mousavizadeh R, Khosravi S, Behzad H, McCormack RG, Duronio V, Scott A (2014) Cyclic strain alters the expression and release of angiogenic factors by human tendon cells. PLoS One 9(5):e97356. doi:10.1371/journal.pone.0097356

Munteanu SE, Barton CJ (2011) Lower limb biomechanics during running in individuals with achilles tendinopathy: a systematic review. J Foot Ankle Res 4:15. doi:10.1186/1757-1146-4-15

Munteanu SE, Scott LA, Bonanno DR, Landorf KB, Pizzari T, Cook JL, Menz HB (2015) Effectiveness of customised foot orthoses for Achilles tendinopathy: a randomised controlled trial. Br J Sports Med 49(15):989–994. doi:10.1136/bjsports-2014-093845

Nagafuchi A (2001) Molecular architecture of adherens junctions. Curr Opin Cell Biol 13(5):600–603

Nourissat G, Berenbaum F, Duprez D (2015) Tendon injury: from biology to tendon repair. Nat Rev Rheumatol 11(4):223–233. doi:10.1038/nrrheum.2015.26

O'Brien M (1992) Functional anatomy and physiology of tendons. Clin Sports Med 11(3):505–520

O'Brien M (1997) Structure and metabolism of tendons. Scand J Med Sci Sports 7(2):55–61

de Oliveira RR, de Lira KD, Silveira PV, Coutinho MP, Medeiros MN, Teixeira MF, de Moraes SR (2011a) Mechanical properties of achilles tendon in rats induced to experimental diabetes. Ann Biomed Eng 39(5):1528–1534. doi:10.1007/s10439-011-0247-z

de Oliveira RR, Lemos A, de Castro Silveira PV, da Silva RJ, de Moraes SR (2011b) Alterations of tendons in patients with diabetes mellitus: a systematic review. Diabet Med 28(8):886–895. doi:10.1111/j.1464-5491.2010.03197.x

Olsen SJ 2nd, Fleisig GS, Dun S, Loftice J, Andrews JR (2006) Risk factors for shoulder and elbow injuries in adolescent baseball pitchers. Am J Sports Med 34(6):905–912. doi:10.1177/0363546505284188

Orchard JW, Blanch P, Paoloni J, Kountouris A, Sims K, Orchard JJ, Brukner P (2015) Cricket fast bowling workload patterns as risk factors for tendon, muscle, bone and joint injuries. Br J Sports Med 49(16):1064–1068. doi:10.1136/bjsports-2014-093683

Paavola M, Kannus P, Paakkala T, Pasanen M, Jarvinen M (2000) Long-term prognosis of patients with achilles tendinopathy. An observational 8-year follow-up study. Am J Sports Med 28(5):634–642

Pedowitz D, Kirwan G (2013) Achilles tendon ruptures. Curr Rev Muscoskelet Med 6(4):285–293. doi:10.1007/s12178-013-9185-8

Pingel J, Fredberg U, Qvortrup K, Larsen JO, Schjerling P, Heinemeier K, Kjaer M, Langberg H (2012) Local biochemical and morphological differences in human Achilles tendinopathy: a case control study. BMC Musculoskelet Disord 13(53). doi:10.1186/1471-2474-13-53

Posthumus M, September AV, O'Cuinneagain D, van der Merwe W, Schwellnus MP, Collins M (2010) The COL5A1 gene is associated with increased risk of anterior cruciate ligament ruptures in female participants. Am J Sports Med 37(11):2234–2240. doi:10.1177/0363546509338266

Rabin A, Kozol Z, Finestone AS (2014) Limited ankle dorsiflexion increases the risk for mid-portion Achilles tendinopathy in infantry recruits: a prospective cohort study. J Foot Ankle Res 7(1):48. doi:10.1186/s13047-014-0048-3

Ramiro-Gonzalez MD, Cano-de-la-Cuerda R, De-la-Llave-Rincon AI, Miangolarra-Page JC, Zarzoso-Sanchez R, Fernandez-de-Las-Penas C (2012) Deep tissue hypersensitivity to pressure pain in individuals with unilateral acute inversion ankle sprain. Pain Med 13(3):361–367. doi:10.1111/j.1526-4637.2011.01302.x

Ranger TA, Wong AM, Cook JL, Gaida JE (2016) Is there an association between tendinopathy and diabetes mellitus? A systematic review with meta-analysis. Br J Sports Med 50(16):982–989. doi:10.1136/bjsports-2015-094735

Reddy GK (2003) Glucose-mediated in vitro glycation modulates biomechanical integrity of the soft tissues but not hard tissues. J Orthop Res 21(4):738–743. doi:10.1016/S0736-0266(03)00006-8

Rees SG, Dent CM, Caterson B (2009) Metabolism of proteoglycans in tendon. Scand J Med Sci Sports 19(4):470–478.doi:10.1111/j.1600-0838.2009.00938.x

Rees JD, Stride M, Scott A (2014) Tendons—time to revisit inflammation. Br J Sports Med 48(21):1553–1557. doi:10.1136/bjsports-2012-091957

Rempel D, Abrahamsson SO (2001) The effects of reduced oxygen tension on cell proliferation and matrix synthesis in synovium and tendon explants from the rabbit carpal tunnel: an experimental study in vitro. J Orthop Res 19(1):143–148. doi:10.1016/S0736-0266(00)00005-X

Reynolds NL, Worrell TW (1991) Chronic achilles peritendinitis: etiology, pathophysiology, and treatment. J Orthop Sports Phys Ther 13(4):171–176. doi:10.2519/jospt.1991.13.4.171

Richards DP, Ajemian SV, Wiley JP, Brunet JA, Zernicke RF (2002) Relation between ankle joint dynamics and patellar tendinopathy in elite volleyball players. Clin J Sport Med 12(5):266–272

Rickert M, Wang H, Wieloch P, Lorenz H, Steck E, Sabo D, Richter W (2005) Adenovirus-mediated gene transfer of growth and differentiation factor-5 into tenocytes and the healing rat Achilles tendon. Connect Tissue Res 46(4-5):175–183. doi:10.1080/03008200500237120

Riley GP (2005) Gene expression and matrix turnover in overused and damaged tendons. Scand J Med Sci Sports 15(4):241–251. doi:10.1111/j.1600-0838.2005.00456.x

Riley G (2008) Tendinopathy—from basic science to treatment. Nat Clin Pract Rheumatol 4(2):82–89. doi:10.1038/ncprheum0700

Riley GP, Harrall RL, Constant CR, Chard MD, Cawston TE, Hazleman BL (1994) Tendon degeneration and chronic shoulder pain: changes in the collagen composition of the human rotator cuff tendons in rotator cuff tendinitis. Ann Rheum Dis 53(6):359–366

Riley GP, Harrall RL, Cawston TE, Hazleman BL, Mackie EJ (1996) Tenascin-C and human tendon degeneration. Am J Pathol 149(3):933–943

Rio E, Moseley L, Purdam C, Samiric T, Kidgell D, Pearce AJ et al (2015) The pain of tendinopathy: physiological or pathophysiological? Sports Med 44(1):9–23. doi:10.1007/s40279-013-0096-z

Roberts TJ (2002) The integrated function of muscles and tendons during locomotion. Comp Biochem Physiol A Mol Integr Physiol 133(4):1087–1099

Robins SP (1988) Functional properties of collagen and elastin. Baillieres Clin Rheumatol 2(1):1–36

Rong C, Chen FH, Jiang S, Hu W, Wu FR, Chen TY, Yuan FL (2012) Inhibition of acid-sensing ion channels by amiloride protects rat articular chondrocytes from acid-induced apoptosis via a mitochondrial-mediated pathway. Cell Biol Int 36(7):635–641. doi:10.1042/CBI20110432

Roquelaure Y, Ha C, Leclerc A, Touranchet A, Sauteron M, Melchior M et al (2006) Epidemiologic surveillance of upper-extremity musculoskeletal disorders in the working population. Arthritis Rheum 55(5):765–778. doi:10.1002/art.22222

Sailly M, Whiteley R, Johnson A (2013) Doppler ultrasound and tibial tuberosity maturation status predicts pain in adolescent male athletes with Osgood-Schlatter's disease: a case series with comparison group and clinical interpretation. Br J Sports Med 47(2):93–97. doi:10.1136/bjsports-2012-091471

Samiric T, Parkinson J, Ilic MZ, Cook J, Feller JA, Handley CJ (2009) Changes in the composition of the extracellular matrix in patellar tendinopathy. Matrix Biol 28(4):230–236. doi:10.1016/j.matbio.2009.04.001

Schatzker J, Branemark PI (1969) Intravital observations on the microvascular anatomy and microcirculation of the tendon. Acta Orthop Scand Suppl 126:1–23

Schubert TE, Weidler C, Lerch K, Hofstadter F, Straub RH (2005) Achilles tendinosis is associated with sprouting of substance P positive nerve fibres. Ann Rheum Dis 64(7):1083–1086. doi:10.1136/ard.2004.029876

Schwartz MA, DeSimone DW (2008) Cell adhesion receptors in mechanotransduction. Curr Opin Cell Biol 20(5):551–556. doi:10.1016/j.ceb.2008.05.005
Scott A, Khan KM, Cook JL, Duronio V (2004) What is "inflammation"? Are we ready to move beyond celsus? Br J Sports Med 38(3):248–249
Scott A, Cook JL, Hart DA, Walker DC, Duronio V, Khan KM (2007) Tenocyte responses to mechanical loading in vivo: a role for local insulin-like growth factor 1 signaling in early tendinosis in rats. Arthritis Rheum 56(3):871–881. doi:10.1002/art.22426
Scott RT, Hyer CF, Granata A (2013) The correlation of Achilles tendinopathy and body mass index. Foot Ankle Spec 6(4):283–285. doi:10.1177/1938640013490019
Scott A, Backman LJ, Speed C (2015a) Tendinopathy: update on pathophysiology. J Orthop Sports Phys Ther 45(11):833–841. doi:10.2519/jospt.2015.5884
Scott A, Zwerver J, Grewal N, de Sa A, Alktebi T, Granville DJ, Hart DA (2015b) Lipids, adiposity and tendinopathy: is there a mechanistic link? Critical review. Br J Sports Med 49(15):984–988. doi:10.1136/bjsports-2014-093989
Screen HR, Lee DA, Bader DL, Shelton JC (2004) An investigation into the effects of the hierarchical structure of tendon fascicles on micromechanical properties. Proc Inst Mech Eng H 218(2):109–119
Screen HR, Shelton JC, Chhaya VH, Kayser MV, Bader DL, Lee DA (2005) The influence of noncollagenous matrix components on the micromechanical environment of tendon fascicles. Ann Biomed Eng 33(8):1090–1099. doi:10.1007/s10439-005-5777-9
Screen HR, Berk DE, Kadler KE, Ramirez F, Young MF (2015) Tendon functional extracellular matrix. J Orthop Res 33(6):793–799. doi:10.1002/jor.22818
Sein ML, Walton J, Linklater J, Appleyard R, Kirkbride B, Kuah D, Murrell GA (2010) Shoulder pain in elite swimmers: primarily due to swim-volume-induced supraspinatus tendinopathy. Br J Sports Med 44(2):105–113. doi:10.1136/bjsm.2008.047282
Seitz AL, McClure PW, Finucane S, Boardman ND 3rd, Michener LA (2011) Mechanisms of rotator cuff tendinopathy: intrinsic, extrinsic, or both? Clin Biomech (Bristol, Avon) 26(1):1–12. doi:10.1016/j.clinbiomech.2010.08.001
September AV, Cook J, Handley CJ, van der Merwe L, Schwellnus MP, Collins M (2009) Variants within the COL5A1 gene are associated with Achilles tendinopathy in two populations. Br J Sports Med 43(5):357–365. doi:10.1136/bjsm.2008.048793
Silbernagel KG, Gustavsson A, Thomee R, Karlsson J (2006) Evaluation of lower leg function in patients with Achilles tendinopathy. Knee Surg Sports Traumatol Arthrosc 14(11):1207–1217. doi:10.1007/s00167-006-0150-6
Silva RS, Nakagawa TH, Ferreira ALG, Garcia LC, Santos JEM, Serrao FV (2016) Lower limb strength and flexibility in athletes with and without patellar tendinopathy. Phys Ther Sport 20:19–25. doi:10.1016/j.ptsp.2015.12.001
Simpson M, Rio E, Cook J (2016) At what age do children and adolescents develop lower limb tendon pathology or tendinopathy? A systematic review and meta-analysis. Sports Med 46(4):545–557. doi:10.1007/s40279-015-0438-0
Snedeker JG, Gautieri A (2014) The role of collagen cross-links in ageing and diabetes—the good, the bad, and the ugly. Muscles Ligaments Tendons J 4(3):303–308
Stecco C, Cappellari A, Macchi V, Porzionato A, Morra A, Berizzi A, De Caro R (2014) The paratendineous tissues: an anatomical study of their role in the pathogenesis of tendinopathy. Surg Radiol Anat 36(6):561–572. doi:10.1007/s00276-013-1244-8
Stepien-Slodkowska M, Ficek K, Kaczmarczyk M, Maciejewska-Karlowska A, Sawczuk M, Leonska-Duniec A et al (2015) The variants within the COL5A1 gene are associated with reduced risk of anterior cruciate ligament injury in skiers. J Hum Kinet 45:103–111. doi:10.1515/hukin-2015-0011
Stilwell DL Jr (1957) The innervation of tendons and aponeuroses. Am J Anat 100(3):289–317. doi:10.1002/aja.1001000302
Teichtahl AJ, Brady SR, Urquhart DM, Wluka AE, Wang Y, Shaw JE, Cicuttini FM (2016) Statins and tendinopathy: a systematic review. Med J Aust 204(3):115–121. e111
Tilley BJ, Cook JL, Docking SI, Gaida JE (2015) Is higher serum cholesterol associated with altered tendon structure or tendon pain? A systematic review. Br J Sports Med 49(23):1504–1509. doi:10.1136/bjsports-2015-095100
Tuite DJ, Renstrom PA, O'Brien M (1997) The aging tendon. Scand J Med Sci Sports 7(2):72–77
Uchiyama Y, Cheng CC, Danielson KG, Mochida J, Albert TJ, Shapiro IM, Risbud MV (2007) Expression of acid-sensing ion channel 3 (ASIC3) in nucleus pulposus cells of the intervertebral disc is regulated by p75NTR and ERK signaling. J Bone Miner Res 22(12):1996–2006. doi:10.1359/jbmr.070805
Visnes H, Bahr R (2013) Training volume and body composition as risk factors for developing jumper's knee among young elite volleyball players. Scand J Med Sci Sports 23(5):607–613. doi:10.1111/j.1600-0838.2011.01430.x
Vogel KG (2004) What happens when tendons bend and twist? Proteoglycans. J Musculoskelet Neuronal Interact 4(2):202–203
Waggett AD, Benjamin M, Ralphs JR (2006) Connexin 32 and 43 gap junctions differentially modulate tenocyte response to cyclic mechanical load. Eur J Cell Biol 85(11):1145–1154. doi:10.1016/j.ejcb.2006.06.002
Wall ME, Banes AJ (2005) Early responses to mechanical load in tendon: role for calcium signaling, gap junctions and intercellular communication. J Musculoskelet Neuronal Interact 5(1):70–84
Wang JH, Li Z, Yang G, Khan M (2004) Repetitively stretched tendon fibroblasts produce inflammatory mediators. Clin Orthop Relat Res 422:243–250
Ward ER, Andersson G, Backman LJ, Gaida JE (2016) Fat pads adjacent to tendinopathy: more than a coinci-

dence? Br J Sports Med. doi:10.1136/bjsports-2016-096174
Weir A, Brukner P, Delahunt E, Ekstrand J, Griffin D, Khan KM et al (2015) Doha agreement meeting on terminology and definitions in groin pain in athletes. Br J Sports Med 49(12):768–774. doi:10.1136/bjsports-2015-094869
Williams IF, McCullagh KG, Silver IA (1984) The distribution of types I and III collagen and fibronectin in the healing equine tendon. Connect Tissue Res 12(3–4):211–227
Witvrouw E, Bellemans J, Lysens R, Danneels L, Cambier D (2001) Intrinsic risk factors for the development of patellar tendinitis in an athletic population. A two-year prospective study. Am J Sports Med 29(2):190–195
Wolf JM, Sturdivant RX, Owens BD (2009) Incidence of de Quervain's tenosynovitis in a young, active population. J Hand Surg [Am] 34(1):112–115. doi:10.1016/j.jhsa.2008.08.020
Xu Y, Murrell GA (2008) The basic science of tendinopathy. Clin Orthop Relat Res 466(7):1528–1538. doi:10.1007/s11999-008-0286-4
Yoon JH, Halper J (2005) Tendon proteoglycans: biochemistry and function. J Musculoskelet Neuronal Interact 5(1):22–34
Zantop T, Tillmann B, Petersen W (2003) Quantitative assessment of blood vessels of the human Achilles tendon: an immunohistochemical cadaver study. Arch Orthop Trauma Surg 123(9):501–504. doi:10.1007/s00402-003-0491-2
Zhang J, Wang JH (2010) Production of PGE(2) increases in tendons subjected to repetitive mechanical loading and induces differentiation of tendon stem cells into non-tenocytes. J Orthop Res 28(2):198–203. doi:10.1002/jor.20962
Zhou Y, Zhou B, Tang K (2015) The effects of substance p on tendinopathy are dose-dependent: an in vitro and in vivo model study. J Nutr Health Aging 19(5):555–561. doi:10.1007/s12603-014-0576-3

Tendon Healing

4

Thierry Pauyo, Elmar Herbst, and Freddie H. Fu

Contents

T. Pauyo, M.D. • E. Herbst, M.D. • F.H. Fu, M.D. (✉)
University of Pittsburgh Medical Center,
3200 South Water, St. Pittsburgh, 15203, PA, USA

4.1 Introduction

The healing process following tendon injury is governed by a plethora of biomechanical factors that has been well studied in the literature from the basic science cellular model to interventions in the clinical setting. Overall, a fully healed tendon is characterized by reduced final mechanical stability (Sharma and Maffulli 2005). In order to optimize the treatment of tendon injury, the treating physician should have a thorough understanding of the principles of tendon healing. The following chapter will discuss tendon pathology, homeostasis, principles of healing, as well as biologic and mechanical factors affecting the healing response.

4.2 Tendon Homeostasis

The maintenance and viability of tendons are largely dependent on the structural molecules that constitute the extracellular matrix (ECM) (Butler et al. 2004). The tenocytes are the primary regulator of the ECM and tendon homeostasis (Galloway et al. 2013). These fibroblast-like cells are interconnected with one another and with adjacent collagen fibers, enabling recognition of mechanical changes in the ECM (Wang 2006). The tenocytes are able to respond to load and mechanical changes by modulating the degradation and formation of ECM (Wang 2006). The preservation of ECM homeostasis is critical

G.L. Canata et al. (eds.), *Muscle and Tendon Injuries*, DOI 10.1007/978-3-662-54184-5_4

in the tendon healing process and its capacity to respond to injury.

The ECM is composed predominantly of type I collagen, which is the primary constituent of the native tendon (Hogan et al. 2011). The longitudinal and parallel arrangement of type I collagen enables the ECM to respond to tensile loads (Karousou et al. 2008). Proteoglycans also play a role in the ECM's capacity to resist tensile and compressive forces (Karousou et al. 2008). Indeed, the collagen network of the ECM is mechanosensitive and is stabilized by mechanical strain (Bhole et al. 2009). Bhole et al. showed, using dynamic differential imaging, that non-strained collagen fibril was resorbed faster than collagen fibrils subjected to strain (Bhole et al. 2009). Normal physiologic loads on the tendon unit are necessary to maintain the ECM homeostasis and structural integrity (Nabeshima et al. 1996; Flynn et al. 2010).

4.2.1 Mechanism of Tendon Injury

The pathophysiology of tendon injury encompasses a wide spectrum of disorders ranging from chronic tendinopathy to the acute complete tendon tear. One school of thought believes that acute tendon injuries are indicative of a chronic underlying tendon disorder (Maganaris et al. 2004). Others believe that acute injury results from one tensile overload, and chronic injury results from repetitive abnormal load over an extended period of time (Galloway et al. 2013; Maganaris et al. 2004; Lin et al. 2004). The viscoelastic properties of tendon allow its capacity to withstand compressive, tensile, and shear loads that are generated from muscle and transmitted to the rigid bone (Bunker et al. 2014). Noyes et al. described three primary failure modes of tendon injuries: (1) failure through the tendon substance, (2) avulsion fracture through the cancellous bone beneath the tendon attachment, and (3) failure at the enthesis (tendon bone interface) (Noyes et al. 1974). While the location of the tear has been well described, the type of abnormal load on the tendon unit plays an integral role in the pathophysiology of tendon injury.

4.2.1.1 Stages of Tendon Healing

The biologic cascade that modulates tendon healing is divided in three distinct stages, each governed by different cell types (Sharma and Maffulli 2006) (Fig. 4.1). The **inflammatory stage** is initiated by the traumatic event surrounding tendon injury, precipitating the hematoma and the agglomeration of platelets, releasing a slew of chemotaxic molecules, cytokines, and growth factors. The phagocytic cells, monocytes, neutrophils, and microphages, migrate to the site of injury via dilated vessels and begin the process of breaking down the blood clot and extracellular matrix. The process of angiogenesis is introduced by macrophages where a new network of vasculature matures in the healing tissue (Gelberman et al. 1992). The ECM is notably stabilized by the increasing amount of collagen type III, which are not yet aligned in parallel. The inflammatory stage lasts between 3 to 7 days following tendon injury. The amount of collagen will steadily increase during the first 5 days where the tendon callus will reach its largest size (Oliva et al. 2011).

The **proliferative stage** follows with an increasing amount of intrinsic fibroblast in the ECM. These cells emerge from the endotenon and epitenon and play a primordial role in resorbing and producing new collagen (Muller et al. 2015). At this stage, the immature healing ECM is still stabilized by a soaring amount of type III collagen, and this phase lasts for about 6 weeks. During the **remodeling stage**, the biomechanical strength of the tendon is at its greatest. The collagen is reorganized in a longitudinal, parallel fashion, while the collagen type III is replaced by collagen type I. The ECM will continue to mature for the next year with a rising amount of longitudinal and cross-linked collagen, while the callus volume of the tendon will decrease and the tendon biomechanical strength will continue to improve (Hogan et al. 2011). The healed tendon is biomechanically weaker than the uninjured tendon, with less cross-linking and smaller diameter collagen, and is more susceptible to reinjury

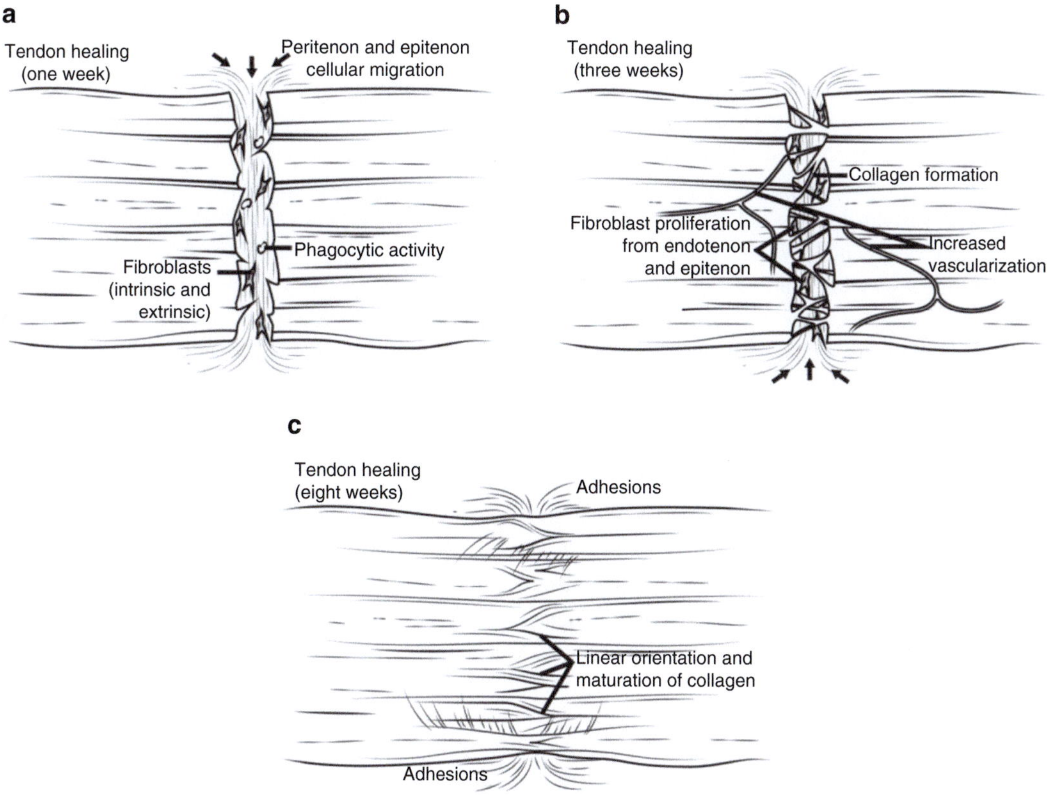

Fig. 4.1 Stages of tendon healing: (**a**) Inflammatory phase. (**b**) Proliferative phase. (**c**) Remodeling phase (Strickland 2000)

(Hyman and Rodeo 2000). Dyment et al. corroborated these findings in a histologic and biomechanical study in the mice model, where they demonstrated that the healed tendon regains 63% of its original strength after an 8-week time period (Dyment et al. 2012).

4.2.1.2 Growth Factors

Growth factors are molecules involved in modulating the tendon healing response, more particularly during the inflammation stages following injury (Molloy et al. 2003; Sciore et al. 1998). The molecules involved include fibroblast growth factor (FGF), vascular endothelial growth factor (VEGF), platelet-derived growth factor (PDGF-β), transforming growth factor-beta (TGF-β), and insulin-like growth factor-1 (IGF-1) (Wurgler-Hauri et al. 2007; Holladay et al. 2016). While these growth factors have been studied extensively in vitro and in vivo, more recently, the attention of the scientific community has gravitated toward platelet-rich plasma (PRP) to augment tendon healing (Filardo et al. 2016). PRP has been studied in patellar tendon, rotator cuff, lateral elbow tendon, and Achilles tendon (Behera et al. 2015; Brkljac et al. 2015; Crescibene et al. 2015; De Carli et al. 2016; Carr et al. 2015). While PRP is widely used in the clinical setting, its efficacy is still controversial in the literature due to the heterogeneity of the study protocols (Filardo et al. 2016). Furthermore, new studies have focused on mesenchymal stem cells and their potential ability to differentiate into tendon cells and promote tendon regeneration (Chen et al. 2009).

4.2.1.3 Tendon Healing of Intrasynovial and Extrasynovial Tendon

As discussed earlier, the healing process following tendon injury is dictated by a multifaceted cellular healing response and is also influenced by the anatomical location of the injured tendon. The intrasynovial tendons, such has flexor tendons of the hand, and extrasynovial tendons, such as Achilles tendon, have different physiological mechanism of healing. The sheathed tendon heals with growth factors secreted from the epitenon and endotenon which passively diffuse through the synovial fluid to the site of injury (Strickland 2000). On the other hand, extrasynovial tendons, lacking the sheaths and synovial fluid, heal via blood flow and growth factors secreted by cells from the paratenon (Molloy et al. 2003; Galvez et al. 2014). The process of tendon healing is further characterized in intrinsic and extrinsic healing. During extrinsic healing, fibroblasts from the paratenon migrate to the site of injury and promote adhesion that potentially inhibit tendon excursion (Sammer and Chung 2014). On the other hand, intrinsic healing is characterized by fibroblasts migrating from the endotenon and epitenon in the synovial sheet, preventing the formation of adhesion with the surrounding tissue, facilitating early mobilization and strength of healing (Sammer and Chung 2014). Gelberman et al., in a study of flexor tendons in a dog model, showed that tendon that is immobilized after injury leads to collagen resorption while promoting adhesion with the surrounding sheath (Gelberman et al. 1983). In contrast, the mobilized tendon had an increase in collagen number and longitudinal orientation while demonstrating a decrease in adhesion with the peripheral soft tissue (Gelberman et al. 1983).

4.3 Rehabilitation

The cellular response during the tendon healing process is greatly influenced by the rehabilitation protocol initiated after injury. While the healed tendon never reaches the original strength of the native tendon (Dyment et al. 2012), there is a need to optimize the rehabilitation factors influencing tendon healing. Schizas et al., in an animal study on Achilles tendons, demonstrated that the immobilized healed tendon had decreased strength, length, collagen diameter and organized orientation (Schizas et al. 2010). Another study exhibited similar finding showing that immobilization impairs tendon healing (Bring et al. 2009). Bring et al., in a histologic study of rat Achilles tendons, demonstrated that immobilized tendon had a decreased amount of angiogenesis, fibroblasts, and production of collagen (Bring et al. 2009). Furthermore, early mobilization has been shown to enhance healed tendon strength and decreased adhesion formation in intrasynovial tendons (Strickland 2000). The translation of basic science to the clinical setting has yielded precious information regarding post-injury rehabilitation protocols. The application of controlled mechanical load should be an integral part of tendon healing to support ECM regeneration and maintenance (Flynn et al. 2010). Valkering et al., in a randomized controlled trial of Achilles tendon rupture, showed that functional weight-bearing enhances early healing response (Valkering et al. 2016). Functional weight-bearing also upregulated the release of metabolites associated with improved healing. The rehabilitation program should emphasize physiologic loading applied to the healing tendon to optimize ultimate tendon function and repair (Galloway et al. 2013).

Conclusion

The mechanisms governing the healing response after tendon injury have been well described in the literature where basic research led to the translation of ideas and innovation in the clinical research setting. While the healing of intrasynovial tendon such as flexor tendons of the hand differs from extrasynovial tendon such as the Achilles tendon, they abide to the same biomechanical healing principles. The current literature seems to support early mobilization along with controlled mechanical loads to maintain the homeostasis of the extracellular matrix. Future research should continue to explore the applications of growth factors and mesenchymal stem cell in order to potentially augment the cellular response in the tendon healing process.

References

Behera P, Dhillon M, Aggarwal S, Marwaha N, Prakash M (2015) Leukocyte-poor platelet-rich plasma versus bupivacaine for recalcitrant lateral epicondylar tendinopathy. J Orthop Surg 23(1):6–10

Bhole AP, Flynn BP, Liles M, Saeidi N, Dimarzio CA, Ruberti JW (2009) Mechanical strain enhances survivability of collagen micronetworks in the presence of collagenase: implications for load-bearing matrix growth and stability. Philos Transact A Math Phys Eng Sci 367(1902):3339–3362

Bring DK, Reno C, Renstrom P, Salo P, Hart DA, Ackermann PW (2009) Joint immobilization reduces the expression of sensory neuropeptide receptors and impairs healing after tendon rupture in a rat model. J Orthop Res 27(2):274–280

Brkljac M, Kumar S, Kalloo D, Hirehal K (2015) The effect of platelet-rich plasma injection on lateral epicondylitis following failed conservative management. J Orthop 12(Suppl 2):S166–S170

Bunker DL, Ilie V, Ilie V, Nicklin S (2014) Tendon to bone healing and its implications for surgery. Muscles Ligaments Tendons J 4(3):343–350

Butler DL, Juncosa N, Dressler MR (2004) Functional efficacy of tendon repair processes. Annu Rev Biomed Eng 6:303–329

Carr AJ, Murphy R, Dakin SG et al (2015) Platelet-rich plasma injection with arthroscopic acromioplasty for chronic rotator cuff tendinopathy: a randomized controlled trial. Am J Sports Med 43(12): 2891–2897

Chen X, Song XH, Yin Z et al (2009) Stepwise differentiation of human embryonic stem cells promotes tendon regeneration by secreting fetal tendon matrix and differentiation factors. Stem Cells 27(6): 1276–1287

Crescibene A, Napolitano M, Sbano R, Costabile E, Almolla H (2015) Infiltration of Autologous Growth Factors in Chronic Tendinopathies. J Blood Transfus 2015:924380

De Carli A, Lanzetti RM, Ciompi A et al (2016) Can platelet-rich plasma have a role in Achilles tendon surgical repair? Knee Surg Sports Traumatol Arthrosc 24(2237):2231–2237

Dyment NA, Kazemi N, Aschbacher-Smith LE et al (2012) The relationships among spatiotemporal collagen gene expression, histology, and biomechanics following full-length injury in the murine patellar tendon. J Orthop Res 30(1):28–36

Filardo G, Di Matteo B, Kon E, Merli G, Marcacci M (2016) Platelet-rich plasma in tendon-related disorders: results and indications. Knee Surg Sports Traumatol Arthrosc. doi:10.1007/s00167-016-4261-4

Flynn BP, Bhole AP, Saeidi N, Liles M, Dimarzio CA, Ruberti JW (2010) Mechanical strain stabilizes reconstituted collagen fibrils against enzymatic degradation by mammalian collagenase matrix metalloproteinase 8 (MMP-8). PLoS One 5(8):e12337

Galloway MT, Lalley AL, Shearn JT (2013) The role of mechanical loading in tendon development, maintenance, injury, and repair. J Bone Joint Surg Am 95(17):1620–1628

Galvez MG, Crowe C, Farnebo S, Chang J (2014) Tissue engineering in flexor tendon surgery: current state and future advances. J Hand Surg Eur Vol 39(1):71–78

Gelberman RH, Chu CR, Williams CS, Seiler JG 3rd, Amiel D (1992) Angiogenesis in healing autogenous flexor-tendon grafts. J Bone Joint Surg Am 74(8):1207–1216

Gelberman RH, Vande Berg JS, Lundborg GN, Akeson WH (1983) Flexor tendon healing and restoration of the gliding surface. An ultrastructural study in dogs. J Bone Joint Surg Am 65(1):70–80

Hogan MV, Bagayoko N, James R, Starnes T, Katz A, Chhabra AB (2011) Tissue engineering solutions for tendon repair. J Am Acad Orthop Surg 19(3):134–142

Holladay C, Abbah SA, O'Dowd C, Pandit A, Zeugolis DI (2016) Preferential tendon stem cell response to growth factor supplementation. J Tissue Eng Regen Med 10(9):783–798

Hyman J, Rodeo SA (2000) Injury and repair of tendons and ligaments. Phys Med Rehabil Clin N Am 11(2):267–288, v

Karousou E, Ronga M, Vigetti D, Passi A, Maffulli N (2008) Collagens, proteoglycans, MMP-2, MMP-9 and TIMPs in human achilles tendon rupture. Clin Orthop Relat Res 466(7):1577–1582

Lin TW, Cardenas L, Soslowsky LJ (2004) Biomechanics of tendon injury and repair. J Biomech 37(6):865–877

Maganaris CN, Narici MV, Almekinders LC, Maffulli N (2004) Biomechanics and pathophysiology of overuse tendon injuries: ideas on insertional tendinopathy. Sports Med 34(14):1005–1017

Molloy T, Wang Y, Murrell G (2003) The roles of growth factors in tendon and ligament healing. Sports Med 33(5):381–394

Muller SA, Todorov A, Heisterbach PE, Martin I, Majewski M (2015) Tendon healing: an overview of physiology, biology, and pathology of tendon healing and systematic review of state of the art in tendon bioengineering. Knee Surg Sports Traumatol Arthrosc 23(7):2097–2105

Nabeshima Y, Grood ES, Sakurai A, Herman JH (1996) Uniaxial tension inhibits tendon collagen degradation by collagenase in vitro. J Orthop Res 14(1):123–130

Noyes FR, DeLucas JL, Torvik PJ (1974) Biomechanics of anterior cruciate ligament failure: an analysis of strain-rate sensitivity and mechanisms of failure in primates. J Bone Joint Surg Am 56(2):236–253

Oliva F, Via AG, Maffulli N (2011) Role of growth factors in rotator cuff healing. Sports Med Arthrosc Rev 19(3):218–226

Sammer DM, Chung KC (2014) Advances in the healing of flexor tendon injuries. Wound Repair Regen 22(Suppl 1):25–29

Schizas N, Li J, Andersson T et al (2010) Compression therapy promotes proliferative repair during rat Achilles tendon immobilization. J Orthop Res 28(7):852–858

Sciore P, Boykiw R, Hart DA (1998) Semiquantitative reverse transcription-polymerase chain reaction analysis of mRNA for growth factors and growth factor receptors from normal and healing rabbit medial collateral ligament tissue. J Orthop Res 16(4):429–437

Sharma P, Maffulli N (2005) Tendon injury and tendinopathy: healing and repair. J Bone Joint Surg Am 87(1):187–202

Sharma P, Maffulli N (2006) Biology of tendon injury: healing, modeling and remodeling. J Musculoskelet Neuronal Interact 6(2):181–190

Strickland JW (2000) Development of flexor tendon surgery: twenty-five years of progress. J Hand Surg Am 25(2):214–235

Valkering KP, Aufwerber S, Ranuccio F, Lunini E, Edman G, Ackermann PW (2016) Functional weight-bearing mobilization after Achilles tendon rupture enhances early healing response: a single-blinded randomized controlled trial. Knee Surg Sports Traumat Arthrosc. doi:10.1007/s00167-016-4270-3

Wang JH (2006) Mechanobiology of tendon. J Biomech 39(9):1563–1582

Wurgler-Hauri CC, Dourte LM, Baradet TC, Williams GR, Soslowsky LJ (2007) Temporal expression of 8 growth factors in tendon-to-bone healing in a rat supraspinatus model. J Shoulder Elbow Surg 16(5 Suppl):S198–S203

Muscle-Tendon Junction Injury

5

William E. Garrett Jr and Mallory S. Faherty

Contents

W.E. Garrett Jr, M.D., Ph.D. (✉)
Department of Orthopaedic Surgery, Duke University, Durham, NC 27708, USA
e-mail: william.garrett@dm.duke.edu

M.S. Faherty, M.S., A.T.C.
Michael W. Krzyzewski Human Performance Laboratory (K-Lab), Department of Orthopaedic Surgery, Duke University, Durham, NC 27708, USA
e-mail: mallory.faherty@duke.edu

5.1 Introduction

Muscle strain injury is one of the most frequently occurring and debilitating injuries in sport and recreation (Glick 1980; Krejci and Koch 1979; Nikolaou et al. 1987; O'Donoghue 1984; Ryan 1969). Both partial and full muscle strain injuries result in significant short-term and long-term consequences (Garrett et al. 1988). These consequences include time lost from work at significant compensation costs and inability to regain pre-injury levels of performance (Garrett et al. 1988). Despite having knowledge of the consequences, the understanding of muscle and tendon injuries is still vastly unknown. The exact anatomical location of damage within the muscle-tendon junction and the predisposing factors for damage in normal, healthy muscle are still unanswered questions surrounding muscle strain injury (Garrett et al. 1988). Our understanding of muscle and tendon injuries has expanded considerably in the last 30 years. Much more is known about the pathophysiology of injury in animal model and in clinical practice. However, much remains to be determined about prevention and treatment.

5.2 Structure

The structural link between the myofilaments and the connective tissues is the muscle-tendon junction (Garrett et al. 1988). The muscle-tendon

G.L. Canata et al. (eds.), *Muscle and Tendon Injuries*, DOI 10.1007/978-3-662-54184-5_5

junction is responsible for aiding in the transmission of tension within the muscle (Garrett et al. 1988). The tendon fibrils insert on the muscle fibers through an elaborate system of folds which increases their surface area (Schwarzacher 1960). The muscle-tendon junction, otherwise referred to as the connecting domain, has a vast number of fine filaments which are oriented approximately perpendicular to the major force vector (Trotter et al. 1981, 1983). These fine filaments connect the terminal myofibrils of the lamina densa to the collagen fibrils of the tendon (Trotter et al. 1981, 1983). These filaments have a diameter of two to seven nanometers (Ajiri et al. 1978; Hanak and Bock 1971; Korneliussen 1973). New sarcomeres are developed at the muscle-tendon junction with growth and development and/or hypertrophy as a result of stretch (Williams and Goldspink 1971, 1973, 1978). The ability to develop new sarcomeres and the plasticity at the terminal sarcomeres, located within the muscle fibers, demonstrate the available plasticity of the skeletal muscle (Williams and Goldspink 1971, 1973, 1978). The plasticity allows for localized change within the muscle-tendon junction, in addition to the possibility of regional structural and functional specializations (Garrett et al. 1988).

Important in the overall structure and function of the muscle-tendon unit are the tendon and ligament. Previous studies have examined the viscoelastic characteristics of tendons and ligaments (Butler et al. 1978; Solveborn 1983). When a tendon or a muscle is loaded with a constant force, the length slowly increases without increase in a time-dependent (therefore viscoelastic) manner (Solveborn 1983; Butler et al. 1978). Elastic structures produce a constant deformation for a constant load (Butler et al. 1978). The length-tension relation changes with load and therefore displays viscoelastic behavior rather than strict elastic behavior (Butler et al. 1978). Increased length in response to a constant force is called creep (Butler et al. 1978). If a muscle or tendon is stretched to a constant length, the measured tension decreases (Butler et al. 1978). The decrease in tension over time is also referred to as stretch relaxation (Solveborn 1983; Butler et al. 1978). Cyclic stretching of the ligament and tendon to the same length results in a decrease in tension with each stretch performed (Butler et al. 1978; Solveborn 1983). Descriptions of the muscle-tendon unit under two types of cyclic repetitive stretching have been provided by previous research (Taylor et al. 1985b, 1990). With repetitive cyclic stretching to the same length, there is an 80% increase in total length during the first four stretches (Taylor et al. 1985b). The stretch relaxation curve following the first stretch is significantly different than the stretch relaxation curve following the second stretch (Taylor et al. 1985b). The third and fourth stretch relaxation curves are also different, but the final six curves demonstrate no differences between them (Taylor et al. 1985b, 1990). Another study, similar to the previously described study, demonstrated that the peak tension decreased with each stretch, in addition to an overall drop in peak tension of 16.6% between the first and tenth stretch (Taylor et al. 1985c). There is a significant decrease in peak tension between the first four stretches, but the peak tension in cycles five through ten do not differ (Taylor et al. 1985c). This information suggests that repetitive stretching will lead to a reduction of load on the muscle-tendon junction at a given length (Taylor et al. 1985c). This effect is independent of any reflex effects or other influences mediated by the central nervous system; reflex effect and central nervous system influences may be involved in addition to the viscoelastic response (Taylor et al. 1985a).

The muscle-tendon unit is viscoelastic (Taylor et al. 1990). The decline in peak tension, which occurs because of the viscoelastic property of stretch relaxation, is associated with the internal changes in the structure of the muscle (Taylor et al. 1990). With each stretch, the relaxation curve for the muscle-tendon unit gradually levels off at higher tensions than the preceding relaxation curve (Taylor et al. 1990). Although a constant amount of tension is not always maintained to cause a length increase, varying amounts of tension up to a maximum lead to elongation (Taylor et al. 1990). This is demonstrative of the creep property of the muscle-tendon junction, forming a curve toward a maximum deformation

(Taylor et al. 1990). Both peak tensile force and absorbed energy are dependent upon the rate of stretch applied (Taylor et al. 1990). Stretch rate dependency is the amount of stress relaxation that occurs in a given amount of time (Taylor et al. 1990). Slower stretches allow for a greater degree of stretch relaxation to occur, resulting in lowered peak forces (Taylor et al. 1990). Energy is absorbed by the muscle-tendon unit during the loading process and is then dissipated during the unloading process (Taylor et al. 1990). During any one stretch, the rate at which the muscle-tendon unit absorbs energy is different from the rate at which it dissipates energy (Taylor et al. 1990). This creates a discrepancy between energy put into the system and the energy released form the system (Taylor et al. 1990). This difference may be explained by heat transfer and/or by internal changes within the ultrastructure of the muscle (Taylor et al. 1990).

5.3 Function

The function of the muscle and muscle-tendon junction has implications for muscle strain injury. The amount of stretch that a muscle may endure impacts the likelihood of having a muscle strain injury (Garrett 1990). Muscles that act on two joints are subjected to more stretch than muscles that act on one joint and are, therefore, more likely to suffer muscle strain injuries (Brewer 1960). The ability to be stretched at more than one joint, based on anatomical location, may play a role in the risk of muscle strain injury associated with these two joint muscles (Brewer 1960; Garrett 1990). These two joint muscles have an intrinsic tightness; in turn they can limit the ability to produce range of motion, but normal physiological joint motion can place the muscles in a position of increased passive tension (Brewer 1960; Garrett 1990). Often times these types of muscles control the regular movement when they are eccentrically contracted (Brewer 1960; Garrett 1990). More specifically, they act to produce joint motion control or decelerate the joint, both actions that are eccentric in nature (Brewer 1960; Garrett 1990).

Normal muscle activated by way of nerve stimulation, which has been previously theorized to lead to muscle strain injury, does not cause complete or incomplete disruption of the muscle (Garrett et al. 1984a). Although force is diminished and there is a failure of the excitation, there is no disruption of the muscle and no muscle strain injury (Garrett et al. 1984a). In order to see any gross microscopic muscle injury, stretch of the muscle is required, as opposed to solely nerve stimulation of the muscle (Garrett et al. 1984a). At the time of muscle failure, the forces produced without muscle activation are several times higher than the maximum isometric force produced by the activated muscles (Garrett et al. 1988). In turn, the passive forces within the muscle may play as much of a role as the active forces that occur in the muscle during muscle strain injury (Garrett et al. 1988).

The passive components of a stretched muscle have the ability to absorb energy, but that potential is greatly increased by active contraction of the muscle (Garrett 1990). This may provide an explanation as to why muscles can be injured when they are incapable of withstanding strain (Garrett 1990). A muscle's ability to withstand strain is a measure of the energy absorbed by the muscle prior to failure (Garrett 1990). Strain energy is represented as the area underneath the curve as it relates stress to strain (Garrett 1990). The two components that compose a muscle's ability to absorb energy include the passive component which is not dependent on the muscle activation and is a property of the connective tissue elements within the muscle, including muscle fiber and the connective tissue in the cell surface and existing between the fibers (Garrett 1990). There is an additional ability to absorb energy based on the contractile ability of the muscle (Garrett 1990). The active muscle components can double the ability of a muscle to absorb energy; therefore, conditions which diminish the ability of a muscle to contract might also diminish the ability of the muscle to absorb energy (Garrett 1990). Muscle fatigue and weakness are considered predisposing factors for muscle injury; this implies that the active ability to absorb the energy is diminished (Garrett 1990).

The ability of a muscle to absorb energy can protect the bone and joint, as well as the muscle itself (Radin et al. 1979). When the muscle is under a low strain, the energy absorption is due to the active component as opposed to the passive component (Radin et al. 1979).

5.4 Injury

A muscle strain is the response of a muscle following forceful stretching in an active or passive manner (Garrett 1990). Muscle strains may be partial or complete (Garrett 1990). These injuries are typically acute and usually a painful event, which is recognized by the patient as the event of injury (Garrett 1990). Two types of muscle strain injuries are possible, direct injury and indirect injury (Garrett 1990). Direct muscle strain injury is characterized by a contusion, which in turn causes an injury based on direct contact to a portion of the muscle (Garrett 1990). An indirect injury is typically at or near the muscle-tendon junction or the tendon-bone junction (Garrett 1990). A complete tear indicates that the muscle is asymmetric when compared to the non-injured contralateral side when the patient is at rest (Garrett 1990). When a complete tear occurs, typically when the muscle is contracted, there is a bulge at the muscle-tendon junction where the muscle is still attached to the bone (Garrett 1990).

Muscle strain injury occurs in two ways, a stretch of the muscle to complete rupture or, more commonly, an incomplete injury in which there is not a complete separate of the tissue to the level of complete tear (Garrett 1990). A strain injury tends to result in bleeding; this bleeding may occur immediately post-injury, but there is a possibility of experiencing a delay prior to the detection of the subcutaneous ecchymosis of one or more days (Garrett 1990). This bleeding is not confined to the muscle proper; the bleeding also escapes through the perimysium and the fascia into the subcutaneous space (Garrett 1990). Computed tomography has confirmed that within the muscle tissue there is also an inflammatory or edematous response that occurs in response to muscle strain injury (Garrett et al. 1989). Ultrasonography of strain injury has demonstrated that bleeding and hematoma can collect between the muscle tissue and the surrounding fascial compartment as a result of the injury (Fornage et al. 1983).

McMaster, in 1993, completed one of the first studies describing injuries at the muscle-tendon junction (McMaster 1933). When there is a normally occurring stretch in the muscle-tendon junction, disruption of the tendon is not present (McMaster 1933). More likely than injuries to the muscle-tendon unit are injuries at the bone-tendon junction, the muscle-tendon junction, and the muscle substance tears (McMaster 1933). Immediate changes are demonstrated in the muscle-tendon junction following a controlled passive strain injury limited to the plastic region of the deformation curve; there is also a limited rupture of the most distal muscle fibers along with hemorrhage (Nikolaou et al. 1987). This is in agreement with previous studies examining the failure properties of the muscle-tendon units under passive extension, demonstrating that the muscle-tendon junction is the site of rupture and therefore the weakest point in the muscle-tendon unit (Nikolaou et al. 1986).

When failure occurs, the muscle fibers near the muscle-tendon junction fail as opposed to a clear separation of the tendon from the muscle fibers; in other words, a small amount of muscle tissue remains attached to the tendon (Garrett et al. 1988). When passive extension is utilized to create muscle strain injuries, those muscle-tendon systems that are deemed normal do not rupture within the tendon (Garrett et al. 1988). The passive extension leads to rupture at the tendon insertion, an avulsion of the muscle organ, a rupture in the muscle belly, a separation of the muscle-tendon junction, or a fracture of the bone (Garrett et al. 1988). During passive extension, the weakest point in the muscle-tendon unit has been identified as the muscle-tendon junction (Garrett et al. 1988). The distal end of the muscle-tendon junction, more specifically, has been identified as the weakest point in the muscle-tendon unit (Garrett et al. 1988). The muscle architecture plays an important role in the failure point, when the muscle is stretched (Garrett et al. 1988). A majority of muscles, regardless of type, fail at the muscle-tendon junction, more specifically at the distal muscle-tendon junction (Garrett et al. 1988). This does not hold true for the gastrocnemius, which is a multipennate muscle (Garrett et al. 1988). The multipennate architecture results in an arrangement of the muscle-tendon junction which is more complicated than other arrangements (Garrett et al. 1988). This architecture diminishes the ability to categorize the distal and proximal tears of the muscle-tendon junction, like can be done with more simplistic muscle architecture types (Garrett et al. 1988). For example, in experiments, 55.5% of gastrocnemius muscles stretched into passive extension have a clear failure point at the distal muscle-tendon junction (Garrett et al. 1988). The remaining percentage of failures occurs between the muscle-tendon junctions, separating the two heads of the gastrocnemius or within each gastrocnemius head along the deep tendon expansions (Garrett et al. 1988). Although these remaining failures cannot be categorized into distal or proximal muscle-tendon junction failures, they still follow a similar pattern of failure when compared to the other muscles tested and still occurred in the muscle-tendon junction (Garrett et al. 1988). Regardless of muscle architecture, when muscles are passively extended, no failures occur mid-belly of the muscle fibers, within the tendon, or at the origin or insertion of the tendon to the bone (Garrett et al. 1988). Ruptures of the muscle-tendon junction do not cleanly separate the tendon from the muscle; during passive extension, when failure occurs, the tendon which is avulsed carries approximately 0.5 mm of the muscle fibers away with it (Garrett et al. 1988).

Rate of strain is necessary to create a strain injury in human muscle and alters where the failure will occur (Garrett et al. 1988). A range of rates is present because of the influence of internal factors including muscle type, muscle architecture, physiologic conditioning, and strength (Garrett et al. 1988). Rate of strain may also be influenced by external factors including warm-up prior to vigorous activity and fatigue (Garrett et al. 1988). During passive extension, regardless of the rate of strain, the point of failure is always the muscle-tendon junction (Garrett et al. 1988). Studies examining passive stretch have demonstrated that disruption within the muscle-tendon junction is predictable within a range of strain rates (Garrett et al. 1984a). This is true for all muscle types during passive stretch; regardless of architectural features and direction of strain, the injury still occurs at the muscle-tendon junction (Garrett et al. 1984a). A stretch of the muscle from either the proximal or distal tendon, without preconditioning or muscle activation, still fails and demonstrates disruption on or near the muscle-tendon junction (Garrett et al. 1984a). The biomechanical response of the muscle when the stretch occurs may be related to the muscle fiber length (Wikiewicz et al. 1983). Muscle strain injury does not occur after a relatively constant muscle fiber strain (Huxley and Peachey 1961). The ends of the muscle fibers near the muscle-tendon junction do not strain as much as the fibers that are in the more central area of the muscle (Huxley and Peachey 1961).

Decreases in contractile ability, which has been measured as maximal isometric tension, come before the decrement of tensile stretch in muscles which undergo strain injury (Noonan et al. 1994). This suggests that structural changes in the muscle affect primarily the contractile apparatus, leaving the connective tissue framework of the muscle essentially unaffected (Noonan et al. 1994). This would cause a decrease in the contractile ability without altering tensile parameters (Noonan et al. 1994). In contrast, it is possible that connective tissue damage does occur before or simultaneously with contractile tissue injury, because the conclusion of unaltered tensile properties is based on the idea that failure properties do not change (Noonan et al. 1994). Functional impairment may occur without a concurrent decrease in tensile strength, which may be clinically important in consideration of muscle strain injury (Noonan et al. 1994). There is a general sense that muscles are injured during powerful eccentric muscle activation (Noonan et al. 1994). During these eccentric contractions, the muscle absorbs energy and continues to function throughout the contraction to aid in prevention of injury (Noonan et al. 1994). If the muscle's contractile ability is impaired, its ability to absorb energy is impaired; this would put the muscle as significant risk of new injury or reinjury (Noonan et al. 1994). In turn, functional impairment even in the face of preserved tensile strength may lead to an increased risk for subsequent more severe muscle injury (Noonan et al. 1994).

In a study by Nikolaou et al., the passive stretch injury in a rabbit's tibialis anterior muscle was stretched to a force equal to 130% of their body weight, which is approximately 80% of the ultimate rupture force of the muscle-tendon unit at a rate of 10 cm/min (Nikolaou et al. 1987). The maximum force generation from a tetanic contraction in the tibialis anterior muscle was 70.5% of the control muscle immediately after the injury; by 24 h post-injury, the tetanic contraction was 51.1% of the control (Nikolaou et al. 1987). By 48 h post-injury, the contraction was 74.5% of the control muscle, and at 7 days, the contraction was 92.5% of the control muscle (Nikolaou et al. 1987). Histology studies showed that there were limited distal fiber rupture and hemorrhage immediately following the muscle strain injury, but within 24 h, there were fiber necrosis, inflammation, and edema (Nikolaou et al. 1987). Forty-eight hours post-injury, there were complete fiber breakdown and more intense inflammation, followed by collagen fibrosis 7 days post muscle strain injury (Nikolaou et al. 1987). In a similar study on rabbit extensor digitorum longus that were stretched at 10 cm/min to deformation, the contractile ability of the muscle was dramatically decreased when tested immediately after the muscle strain injury (Taylor et al. 1986). The muscle strain injury caused a statistically significant decrease reported in the total deformation and the load to failure (Taylor et al. 1986).

Clinical findings have indicated that muscle injuries occur most often during powerful eccentric contractions (Glick 1980; Peterson and Renstrom 1986; Zarins and Ciullo 1983). This has been evaluated in the research setting while stretching muscles to failure under three conditioning of motor nerve activation (Garrett et al. 1987). The conditions tested included tetanically stimulated, submaximally stimulated, and unstimulated (Garrett et al. 1987). In the groups that failed and a muscle strain injury was produced, only 15% higher forces were generated in the stimulated muscles (Garrett et al. 1987). Between all of the groups, the location of failure, which was at or near the muscle-tendon junction, did not change (Garrett et al. 1987). In contrast, muscles that were stretched to failure while activated had energy absorptions rates that were about 100% greater (Garrett et al. 1987).

Eccentric contractions, which stretch or lengthen the muscle, have the potential to produce contractions of much higher force when compared to other contraction types, including when the muscle stays at a constant length (isometric contraction) and when the muscle is allowed to shorten (concentric contraction), which shortens the muscle (Garrett 1990). Therefore, the development of excessive force within the muscle-tendon unit is increased (Stauber 1989). During eccentric contraction, the passive elements of the muscle, which include the connective tissue, provide a low level of force throughout the contraction (Elftman 1966). In order for these passive elements to provide resistance, there must be enough stretch applied to the muscle; prior to the stretch or prior to this threshold of stretch, there is no resistance or very little resistance provided by these passive elements (Elftman 1966). In the muscle-tendon unit, passive forces do provide some limit to range of motion (Garrett 1990). The role of passive forces means that there is an association between excess strain, which causes muscle strain injury, and eccentric muscle contraction, which by definition is associated with muscle stretch (Garrett 1990).

5.5 Recovery

Functional recovery of muscle can be identified through physiological testing which includes maximal force production in response to a nerve stimulation (Nikolaou et al. 1987; Garrett 1990). Following acute injury, muscles produce 70% of their normal force production (Nikolaou et al. 1987). Within 24 h of initial injury, the force production of a muscle declines to about 50% of the normal force production of the muscle; the comparison is the force production of the healthy, non-injured muscle (Nikolaou et al. 1987). Seven days following the initial injury, the force production of the muscle is greatly improved, with measures up to 90% of the normal force production of the muscle (Nikolaou et al. 1987). This represents recovery of contractile ability, which is relatively rapid (Nikolaou et al. 1987). Even when the contractile ability is initially diminished, it returns to its normal strength within 7 days of the initial acute injury (Nikolaou et al. 1987).

Recreation of a nondisruptive muscle strain injury has been accomplished by stretching an unstimulated muscle and observing the force-displacement relationship (Nikolaou et al. 1987). If the slope is no longer linear and the muscle is considered to have undergone a "plastic" deformation, the resulting alterations are a material structure (Nikolaou et al. 1987). The ability of the muscle to recover has been demonstrated through physiology and histology studies (Nikolaou et al. 1987). These types of injuries can be recreated by stretching the muscle to 80% of the force necessary to disrupt the contralateral muscle (Nikolaou et al. 1987). The histological studies show that injuries nondisruptive to the whole muscle can cause a disruption of a small number of muscle fibers near the muscle-tendon junction (Nikolaou et al. 1987). The fibers do not actually tear at muscle-tendon junction; rather they tear within the fibers a short distance from the tendon; rarely does the tear occur near the middle of the muscle fiber (Nikolaou et al. 1987). When these types of injuries are demonstrated acutely, there is some hemorrhage within the muscle which is a mark of the distribution that has occurred (Nikolaou et al. 1987). Within 1 to 2 days, the inflammatory reaction becomes more pronounced, there is an invasion of inflammatory cells, and the edema is now present (Nikolaou et al. 1987). When the injury reaches day seven, the inflammation reaction is being replaced by an increase in the fibrous tissue near the region of the actual injury; although some of the muscle fibers have begun the regeneration process, normal histology is not restored at this point, and the scar tissue is still present (Nikolaou et al. 1987).

Speed is also a consideration for recovery following muscle strain injury (Nikolaou et al. 1987). There are no differences in force or elongation to failure when examining the speed at which muscles are pulled to failure at speeds of 10 cm/min and 100 cm/min (Nikolaou et al. 1987). Biomechanical studies on rabbits demonstrated that passively strained muscle can recover function within 48 h, in contrast to the histological findings at 48 h, which demonstrate inflammation and active healing (Nikolaou et al. 1987). In patients with acute muscle strain, decreased function is observed at periods of up to 48 h following injury (Nikolaou et al. 1987). This decreased function is not due to the further degradation of contractile function of the injured muscle, but due to the edema and the increased pain caused by the inflammatory nature of the healing process (Nikolaou et al. 1987). The formation of scar and localized fibrosis seen at 7 days may also play an important role in the tendency for these muscle strain injuries to reoccur (Nikolaou et al. 1987).

5.6 Clinical Implications

Muscle strain injury has a significant impact on sport and recreation (Garrett 1990). Sports requiring large amounts of sprints and bursts of speed and/or rapid acceleration have a high likelihood of muscle strain injury (Peterson and Renstrom 1986). These sports include speed athletes, those who participate in American football, basketball, rugby, and soccer (Peterson and Renstrom 1986). In addition to requirements for sport participation, intrinsic factors also influence risk of muscle strain (Garrett et al. 1984b). Generally, the injured muscles are more superficial and cross two or more joints (Garrett et al. 1984b). These muscles also tend to have a relatively high percentage of type II, fast-twitch muscle fiber (Garrett et al. 1984b). Muscles that have a high percentage of fast-twitch, type II muscle fiber require faster contractions within the muscle (Garrett et al. 1984b). Because of this requirement for faster contractions, kinesiology, and the high speeds that the contractions can reach, these muscles are predisposed to injury during sport participation (Garrett et al. 1984b).

Establishing the effectiveness of commonly used clinical modalities is important for the prevention and treatment of muscle strain injury (Noonan et al. 1994). The effects of commonly utilized modalities such as stretching have been previously evaluated (Noonan et al. 1994). It may be most appropriate to evaluate injury prevention through testing the ability to prevent or minimize a smaller-scale injury instead of a complete rupture injury (Noonan et al. 1994). This would indicate that the injury is closer to the injury threshold, as opposed to being at the extreme end of total rupture and total failure (Noonan et al. 1994). A 30% stretch has been identified as the point in which there is a failure of force within the muscle, translating to a loss of the ability of the muscle to contract following the stretch (Noonan et al. 1994). In contrast, muscle-tendon junctions stretched to 20% of failure force suffered no decrement in contractile ability (Noonan et al. 1994). This suggests that there may be a threshold for passive stretch injury in the muscle-tendon junction (Noonan et al. 1994). This is supported by histologic examinations; fiber disruption and hemorrhage are only found in muscles stretch to 30% of the force failure (Noonan et al. 1994). This information is meaningful because the identification of a threshold may be useful for evaluating the effect of various treatments or routines on passive stretch-induced muscle injury (Noonan et al. 1994). By finding this threshold for injury, there are, perhaps, exact mechanisms by which passive stretch-induced injury occurs can be elucidated (Noonan et al. 1994).

The inclusion of warm-up periods prior to an exercise task has been debated, due to the performance and injury prevention benefits warm-ups may provide (Safran et al. 1988; Asmussen, Boje 1945; DeBruyn-Prevost 1980; Genovely and Stamford 1982; Ingjer and Stromme 1979; Karpovich and Hale 1956). The intention of a warm-up period is to improve performance and reduce risk of injury, although this has not been demonstrated (Asmussen and Boje 1945; DeBruyn-Prevost 1980; Genovely and Stamford 1982; Ingjer and Stromme 1979; Karpovich and Hale 1956; Safran et al. 1988). The warm-up period should include stretching and active muscle contractions, increasing the range of motion of the joints and muscle-tendon units, in addition to increasing the temperature of the muscles and the efficiency of the contracts that the muscles produce (Kulund and Tottossy 1983; Beaulieu 1981; Williford et al. 1986). The protective effect that the warm-up period may have has been attributed to the increased range of motion and reduced stiffness that is a direct result of the increase in muscle temperature (Safran et al. 1988). With a four-degree increase in the temperature of the muscle, the amount of elongation which can occur without subsequent rupture is increased (Strickler et al. 1990). Evidence is available to show that greater force and increased length are needed to tear isometrically preconditioned muscle or muscle that has gone through a warm-up period (Safran et al. 1988). Regardless of the muscle having gone through a warm-up period, the site of failure is always the muscle-tendon junction (Safran et al. 1988). Muscles which have not gone through a warm-up period appear to be inelastic when the length of the muscle is increased (Safran et al. 1988). This is the biomechanical evidence necessary to prove that warm-up periods may reduce the incidence of muscle strain injury (Safran et al. 1988).

Conclusion

This chapter has reviewed the nature of muscle strain injury in animal model and correlated with clinical studies on muscle strain injury. It is known that most indirect muscle injuries occur in response to stretch and usually while the muscles are activated, therefore resisting stretch. Injury locations are not random in the muscle belly, but rather in the muscle-tendon junction. Most of the research presented was studied utilizing specialized equipment requiring incisions of the tendon. Recent advances in technique allow for the creation of injury in a nondisruptive manner that allows for the study of treatment therapies and general recovery. Muscle injuries cause a great deal of time loss and disability. Much remains in our understating of muscle strain injury.

References

Ajiri T, Kimura T, Ito R, Inokuchi S (1978) Microfibrils in the myotendon junctions. Acta Anat (Basel) 102(4):433–439

Asmussen E, Boje O (1945) Body temperature and capacity of work. Acta Physiol Scad 10:1–2

Beaulieu JE (1981) Developing a stretching program. Phys Sportsmed 9(11):59–69. doi:10.1080/00913847.1981.11711207

Brewer B (ed) (1960) Instructional lecture American Academy of Orthopaedic Surgeons

Butler DL, Grood ES, Noyes FR, Zernicke RF (1978) Biomechanics of ligaments and tendons. Exerc Sport Sci Rev 6:125–181

DeBruyn-Prevost P (1980) The effects of various warming up intensities and durations upon some physiologic variables during exercise corresponding to the WC10. Eur J Appl Physiol 43:93–100

Elftman H (1966) Biomechanics of muscle with particular application to studies of gait. J Bone Joint Surg Am 48(2):363–377

Fornage BD, Touche DH, Segal P, Rifkin MD (1983) Ultrasonography in the evaluation of muscular trauma. J Ultrasound Med 2(12):549–554

Garrett WE Jr (1990) Muscle strain injuries: clinical and basic aspects. Med Sci Sports Exerc 22(4):436–443

Garrett WEJ, Almenkinders L, Seaber A (1984a) Biomechanics of muscle tears in stretching injuries. Trans Orthop Res Soc 9:384

Garrett WE Jr, Califf JC, Bassett FH 3rd (1984b) Histochemical correlates of hamstring injuries. Am J Sports Med 12(2):98–103

Garrett WE Jr, Nikolaou PK, Ribbeck BM, Glisson RR, Seaber AV (1988) The effect of muscle architecture on the biomechanical failure properties of skeletal muscle under passive extension. Am J Sports Med 16(1):7–12

Garrett WE Jr, Rich FR, Nikolaou PK, Vogler JB 3rd (1989) Computed tomography of hamstring muscle strains. Med Sci Sports Exerc 21(5):506–514

Garrett WE Jr, Safran MR, Seaber AV, Glisson RR, Ribbeck BM (1987) Biomechanical comparison of stimulated and nonstimulated skeletal muscle pulled to failure. Am J Sports Med 15(5):448–454

Genovely H, Stamford BA (1982) Effects of prolonged warm-up exercise above and below anaerobic threshold on maximal performance. Eur J Appl Physiol Occup Physiol 48(3):323–330

Glick JM (1980) Muscle strains: prevention and treatment. Phys Sportsmed 8(11):73–77. doi:10.1080/00913847.1980.11710969

Hanak H, Bock P (1971) Die Feinstruktur det muskelschnenverbindung von skelettund herzmusk. J Ultrastr 36:150–165

Huxley AF, Peachey LD (1961) The maximum length for contraction in vertebrate straiated muscle. J Physiol 156:150–165

Ingjer I, Stromme S (1979) Effects of active, passive or no warm-up on hte physiological response to heavy exercise. Eur J Appl Physiol 40:273–282

Karpovich P, Hale C (1956) Effect of warm up on physical perforamnce. JAMA 162:1117–1119

Korneliussen H (1973) Ultrastructure of myotendinous junction in Myxine and rat specializations between the plasma membrane and the lamina densa. Z Anat Entwickl Gesch 142(1):19–101

Krejci V, Koch P (1979) Muscle and tendon injuries in athletes. Year Book Medical Publishers, Chigaco

Kulund DN, Tottossy M (1983) Warm-up, strength, and power. Orthop Clin North Am 14(2):427–448

McMaster P (1933) Tendon and muscle ruptures. J Bone Joint Surg 15:705–722

Nikolaou P, Macdonald B, Glisson R (eds) (1986) The effect of architecture on the anatomical failure site of skeletal muscle. Trans Orthop Res Soc 11. 228

Nikolaou PK, Macdonald BL, Glisson RR, Seaber AV, Garrett WE Jr (1987) Biomechanical and histological evaluation of muscle after controlled strain injury. Am J Sports Med 15(1):9–14

Noonan TJ, Best TM, Seaber AV, Garrett WE Jr (1994) Identification of a threshold for skeletal muscle injury. Am J Sports Med 22(2):257–261

O'Donoghue D (1984) Treatment of athletic injuries. WB Saunders, Philadelphia

Peterson L, Renstrom P (1986) Sports injuries: their prevention and treatment. Year Book Medical Publishers, Chicago

Radin E, Simon S, Rose R, Paul I (1979) Practical biomechanics for the orthopaedic surgeon. A Wiley Medical Publication, New York

Ryan A (1969) Quadriceps strain, rupture, and charlie horse. Med Sci Sports 1:106–111

Safran MR, Garrett WE Jr, Seaber AV, Glisson RR, Ribbeck BM (1988) The role of warmup in muscular injury prevention. Am J Sports Med 16(2):123–129

Schwarzacher H (1960) Untersuchungen uber die skeletmuskel—schnenverbindung. Acta Anatomia 40:49–86

Solveborn S (1983) The book about stretching. Japan Publications, Tokyo

Stauber WT (1989) Eccentric action of muscles: physiology, injury, and adaptation. Exerc Sport Sci Rev 17:157–185

Strickler T, Malone T, Garrett WE (1990) The effects of passive warming on muscle injury. Am J Sports Med 18(2):141–145

Taylor D, Seaber A, Garrett W Jr (1985a) Cyclic repetitive stretching of muscle-tendon units. Surg Forum 36:339–541

Taylor D, Seaber A, Garrett W Jr (1985b) Repetitive stretching of muscles and tendons to a specific tension. Trans Orthop Res Soc 10:41

Taylor D, Seaber A, Garrett W Jr (1985c) Response of muscle-tendon units to cyclic repetitive stretching. Trans Orthop Res Soc. 10:84

Taylor D, Seaber A, Garrett W Jr (1986) Immediate response of muscle to traumatic stretching. Surg Forum 37:547–549

Taylor DC, Dalton JD Jr, Seaber AV, Garrett WE Jr (1990) Viscoelastic properties of muscle-tendon units. The

biomechanical effects of stretching. Am J Sports Med 18(3):300–309
Trotter JA, Corbett K, Avner BP (1981) Structure and function of the murine muscle-tendon junction. Anat Rec 201(2):293–302. doi:10.1002/ar.1092010209
Trotter JA, Eberhard S, Samora A (1983) Structural domains of the muscle-tendon junction. 1. The internal lamina and the connecting domain. Anat Rec 207(4):573–591. doi:10.1002/ar.1092070406
Wikiewicz T, Roy R, Powell P (1983) Muscle architecture in the human lower limb. Clin Orthop 179:275–283
Williams PE, Goldspink G (1971) Longitudinal growth of striated muscle fibres. J Cell Sci 9(3):751–767
Williams PE, Goldspink G (1973) The effect of immobilization on the longitudinal growth of striated muscle fibres. J Anat 116(Pt 1):45–55
Williams PE, Goldspink G (1978) Changes in sarcomere length and physiological properties in immobilized muscle. J Anat 127(Pt 3):459–468
Williford HN, East JB, Smith FH, Burry LA (1986) Evaluation of warm-up for improvement in flexibility. Am J Sports Med 14(4):316–319
Zarins B, Ciullo JV (1983) Acute muscle and tendon injuries in athletes. Clin Sports Med 2(1):167–182

MRI of Muscle and Tendon Pathology

6

Giuseppe Monetti, Gianluca Rampino, and Giuseppe Rusignuolo

Contents

G. Monetti (✉)
Dipartimento di Diagnostica per Immagini, Ospedale Privato Accreditato Nigrisoli,
Viale Ercolani, 9, Bologna, Italy
e-mail: info@muskultrasound.it

G. Rampino
Unità operativa di Diagnostica per Immagini Friuli Coram di Udine, Udine, Italy

G. Rusignuolo
Struttura Complessa di Radiologia Azienda Ospedaliera Santa Maria di Terni, Terni, Italy

6.1 Introduction

Magnetic resonance imaging (MRI) plays a large role in the evaluation of muscle pathology. This role is shared with dynamic ultrasound (US), which is still the gold standard method.

A key advantage of MRI in assessing muscle conditions is its multiplanar capability, which affords visualization of structures in the three spatial planes: sagittal, axial, and coronal.

Another major strength of MRI is its ability to provide panoramic views, which allow visualization of a whole limb in a single sequence, something that is extremely difficult to achieve with US.

MRI is the method of choice to examine all body structures—muscles, tendons, ligaments, vessels, bone, etc.—because it provides a wide range of sequences that meet most diagnostic requirements.

A further advantage of MRI is its non-invasive nature, especially compared with computed tomography (CT) and standard radiography.

Its single drawback is related to metal materials, especially metals other than titanium, which generate significant artefacts that severely impair scan evaluation.

G.L. Canata et al. (eds.), *Muscle and Tendon Injuries*, DOI 10.1007/978-3-662-54184-5_6

6.2 Standard MRI

Standard or tunnel MRI, which is by far the most widely used MRI technique, employs a broad range of magnetic fields which in human imaging range from 0.25 to 3 Tesla.

Especially in high-field magnets, a range of available sequences allow selecting the one that is more appropriate to the structure and condition being examined.

T1-weighted sequences provide a morphological image of muscle (Fig. 6.1a).

T2-weighted sequences, which generate high-contrast images, afford functional assessment by clearly depicting inflammatory processes, fluid, or overtly liquid components in muscle (Fig. 6.1b).

An especially useful sequence in assessing muscle is the fat-suppression sequence, which removes the signal from adipose tissue, thus providing accurate information on lipomas.

6.2.1 Contrast-Enhanced MRI

Contrast agents are employed when very high definition is needed. They can contribute to differential diagnosis, particularly in the case of degenerative conditions, by differentiating among benign neoplasms or, more importantly, malignancies (Fig. 6.2a–b)

Paramagnetic contrast agents better tolerated than non-iodinated agents, especially where anaphylactic shock is concerned.

6.2.2 Magnetic Resonance Angiography

Magnetic resonance angiography (MRA) provides highly detailed images of the arterial and venous network. Its limited invasiveness is highly valuable to assess upper and lower limb muscle pathology.

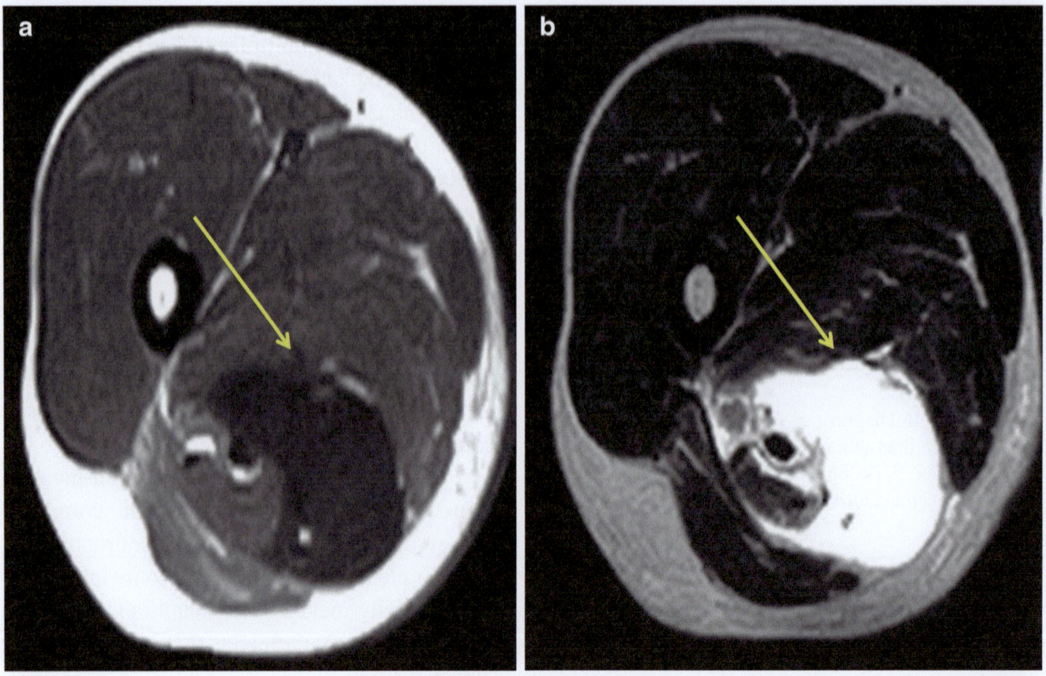

Fig. 6.1 (**a**) Axial image acquired at the level of the thigh with a T1-weighted (morphological) sequence showing a large haematoma due to complete ischiocrural muscle rupture. (**b**) Image acquired using a high-contrast sequence like STIR. The functional information and the hyperintense fluid component are very clearly depicted

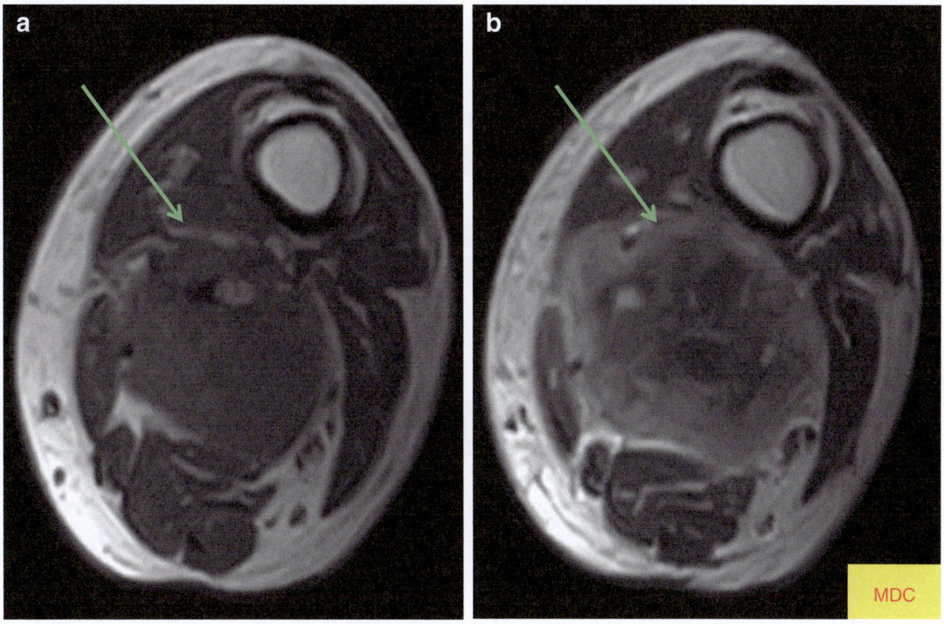

Fig. 6.2 (**a**) New, space-occupying, malignant formation involving the medial distal third of the thigh, where unenhanced T1-weighted sequences afford poor definition of the mass compared with adjacent muscle. (**b**) Same lesion as in A. Marked though inhomogeneous enhancement in the peripheral and central portion of the lesion obtained with a contrast-enhanced sequence

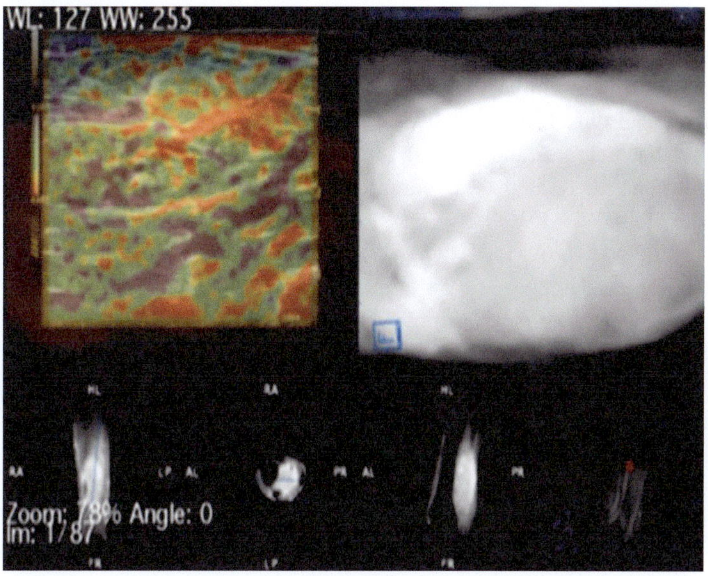

Fig. 6.3 Fusion technology allows overlaying MRI, CT, and US scans also when using colour and power Doppler or, in this case, elastography

6.2.3 Fusion Technology

This approach allows MRI scans to be superimposed on images acquired with other modalities such as US and CT.

Fusion technology is particularly valuable in the follow-up of malignancies and post-traumatic conditions, since it affords accurate monitoring of lesion resolution and progression (Fig. 6.3).

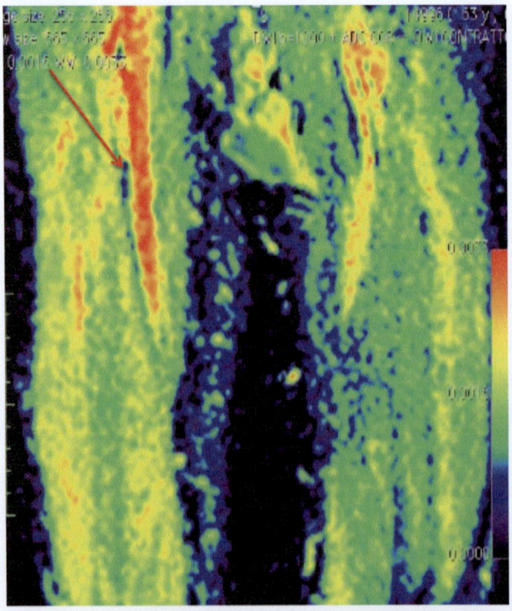

Fig. 6.4 DWI with ADC map provides high-definition images of muscle lesions based on the motion of hydrogen molecules

6.2.4 Diffusion MRI

This approach detects the abnormal motion of water molecules, providing very clear images of trauma-induced muscle lesions, such as haemorrhage and haematoma, and critical information on signal changes related to metabolic muscle disorders.

The method provides two techniques: diffusion-weighted imaging (DWI) and diffusion tensor imaging (DTI).

With DWI, the more widely used, ADC maps enable a more clear visualization of tissue pathology (Fig. 6.4).

DTI (tractography) provides a detailed image of the whole course of structures such as peripheral nerves (Fig. 6.5).

6.2.5 MR Elastography

A further application of the MR technology, MR elastography, uses fast DWI sequences to depict muscle during contraction and relaxation.

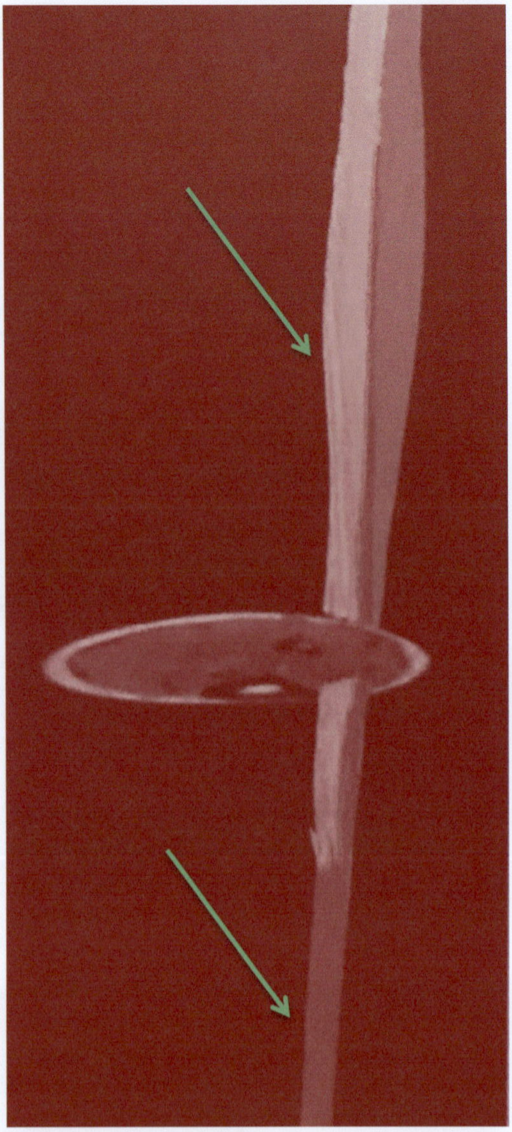

Fig. 6.5 With DTI, the course of individual nerves can be extrapolated from surrounding structures using image subtraction sequences

6.2.6 Upright MRI

Even though upright MRI has been available for some years, manufacturers are still few.

The method has considerable added value in the examination of musculoskeletal conditions, since it affords accurate assessment of structures, especially in relation to patient posture, which clearly is mostly upright.

In particular, upright MRI allows resolving some differential diagnostic queries that cannot be decided on scans obtained with standard MRI.

6.2.7 Dynamic MRI

Our diagnostic imaging department has been the first to develop dynamic MRI at the international level, using the ESAOTE G-scan Brio magnet (Genova, Italy). The method is proving highly successful both in orthopaedic and neurosurgical applications.

The generation of dynamic scans while the patient is making movements in slow motion (internal and external rotation, flexion, and extension, to mention just a few) allows ideal assessment of the movement of each joint and muscle group, as dynamic US has been doing for some years. The panoramic views offered by MRI are a major advantage that enables very accurate diagnoses.

Our radiology technicians, Alessia Principe and Filippo De Carli, have been working to develop this important innovation with great professionalism and enthusiasm.

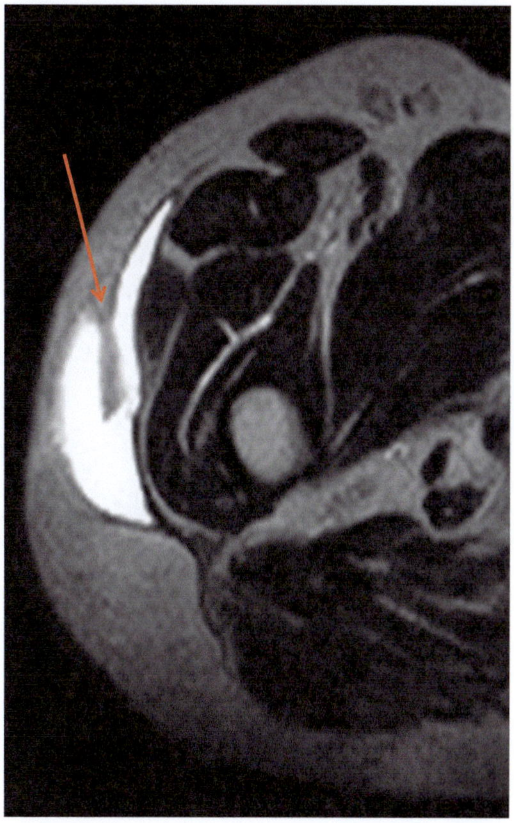

Fig. 6.6 Grade 3 Morel-Lavallée lesion involving the subcutaneous fat adjacent to the tensor fasciae latae muscle of the right thigh; the underlying muscle is unaffected

6.3 Muscles

6.3.1 Trauma-Related Conditions

Trauma-induced muscle injuries are among the most common musculoskeletal conditions.

Traumas can be divided into minor and major.

6.3.1.1 Minor Traumas

Injury to subcutaneous adipose tissue (crush injury) can be divided into lymphoedema, fat necrosis, and fascial shearing injury. The latter condition induces subcutaneous and suprafascial haematomas and is known as Morel-Lavallée syndrome (grade 1, 2, and 3, respectively) (Fig. 6.6).

MRI is indicated only in patients with extensive Morel-Lavallée syndrome, since US examination is easier to perform and sometimes conclusive.

Muscle injuries include contracture, elongation, and contusion.

Contractures and elongations are induced by an indirect mechanism—they thus lack tears of intrinsic muscle fibres and are characterized by oedema.

Contusions induce muscle changes due to direct trauma; the main injury often involves the deep muscle plane, where the propagation of the force vector is halted by bone.

In patients with contractures and elongations, MRI can depict changes in signal intensity related to oedema formation. Its characteristic high signal intensity and inhomogeneous distribution are easier to see using high-contrast sequences.

A typical minor muscle injury, delayed-onset muscle soreness (DOMS), is due to perifascial

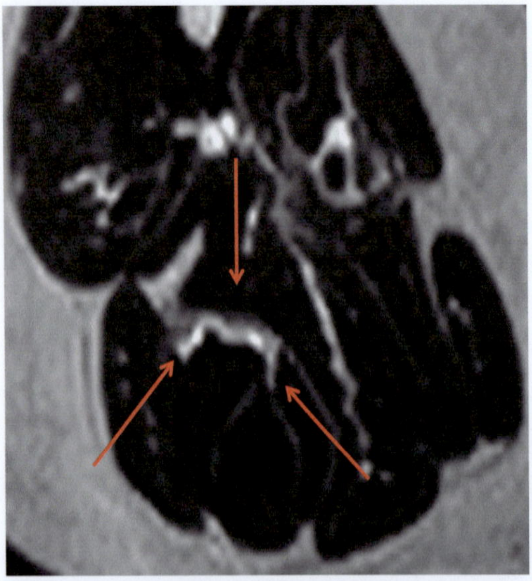

Fig. 6.7 Clear involvement of myofascial components in a patient with DOMS

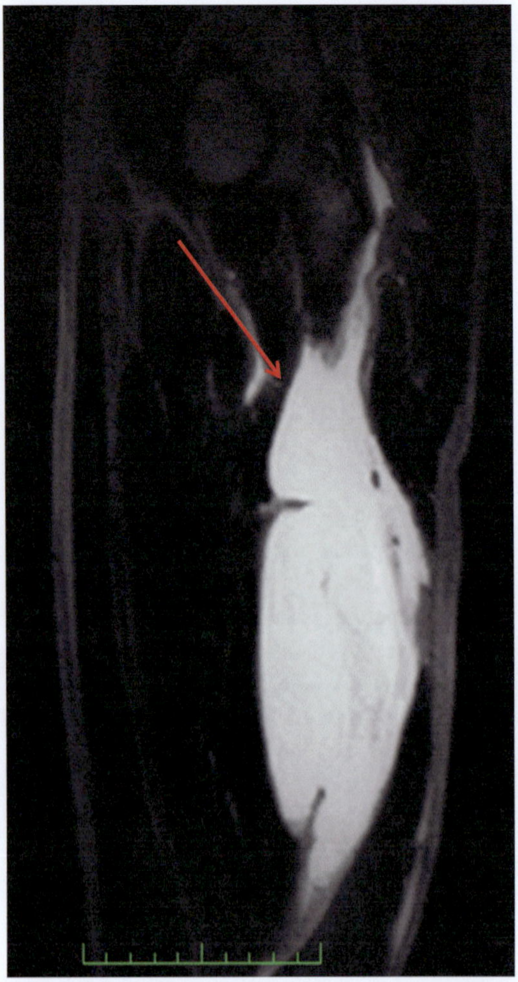

Fig. 6.8 Subacute phase of the lesion, assessed about 72 h from the trauma (methaemoglobin phase). Complete colliquation of the haematoma allows appreciating its actual extent also in view of its evacuation

oedema. Again, high-contrast sequences, especially STIR, are the most suitable (Fig. 6.7).

6.3.1.2 Major Traumas

Major muscle traumas are divided by their severity into partial and complete rupture.

Injury grading and the definition of distraction should be reserved to clinical settings, whereas the MRI report should describe the lesion in terms of extent, compartment, and extra-compartmental extension, as appropriate.

Partial ruptures are often fairly difficult to diagnose if they involve minor injury. MRI is eminently suitable to monitor haematoma evolution. Haematomas are found in partial as well as complete lesions, because they are related to fibre tearing.

Haematomas form in the first few hours after the trauma, in the hyperacute phase, which lasts ca. 12 h, and show inhomogeneous signal intensity due to the erythrocyte fraction (oxyhaemoglobin phase).

The acute phase, marked by erythrocyte lysis, usually takes place from 24 to 48 after the injury (deoxyhaemoglobin phase).

The subacute stage—from ca.48 to 72 h post-trauma—is related to complete colliquation of the haematoma (methaemoglobin phase) (Fig. 6.8).

Finally, the last stage (chronic phase) involves organization of the haematoma, if it is not treated, due to haemosiderin degradation processes.

In this phase, the haematoma may undergo calcification, which in the most severe cases may evolve to metaplastic ossification.

The main advantages of MRI over US in this setting are related to site, extension, signal, course, and morphology.

Site: muscle lesions may be found in anatomical areas that are difficult to assess by US, in particular the pelvic muscles such as the internal and external obturators, the iliopsoas, and the quadratus femoris, which are not clearly visualized by US.

Extension: it relates to the multiplanar ability and, especially, the panoramic views offered by MRI.

Signal: MRI accurately depicts the changes related to the trophism of muscle components, particularly fatty replacement of muscle fibres, which may be due to trauma or, more often, neuromuscular disease (Fig. 6.9).

Course and morphology: these advantages make MRI the imaging modality of choice to study large, flat muscles such as the dorsal muscles and pelvic muscles like the piriformis, where the absence of a thick layer prevents US from supplying useful findings.

Since MRI involves scanning in the coronal plane, it provides an optimal depiction of these changes, besides the panoramic views that enable comparing a structure to the contralateral one.

Organized haematomas deserve special attention, since they often have the same appearance as tumours, both benign and malignant.

The workup of these patients should include imaging with a paramagnetic contrast agent, power and colour Doppler examination, and, where appropriate, also a dynamic MRI scan, which provides a clearer definition of the involvement of adjacent structures by the lesion.

Fusion technology, which involves overlaying MRI and US scans, supplies valuable information in the follow-up of these lesions.

Patients with muscle injuries often suffer from concomitant vascular lesions, since wide tears and extensive haematomas may also involve dislocation or compression of adjacent vascular and nerve structures.

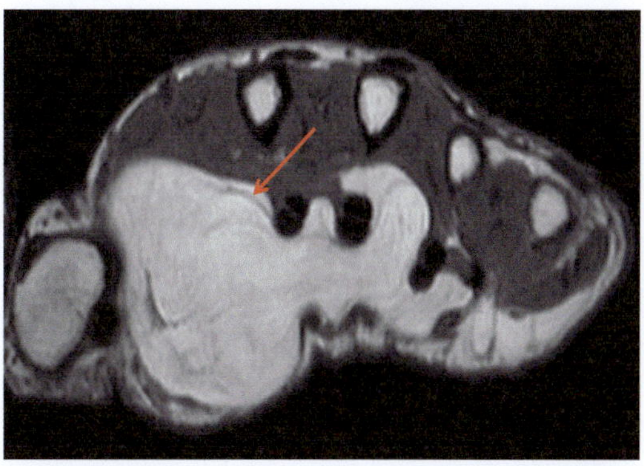

Fig. 6.9 MRI provides optimal definition of the interface among different tissues, in particular muscle and fat, as in this giant cell tumour, whose fibroadipose tissue component is clearly outlined against adjacent muscle

6.3.2 Myofascial Disinsertion

Myofascial disinsertion often poses a diagnostic challenge, be it assessed by dynamic US or by MRI.

However, MRI is clearly the superior modality, since it allows comparison with the healthy contralateral limb using panoramic views and accurately demonstrates the distinctive hyperintense, crescent-like signal of these injuries in high-contrast sequences.

Dynamic MRI is a further highly useful approach to diagnose these lesions.

6.3.3 Myotendinous Avulsion

We feel that the diagnostic role of MRI in these injuries is ancillary, because especially in the acute phase, standard X-rays, associated where necessary with 3D CT reconstruction, are still the method of choice.

MRI and US are effectively employed at a later stage, when the involvement of musculotendinous structures is assessed in view of the treatment selection.

6.3.4 Lesions Due to Compression Injury

In these lesions, MRI plays a crucial role, since it affords accurate and thorough evaluation of the involvement of neighbouring anatomical structures.

Dynamic MRI is currently the most informative technique, since the interpretation of the partial or complete involvement of large muscle groups using static MRI is sometimes inconclusive.

Dynamic MRI, which evaluates structures under active and passive contraction and relaxation, consistently provides to the surgeon a detailed map of muscle involvement by the lesion.

6.3.5 Post-traumatic Degenerative Conditions

Post-traumatic degenerative conditions comprise several changes, first of all scar fibrosis, which always follows a lesion.

Other common conditions include metaplastic ossification, rhabdomyolysis, compartmental syndrome, and, less frequently, conditions such as cysticercosis and echinococcosis.

6.3.5.1 Post-traumatic Fibrosis

These conditions should be subdivided into fibrosis resulting from partial/complete muscle rupture in the injured area and generalized fibrosis, which is a sequela of extensive contusions involving large muscle tracts.

Scar fibrosis is the most common degenerative event after a trauma, since the repair of torn muscle fibres always involves formation of a scar of variable extent (Fig. 6.10).

The imaging modalities of choice for this type of processes are power and colour Doppler and elastography, which afford optimal assessment of the lesion and, especially, depict any ongoing neoangiogenesis or lesion recurrence. MRI therefore plays a limited role.

MRI may usefully be employed to assess the contralateral limb, especially in patients with

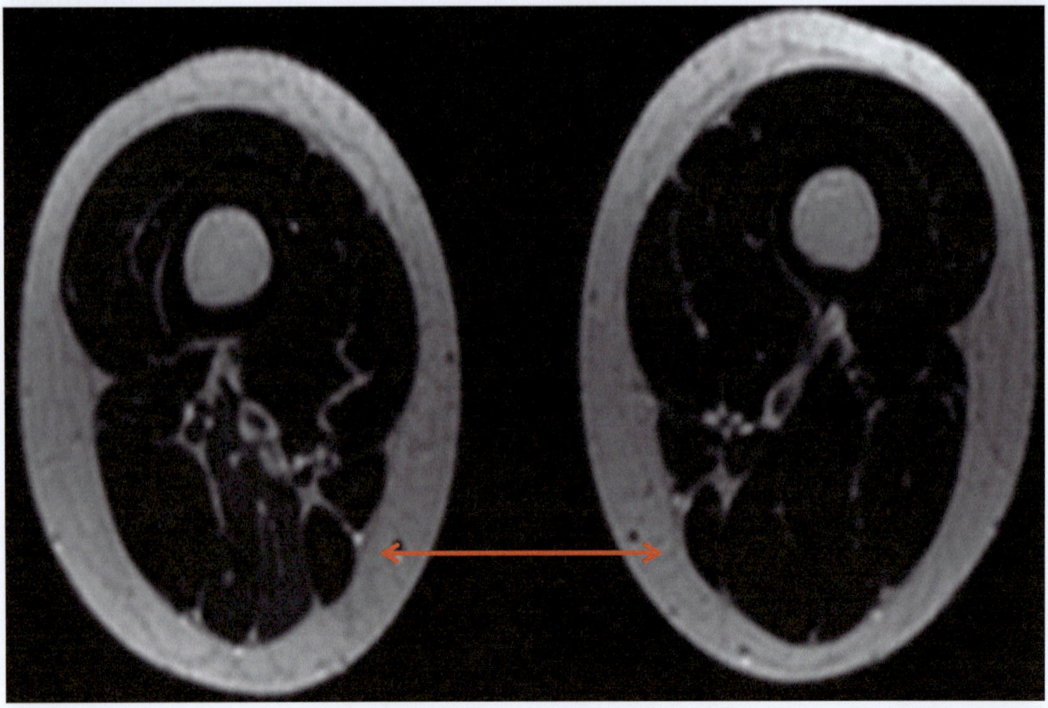

Fig. 6.10 The high-definition image provided by this bilateral MRI scan enables assessing muscle trophism. On the *right*, note the markedly hypotrophic ischiocrural muscles, whose signal indicates the beginning of fibroadipose replacement as a result of the nerve injured

hypotrophy/hypertrophy of the muscle components involved, and to depict fatty replacement in injured muscles.

6.3.5.2 Metaplastic Ossification

Haematomas, which are often due to compression injury, may undergo degeneration if they are not appropriately treated. In metaplastic ossification (myositis ossificans), muscle is replaced by calcified tissue.

Standard radiography and CT are the imaging methods of choice, especially in overt pathology.

MRI does not play a large role and is usefully supplemented by US scanning, especially in the early phase, when US is capable of detecting calcium deposits in the haematoma already on the third to fourth day.

6.3.5.3 Rhabdomyolysis

Muscle rhabdomyolysis may be due to a variety of causes, among them metabolic disorders such as post-traumatic fatigue.

Excessive loading induces muscle fibre degeneration, which involves an acute and a chronic stage.

The diagnosis is strictly haematochemical (by determination of muscle enzymes), or it may also include needle biopsy or electron microscopic examination. The typical acute-phase MRI and US finding is a disrupted architecture of muscle bundles, which consist of a fibrous stroma and of parallel fibres forming tertiary bundles.

The acute phase, which is accompanied by cramps and stiffness, lasts 8–10 days.

In the majority of patients, the condition resolves slowly, although the tissues may still show signal changes due to residual areas of fibrosis.

6.3.6 Compartmental Syndromes

Compartmental syndromes are common in anatomical districts where vascular and nerve structures can be trapped by hypertrophic muscles (as in body builders), large haematomas, or space-occupying lesions.

In these patients, MRI is capable of depicting direct and indirect signs of compression.

Direct signs are changes in normal muscle architecture and signal alterations due to ischaemic processes involving the muscle.

Indirect signs are often related to extensive lymphoedema of adjacent subcutaneous adipose tissue.

An anatomical area that is particularly prone to compartmental syndrome is the anterior tibial region, where vascular and nerve structures are compressed by bone in the deep plane and by retinacula and aponeuroses in the superficial plane (Fig. 6.11).

Also in these cases, dynamic MRI provides a useful adjunct, since it often supplies high-definition images of the compressed area.

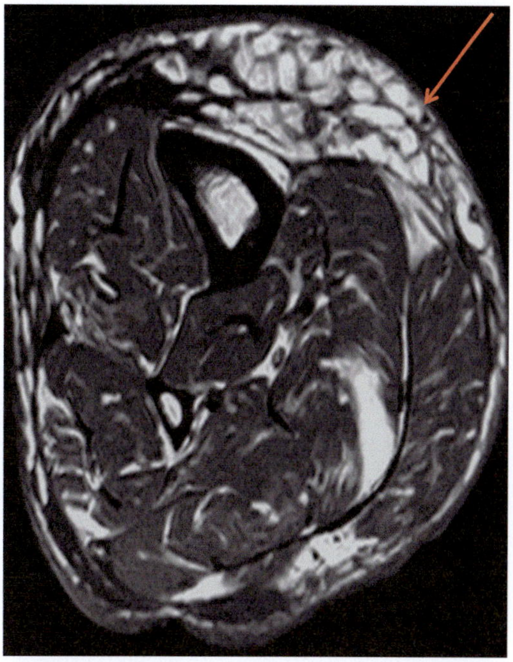

Fig. 6.11 Marked subcutaneous lymphoedema involving the anteromedial aspect of the leg due to early acute-phase compartmental syndrome

In the immediate post-trauma period, power and colour Doppler afford accurate examination of vascular and nerve compression injuries.

6.3.6.1 Muscle Hernias

Muscle herniation occurs when tearing allows muscle protrusion through a superficial aponeurotic fascia.

Hernias, which include the so-called sports hernias, typically occur in the anteromedial aponeurotic fascia at the level of the tibia and at paraumbilical and inguinal sites.

MRI is not the imaging modality of choice for their evaluation. A dynamic US scan taken during a Valsalva manoeuvre clearly depicts the hernia by showing fascial discontinuity.

A differential diagnosis is often required with pseudohernias, which are determined by muscle compression due to a lax aponeurotic fascia.

Here, too, MRI is not indicated, except to depict the muscle compression at the level of the aponeurotic fascia (with dynamic MRI) during muscle contraction and relaxation or during a Valsalva manoeuvre.

Accessory muscles, especially the soleus and the anconeus epitrochlearis accessory muscle, are not uncommon and should always be kept in mind, because they partially alter the morphology of the district and require examination of the contralateral limb.

The panoramic views and its ability to provide scans under muscle contraction and relaxation make dynamic MRI the imaging method of choice for these lesions, in conjunction with US.

6.3.6.2 Neuromuscular Conditions

There are several neuromuscular disorders, involving the first and second motor neurons and the nervous system, whose diagnosis is not within the remit of the radiologist.

The task of MRI, and where appropriate of US, is to monitor, at the behest of the neurologist, a situation that has clearly been characterized at the clinical and instrumental level, and to document any change in muscle involvement, be it an improvement, a stationary situation, or a progression.

The key finding in such disorders is progressive muscle replacement by fibroadipose tissue.

In the various body compartments, MRI accurately depicts hypotrophic muscle components, especially their signal alteration. In morphological sequences, muscle shows diffuse hyperintensity due to progressive fibroadipose tissue replacement: the more severe diseases, such as Duchenne muscular dystrophy, involve a near inversion of the normal 1:7 ratio (ca. 7:1).

MRI and US are highly useful in identifying the districts less severely involved, where collection of tissue biopsies can help refine the diagnosis and therapeutic management.

6.3.7 Neoplastic Disease

This is the field where diagnostic imaging provides crucial information on lesion extension and the involvement of extra-compartmental structures, since the diagnosis of tumour type is made on biopsy specimens.

In addition, MRI provides information which in relation to the signal changes, the district involved, patient age and gender, and symptom characteristics helps improve the surgical or chemotherapeutic approach.

In these patients, MRI with a paramagnetic contrast agent, MRA, and sometimes dynamic MRI provide valuable data to assess the spatial and locoregional extension of the lesion (Fig. 6.12).

6.4 Tendons

Tendons are divided into muscle anchoring and gliding.

Both consist of three types of bundles—primary, secondary, and tertiary—and are covered by the peritenon or paratenon.

Gliding tendons are also covered by a synovial sheath, made up of a visceral and a parietal layer, which enables safe gliding on fibro-osseous structures and in the narrower anatomical grooves and tunnels.

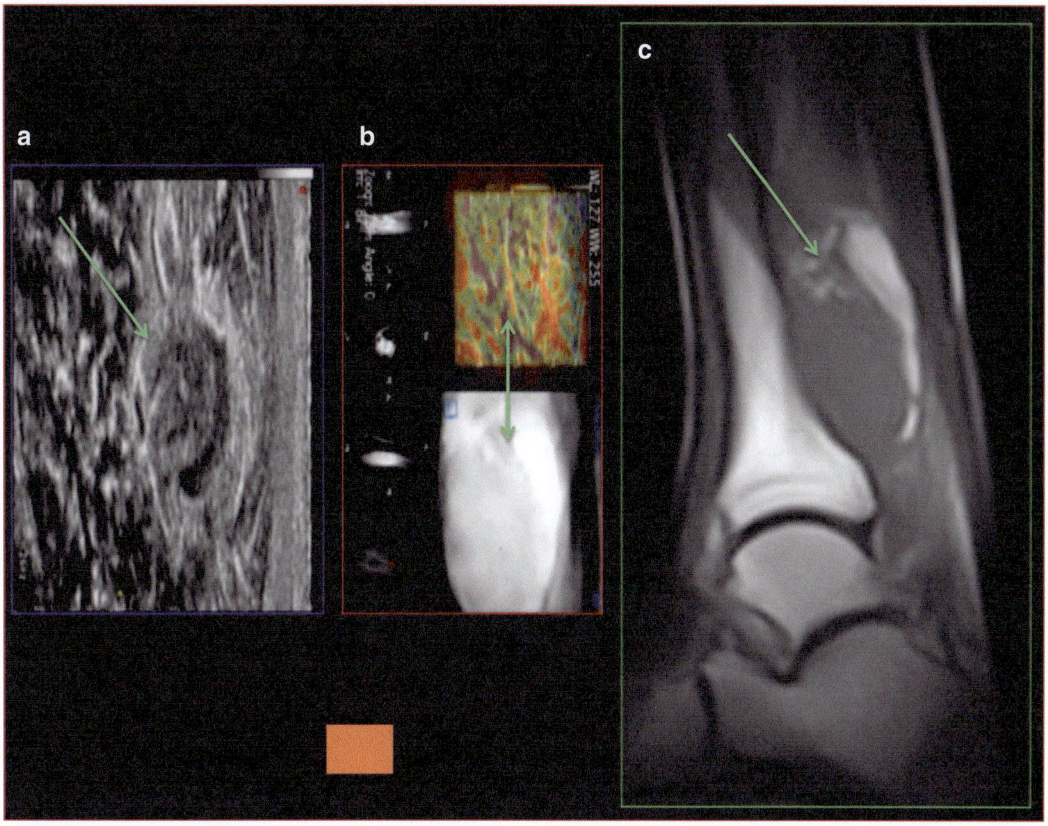

Fig. 6.12 The US scan (**a**), fusion image (**b**), and MRI scan (**c**) allow a new, large, space-occupying formation to be diagnosed as a muscle sarcoma

In turn, the tendon attachments (entheses) are characterized by a synovial bursa that protects the tendons at their insertion into bone.

Unlike muscles, tendons have poor elongation potential and are generally taut, since they anchor muscles to fibrocartilage and bone.

Tendon pathology includes peritendinitis, insertional and non-insertional degenerative tendinopathy (tendinosis), partial- and full-thickness rupture, myotendinous disinsertion, musculotendinous avulsion, and tenosynovitis, the latter affecting gliding tendons.

6.4.1 Peritendinitis

These disorders are characterized by inflammatory processes involving the tendon sheath (peritenon).

Often, particularly when Achilles tendon is involved, inflammation is accompanied by bursitis (in the case of Achilles tendon, inflammation of the deep retrocalcaneal bursa).

These patients may exhibit a concomitant inflammation of the Kager fat pad in Kager's triangle (Achilles tendon) or of Hoffa's fat pad (patellar tendon).

The imaging method of choice to assess tendon pathology is colour and power Doppler, specifically elastography.

MRI plays a useful role in depicting the extent of the tendon damage, since it provides accurate information on the course of the whole tendon.

Dynamic MRI plays a key role, because it affords optimal visualization of tendon behaviour and of the musculotendinous junction of the homonymous muscle.

6.4.2 Degenerative Tendinopathy

These disorders are divided into insertional (enthesopathy) and non-insertional.

Patients with enthesopathy often have multiple calcifications in the tendon insertion that are not clearly visualized by MRI because, like the tendon, they are characterized by low signal intensity.

US is again the more informative imaging modality.

In non-insertional tendinopathy, the tendon often displays fusiform, thickened tracts that may be several centimetres long; the panoramic views make MRI ideal to visualize their extension.

The evaluation of tendon xanthomatosis deserves a specific mention. Xanthomas are determined by metabolic changes in patients with hypercholesterolaemia and hyperlipidaemia, which induce intrinsic degeneration of tendon fibres with formation of vacuoles and ultimately calcific degeneration. Unless prompt and appropriate treatment is applied, the tendon may undergo severe tearing.

MRI provides useful information on calcific tendinopathy, which is characterized by extensive metaplastic ossification that is not clearly depicted by US.

In such cases, dynamic MRI affords optimal assessment of large calcium deposits.

6.4.3 Partial Tears

Partial tendon rupture is more common at attachment sites. Lesion morphology closely depends on the tendon region involved.

In the case of torn rotator cuff tendons, highly accurate information on lesion side, bursal, interstitial, or articular, maximizes treatment effectiveness.

Dynamic US affords optimal evaluation of these lesions, and dynamic MRI is a useful adjunct.

Notably, degenerative tendinopathy and partial tears share very similar symptoms.

In such patients, it is useful to make a thorough assessment of any associated areas of inflammation, especially for medicolegal purposes.

Although US is clearly more informative than MRI, the latter clearly depicts chronic tendon tears, whereas significant tendon retraction is not equally well visualized by US.

6.4.4 Complete Tears

The diagnosis of full-thickness tendon rupture is almost exclusively clinical and does not commonly require imaging.

MRI and US are needed to assess lesion severity; they also provide key information on the surgical approach to be adopted and on the convenience of using heterologous materials in case of severe, extensive injury.

MRI is the imaging modality of choice for preoperative tendon assessment, since it provides accurate information on the amount of upstream and downstream stump retraction and on the involvement of neighbouring structures such as muscles, ligaments, fasciae, and bone.

Moreover, dynamic MRI provides key information by precisely demonstrating lesion extension, especially compared with static MRI, where high-contrast sequences may overestimate the lesion.

6.4.5 Tenosynovitis

Tenosynovitis affects tendons with a synovial sheath and is divided into exudative and dry, the latter being more frequently related to traumatic injury.

Exudative tenosynovitis is typical of rheumatic disorders, where the inner synovial sheath is usually thickened and hypertrophic.

Finally, stenosing tenosynovitis affects tendons that pass through narrow tunnels or fibro-osseous grooves, like those of the fingers, where hypertrophic pulleys hamper tendon gliding and give rise to trigger finger (typically the thumb and index, middle, and ring fingers).

The more suitable MRI sequences are the high-contrast sequences, i.e. T2 weighted and especially STIR.

Dynamic MRI accurately depicts stump retraction.

This is particularly needed in patients with exudative tenosynovitis due to rheumatic disorders and in those with tendon entrapment due to Dupuytren syndrome, where the nodules in the palmar aponeurosis tend to incarcerate the tendons.

6.4.6 Tenorrhaphy

The follow-up of tendon surgery is carried out no earlier than 3 months postoperatively, since scar fibrosis generates significant artefacts.

The tendon is thickened, often inhomogeneously so, due to the operation.

In such patients, complementary MRI and US examination is essential and very useful.

By enabling superimposition of MRI and US scans, fusion technology provides highly precise information.

Also in this case, dynamic MRI clearly depicts any adhesions or fibrous scars that hamper tendon extension.

Suggested Reading

Basford JR, Jenkin TR, An KN et al (2002) Evaluation of healthy and diseased muscle with magnetic resonance elastography. Arch Phys Med Rehabil 83(11):1530–1536

Bousquet G (1982) Il ginocchio illustrato. Ermes Medica Drommi, Roma

Di Giacomo G, Pouliart N, Costantini A (2008) Atlas of functional shoulder anatomy. Springer-Verlag, Italia

Dresner MA, Rose G, Rossman PJ et al (2001) Magnetic resonance elastography of skeletal muscle. J Magn Reson Imaging 13(2):269–276

Heers G, Jenkyn T, Dresner MA et al (2003) Measurement of muscle activity with magnetic resonance elastography. Clin Biomech 18(6):537–542

Jacobson JA (1999) Musculoskeletal sonography and MR imaging: a role for both imaging methods. Radiol Clin N Am 37(4):713–735

Jenkin TR, Ehman RL, An KN (2003) Noninvasive muscle tension measurement using the novel technique of magnetic resonance elastography (MRE). J Biomech 36(12):1917–1921

Jost B, Koch PP, Gerber C (2000) Anatomy and functional aspects of the rotator interval. J Shoulder Elb Surg 9(4):336–341

Lauren MS, Garry EG (2012) MRI of weight-bearing and movement. Osteoarthritis Cartilage 20(2):69–78

Manaster DJ, Andrews CL, Crim J, Grossman JW, Miller TT, Petersilge CA, Roberts CC, Rosenberg ZS (2006) Diagnostic and surgical imaging anatomy musculoskeletal. Amirsys Inc

Monetti G, Pistolesi GF (1994) L'Imaging delle articolazioni, Ed. Gnocchi.

Monetti G, Bazzocchi M (1994) Muscoli e tendini, Ed. Gnocchi.

Monetti G (2011) Risonanza Magnetica dell'apparato muscolo-scheletrico. RM Orto—Clino. Timeo editore, Bologna

Pirola V (2004) Cinesiologia. Edi-Ermes

Pope TL Jr (2009) Diagnostica per immagini in traumatologia muscolo-scheletrica. Elsevier, Milano

Porcellini G, Castagna A (2014) La Spalla, seconda edizione. Verduci editore

Reiser M, Baur-Melnyk A, Glaser C (2009) Imaging muscolo-scheletrico, CIC ed

Reiser MF (2014) Magnetic resonance imaging of the skeletal musculature, Marc Andrè Weber Editor (Springer)

Resnick D, Kang HS (1997) Shoulder. In: Resnick D, Kang HS (eds) Internal derangement of joints: emphasis on MR imaging. WB Saunders, Philadelphia

Roh MS, Wang VM, April EW, Pollock RG, Bigliani LU, Flatow EL (2000) Anterior and posterior musculotendinous anatomy of the supraspinatus. J Shoulder Elbow Surg 9 (September–October 5)

Stoller DW (2008) Stoller's Atlas of orthopaedics and sports medicine, Wolters Kluwer-Lippincott Williams & Wilkins

Thompson JC (2004) Atlante di anatomia ortopedica di Netter. Ed. Masson

Ultrasound of Muscle and Tendon Pathology

7

Giuseppe Monetti, Marco Fogli,
and Gianluigi Mele

Contents

7.1 Introduction

Ultrasound (US) is the method of choice for assessing muscles and tendons. Its chief advantages are the ability to provide dynamic scans, low cost, and a practical approach to the patient.

However, US is by no means easy to perform, since although it provides highly satisfactory results and offers countless diagnostic possibilities, pitfalls are quite numerous.

7.2 B-Mode Ultrasound

B-mode scanning, the most common US technique, uses probes ranging from 2.5 to 20 MHz.

Intermediate frequency (7.5–14 MHz) linear transducers are the most suitable to assess musculoskeletal structures.

It is worth stressing that high-frequency probes, though ideal to evaluate very superficial structures, do not go deeper than 2.5–3 cm and fail to provide a panoramic view.

G. Monetti (✉)
Dipartimento di Diagnostica per Immagini, Ospedale Privato Accreditato Nigrisoli,
Viale Ercolani, 9, Bologna, Italy
e-mail: info@muskultrasound.it

M. Fogli
Dipartimento di Scienze Biomediche e Chirurgiche, Scuola di Specializzazione in Scienze Motorie, Ferrara, Italy

G. Mele
Centro di Diagnostica Sportiva D-lab di Bologna, Bologna, Italy

G.L. Canata et al. (eds.), *Muscle and Tendon Injuries*, DOI 10.1007/978-3-662-54184-5_7

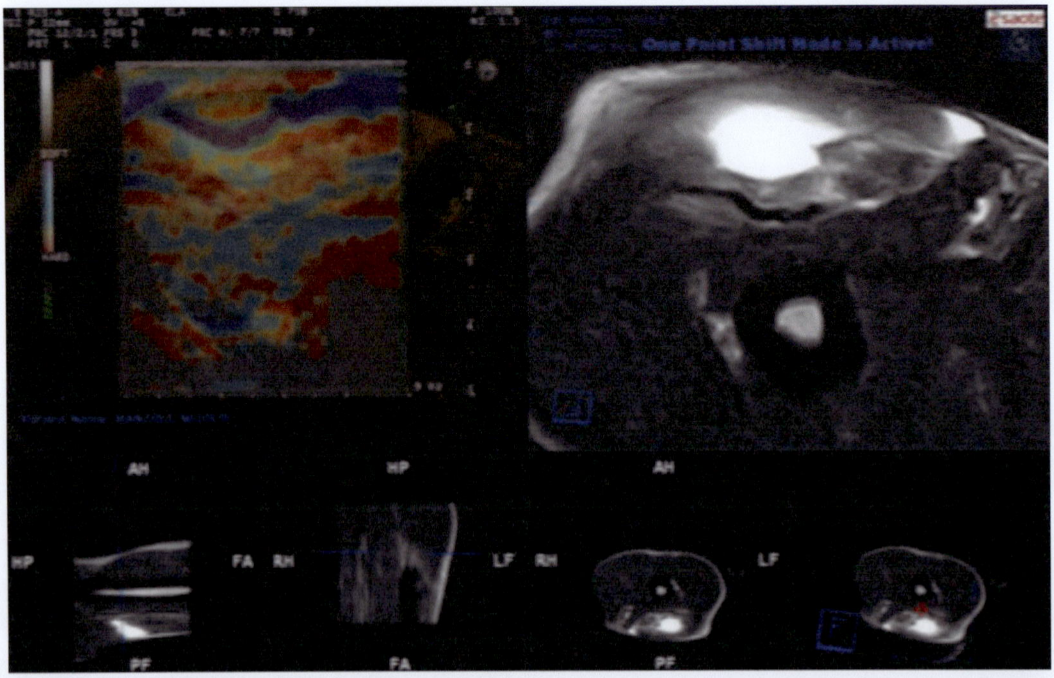

Fig. 7.1 Fusion technology is extremely useful, especially in following up lesions, since the overlay of the initial US and MRI scans enables superimposition of further scans and demonstration of any changes

Convex probes are useful to assess deep, space-occupying lesions of a different nature, which are poorly depicted by linear probes.

Colour and power Doppler sonography is a valuable technique that affords excellent visualization of arteries and veins and of small-size nerve structures, where it depicts pulsating vessels.

Intravenous contrast agents may provide useful information, especially in patients suffering from the inflammatory and degenerative processes related to rheumatic disorders; in rare cases they also help assess new formations that are suspicious for malignancy.

7.3 Ultrasound Fusion

Fusion technology enables US scans to be superimposed on magnetic resonance imaging (MRI) scans, providing valuable information, especially when following up patients with traumatic or neoplastic lesions.

A major weakness of US is its poor reproducibility, even when examinations are performed by the same operator.

After superimposing the initial US and MRI scans, follow-up US scans can be superimposed on the first MRI scan as they are acquired, providing accurate information on any intervening variations (Fig. 7.1).

7.4 Elastography

Elastography is currently available in all ultrasound scanners. It is based on the principle that a distinctive vibration is associated with the degree of elasticity of the tissue being examined. The vibration, obtained by moderate tissue compression with the probe, is translated by the software into a colour map (Fig. 7.2a–b).

Elastography allows excellent follow-up assessment of muscle and tendon lesions by demonstrating the recovery of elasticity in areas that have suffered injury.

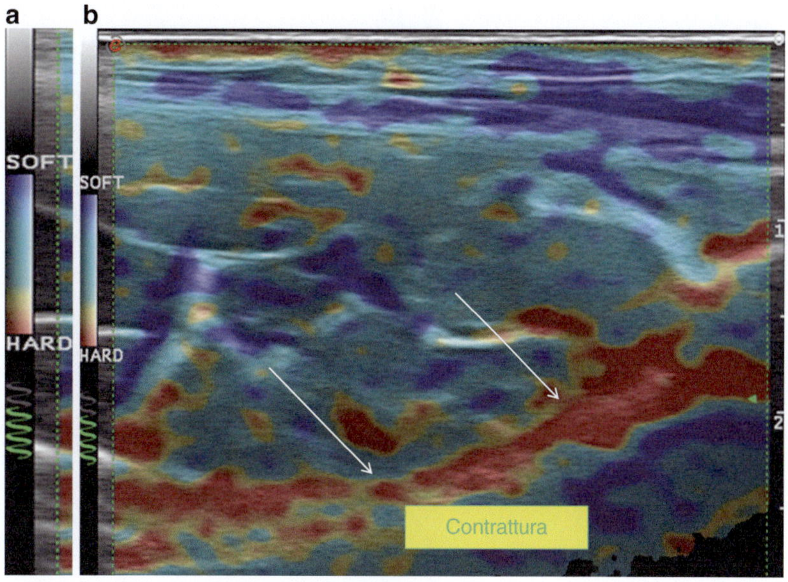

Fig. 7.2 (a–b) Elastography is a useful technique to assess musculoskeletal conditions, thanks to the vibrating probe and the generation of a colour map reporting the degree of tissue elasticity (from soft to hard). Note the altered elasticity due to contracture of the left anterior rectus abdominis muscle

The technique can be applied to all anatomical structures, including cartilage, ligaments, vessels, and bone.

Notably, second-generation machines are endowed with electronic control, which eliminates artefacts due to differences in tissue compression by the operator.

7.5 Muscles

7.5.1 Trauma-Related Conditions

Muscle traumas are divided into minor and major.

7.5.1.1 Minor Traumas

Minor muscle traumas include elongations, contusions, and contractures as well as crush injury involving subcutaneous adipose tissue, such as lipodystrophy, lymphoedema, and fat necrosis.

In the latter three conditions, US plays a key role: dynamic US provides a highly accurate and detailed assessment of the involvement of subcutaneous fat tissue and of blood extravasation, to exclude subfascial involvement, while vascular injuries are assessed with colour and power Doppler.

Elastography is a key technique, since it allows monitoring the possible loss of elasticity of subcutaneous adipose tissue due to injury (Fig. 7.3).

B-mode US does not play a large role in assessing elongations and contractures, because the absence of fibre lesions entails that there forms no haematoma but only a moderate and diffuse intramuscular oedema.

Oedema is not clearly depicted by US, but power Doppler accurately shows obvious vascular injuries, at least compared with the contralateral muscles (Fig. 7.4a).

Elastography is the method of choice to assess contractures and elongations, since it clearly demonstrates the actual loss of elasticity of muscle component during compression.

As regards contusions, US is not very informative, whereas elastography demonstrates increased tissue elasticity related to the diffuse oedema (Fig. 7.4b).

Elastography is conclusive in patients with delayed-onset muscle soreness (DOMS) (Fig. 7.5).

7.5.1.2 Major Traumas

Major muscle traumas are divided into partial and complete ruptures.

The US report should always provide a detailed and accurate description of the lesion, its extent, and any involvement of adjacent structures.

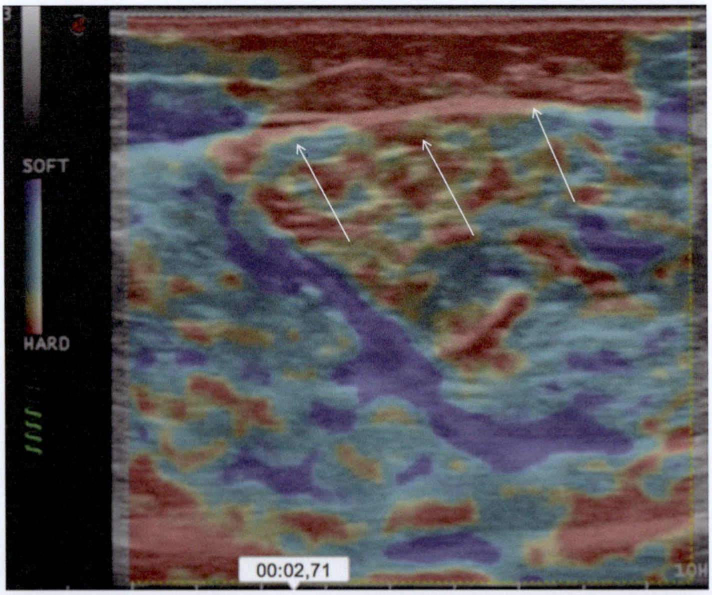

Fig. 7.3 Typical loss of subcutaneous adipose tissue elasticity due to contusion and compression

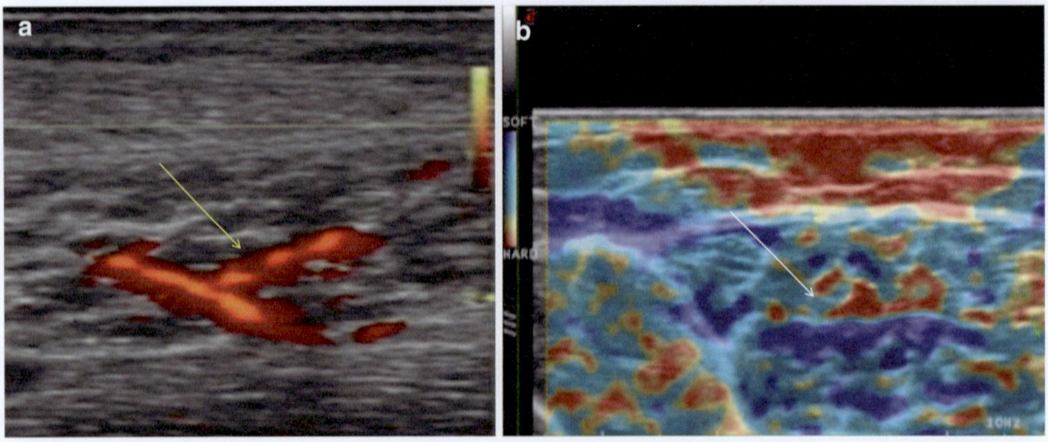

Fig. 7.4 (**a**) A power Doppler scan always shows hypervascularity in the area affected by minor traumas like elongations and contractures. (**b**) Elastography documents a high degree of tissue elasticity at the site of the injury, due to reactive oedema

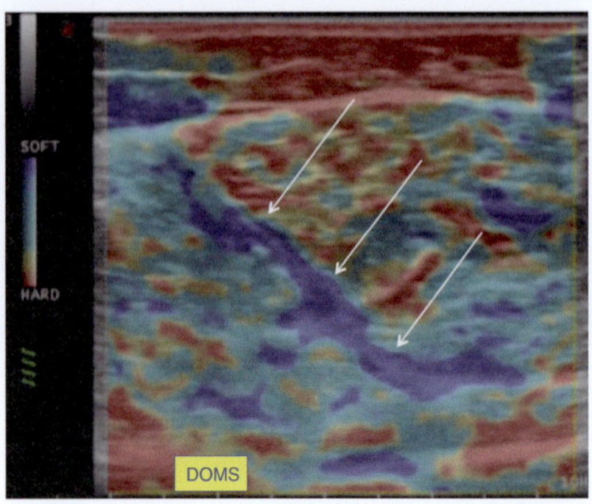

Fig. 7.5 Elastography is the method of choice to assess DOMS, because it depicts the area characterized by a higher degree of elasticity due to haematoma formation and fluid infiltration through the fascia

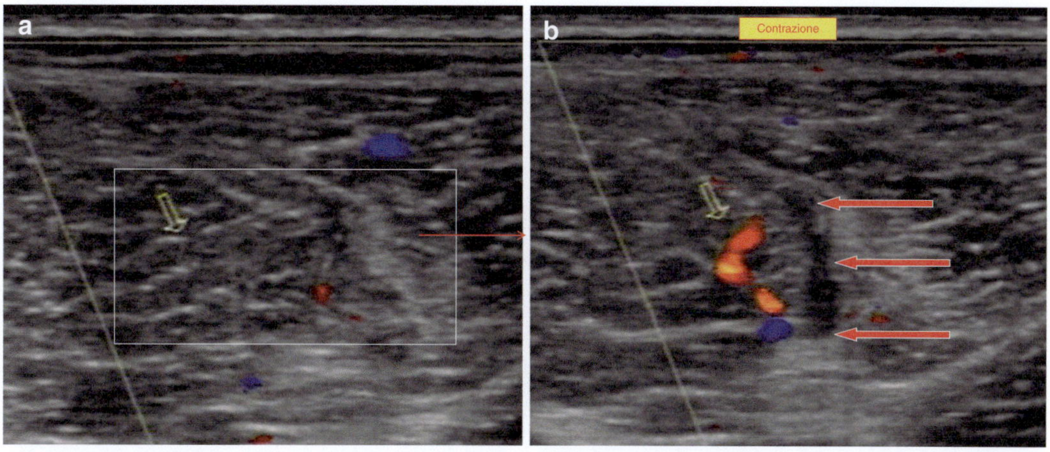

Fig. 7.6 (**a–b**) In patients with minor partial lesions, dynamic US provides key diagnostic information by demonstrating stump retraction during muscle contraction, whereas the bundling up of muscle fascicles in static US scans may lead to misdiagnosis

Partial ruptures are divided into grade 1 and 2.

In grade 1 lesions, the US scan is sometimes poorly informative, because a small lesion may be barely identifiable in patients with extensive injury. In such cases, the partial lesion is more clearly demonstrated by MRI and elastography.

Grade 2 ruptures should be assessed by dynamic US, because in patients with limited injury extension static, US may fail to depict a small lesion, due to the bundling up of muscle fascicles.

If a lesion is indeed present, dynamic US affords optimal evaluation, because during the contraction phase, the muscle fibres separate, and the haematoma is clearly visualized (Fig. 7.6a–b).

In such cases, elastography shows an area of higher elasticity related to haematoma colliquation.

7.5.2 Complete Ruptures

Complete muscle ruptures are full-thickness, grade 3 lesions that may extend predominantly in longitudinal or vertical direction.

Timely US diagnosis is of crucial importance, because full-thickness lesions with a predominantly vertical pattern can be repaired if surgery is promptly performed (Fig. 7.7).

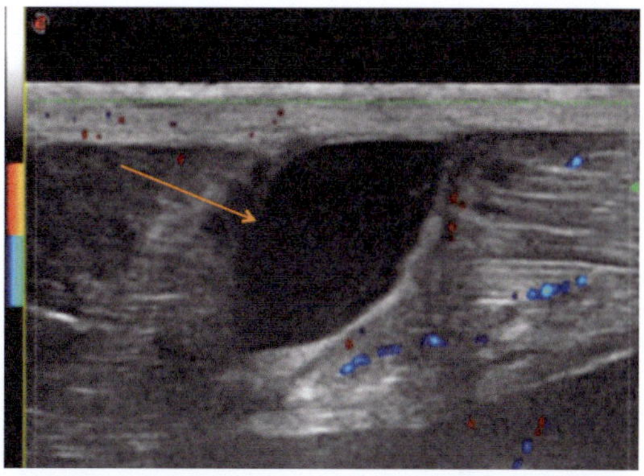

Fig. 7.7 Nearly complete rupture of the triceps brachii muscle assessed ca. 12 h after the trauma (acute phase). The lesion is predominantly vertical and is thus amenable to repair, if surgery is promptly performed

Lesions that extend longitudinally over several centimetres are rarely amenable to surgery.

On US examination, complete lesions always have the classic "bell clapper" appearance, due to retraction of the muscle stumps in opposite directions (Fig. 7.8).

The US and MRI scan of the haematoma share several similarities, depicting the haemoglobin phases from the early stage of formation to its organization (Fig. 7.9).

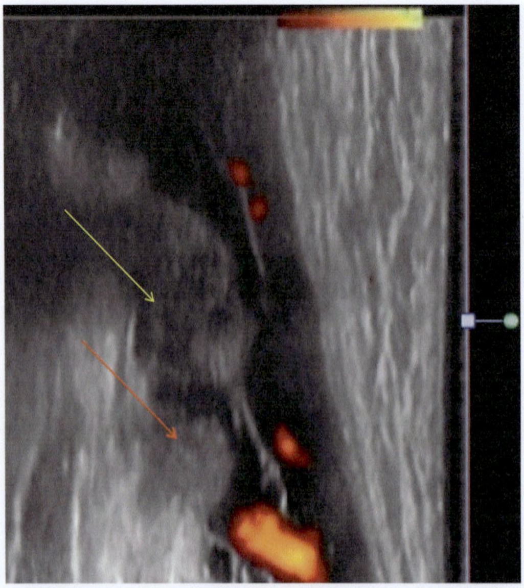

Fig. 7.8 Distinctive "bell clapper" sign due to muscle retraction as a result of complete rupture associated with haematoma and marked vascular inflammation, demonstrated by power Doppler

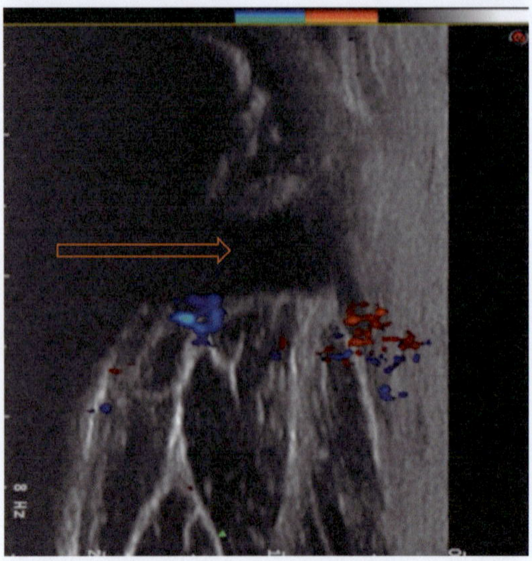

Fig. 7.9 Acute musculotendinous disinsertion at the level of the proximal insertion of the adductor longus tendon. Note the haematoma between the stumps

US examination of partial and complete ruptures should be performed within 48–72 h of the trauma, because after this time the acute oedema makes it more difficult to evaluate the extent of the lesion.

7.5.3 Myotendinous Disinsertion

Muscle lesions do not always occur within the muscle belly.

In those at the level of the myotendinous junction, US plays a key role, since prompt and accurate examinations are crucial for successful surgical repair.

The US scans show the typical downstream retraction of the tendon stump; the retracted, tapering muscle; and a large interposed haematoma.

Elastography is extremely useful, since it depicts the complete loss of tendon tension and the increased, marked elasticity of the muscle due to retraction and the haematoma.

7.5.4 Myofascial Disinsertion

Myofascial disinsertions are often difficult to detect by US, because if they are extensive and, especially, they are assessed in the acute phase, it may underestimate their extent.

In such cases, elastography provides key information by depicting the altered elasticity of the myofascial components at the lesion site. MRI is conclusive, because it demonstrates lesion extension and the detached muscle fibres at the site of the injury.

7.5.5 Myotendinous Avulsion

US does not play a primary role in the assessment of these lesions, due to the frequent presence of periosteal fragments.

In these patients, US examination is hampered by the common presence of tendon changes that date back to adolescence, where ossification centres on both sides hamper the differential diagnosis.

The imaging method of choice is still conventional radiography, associated as necessary with 3D computed tomography reconstruction.

US, elastography, and MRI play an important role at a later time, by depicting the myotendinous junction, which is frequently involved.

7.6 Post-traumatic Degenerative Conditions

The most frequent alterations induced by degenerative conditions due to muscle trauma include fibrosis, metaplastic ossification, rhabdomyolysis, and compartmental syndromes.

7.6.1 Fibrosis

US is without any doubt the method of choice to study and follow-up muscle lesions and provides critical information on the patient's ability to return to competitive sports.

The typical sequela of muscle injury is the formation of scar fibrosis.

Monitoring of lesion evolution with dynamic US during treatment supplies decisive information.

In such cases elastography is crucial, since it provides not only morphological information but also functional data on the extent of fibrosis and the loss or recovery of muscle fibre elasticity.

Colour and power Doppler affords optimal assessment of the typical reparative neoangiogenesis processes of the fibrotic evolution as well as identification of lesion recurrence.

7.6.2 Metaplastic Ossification

Metaplastic ossification (myositis ossificans) is caused by calcium salt deposition in traumatic lesions with large haematomas which, unless treated, evolve first to calcifications and eventually to ossifications.

The method of choice in the overt phase is still standard radiography integrated, as appropriate, by 3D CT reconstruction.

US plays a crucial role in the acute phase, since calcium salts are deposited in a haematoma already on the third to fourth day.

This means that US is capable of identifying, before any other imaging method, the early microcalcifications that form in the haematoma and that, unless promptly treated, may evolve to metaplastic ossification.

The most critical phase is when moderate ossifications have already formed and produce an acoustic shadow that may hamper the assessment of the actual extension of the ossifications.

Consequently, the US scan always needs radiographic confirmation, since calcifications are easily detected by US but are wholly non-specific.

Large calcifications may be seen in patients with *Echinococcus* cysts, cysticercosis, and a number of benign and malignant neoplasms.

Elastography depicts a marked loss of elasticity in muscle areas involved by fibrosis and ossification.

7.6.3 Rhabdomyolysis

In patients with rhabdomyolysis, US examination—though not conclusive—can however depict changes in the muscle components, which during the acute phase consistently display nearly complete disruption of morphological structures.

The diagnosis is not made by imaging but by determination of muscle enzymes. Needle biopsy may also be performed and, if necessary, electron microscopic examination.

The chronic phases of rhabdomyolysis are depicted by US as nearly complete tissue recovery, with diffuse inhomogeneous areas related to the organization of the muscle lesion.

7.6.4 Compartmental Syndrome

Compartmental syndrome arises in anatomical districts where vascular and nerve structures running through osseous tunnels are compressed by hypertrophic muscles, large haematomas, or space-occupying lesions.

A commonly involved district is the anteromedial leg region, where the tibia and fibula provide an impassable barrier in the deep plane, and the aponeurotic fasciae and the robust retinacula compress the underlying muscle.

In patients with complete muscle rupture, the associated large haematoma is the main cause of the vascular and nerve compression that induces the compartmental syndrome.

In such cases, prompt and detailed colour and power Doppler examination affords optimal assessment of any vascular compression injuries and of the involvement of nerve structures.

Elastography is also very helpful, since it depicts an altered elasticity of the muscle components.

7.7 Muscle Hernias

Dynamic US is the modality of choice to evaluate muscle hernias, which are clearly visualized as a discontinuous area in the superficial aponeurotic fascia.

A dynamic US scan taken during a Valsalva manoeuvre may depict a greater protrusion of the hernia, especially in the case of umbilical, para-umbilical, and abdominal lesions.

The hernia disappears during muscle contraction and then reappears with muscle relaxation.

Dynamic US is also very useful in the case of pseudo-hernias, where strong compression of muscular components against the aponeurotic wall is not however associated with fascia discontinuity.

In these cases, colour and power Doppler provides valuable data due to the presence of associated inflammatory processes.

7.7.1 Accessory Muscles

Accessory muscles are a fairly frequent finding; the most common is the soleus accessory muscle.

In such cases, dynamic US shows the absence under Achilles tendon of the Kager fat pad and its replacement by a muscle that contracts and relaxes in the active and passive phase of dynamic US.

7.7.2 Neuromuscular Conditions

The neuromuscular disorders examined herein are those related to first and second motor neuron pathology and to the neurological syndromes related to the central nervous system, where imaging, especially US, does not play a key role in diagnosis but rather in monitoring disease evolution.

A typical finding in such patients is progressive replacement of muscle with fibroadipose tissue, which in Duchenne muscular dystrophy, the most severe condition, involves a near inversion of the normal 1:7 ratio (ca. 7:1).

Besides, US is very useful to identify the areas less severely involved, where tissue biopsies may be collected to help refine the diagnosis.

US monitoring is performed at the behest of the neurologist, in patients with a clear diagnosis.

Elastography demonstrates a strongly reduced elasticity of the muscle components due to significant fibroadipose tissue replacement.

7.7.3 Neoplastic Disease

These conditions would deserve an extensive discussion.

It is important to stress that diagnostic imaging in such patients should be confined to describing the lesions and the possible involvement of extra-compartmental structures, besides raising diagnostic suspicion. However, making a diagnosis is often impossible and is the task of histology and biopsy.

US may be the first imaging study to depict new formations that escape clinical detection in muscle or subcutaneous adipose tissue.

It should however be noted that it is difficult to distinguish by US a long-standing, well-organized, and inhomogeneous haematoma from an intramuscular neoplasm.

7.8 Tendons

Tendons are commonly divided into muscle anchoring and gliding.

All consist of primary, secondary, and tertiary bundles and are covered by the peritenon.

The attachment sites (entheses) of muscle-anchoring tendons are protected by a synovial bursa at the level of their bone insertion.

Gliding tendons are covered with a synovial sheath consisting of a visceral and a parietal layer, between which a thin film of synovial fluid moistens and nourishes the tendon structures and their few vessels.

The conditions affecting muscle-anchoring tendons include peritendinitis, insertional degenerative tendinopathy (enthesitis), non-insertional degenerative tendinopathy, and partial and complete tears.

7.8.1 Peritendinitis

By virtue of its ability to demonstrate even minute peritenon changes with extreme accuracy, US is the method of choice to assess tendon pathology.

Tendons are poorly vascularized and most vessels supply the peritenon.

Inflammation always involves the peritenon, most frequently its deep portion; the bursa is almost constantly involved too (in the case of Achilles tendon, the deep retrocalcaneal bursa).

Peritendinitis is often associated with inflammation of the fat pads, such as the one in Kager's triangle (Achilles tendon) or Hoffa's fat pad (patellar tendon).

7.8.2 Insertional Tendinopathy (Enthesopathy)

Enthesopathy affects the distal tendon insertion, where intrinsic tendon degeneration is often accompanied by multiple microcalcifications.

In such cases, power Doppler proves extremely useful in assessing the degree of inflammation.

Elastography demonstrates altered tendon elasticity due to the oedema.

In non-insertional tendinopathy, the tendon displays long, fusiform, thickened tracts often characterized by high structural homogeneity.

This finding should not be underrated, since it is often associated with increased tendon elasticity, a sign of tissue softening due to significant oedema that in the case of severe trauma can lead to spontaneous rupture (Fig. 7.10).

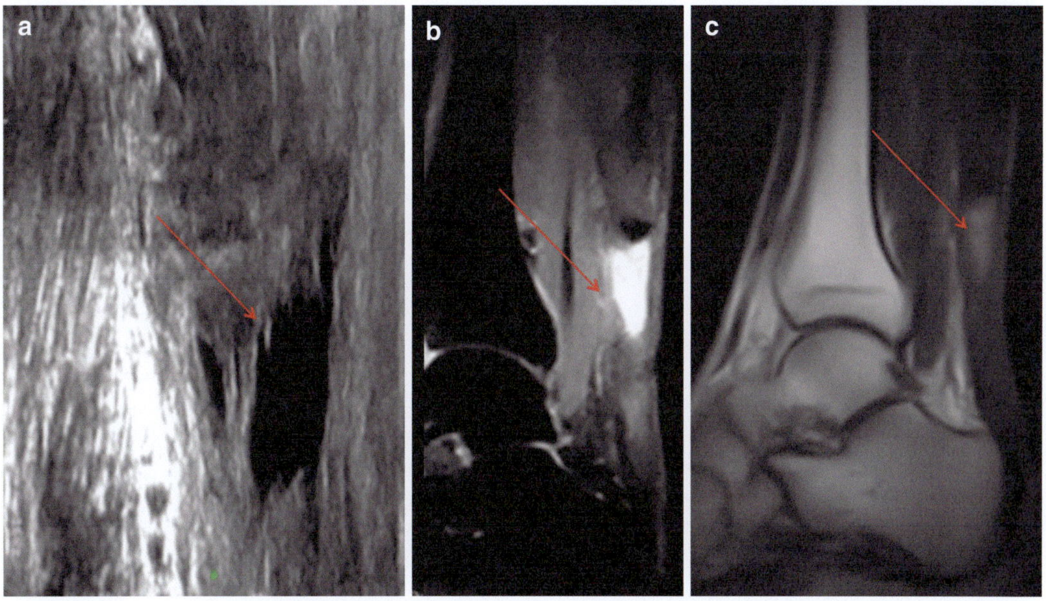

Fig. 7.10 In complete tendon ruptures, particularly those of Achilles tendon, dynamic US (**a**) and upright MRI (**c**) provide superior information on lesion extent compared with standard MRI (**b**), especially standard MRI with high-contrast sequences, which excessively magnify the lesion

Xanthomatosis deserves a specific mention. This degenerative tendinopathy mainly affects patients with hypercholesterolaemia and hyperlipidaemia. It induces formation of large vacuoles in tendons, especially Achilles tendon, and diffuse microcalcifications that in the absence of appropriate treatment may lead to spontaneous tendon rupture.

US demonstrates high-grade degenerative tendinopathy associated with multiple calcifications along the tendon course, whose correlation with laboratory data allows a diagnosis of xanthomatosis.

7.8.3 Partial Tears

In partial tendon tears, dynamic US clearly evaluates the actual lesion extension.

Elastography is very informative, depicting the loss of tendon tension related to the partial lesion.

Different anatomical structures are associated with different US findings.

A typical example is the rotator cuff of the shoulder: in case of surgical repair, accurate US examination is needed to determine whether the tear affects the bursal, articular, or interstitial side.

7.8.4 Complete Tears

In case of full-thickness tendon tears, prompt US examination supplies information that allows selecting the most appropriate treatment option: surgery or physical therapy (Fig. 7.10a–c).

In such cases, US is far superior to MRI, which especially in high-contrast sequences tends to overestimate the extent of the lesion.

Dynamic US, associated with dynamic MRI, affords very accurate assessment (Fig. 7.11a–c).

7.8.5 Tenorrhaphy

US monitoring should be performed no earlier than 2–3 months after surgical repair, since scar fibrosis generates major acoustic shadowing, preventing correct assessment.

Such tendons, particularly Achilles tendon, often show a mixed structural inhomogeneity, since sutures are interspersed with microcalcifi-

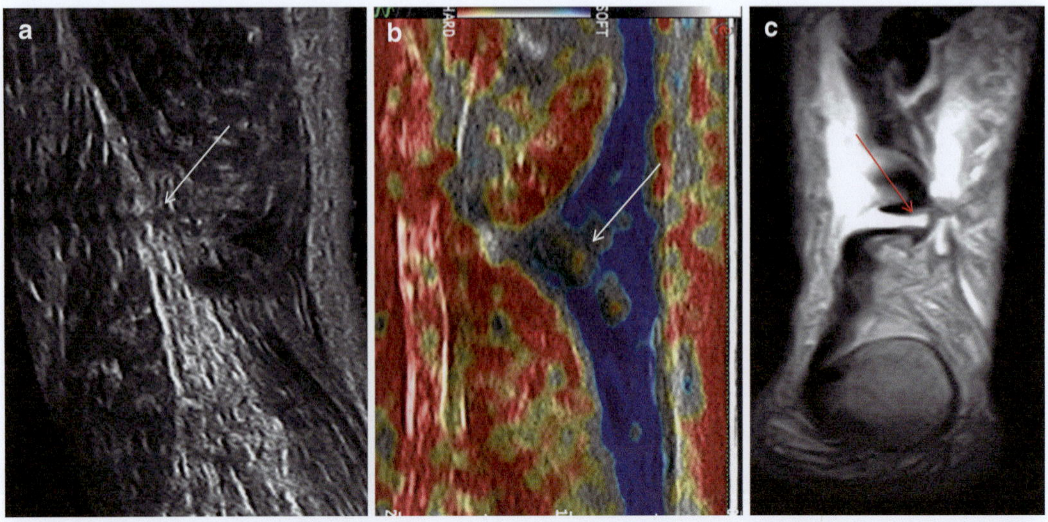

Fig. 7.11 The coronal views, which are seldom used in the sonographic assessment of Achilles tendon, may however not allow to make a correct diagnosis. (**a**) A complete tear of the intermediate tract of the tendon is clearly depicted by the coronal MRI scan acquired with a STIR sequence (**c**) and is confirmed by elastography, which shows highly elastic tissue at the site of the lesion, due to the presence of a large haematoma (**b**)

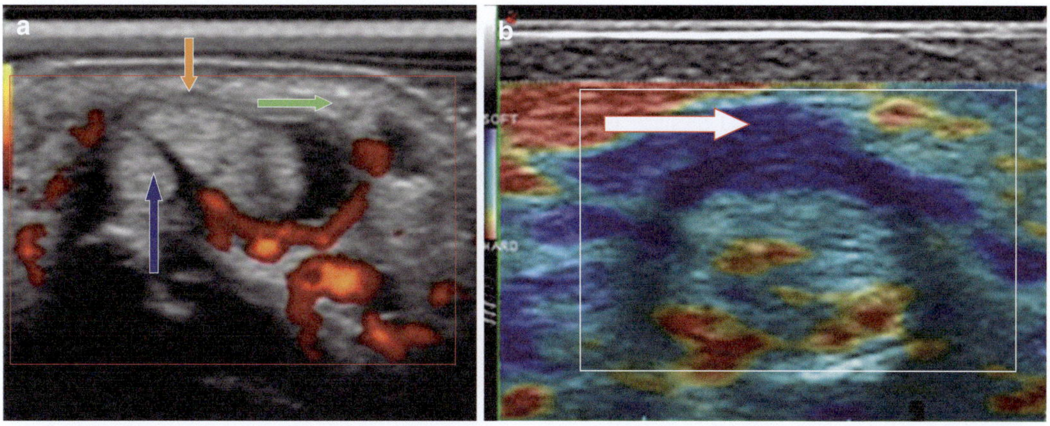

Fig. 7.12 Stenosing tenosynovitis characteristic of de Quervain's disease at the level of the carpal tunnel tract of the extensor brevis and abductor longus; these tendons are covered by a common sheath and pass through the same fibrous pulley, separated by a clear septum (**a**) intimate connection with the sensitive radial nerve, which at times induces severe neuropathy at this level (**b**) on elastography, the fibrous pulley is markedly hypertrophic although still considerably elastic and does not therefore require urgent surgery

cations, which are the sequelae of the postoperative haematoma.

Such tendons are three to four times thicker than normal tendons.

In case of suspected recurrence, dynamic US allows assessing any recurrent tears.

Elastography provides important postoperative information on the recovery of normal tendon tension, a key factor in the decision to allow patients to return to competitive sports.

7.8.6 Tenosynovitis

Tenosynovitis includes various forms: exudative, chiefly related to inflammatory conditions; dry, associated with post-traumatic conditions; proliferative, mostly related to rheumatic disorders; and stenosing, caused by the involvement of the tendon reflection pulleys, typically found in patients with trigger finger.

US, especially power and colour Doppler, provides accurate information on exudative tenosynovitis.

The same is true of proliferative tenosynovitis, which typically affects patients with rheumatic disorders, where the synovial sheath is frequently thickened and hypertrophic. Power Doppler and especially imaging with an intravenous contrast agent document marked inflammation.

In stenosing tenosynovitis, such as de Quervain's disease and trigger finger, US should be associated with elastography, since loss of elasticity and tendon tension are often indications for prompt surgery (Fig. 7.12a–b).

Suggested Reading

Balconi G, Monetti G, De Pra L (1995) Joints ultrasound of superficial structures. In: Solbiati L, Rizzatto G (eds), Churchill Livingstone, Edimburgh

Beggs I (2006, July) Ultrasound of the shoulder and elbow. Orthop Clin N Am 37(3):277–285

Bianchi S, Martinoli C (2007) Ultrasound of the musculoskeletal system. Springer, Berlin, Heidelberg

Bousquet G (1982) Il ginocchio illustrato. Ermes Medica Drommi, Roma

Bradley M, O'Donnell P (2002) Atlas of musculoskeletal ultrasound anatomy-GMM

De Marchi A, Pozza S, Faletti C (2007) Atlante di Ecografia Muscolotendinea - Tecnica -Anatomia - Quadri Patologici-Utet

Di Giacomo G, Pouliart N, Costantini A (2008) Atlas of functional shoulder anatomy. Springer-Verlag, Italia

Fornage BD (1988) Ultrasonography of muscles and tendons. Examination technique and atlas of normal anatomy of the extremities. Springer Verlag, New York

Jacobson JA (1999) Musculoskeletal sonography and MR imaging: a role for both imaging methods. Radiol Clin N Am 37(4):713–735

Jost B, Koch PP, Gerber C (2000) Anatomy and functional aspects of the rotator interval. J Shoulder Elb Surg 9(4):336–341

Khurana A, Dahiya N (2004) 3D & 4D ultrasound—a text and atlas. Jaypee Anshan, Tunbridge Wells Kent, UK

Lin CD, Nazarian LN, O'Kane PL et al (2002) Advantages of real-time spatial compound sonography of the musculoskeletal system versus conventional sonography. AJR Am J Roentgenol 171:1629–1631

Manaster BJ et al (2006) Diagnostic and surgical imaging anatomy: musculoskeletal, Amirsys, Salt Lake City

Martino F, Silvestri E, Grassi W, Garlaschi G (2006) Ecografia dell'Apparato Osteoarticolare, Anatomia, Semeiotica e Quadri Patologici. Springer-Verlag

McNally EG (2005) Practical musculoskeletal ultrasound. Elsevier—Churchill—Livingstone, Philadelphia

Monetti G (1988) L'impiego degli ultrasuoni nella diagnostica della patologia neuromuscolare, Ultrasonica, vol. 3

Monetti G (1989) Ecografia muscolo-tendinea e dei tessuti molli. Solei Ed., Milano

Monetti G (1994a) Ecografia osteo-articolare e muscolotendinea. Gnocchi Editore, Napoli

Monetti G, Pistolesi GF (1994) L'Imaging delle articolazioni, Gnocchi Ed

Monetti G, Bazzocchi M (1994) Muscoli e tendini, Gnocchi Ed

Monetti G (2000) Ecografia muscolo-scheletrica imaging integrato. Idelson-Gnocchi

Monetti G (2009) Ecografia muscolo-scheletrica Vol. I. Tecnica, anatomia ed imaging integrato. Timeo Editore, Bologna

Monetti G (2010a) Ecografia muscolo-scheletrica Vol. II. Patologia ed imaging integrato di muscoli, tendini e tecniche speciali. Timeo Editore, Bologna

Monetti G (2010b) Ecografia muscolo-scheletrica Vol. III. Patologia ed imaging integrato delle articolazioni. Timeo Editore, Bologna

Monetti G (2011a) Ecografia Muscolo-scheletrica—Elastosonografia. Timeo editore, Bologna

Monetti G (2011b) Ecografia Muscolo-scheletrica—3D–4D. Timeo editore, Bologna

Monetti G, Santoli G, Monteduro F (1993) Arto superiore. Trattato italiano di ecografia, Poletto Edizioni

Monetti G, Ziviello M, Bazzocchi R (1994) Le articolazioni in ecografia. Gnocchi Ed.

O'Neill J (2008) Musculoskeletal ultrasound anatomy and technique. Springer

Peetrons P, Chhem R (2000) Atlas D'Echographie du Systeme Locomoteur. Tome 1: Le membre superieur. Tome 2: Le membre inferieur. Sauramps Medical

Pope TL Jr (2009) Diagnostica per immagini in traumatologia muscolo-scheletrica. Elsevier, Milano

Porcellini G, Castagna A (2014) La Spalla, seconda edizione. Verduci editore

Reiser M, Baur-Melnyk A, Glaser C (2009) Imaging muscolo-scheletrico, CIC ed

Roh MS, Wang VM, April EW, Pollock RG, Bigliani LU, Flatow EL (2000) Anterior and posterior musculotendinous anatomy of the supraspinatus. J Shoulder Elbow Surg; 9 (September–October 5)

Stoller DW (2008) Stoller's atlas of orthopaedics and sports medicine, Wolters Kluwer-Lippicott Williams & Wilkins

Thompson JC (2004) Atlante di anatomia ortopedica di Netter. Ed. Masson

The Dynamic Magnetic Resonance Imaging

8

Giuseppe Monetti, Gianluca Rampino, and Giuseppe Rusignuolo

Content

Our research center D-LAB in Bologna is the first ever to utilize the dynamic MRI investigation.

The MRI scanner employed is constituted of the latest-generation Esaote G-Scan Brio, which allows for dynamic sequences through the 2D HYCE S technique, acquired in a single layer, by means of delayed sequences, which allow the correct acquisition by the MRI scanner itself.

The examination setting is carried out as the clinostatic MRI investigation, compared with the orthostatic investigation, in order to enable the perception of possible changes of asset between the sequence of the supine and the upright weight-bearing position of the patient.

Afterward we incorporate the dynamic sequences, which vary necessarily from patient to patient, in relation to the type of the reported pathology.

During the mentioned investigation, maneuvers of flexed extension, abduction, external rotation, inversion, and eversion are performed to evoke possible disorders otherwise not demonstrable in static sequences and at times not demonstrable neither in clino- nor in orthostatism.

It proves important to underline the actual existing differentiation related to the cine-MRI investigations carried out up to this day, being these no different from the reassembly of various frames gained from different angles and put together by the means of animation.

G. Monetti (✉)
Dipartimento di Diagnostica per Immagini, Ospedale Privato Accreditato Nigrisoli,
Viale Ercolani, 9, Bologna, Italy
e-mail: info@muskultrasound.it

G. Rampino
Unità operativa di Diagnostica per Immagini Friuli Coram di Udine, Udine, Italy

G. Rusignuolo
Struttura Complessa di Radiologia Azienda Ospedaliera Santa Maria di Terni, Terni, Italy

G.L. Canata et al. (eds.), *Muscle and Tendon Injuries*, DOI 10.1007/978-3-662-54184-5_8

The dynamic investigation, on the contrary, consists of actual movements of each joint and limb, so to actually evoke the different postures and the potentially pathological behavior of muscles, tendons, and joints.

The survey can be carried out on any area of the body; therefore in this case, dealing with the muscle tendon pathology, more frequently the upper and lower limbs at the level of their muscular components are taken into account.

Figure 8.1 represents a series of sequences depicting the different moments of the brachial biceps and triceps muscle contraction, in physiological conditions.

The dynamic investigation arises as very useful during ongoing muscle injuries with large hematomas, which at times are not well definable in their extension and therefore can be placed in the differential diagnosis together with any growths of benign or malignant nature.

That is the case of Fig. 8.2, in which various sequences performed by dynamic ultrasound, elastosonography, and MRI are featured, demonstrating a large lesion partly colliquated and

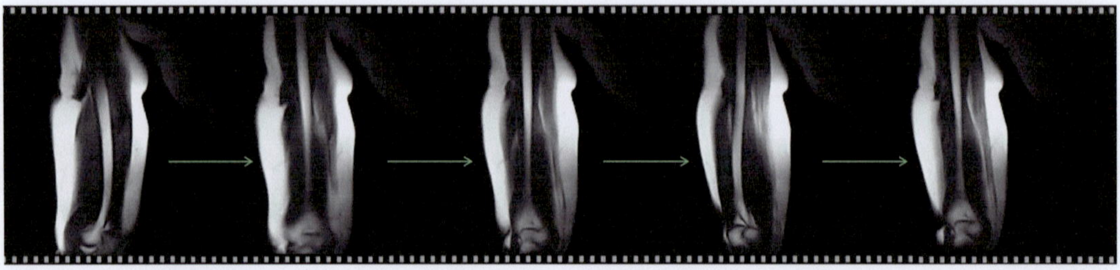

Fig. 8.1 Dynamic MRI scan acquired at the level of the arm during flexion/extension

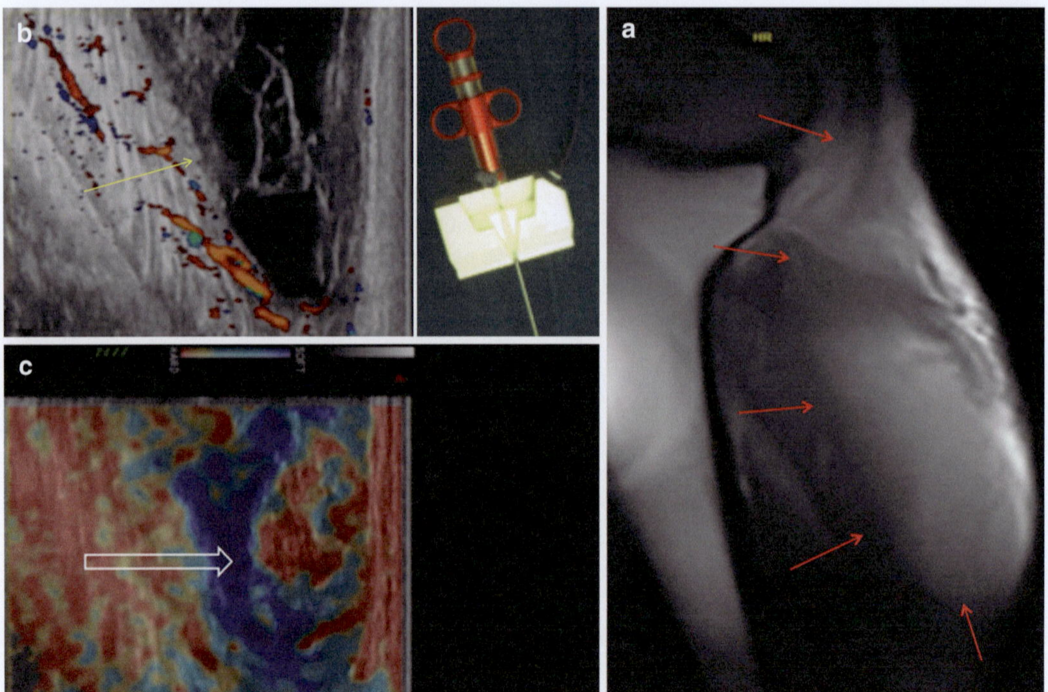

Fig. 8.2 Dynamic MRI (**a**) clearly documents the actual extent of a muscle lesion, be it due to a tumor or, as in this case, to a large posttraumatic hematoma. The additional detail provided by US, using power Doppler (**b**) or elastography (**c**), can guide needle biopsy aspiration if required

partly structured, referring to a possible space-occupying lesion.

In Fig. 8.3, it becomes fully highlighted, during the dynamic phases of contraction and flexed extension of the lower limb that the mentioned lesion is constituted by a large hematoma involving the medial twin head muscle, surely more perceivable during the dynamic phases.

Another extremely useful application of the mentioned method is provided through the fusion method (Fig. 8.4), which allows the overlap even in dynamic with the ultrasound investigation performed in real time.

Thus it is possible to check in a more accurate manner the possible alterations not underlined by either method and, above all, to use this method during the follow-up, in order to examine and better assess the evolution of the clinical picture.

Certainly a suitable utilization is carried out at the level of the extensive muscle lesions, during which at times the ultrasound examination does not allow a panoramic picture, so to provide

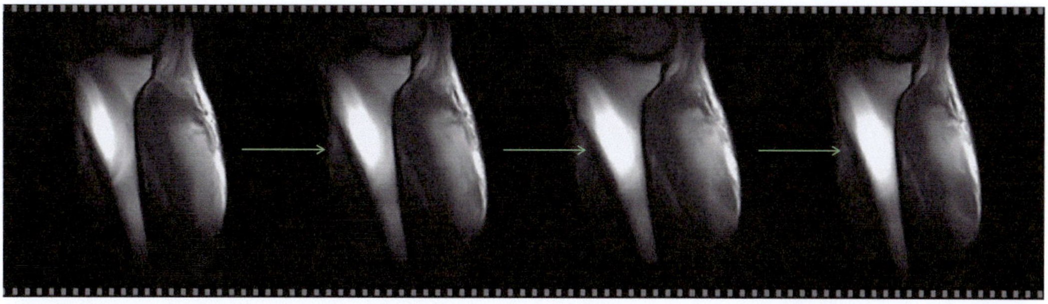

Fig. 8.3 Dynamic MRI demonstrates the different morphology of the mass during muscle contraction as the leg is flexed/extended

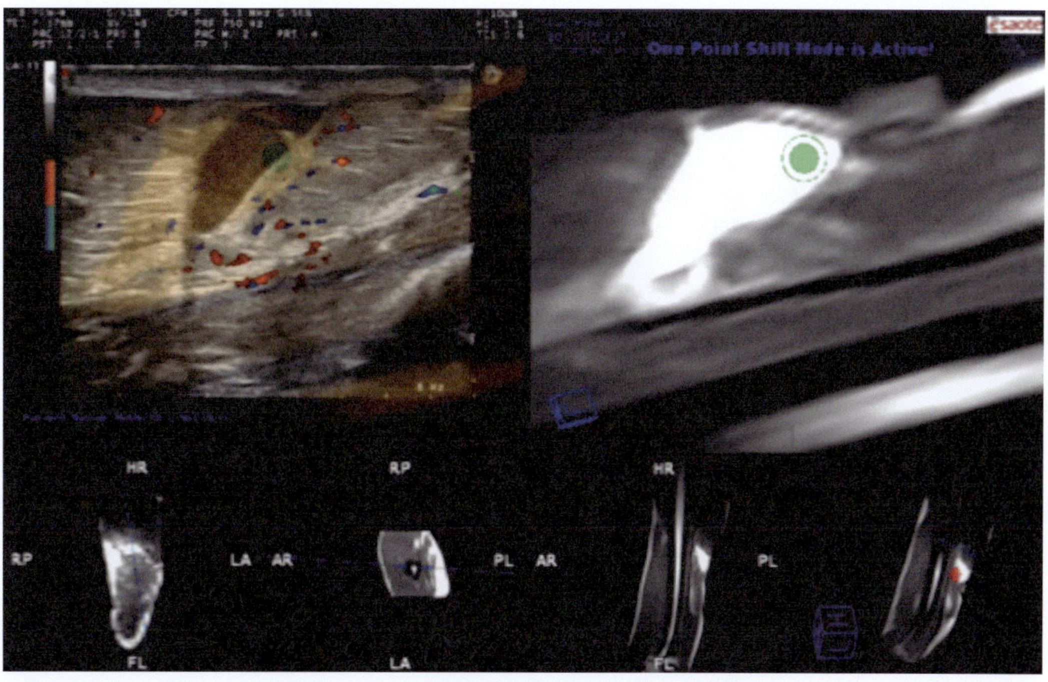

Fig. 8.4 Fusion technology affords optimal follow-up of muscle lesions through the overlay of US and MRI scans

certain and well-defined details of the extension of the mentioned lesion.

During the active and passive contraction phases, the presence of a partial lesion of the quadriceps muscle of the femur at the distal insertion is featured in Fig. 8.5, with evident greater retraction during the active contraction phase.

The employment of the dynamic method proves to be equally useful in ongoing plotted detachments of the osteotendon junction, such as the case of the anterior inferior iliac spine investigated through computed tomography plus 3D reconstruction (Fig. 8.6a) and better defined by the means of the dynamic MRI method, which during the phase of contraction shows in a more accurate manner the diastasis of the bone fragment retracted through the contraction of the adjacent muscle components (Fig. 8.6b).

The employment of the dynamic method in ongoing lesions caused by compression proves to be of fundamental importance, which can be difficult to approach by the means of the ultrasound investigation, especially in relation to the formation of a wide groove which does not allow a suitable probe support.

In the case of Fig. 8.7, the presence of a mass lesion of the brachial triceps muscle is evident, which during the dynamic stage of the contraction enables to highlight the presence of a minimum quantity of un-interrupted muscle fibers to allow plastic reconstruction of the muscle itself by the surgeon.

The use of the dynamic study proves relevant also at the myotendinous junction level of the structures of the lower and upper limbs, especially related to the Achilles tendon, when the

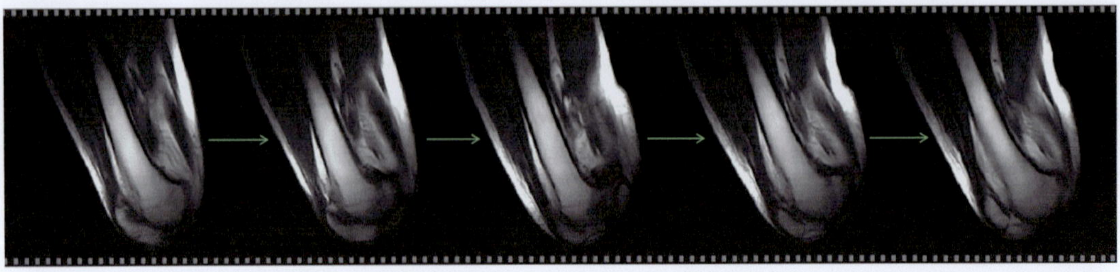

Fig. 8.5 Dynamic MRI scan obtained at several degrees of quadriceps flexion/extension and contraction, clearly demonstrating the partial retraction of the injured muscle

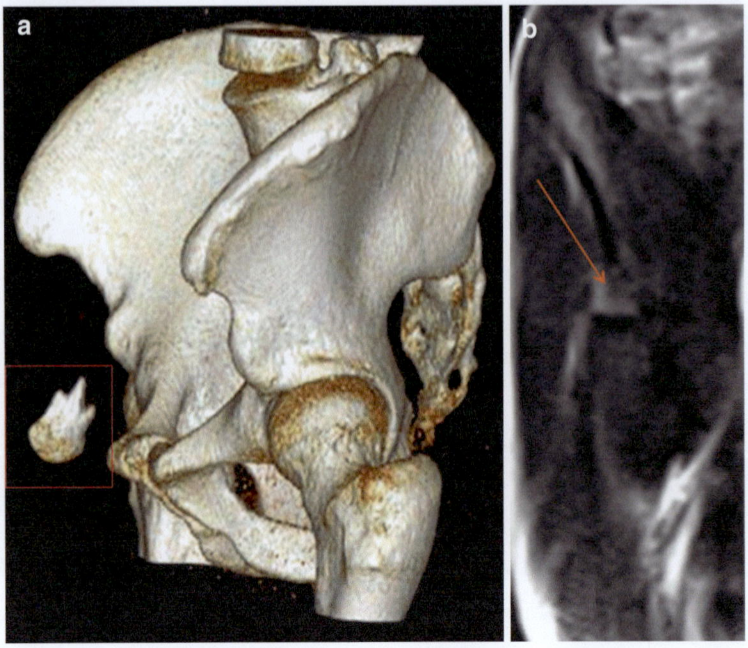

Fig. 8.6 (**a**) 3D CT reconstruction demonstrating complete traumatic avulsion of the anterior inferior iliac spine. (**b**) Dynamic MRI image acquired during muscle contraction

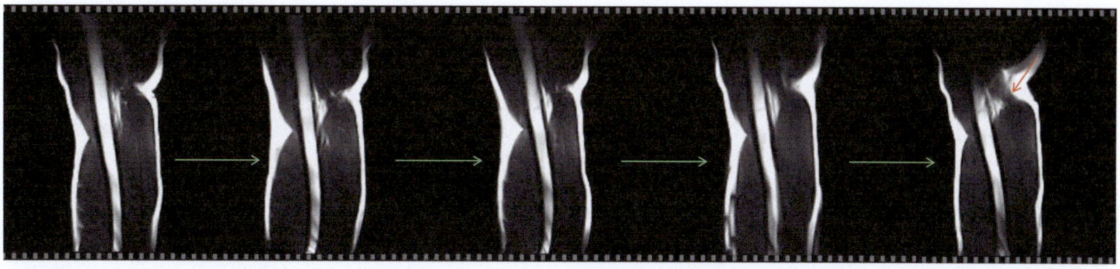

Fig. 8.7 Severe compression of the long head of the triceps muscle documented by dynamic MRI during muscle contraction. The intact fibers (*orange arrow*) indicate that the lesion is amenable to surgical reconstruction

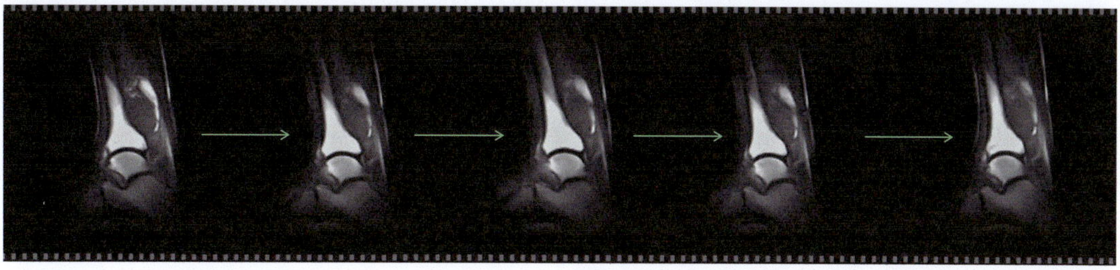

Fig. 8.8 Dynamic MRI scan of the gastrocnemius muscles acquired in the sagittal plane during flexion/extension. Excellent demonstration of the partial alteration of the Achilles tendon musculotendinous junction

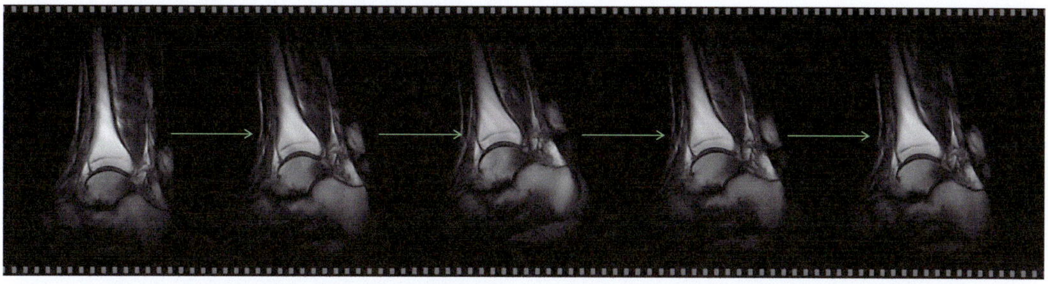

Fig. 8.9 The dynamic MRI scan affords a more exhaustive assessment of the tendon by showing large calcifications and ossifications during flexion/extension

lesions very often occur at the myotendinous junction level and are difficult to assess through the ultrasound approach.

In case of Fig. 8.8 in various sequences carried out by flexing and contracting, the twin heads of the gastrocnemius muscle are perceptible, in the case of a myotendinous high-grade lesion.

A further circumstance in which the dynamic magnetic resonance allows a higher assessment accuracy is that of gross ossifications related to miotendon structures, in which the ultrasound would encounter considerable difficulties due to the large shadow cone determined by the ossification itself, thus not allowing a proper assessment of the underlying structures.

In Fig. 8.9 a gross bone calcification along the course of the Achilles tendon at the level of the myotendinous junction is clearly noticeable, which during the dynamic phases of the contraction and flexed extension of the lower limb highlights perfectly the different assets acquired.

Further extremely brilliant employment resides in the study of the upper limb muscle and tendon components, with particular reference to the tendons constituting the rotator cuff, when in addition to the dynamic investigation, we provide the patient with weights varying from 1 to 4 kg, which allow for a further strain of the tendon components in ongoing partial or complete ruptures, not properly identified by the static MRI investigation, yet fully underlined in the dynamic sequences (Fig. 8.10).

The possible massive lesion of the rotator cuff is equally well detectable, where the static investigation had not been able to identify the extent of the damage.

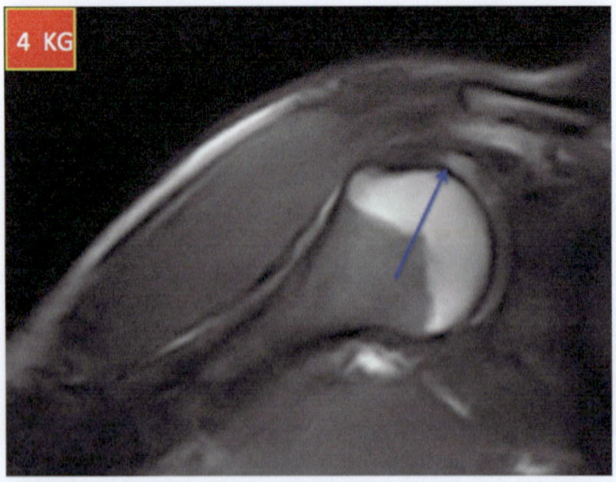

Fig. 8.10 This dynamic MRI scan acquired during abduction and external rotation with application of 4 kg depicts a wide lesion in the pre-insertional area of the supraspinatus that would not be shown by standard MRI

Providing the patient with weights that vary from 2 to 4 kg, a complete retraction of the muscular components is obtainable, referring to a massive retraction and a fibroadipose replacement.

The use of T2 and STIR sequences by means of high-field scanners at times tends to emphasize the extent of the damage, as in the case of Fig. 8.11, in which is perceptible a hyperintense alteration caused by the lesion of the myotendinous junction of the Achilles tendon, in reference to the mentioned method, interpretable as a mass lesion.

The dynamic investigation, carried out in orthostatism and in contraction, allows for a better demonstration of the true extent of the damage, certainly of a high degree, but not total, in which several fibers are still perceptible, thus allowing a proper assessment of the type of operation to be performed by the surgeon (Fig. 8.11).

Further superb employment comes from dynamic investigations carried out on both flexor and extensor tendons of the hand, where,

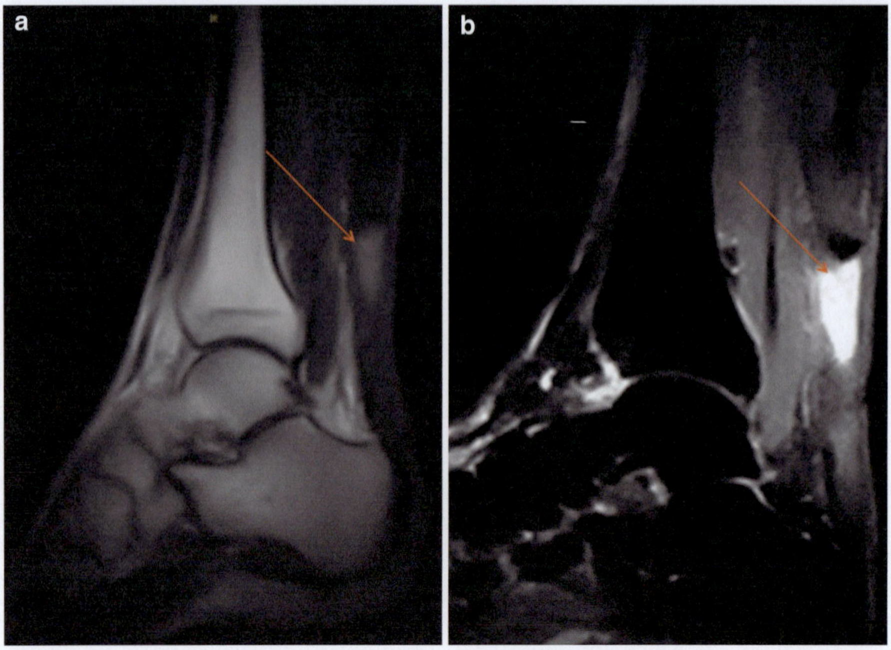

Fig. 8.11 (**a–b**) Dynamic MRI allows to determine the actual extent of an interstitial lesion of Achilles tendon more accurately than standard MRI. High-contrast sequences tend to magnify the actual injury

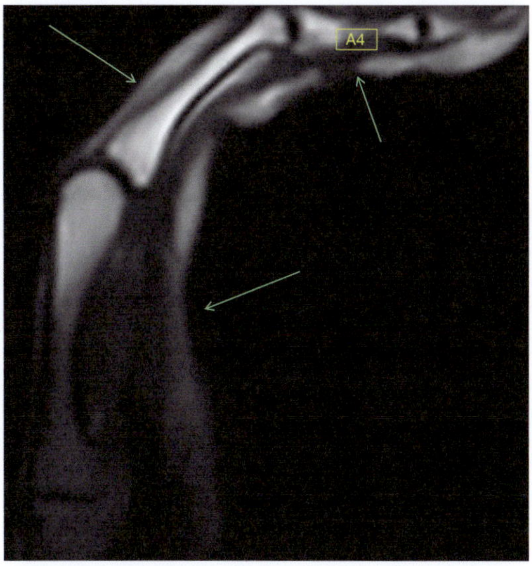

Fig. 8.12 Dynamic MRI scan depicting the marked involvement of the flexor pulley system (in this case the A 4 pulley) in a patient with trigger finger

in ongoing high-grade lesions, partial or complete, sometimes the ultrasound examination is not resolutive, being that the case of Fig. 8.12.

Analyzing the above, it is clear that the MRI dynamic investigation is at times resolutive during the assessment of a partial or complete damage, otherwise difficult to assess using static high-field MRI, at times even when a single orthostatic resonance is solely employed.

The use, as mentioned above, of any weights for the study of the upper limb muscles enables additional better definition of the extent of the damage.

These concepts are not to be interpreted as a replacement of the standard MRI investigation but as a complement and completion in required circumstances, for the purpose of a correct therapeutic assessment, either conservative or surgical, therefore if surgical, of even greater utility, in order to better identify the type of surgery to choose.

Suggested Reading

Bousquet G (1982) Il ginocchio illustrato. Ermes Medica Drommi, Roma

Di Giacomo G, Pouliart N, Costantini A (2008) Atlas of functional shoulder anatomy. Springer-Verlag, Italia

Jacobson JA (1999) Musculoskeletal sonography and MR imaging: a role for both imaging methods. Radiol Clin N Am 37(4):713–735

Jost B, Koch PP, Gerber C (2000) Anatomy and functional aspects of the rotator interval. J Shoulder Elb Surg 9(4):336–341

Lauren MS (2012) MRI of weight-bearing and movement, Osteoarthritis Cartilage 20(2):69–78

Manaster DJ et al (2006) Diagnostic and surgical imaging anatomy musculoskeletal. Amirsys, Salt Lake City

Monetti G, Pistolesi GF (1994) L'Imaging delle articolazioni, Ed. Gnocchi

Monetti G (2011) Risonanza Magnetica dell'apparato muscolo-scheletrico. RM Orto–Clino. Timeo editore, Bologna

Pope TL Jr (2009) Diagnostica per immagini in traumatologia muscolo-scheletrica. Elsevier, Milano

Porcellini G, Castagna A (2014) La Spalla, seconda edizione. Verduci Editore

Reiser M, Baur-Melnyk A, Glaser C (2009) Imaging muscolo-scheletrico, CIC ed

Reiser MF (2014) Magnetic resonance imaging of the skeletal musculature, Marc-Andrè Weber (ed). Springer

Resnick D, Kang HS (1997) Shoulder. In: Resnick D, Kang HS (eds) Internal derangement of joints: emphasis on MR imaging. WB Saunders, Philadelphia

Roh MS, Wang VM, April EW, Pollock RG, Bigliani LU, Flatow EL (2000) Anterior and posterior musculotendinous anatomy of the supraspinatus. J Shoulder Elbow Surg; 9 (September–October 5)

Stoller DW (2008) Stoller's atlas of orthopaedics and sports medicine, Wolters Kluwer-Lippincott Williams & Wilkins

Thompson JC (2004) *Atlante di anatomia ortopedica di Netter*. Ed. Masson

Classification of Muscle Lesions

9

Nicola Maffulli, Rocco Aicale,
and Domiziano Tarantino

Contents

N. Maffulli, M.D., M.S., Ph.D., FRCS (Orth.) (✉)
Department of Musculoskeletal Disorders, School of Medicine and Surgery, University of Salerno, Salerno, Italy

Queen Mary University of London, Barts and the London School of Medicine and Dentistry, Centre for Sports and Exercise Medicine, Mile End Hospital, 275 Bancroft Road, London, E1 4DG, UK
e-mail: n.maffulli@qmul.ac.uk

R. Aicale • D. Tarantino
Department of Musculoskeletal Disorders, School of Medicine and Surgery, University of Salerno, Salerno, Italy
e-mail: aicale17@gmail.com; domiziano22@gmail.com

9.1 Introduction

Muscle injuries are frequent in athletes, accounting for 10 to 55% of all acute sport injuries (Chan et al. 2012). Despite their high incidence and improvement in clinical diagnostic criteria and imaging, their optimal management and rehabilitation strategies are still debated in literature. The reinjury rate is high after a muscle lesion, and improper treatment or attempts at too early return to sport increase the rate of reinjury and complications.

Most muscle injuries are mainly managed conservatively with excellent results, while surgery is reserved only for larger tears.

The most commonly involved muscles and muscle groups are the hamstrings, the rectus femoris, and the medial head of the gastrocnemius.

The diagnosis is usually clinical; imaging tools are often used to better identify the extent and site of lesion, the relevant prognostic factors predictive of recovery time, the return to pre-injury sport activity, and risk of recurrence (De Smet and Best 2000).

Based on anatomy, biomechanics, and imaging features of muscle injury, a new classification system has been proposed.

Traumatic lesions depend on the direction and angle of the movements generated by the applied forces. When the trauma is direct, an external force is applied to the muscle, and external and internal structures are squeezed against each other. The injury depends on the impact intensity,

G.L. Canata et al. (eds.), *Muscle and Tendon Injuries*, DOI 10.1007/978-3-662-54184-5_9

state of contraction of the muscle, traumatic moment, and the muscle injured (Walton and Rothwell 1986). When the trauma is indirect, there is no external traumatic force, and the main cause of injury is an eccentric contraction of the muscle.

9.2 Epidemiology

In professional soccer players, muscle injuries represent 31% of all injuries and are responsible for 25% of days of absence from training and competition. Most of these injuries (96%) are indirect and mostly affect the hamstrings and rectus femoris; also, the adductor and quadriceps may be involved, especially when the athlete attempts to kick the ball (Corazza et al. 2014). In other sports, the incidence of muscle injuries is variable: 11% in rugby, 16% in running sports, and 18% in basketball. In these sports, the hamstrings, quadriceps, and adductor muscles are the most frequently affected (Malliaropoulos et al. 2010; Borowski et al. 2008; Lopez et al. 2012).

These injuries are less frequent in young athletes: the injury incidence is 1.19 per 1000 h of training activity in soccer players younger than 22 years and 1.63 for those older than 30 years. The incidence is 6.6 per 1000 h of competition in younger athletes and 9.5 in older soccer players (Ekstrand et al. 2011).

9.3 Anatomy and Mechanism of Injury

Skeletal muscles are composed of individual muscle cells, the myocytes. Myocytes are formed from the fusion of myoblasts to assemble long, cylindrical, and multinucleated cells. Single muscle fibres are grouped into fascicles surrounded by connective tissue, the perimysium; each fibre is surrounded by a single layer of connective tissue, the endomysium (Falcieri 2014). A motor unit is composed of an alpha motor neuron and the skeletal muscle fibres. It innervates muscle fibres which can be slow (S) or fast (F). Fast fibres can be fatigue-resistant (FR) fibres, fast-twitch fatigable (FF) fibres, and fast contraction fibres with intermediate features.

The musculotendinous junction (MTJ) connects the skeletal muscle to its tendon, forming, with the muscle, a complex biomechanical unit. The MTJ is located at the extremities of the muscle fibres, where they end and where tendons fibre link. This is the main site in which the force produced by muscle contraction is transmitted (Charvet et al. 2012). In this region, the muscle enormously increases the contact area with the tendon, via deep interdigitations of the cell membrane, allowing the junction to resist to muscle contraction, from 1.8 to 3.5 × 104 N/m^2 (Charvet et al. 2012).

These interdigitations transmit the force developed by the joint and bone in a tangential direction to the tendon fibres. Physical exercise may modify the architecture of the fibres increasing these interdigitations and the tension developed by the unit (Brancaccio et al. 2013).

Muscle injuries can occur with different mechanisms, depending on the age of the subject (Keller and Engelhardt 2014); the weak link in the muscle-tendon-bone chain changes with age (Boutin et al. 2002):

- In children, the weakness of the apophyseal growth plates may lead to apophyseal avulsion fractures, when excessive tensions are applied on the muscle-tendon-bone chain.
- In young adults, mechanical failure usually occurs at the muscle-tendon interface.
- In older adults, coexistent tendinopathy and an overload of the musculotendinous unit may contribute to the tearing process (Pomeranz and Heidt 1993).

When the trauma to the muscle is direct, the lesion occurs at the site of the impact, at the MTJ, while an indirect trauma occurs at the end of the muscle belly. The structural damage to the muscle fibres may be caused by a single contraction or by the cumulative effect of several contractions. An eccentric contraction is a major cause of injury, probably as a consequence of the forces produced by eccentric contractions compared to the forces produced by isometric or concentric contractions (Garrett 1990; Jarvinen et al. 2005).

Eccentric strengthening may prevent the occurrence of injury of the muscle-tendon unit, increasing the ability of the muscle to absorb loads (Melegati et al. 2014; Isner-Horobeti et al. 2013); it also reduces muscle stiffness and the viscoelasticity of the system.

Overall, strains and complete tears occur mostly at the MTJ, the weakest link within the muscle-tendon unit (De Smet and Best 2000; Garrett et al. 1987), where the tendon arises from the muscle belly (musculotendinous junctions) and myotendinous junction (Koh and McNally 2007).

In eccentric muscle movements, when the tension increases suddenly, the damage may occur in the area beneath the epimysium and the site of muscle attachment to the periosteum (Garrett 1990; Koh and McNally 2007).

The adjacent region to the MTJ is the most injury-susceptible area of the muscle unit, independently from type and direction of applied forces and muscle architecture (El-Khoury et al. 1996). In this area, even a minor strain, by inducing an incomplete disruption which could be only microscopically evident, may weaken it and predisposes it to further injuries. At microscopy, haemorrhage is evident at the disruption sites (<24 h after disruption), while an inflammatory reaction becomes evident later, usually after 2 days (Shellock et al. 1991). The laying down of fibrous tissue and scar tissue starts after 7 days (Garrett 1996; Nikolaou et al. 1987) and becomes visible as early as 14 days following the initial insult (Greco et al. 1991). After 2 weeks, the muscle gains over 90% of its original function, but the presence of fibrous tissue alters the muscle's optimal length, and it may impair maximal contraction and predispose to further injuries (Jonhagen et al. 1994).

According to the mechanisms of trauma, muscle injuries can be classified as direct and indirect.

9.3.1 Direct Trauma

A direct muscle trauma can cause:

- Contusion through a contact against an opponent or a sport-related tool; it may be classified as mild, moderate, and severe according to the functional disability that they produce.
- *Lacerations* arise from an impact against a sharp surface, and they are not further classified.

9.3.2 Indirect Trauma

There is no impact against the opponent or against any sharp or blunt surface. It is classified as nonstructural and structural (Mueller-Wohlfahrt et al. 2013). In nonstructural injuries, muscle fibres do not present an anatomically evident lesion, while structural injuries present an anatomically defined lesion.

Nonstructural injuries: they are the most common kind of injuries, representing a 70% of all muscle injuries in soccer players (Corazza et al. 2014). Even if lesions may not be readily recognized, they cause more than 50% of days of absence away from sport activity and training. Nonstructural injuries can become structural injuries.

- Type 1A injury caused by fatigue and changes in training protocols, running surfaces, and high-intensity activities.
- Type 1B injury may result from excessive and prolonged eccentric contractions.
- Type 2A injury is mainly associated with spinal disorders, often misdiagnosed, as in minor intervertebral disorders which irritate the spinal nerve, altering the control of the muscle tone of the 'targeted' muscle.
- Type 2B injury is caused by an unbalanced control of the neuro-musculoskeletal system, mostly of the mechanism of mutual inhibition coming from the muscle spindles, and it can compromise the control of the muscle tone and induce muscle disorders; this happens

when the inhibition system of agonist muscles is altered and they are excessively contracted for compensation.

Structural injuries: they are divided into three subgroups according to the severity of the lesion within the muscle.

- Type 3A injury is a minor partial lesion involving one or more primary fascicles within a secondary bundle.
- Type 3B injury is a moderate partial lesion involving at least a secondary bundle, with less than 50% of breakage surface.
- Type 4 injury is a subtotal tear with more than 50% of breakage surface or a complete tear of the muscle, involving the muscle belly or the musculotendinous junction.

Structural injuries may be proximal (P), middle (M), and distal (D). The prognosis of proximal lesions occurring in hamstring muscles and rectus femoris is worse than those occurring at the middle or distal portions. In the triceps surae, distal injuries present the worst prognosis.

9.4 Classifications

Acute muscle injuries are commonly classified as strains (Grade I), partial tears (Grade II), and complete tears (Grade III) (Garrett et al. 1987; Brandser et al. 1995; Palmer et al. 1999). The traditional classification system described earlier does not take into account the exact location of the injury; with the advent of MRI and ultrasound imaging, location can now be exactly identified.

Therefore, to stress the concept that an ideal classification system should inform on extent, size, and exact location of a muscle injury (Armfield et al. 2006), a system has been proposed which takes into account the MRI and US imaging features of acute muscle strain injuries (Tables 9.1 and 9.2).

This classification identifies muscle injuries according to their anatomical site. Most practitioners are able to diagnose relevant injuries based on physical examination and to plan an appropriate management. Imaging can give important information which may form the basis for longitudinal studies on the evolution of such injuries.

Table 9.1 Classic classification system and relationship with imaging features of muscles injuries

Imaging grading	MRI finding	US findings
I (strain)	Less than 5% of fibre disruption; feathery oedema-like pattern, intramuscular high signal on the fluid-sensitive sequences	Normal appearance, focal or general increased echogenicity; no architectural distortion
II (partial tear)	Oedema and haemorrhage of the muscle or MTJ may extend along the fascial planes, between muscle groups Fibres, which are disorganized and thin, are surrounded by haematoma and perifascial fluid. If haemosiderin or fibrosis is present, T2-weighted images have low signal intensity. The small calibre of the fibres at the site of injury may be also expression of incomplete healing. In high-performance athletes, MRI findings, particularly the measure of the cross-sectional area of injury, are relevant to define the rehabilitation	Muscle fibres are discontinuous; the disruption site is hypervascularized and altered in echogenicity in and around, with no perimysial striation of the area adjacent to the MTJ
III (complete tear)	Complete discontinuity of muscle fibres, haematoma, and retraction of the muscle ends	Comparable with MRI

Table 9.2 Proposed classification system

Site of lesion		
Proximal MTJ		
Muscle	• Proximal • Middle • Distal	• Intramuscular • Myofascial • Myofascial/perifascial • Myotendinous • Combined
Distal MTJ		

9.4.1 Classic Classification System

- Grade I injury (strain): the tear involves few muscle fibres; swelling and discomfort are evident with maintenance or minimal impairment of strength and function.

  At MR imaging, a classic 'feathery' oedema-like pattern visible on fluid-sensitive sequences may be associated with some fluid in the central portion of the tendon and, at times, along the perifascial intermuscular region (De Smet and Best 2000), with no discernible muscle fibre disruption or architectural distortion (Kneeland 1997).

  US is often normal and may show the presence of focal or general increased echogenicity (Koh and McNally 2007). Perifascial fluid is present in almost 50% of patients.
- Grade II injury (partial tear): some continuity of fibres is maintained at the injury site. Less than one-third of muscle fibres are torn in low-grade injuries, from one-third to two-thirds in moderate ones and more than two-thirds in high-grade injuries (Connell et al. 1999). Muscle strength and high-speed/high-resistance athletic activities are usually impaired, with marked loss of muscle function.

  At MRI, the appearance of the lesion changes with both intensity and severity of the partial tear; changes are time dependent, and oedema and haemorrhage of the muscle or MTJ may extend along the fascial planes, between muscle groups. Fibres, which are disorganized and thin, are surrounded by haematoma and perifascial fluid (El-Khoury et al. 1996; Palmer et al. 1999). The MRI findings may be used as an estimate of time for rehabilitation (Bianchi et al. 2002; Cross et al. 2004; Slavotinek et al. 2002), and they can sometimes predict how much time high-performance athletes will be away from play (Pomeranz and Heidt 1993; Taylor et al. 1993).

  At US, muscle fibres are discontinuous, the disruption site is hypervascularized, and echogenicity is altered in and around the lesion (Lee and Healy 2004), with no perimysial striation of the area adjacent to the MTJ (Koh and McNally 2007). Intramuscular fluid and a surrounding hyperechoic halo may also be appreciated (Koh and McNally 2007; Lee and Healy 2004).
- Grade III injury (complete tear): at US and MR imaging, these injuries show complete discontinuity of muscle fibres, haematoma, and retraction of the muscle ends (Lee and Healy 2004); at clinical assessment, muscle function is lost (Palmer et al. 1999; El-Khoury et al. 1996; Agre 1985; Connell et al. 2004).

When extensive acute oedema and haemorrhage fill the defect between the torn edges, it is difficult to distinguish partial from complete tears, whereas real-time dynamic US imaging may be helpful (Koh and McNally 2007). If complete tears are not treated surgically, the ends of the muscle can become rounded and may tether to adjacent muscles or fascia (Koh and McNally 2007).

9.4.2 New Classification System Proposed

Anatomically, muscles have an origin, proximal and distal tendons, proximal and distal MTJs, one or more muscle bellies, and an insertion. Since injuries may involve all these sites, it is proposed to distinguish muscular, MTJ (proximal and distal), and tendon injuries (proximal and distal). Muscular lesions can be further classified as intramuscular, myofascial, myofascial/perifascial, musculotendinous, or a combination. According to the site of injury, muscle injuries are classified as proximal, middle, and distal.

Some studies suggest that the extent of a muscle injury is a prognostic factor for recovery time (Slavotinek et al. 2002; Connell et al. 2004) and variables such as the percentage cross-sectional area of abnormal muscle (typically measured on fat-suppressed images in the transverse plane), the cranio-caudal length of muscle abnormality adjacent to the MTJ (obtained from longitudinal images), and the approximate volume of muscle injury have all been proposed to estimate severity.

9.5 Imaging

US and MRI are the main methods to perform imaging assessment, relate them to patient's clinical features, and identify possible comorbidities and any history of a previous sport injury.

Ultrasound Scanning: it can be used as a first-level diagnostic tool, and it is useful to monitor the healing process of the lesion. US allows to diagnose a structural injury of the muscle 36 to 48 h after the trauma, as the peak of haemorrhagic oedematous collection is observed after 24 h when it starts to decrease (Lee and Healy 2004). US monitoring can be performed 2, 4, or 5 days after the trauma.

Dynamic US examination is useful for the assessment of both elongation and dislocation of tertiary bundles and the extent of the lesion (Koh and McNally 2007).

Colour Doppler and power Doppler can be used to visualize the course of arteries and veins and to show that the hypervascularity within the scar tissue of the lesion is unstable.

Magnetic Resonance Imaging: it is a multiparametric diagnostic tool, used for detection of also minimal changes (Ehman and Berquist 1986). It has a 92% sensitivity for nonstructural injuries (Kneeland 1997). MRI allows wide evaluation of deeper muscles than to US examination (Koh and McNally 2007). Gadolinium can be useful to monitor the stability of the scar tissue after structural injury.

Indications are:

- Prognosis of nonstructural injuries
- Exclusion of a structural injury when clinical and US finding are discordant
- Assessment of muscles which are difficult to examine at US
- In subtotal or complete muscle lesions with suspect tendon involvement or bone-tendon avulsions

9.6 Imaging Features

Nonstructural injuries:

US: often negative; transient hyperechoic or hypoechoic changes at times, after 35 days

Power Doppler US: negative

MRI: negative; evidence of limited oedema at times (Mueller-Wohlfahrt et al. 2013)

Structural injuries:

Patients should be informed that it may be difficult to differentiate mild from moderate partial injuries, especially when the lesion is small. Given the presence of liquid, MRI may overestimate the entity of the injury (Mueller-Wohlfahrt et al. 2013).

Type 3A

US: slightly hyperechoic area which later becomes inhomogeneous and hypoechoic, focalized, with some structural disarray; it is possible to detect a small anechoic area in the context of the muscle.

MRI: oedema imbibition and mild inhomogeneous signal hyperintensity because of the interstitial and perifascial oedema or small haemorrhagic extravasation.

Type 3B

US: hyperechoic area which becomes markedly inhomogeneous, with evidence of structural disarray, and a wide anechoic area within and outside the muscle.

MRI: the muscle is enlarged because of oedema, with inhomogeneous signal hyperintensity related to interstitial and perifascial oedema or haemorrhagic extravasation.

Type 4

US: severe inhomogeneous and disorganized areas, iso- or hyperechoic. Successively, inhomogeneity and marked structural changes, retraction of the ends of the torn muscle, and wide anechoic area within and between muscles.

MRI: muscle end retraction and hyperintense fluid caused by haemorrhagic extravasation between the two muscle ends.

References

Agre JC (1985) Hamstring injuries. Proposed aetiological factors, prevention, and treatment. Sports Med 2:21–33

Armfield DR, Kim DH, Towers JD et al (2006) Sports-related muscle injury in the lower extremity. Clin Sports Med 25:803–842

Bianchi S, Martinoli C, Waser NP et al (2002) Central aponeurosis tears of the rectus femoris: sonographic findings. Skelet Radiol 31:581–586

Borowski L, Yard E, Fields S et al (2008) The epidemiology of US high school basketball injuries, 2005–2007. Am J Sports Med 36:2328–2335

Boutin RD, Fritz RC, Steinbach LS (2002) Imaging of sports related muscle injuries. Radiol Clin N Am 40:333–362

Brancaccio P, Somma F, Provenzano F et al (2013) Changes in muscular pennation angle after crenotherapy. Muscles Ligaments Tendons J 9(3):112–115

Brandser EA, El-Khoury GY, Kathol MH et al (1995) Hamstring injuries: radiographic, conventional tomographic, CT, and MR imaging characteristics. Radiology 197:257–262

Chan O, Del Buono A, Maffulli N et al (2012) Acute muscle strain injuries: a proposed new classification system. Knee Surg Sports Traumatol Arthrosc 20: 2356–2362

Charvet B, Ruggiero F, Le Guellec D (2012) The development of the myotendinous junction. A review. Muscles Ligaments Tendons J 2:53–63

Connell DA, Potter HG, Sherman MF et al (1999) Injuries of the pectoralis major muscle: evaluation with MR imaging. Radiology 210:785–791

Connell DA, Schneider-Kolsky ME, Hoving JL et al (2004) Longitudinal study comparing sonographic and MRI assessments of acute and healing hamstring injuries. AJR Am J Roentgenol 183:975–984

Corazza A, Orlandi D, Baldari A et al (2014) Thigh muscles injuries in professional soccer players: a one year longitudinal study. Muscles Ligaments Tendons J 24(3):331–336

Cross TM, Gibbs N, Houang MT et al (2004) Acute quadriceps muscle strains: magnetic resonance imaging features and prognosis. Am J Sports Med 32:710–719

De Smet AA, Best TM (2000) MR imaging of the distribution and location of acute hamstring injuries in athletes. AJR Am J Roentgenol 174:393–399

Ehman RL, Berquist TH (1986) Magnetic resonance imaging of musculoskeletal trauma. Radiol Clin N Am 24:291–319

Ekstrand J, Hägglund M, Waldén M (2011) Epidemiology of muscle injuries in professional football (soccer). Am J Sports Med 39:1226–1232

El-Khoury GY, Brandser EA, Kathol MH et al (1996) Imaging of muscle injuries. Skelet Radiol 25:3–11

Falcieri E (2014) Basic science & clinic around skeletal muscles. Muscles Ligaments Tendons J 24(3):253

Garrett WE Jr (1990) Muscle strain injuries: clinical and basic aspects. Med Sci Sports Exerc 22:436–443

Garrett WE (1996) Muscle strain injuries. Am J Sports Med 24:S2–S8

Garrett WE, Safran MR, Seaber AV et al (1987) Biomechanical comparison of stimulated and non-stimulated skeletal muscle pulled to failure. Am J Sports Med 15:448–454

Greco A, McNamara MT, Escher RM et al (1991) Spin-echo and STIR MR imaging of sports-related muscle injuries at 1.5T. J Comput Assist Tomogr 15: 994–999

Isner-Horobeti M, Dufour S, Vautravers P et al (2013) Eccentric exercise training: modalities, applications and perspectives. Sports Med 43:483–512

Jarvinen TA, Jarvinen TL, Kaariainen M et al (2005) Muscle injuries: biology and treatment. Am J Sports Med 33:745–764

Jonhagen S, Nemeth G, Eriksson E (1994) Hamstring injuries in sprinters. The role of concentric and eccentric hamstring muscle strength and flexibility. Am J Sports Med 22:262–266

Keller K, Engelhardt M (2014) Strength and muscle mass loss with aging process. Age and strength loss. Muscles Ligaments Tendons J 24(3):346–350

Kneeland JP (1997) MR imaging of muscle and tendon injury. Eur J Radiol 25:198–208

Koh ES, McNally EG (2007) Ultrasound of skeletal muscle injury. Semin Musculoskelet Radiol 11:162–173

Lee JC, Healy J (2004) Sonography of lower limb muscle injury. AJR Am J Roentgenol 182:341–351

Lopez V, Galano G, Black C et al (2012) Profile of an American amateur rugby union sevens series. Am J Sports Med 40:179–184

Malliaropoulos N, Papacostas E, Maffulli N et al (2010) Posterior thigh muscle injuries in elite track and field athletes. Am J Sports Med 38:1813–1819

Melegati G, Tornese D, Gevi M et al (2014) Reducing muscle injuries and reinjuries in one Italian professional male soccer team. Muscles Ligaments Tendons J 24(3):324–330

Mueller-Wohlfahrt HW, Haensel L, Mithoefer K et al (2013) Terminology and classification of muscle injuries in sport: the Munich consensus statement. Br J Sports Med 47:342–530

Nikolaou PK, Macdonald BL, Glisson RR et al (1987) Biomechanical and histological evaluation of muscle after controlled strain injury. Am J Sports Med 15:9–14

Palmer WE, Kuong SJ, Elmadbouh HM (1999) MR imaging of myotendinous strain. AJR Am J Roentgenol 173:703–709

Pomeranz SJ, Heidt RS (1993) MR imaging in the prognostication of hamstring injury. Work in progress. Radiology 189:897–900

Shellock FG, Fukunaga T, Mink JH et al (1991) Exertional muscle injury: evaluation of concentric versus eccentric actions with serial MR imaging. Radiology 179:659–664

Slavotinek JP, Verrall GM, Fon GT (2002) Hamstring injury in athletes: using MR imaging measurements to compare extent of muscle injury with amount of time lost from competition. AJR Am J Roentgenol 179:1621–1628

Taylor DC, Dalton JD Jr, Seaber AV et al (1993) Experimetal muscle strain injury. Early functional and structural deficits and the increased risk for reinjury. Am J Sports Med 21:190–194

Walton M, Rothwell A (1986) Reactions of thigh tissues of sheep to blunt trauma. Clin Orthop Relat Res 176:273–281

Prevention of Musculotendinous Pathologies

10

Peter Myers, Joanne Bullock-Saxton, and John Fitzgerald

Contents

P. Myers, AM, MBBS, FRACS, FA.Orth.A (✉)
Brisbane Orthopaedic and Sports Medicine Centre, Brisbane, Australia
e-mail: p.myers@bosmc.com.au

J. Bullock-Saxton, Ph.D.(Physio.), M.Phty.(Manip.)
J. Fitzgerald, B.Phty., B.Sc.(Hons.), APAM
Active Rehabilitation Physiotherapy, Brisbane, Australia

10.1 Introduction

Musculotendinous (MT) injury and tendinopathy occur for a wide variety of reasons. The pathophysiology of injury and the principles of rehabilitation have been addressed by other authors of this text. This chapter focuses on what evidence exists for prevention of musculotendinous injury.

The clinician must be mindful that there are many variables that may interact to make a patient susceptible to the development of MT injury. In addition, the properties of the muscle, tendon and enthesis tissue vary widely, and the tissue mechanical characteristics will generally determine the type of injury sustained. Injury patterns can include a strain, a partial tear, an intrasubstance tear, a complete disruption or a low-grade overuse inflammatory response.

Predicting MT injury with the goal of being able to prevent it is an imprecise science and relies on the skill, experience and intuition of the clinician. Such a prediction requires an awareness of the potential for injury and bringing together information relating to medical history (Lin et al. 2004) (Magnaris et al. 2004) medication use, comorbidities such as diabetes or inflammatory conditions, activity level, skill repetition and nature of activity, external environmental factors as well as intrinsic collagen qualities and physical biomechanical characteristics. It is beyond the scope of this chapter to explore each of these potential areas in detail; however, we will attempt to highlight known

G.L. Canata et al. (eds.), *Muscle and Tendon Injuries*, DOI 10.1007/978-3-662-54184-5_10

factors which should alert a clinician to the fact that damage to the MT unit may ensue. In addition, while many of the underlying principles discussed can be applied to many parts of the body, this chapter will restrict itself to lower limb injury.

10.2 General Principles of Injury Prevention

Acute MT injuries classically result from a single tensile overload incident. Chronic injuries however result from repetitive excessively loaded events (Sandrey 2003) (Magnaris et al. 2004). It has been suggested that acute injuries may indicate the presence of a chronic pathology predisposing to the injury (Magnaris et al. 2004).

Historically, prevention of MT injury during sports participation has centred on stretching, strengthening and the preparticipation warm-up. This has developed to include specific exercises such as plyometrics, eccentric training and neuromuscular stretching among others along with the use of anatomical modifying aids such as orthotics, taping and bracing. An association between static stretching exercises and a reduced incidence of MT injuries were reported in college football players (Cross and Worrell 1999), and in a prospective cohort study of male soccer players, those with less hamstring flexibility were more likely to sustain a hamstring MT injury (Witvrouw et al. 2003). Many ailments associated with running can readily be explained by anatomy and biomechanics. Gallo et al. in a recent review (Gallo et al. 2012) found little evidence for stretching and conditioning for prevention of lower limb soft tissue running injuries. Overall, evidence that interventions could reduce lower limb pain and injury after intense running was considered weak. However, their continued use does not appear to cause harm and probably aids in athletic performance in many individuals and may therefore reduce risk of injury in some.

Genetic. It has been shown (Baumert et al. 2016) that certain gene variations, or polymorphisms, are associated with a propensity to exercise induced muscle soreness and possibly to an increased risk of delayed recovery or even of MT disruption. This knowledge may not benefit the majority of athletes but certainly could assist elite athletes in planning their training schedules to maximise recovery and reduce overload injuries.

Traumatic. It is known that concentric exercises can lead to an increased likelihood and degree of exercise-induced muscle damage (EIMD) and that this can be reduced by eccentric exercises. As it is known that EIMD may in turn predispose to MT injury, it is important that eccentric exercises be incorporated into a preparticipation exercise program. Concentric exercises enable strength and enhance joint stability, but most MT injuries occur during eccentric load, thus emphasising that eccentric exercises should form a part of a regular training session (Gleeson et al. 2003).

Fatigue has been implicated in many sports injuries. In English professional soccer, significantly more hamstring tears occur towards the end of both halves suggesting fatigue to be a factor (Woods et al. 2004). While muscles are injured at the same length, regardless of fatigue, fatigued muscles are less able to absorb energy, in eccentric load, before reaching the degree of elongation which causes the injury (Petersen and Holmich 2005). Thus, endurance training is an important factor in aiming to prevent MT injuries.

Dietary and Body Habitus. Apart from causing obesity, which is in itself a risk factor for MT injury, excessive intake of lipid can cause a dyslipidaemia which can weaken tendons biologically. This is a theoretical and uncommon problem but may be relevant in the elite athlete with altered lipid metabolism (Scott et al. 2015)

Patients with a body mass index (BMI) of 25 or more have an increased risk of Achilles or posterior tibial tendinopathy (Frey and Zamora 2007). Elevated BMI is also associated with MRI evidence of patellar tendon pathology (Scott et al. 2015). Rupture of the tibialis posterior tendon has been shown to be associated with hypertension, diabetes and obesity (Holmes and Mann

1992). Each of these conditions should be managed medically before the patient begins an activity which would risk developing a tendinopathy.

10.2.1 Around the Hip

Gluteal Tendinopathy. While this condition is uncommon in athletes, it can occur as an overuse injury. An association with increased acetabular anteversion has been suggested by MRI study (Moulton et al. 2015). This would support abnormal biomechanics along with overuse as causative factors in this injury. Prevention would therefore rely on awareness of altered hip biomechanics and appropriate training schedules for the individual athlete.

10.2.2 Hamstrings

Injuries to the hamstring tendons are the most prevalent of all MT injuries resulting from sports participation. These can be disabling, recurrent and slow to recover from. Despite their prevalence, there is no recognised reliable protocol for prevention of hamstring injuries. Fiorentino and Blemker (Fiorentino and Blemker 2014) in a very elegant study have shown that an individual's muscle-tendon dimensions can contribute to strain injury susceptibility especially in the biceps femoris long head. They have shown that peak tissue strain occurs at the proximal myotendinous junction and increases as the aponeurosis width narrows and the muscle width widens. Again, this may not be relevant to most active people; however, it is very relevant to an elite level sprinter. This information is relevant for strength and conditioning trainers who, ideally, should guide athletes to a slow progression of hamstring strength development in the hope that muscle-tendon dimension imbalance does not occur.

A systematic review by Hibbert et al. did suggest that eccentric hamstring training is effective in prevention of hamstring strains but noted that poor methodology and the heterogeneity of studies limited their ability to recommend clinical protocols (Hibbert et al. 2008).

10.2.3 Quadriceps

10.2.3.1 Quadriceps Tendon

Ruptures of the quadriceps tendon classically occur in males in their sixth decade from a sudden eccentric contraction (Clayton and Court-Brown 2008). The classic site is in the hypovascular zone 2–3 cm proximal to the patella (Ilan et al. 2003). There may be predisposing factors present such as obesity, diabetes, inflammatory arthropathy and quinolone or steroid use, but this is uncommon. Partial tears are rare and generally do not require surgery, whereas complete tears are best managed surgically. Apart from avoiding the injury situation, there is no means of preventing such an injury.

10.2.3.2 Rectus Femoris

MT injuries of the rectus femoris are uncommon in American football (Gamradt et al. 2009) but more common in Australian rules football most likely because of the high frequency of kicking and a fatigue factor with running (Orchard 2001). Surgery is rarely required but recovery can be slow. There is a high incidence of recurrent injury in those who return to sport (Orchard 2001). There has been a case report of bilateral rectus femoris rupture in a patient receiving quinolone therapy (Karistinos and Paulos 2007). Prevention is best achieved by appropriate strength, flexibility and endurance of the quadriceps mechanism in preparation for sports activity.

10.2.4 Patellar Tendon

Patellar tendonitis (PT)—classically referred to as jumper's knee—is a very troublesome condition for an athlete. While most can tolerate the condition and adjust for it to a degree, athletes cannot perform at their peak level while this condition remains painful. The capacity of the lower limb to absorb the ground reaction forces at the point of landing from a jump or decelerating is the key to understanding, treating and preventing this condition (Van der Worp et al. 2014). This involves flexibility of all joints of the lower limb along with strength and endurance of the muscles controlling those joints. Another issue in the pathogenesis of PT is the change in the angle between the patella and the patellar tendon with knee flexion. The effect of this change in angle is most marked in the deeper more central fibres of the tendon. The angle change increases with deeper knee flexion and is even more increased in patients with patella alta. These patients are more prone to a variant of PT which involves the proximal fat pad.

A patient's susceptibility to PT has been shown to be related to a stiffer movement pattern at the point of landing resulting in a shorter landing time. The authors recommended a more flexible landing pattern as a means of possibly preventing PT (Van der Worp et al. 2014). The same authors assess age, playing at the national level and volleyball (compared with basketball) to be positive risk factors for PT (Van der Worp et al. 2012). Also, in volleyball players, the total amount of jumping (number and frequency) rather than total training volume appears to be a more important risk factor for PT (Bahr and Bahr 2014).

Others have shown that the relationship between hip and knee flexion with landing can be a predictor of the presence and severity of patellar tendon injury (Mann et al. 2013). It has previously been shown that a deeper knee flexion angle can accurately predict the presence of PT in volleyball players (Richards et al. 1996). This is not surprising in the light of current knowledge as the pain of the condition would have caused weakness of the quadriceps thus requiring further flexion at both the hip and the knee in order to absorb the ground reaction forces.

10.2.5 Calf

Strain injuries of the medial head of gastrocnemius are a fairly common injury making up some 3.6% of soccer injuries. The differing functions and anatomical attachments of the gastrocnemius and soleus with the fast twitch type IIb fibres of gastrocnemius spanning two joints by joining with the slow twitch type I fibres of soleus spanning only one joint predispose this construct to injury at the attachment area. Injury is classically caused by sudden dorsiflexion of the plantar flexed foot with the knee in extension or sudden knee extension with the ankle dorsiflexed. Middle-aged and poorly conditioned athletes engaged in an unaccustomed more strenuous activity are more prone to this injury (Gallo et al. 2012).

Considering the anatomical and causative factors, this injury is almost impossible to prevent. Appropriate calf strengthening and stretching along with an awareness of the potential for injury during unaccustomed overloaded activity may help to reduce the risk of this injury.

10.2.6 Achilles Tendon

The Achilles tendon (AT) is an amazing anatomical structure. It can withstand enormous forces up to 12.5 times body weight as a result of the energy absorption of the gastrocnemius-soleus complex and the spiralling of the tendon fibres (Maffulli 1999). It can elongate up to 4% before microscopic damage occurs, while ruptures can occur at or over 8% (O'Brien 1992). There are many factors which have been associated with pathology of the AT. These include intrinsic factors such as hypovascularity, endocrine or metabolic disorders and innumerable extrinsic factors such as overuse, poor flexibility, training errors, lateral heel strike, foot pronation, inappropriate footwear, running surface irregularity, reduced ankle dorsiflexion range (Whitting et al. 2011), altered knee kinematics and reduced proximal muscle activity (Gallo et al. 2012). Such associations are not necessarily proven as cause and effect, and correction of any of these in isolation is not proven to be an effective prevention of AT pathology.

Some of these factors, such as overtraining with resultant muscle and tendon fatigue along with overpronation, can be recognised and managed appropriately, and hopefully, the injury risk will be reduced. If mechanical factors and trauma have been excluded as a cause of AT pain, then an inflammatory cause, such as ankylosing spondylitis, should be suspected and investigated (Jarrot et al. 2015). Patients with inflammatory arthropathy should have this managed appropriately before proceeding with aggressive agility activities.

10.3 Iatrogenic Causes

Medications. There are four drug groups associated with tendinopathy. While drug-associated tendinopathy is in itself a rare side effect, the more common associations are with quinolones and long-term glucocorticoid use, while statins and aromatase inhibitors are less common. The mean time to onset of symptoms is said to be only a few days for fluoroquinolones, several months for statins and up to years for glucocorticoids (Kirchgesner et al. 2014). The Achilles tendon is the most commonly affected with 5.8% of patients treated with quinolones in one series suffering symptoms including tendonitis and rupture (Barge-Caballero et al. 2008).

A systematic review by Teichtahl (Teichtahl et al. 2016) in 2016 showed very poor evidence that statins were a significant risk factor for tendon rupture. However, there are definite reports that a subset of patients treated with statins can develop tendinopathies or even rupture and a proposed molecular method for this tendinopathy (Tsai et al. 2016). Clearly more studies are needed.

In order to prevent these iatrogenic tendon pathologies, the treating physician must be aware of the possibility of tendon pathology occurring in patients being treated with these medications. There is comorbidity with multiple drugs, hypertension, diabetes and increased age. These patients must be cautioned against physical activity which may overload their tendons until well after the cessation of the medication.

Injections. Apart from short-term symptomatic improvement, there does not appear to be a benefit of injection therapy over placebo for Achilles tendon injury (Coombes et al. 2010). Indeed, there is strong evidence that glucocorticoid injection is associated with significant ongoing harm to tendon tissue and cells (Dean et al. 2014). Therefore, there is no place for any form of injection either in or around a tendon as a preventative treatment.

10.4 Specific Preventative Measures

From the preceding text along with a general understanding of the structure and function of the MT unit, some advice can be offered with the intention of prevention of MT injuries. This advice can be offered to patients by their trainer, physiotherapist, sports doctor or orthopaedic surgeon. Primary among these is the importance of being aware of the potential for MT injury and thus planning to avoid it.

Exercise programs. A patient beginning an exercise program must firstly develop the correct technique for that exercise and then the specific muscular strength, endurance and control to progress the intensity and agility of that specific exercise or activity. Factors which need to be considered when adjusting a specific program for a particular patient include their age, weight, pre-existing problems and other medical issues such as diabetes, hypertension and medications.

Running technique training along with a graded progression of endurance, speed and inclination will help prevent many running-associated injuries such as gluteus medius strain, ilio-tibial band friction syndrome, patellar tendonitis and medial calf tears (Gallo et al. 2012). Developing a controlled and flexible landing pattern and building the intensity, frequency and overall volume of activity in a gradual manner should reduce the risk of patellar tendonitis (Van der Worp et al. 2014).

10.4.1 Physical Agents

Patients with a definite abnormality of foot structure such as dynamic pes planus, painful pes cavus and hindfoot inversion may benefit from a custom-fitted orthotic (Kaufman et al. 1999). Patients with plantar fasciitis may benefit from the use of an orthotic although this is not necessarily preventative (Yu et al. 2016).

Incorrect bike fit can play a role in MT injuries incurred during cycling (Deakon 2012) which include patellar tendonitis, ITB friction syndrome and Achilles tendonitis. These can be reduced or even prevented with appropriate bike geometry and individual fitting.

The stiffness of flooring is important in activities such as ballet dancing and gymnastics. Hackney et al. (Hackney et al. 2015) showed significant decreases in maximum knee angle at landing with low stiffness flooring, suggesting a possible means of reduction of landing-related injuries in ballet dancers.

Conclusions

In attempting to prevent musculotendinous injury, the clinician must firstly have an awareness of the potential for injury to which their patient may be exposed. The intrinsic factors related to the patient must be matched with the extrinsic factors related to the specific activity and the environment in which it takes place. Unfortunately most injuries are not preventable, but some could be if we are able to advise our patients beforehand regarding the possibilities for minimising injury risk. Even with the best training program, the most skilful execution of the activity and optimal patient compliance, the biology must still match up to the physical forces of the activity, and unfortunately sometimes the biology is not up to the contest. It is this challenge which is integral to the appeal of many sports and activities and part of the enjoyment and satisfaction of participation.

References

Bahr MA, Bahr R (2014) Jump frequency may contribute to risk of jumper's knee: a study of individual and sex differences in a total of 11,943 jumps video recorded during training and matches in young elite volley ball players. Br J Sports Med 48(17):1322–1326

Barge-Caballero E et al (2008) Quinolone related Achilles tendinopathy in heart transplant patients: incidence and risk factors. J Heart Lung Transplant 27(1):46–51

Baumert P et al (2016) Gentic variation and exercise-induced muscle damage: implications for athletic performance, injury and ageing. Eur J Appl Physiol 116:1595–1625

Clayton RA, Court-Brown CM (2008) The epidemiology of musculoskeletal tendinous and ligamentous injuries. Injury 39(12):1338–1344

Coombes BK, Bisset L, Vincenzino W (2010) Efficacy and safety of corticosteroid injections and other injections for management of tendinopathy: a systematic review of randomised controlled trials. Lancet 376(9745):1751–1767

Cross KM, Worrell TW (1999) Effects of a static stretching program on the incidence of lower extremity musculotendinous strains. J Athl Train 34(1):11–14

Deakon RT (2012) Chronic musculoskeletal conditions associated with the cycling segment of the triathlon; prevention and treatment with an emphasis on proper bicycle fitting. Sports Med Arthrosc Rev 20(4):200–205

Dean BJF et al (2014) The risks and benefits of glucocorticoid treatment for tendinopathy: a systematic review of the effects of local glucocorticoid on tendon. Semin Arthritis Rheum 43(4):570–576

Fiorentino NM, Blemker SS (2014) Musculotendon variabilityinfluences tissue strains experienced by the biceps femoris long head muscle during high-speed running. J Biomech 47(13):3325–3333

Frey C, Zamora J (2007) The effect of obesity on orthopaedic foot and ankle pathology. Foot Ankle Int 28(9):996–999

Gallo RA, Plakke M, Silvis ML (2012) Common leg injuries of long distance runners, Anatomical and biomechanical approach. Res Sports Med 4(6): 485–495

Gamradt SC et al (2009) Nonoperative treatment for proximal avulsion of rectus femoris in professional American football. Am J Sports Med 37(7):1370–1374

Gleeson N, Eston R, Marginson V, McHugh M (2003) Effects of prior concentric training on eccentric exercise induced muscle damage. Br J Sports Med 37:119–125

Hackney J, Brummel S, Newman N (2015) Effect of reduced stiffness dance flooring on lower extemity joint angular trajectories during a ballet jump. J Dance Med Sci 19(3):110–117

Hibbert O et al (2008) A systematic review of the effectiveness of eccentric strength training in the prevention of hamstring muscle strains in otherwise healthy individuals. N Am J Sports Phys Ther 3(2):67–81

Holmes GB, Mann RA (1992) Possible epidemiological factors associated with rupture of the posterior tibial tendon. Foot Ankle Int 13(2):70–79

Ilan DI, Tejwani N, Keschner M, Leibman M (2003) Quadriceps tendon rupture. J Am Acad Orthop Surg 11(3):192–200

Jarrot PA, Leone J, Brochot P, Pennaforte JL (2015) Achilles tendonitis in systemic lupus erythematosus: search for an associated inflammatory disease. Lupus 24(12):1318–1320

Karistinos A, Paulos L (2007) "Ciprofloxacin induced" bilateral rectus femoris tendon rupture. Clin J Sports Med 17(5):406–407

Kaufman KR, Brodine SK, Shaffer RA (1999) The effect of foot structure and range of motion on musculoskeletal overuse injuries. Am J Sports Med 27(5):585–593

Kirchgesner T, Larbi A, Omoumi P, Malghem J (2014) Drug induced tendinopathy: from physiological to clinical applications. Joint Bone Spine 81(6):485–492

Lin TW, Cardenas L, Soslowsky LJ (2004) Biomechanics of tendon injury and repair. J Biomech 37(6): 865–877

Maffulli N (1999) Rupture of the Achilles tendon. J Bone Joint Surg Am 81-A(7):1019–1036

Magnaris CN, Narici MV, Almekinders LC, Maffulli N (2004) Biomechanics and pathophysiology of overuse tendon injuries: ideas on insertional tendinopathy. Sports Med 34(14):1005–1017

Mann KJ, Edwards S, Drinkwater EJ, Bird S (2013) A lower limb assessment tool for athletes at risk of developing patellar tendinopathy. Med Sci Sports Exerc 45(3):527–533

Moulton KM, Aly AR, Rajasekaran S, Shepel M (2015) Acetabular anteversion is associated with gluteal tendinopathy at MRI. Skelet Radiol 44(1):47–54

O'Brien M (1992) Functional anatomy and physiology of tendons. Clin Sports Med 11:505–520

Orchard JW (2001) Intrinsic and extrinsic risk factors for muscle strains in Australian football. Am J Sports Med 23(3):300–303

Petersen J, Holmich P (2005) Evidence based prevention of hamstring injuries in sport. Br J Sports Med 39(6):319–323

Richards DP, Ajemian SV, Wiley JP (1996) Kneejoint dynamics predict patellar tendinitis in elite volleyball-players. Am J Sports Med 24(5):676–683

Sandrey MA (2003) Acute and chronic tendon injuries: factors affecting the healing reesponse and treatment. J Sport Rehabil 12:70–91

Scott A et al (2015) Lipids, adiposity and tendinopathy: is there a mechanistic link? Critical review. Br J Sports Med 49(15):984–988

Teichtahl AJ, Brady SR, Urquhart DM (2016) Statins and tendinopathy: a systematic review. Med J Aust 204(3):115–121

Tsai WC et al (2016) Prevention of Simvastation-Induced inhibition of tendon cell proliferation and cell cycle progression by geranylgeranyl pyrophosphate. Toxicol Sci 149(2):326–334

Van der Worp H, De Poel HJ, Diercks RL (2014) Jumper's knee or lander's knee? A systematic of the relation between jump biomechanics and patellar tendinopathy. Int J Sports Med 35(8):714–722

Van der Worp H, van Ark M, Zwerver J, van den Akker-Scheek I (2012) Risk factors for patellar tendinopathy in basketball and volleyball players: a cross sectional study. Scand J Med Sci Sports 22(6):783–790

Whitting JW, Steele JR, Kcghee DE (2011) Dorsiflexion capacity affects achilles tendon loading during drop landings. Med Sci Sports Exerc 43(4):706–713

Witvrouw E, Danneels L, Asselman P et al (2003) Muscle flexibility as a risk factor for developing muscle injuries in male professional soccer players. A prospective study. Am J Sports Med 31:41–46

Woods C et al (2004) The Football Association Medical Research Programme: an audit of injuries in professional football—analysis of hamstring injuries. Br J Sports Med 38:36–41

Yu H, Randhawa K, Côté P (2016) The effectiveness of physical agents for lower limb soft tissue injuries: a systematic review. J Orthop Sports Phys Ther 46(7):523–554

11 Why the Tendon Tears and Doesn't Like to Heal

Pietro Simone Randelli, Luca Pulici,
Nicolò Cosmelli, and Alessandra Menon

Contents

P.S. Randelli (✉) • L. Pulici • N. Cosmelli
Department of Biomedical Sciences for Health, University of Milan, Milan, Italy

1st Department, Azienda Socio Sanitaria Territoriale Centro Specialistico Ortopedico Traumatologico Gaetano Pini-CTO, Milan, Italy
e-mail: pietro.randelli@unimi.it

A. Menon
1st Department, Azienda Socio Sanitaria Territoriale Centro Specialistico Ortopedico Traumatologico Gaetano Pini-CTO, Milan, Italy

Abbreviations

AGEs Advanced glycation end products
HP Hyperparathyroidism
NSAIDs Nonsteroidal anti-inflammatory drugs
PTH Parathyroid hormone

11.1 Introduction

Tendons are part of the musculotendinous unit, and their main function is to transfer the muscular tension to the bone levers.

The homeostasis of tendons is a critical aspect. An unbalanced relation between regenerative and degenerative processes can predispose to tendon tears (Sharma and Maffulli 2005), which are common conditions that every physician treating musculoskeletal system disorders will face throughout his career (Paavola et al. 2005).

Numerous intrinsic and extrinsic factors can interfere with tendon homeostasis, creating a disequilibrium and leading to tendon weakening.

Some of these factors are irreversible; others can be modified by a correct medical approach. In order to properly treat such patients with weakened tendons, a complete knowledge of the matter is therefore crucial.

G.L. Canata et al. (eds.), *Muscle and Tendon Injuries*, DOI 10.1007/978-3-662-54184-5_11

11.2 Intrinsic or Extrinsic Factors Leading to Tendon Tears

11.2.1 Intrinsic Factors

11.2.1.1 Anatomical Factors

The mechanical forces generated by muscle contraction are transmitted to the bones via tendons. Sheets of connective tissue, surrounding tendon components, define the tendon structure (Benjamin et al. 2008; Franchi et al. 2007; Maffulli et al. 2005).

This complex and hierarchical structure guarantees an appropriate transmission of pulling forces to rigid collagen fibers through elastic elements. As a result, tendons are remarkably strong and can withstand high tensions (Nickisch 2009).

Tendons have relatively low cellularity. There are two different mature cell types located between the collagen bundles: tenocytes and tenoblasts.

The vascularization also plays a key role in the pathophysiology of the tissue and is very variable. The three different areas of the tendon have different blood supply (Maffulli et al. 2005; Arverud et al. 2016). The musculotendinous junction is vascularized by separated arteries that provide blood flow to both tendon and muscle tissues. There are no anastomoses between these branches. Arteries and veins run transversally to the long axis in the paratenon and vascularize the midpart of the tendon via endotenon through arterioles and venules (Arverud et al. 2016).

There is a fibrocartilaginous layer interposing between the different tissues of the tendon-to-bone junction, and there is no straight communication among the different tissues.

Different tendons show different weak points according to their vascularization pattern. The Achilles tendon, for example, presents an area of lowest blood supply from 2 to 6 cm proximally to its bone insertion. Tendon tears usually occur in this area (Arverud et al. 2016; Knobloch 2008).

The area of deficiency in the rotator cuff is generally situated 7–10 mm far from the tendon-to-bone junction, where there is a lack of communication between the vascularization systems (Ling et al. 1990).

Due to vascularization flaws, low cellularity, and the great forces involved, it is anatomo-physiologically evident how the balance between regenerative and degenerative processes can be compromised (Sharma and Maffulli 2005; Maffulli et al. 2005; Arverud et al. 2016; Ling et al. 1990; Aström and Westlin 1994).

11.2.1.2 Aging

Tendon tears usually occur in middle-aged and older patients when the involved forces exceed the tolerated ones (Paavola et al. 2005). A physiological deterioration is expected in aging tendons resulting in weakened structure and function that can lead to tendon stiffness. It is a universal process that involves the different components of the tissue (Tuite et al. 1997; Kubo et al. 2001). During aging fibroblastic activity of tenoblasts is decreased, as the number of total cells (Nakagawa 1996).

In some cases, calcification could further weaken the tendon tissue and contribute to ruptures. In effect, some authors well described the progression of calcifying tendinitis to rotator cuff tears (Gotoh et al. 2003; Hsu et al. 1994; Uhthoff and Sano 1997). The effect of aging on the vascularization of the tendon is a reduction of vessels per unit of surface area (Tuite et al. 1997).

When the patient ages, the physical requests to the musculoskeletal system decrease. This mimics the disuse of tendons (reduced loading), thus a physiological weakening due to a catabolic state (Waugh et al. 2012; Dideriksen et al. 2016).

Such a mixture of depletions makes the tendon more vulnerable to damages.

11.2.1.3 Pathologies

Several pathologies have been associated with tendinopathy and tendon tears. The most accurately described ones are hyperparathyroidism, gout, obesity, diabetes, and vasculopathies (Ackermann and Hart 2016).

Hyperparathyroidism (HP) is a multisystemic disease caused by an excessive release of parathyroid hormone (PTH). The consequences are abnormal blood values of calcium and phosphate. It compromises the renal and neurological functioning, and musculoskeletal manifestations are often described (Pappu et al. 2016). Calcium deposits imply manifestations such as condrocalcinosis, arthralgias, and calcifying tendinitis that can be the cause of tendon tears (Pappu et al. 2016; Gao et al. 2013).

The correlation between high level of uric acids and consequently monosodium urate crystal deposition of gout and tendinopathies has been recently investigated by Andia and Abate (2016). The inflammatory response ruled by the IL-1β can interfere with tendon homeostasis, but further investigations, regarding the effects of crystals on tendon cells and innate immunity, still need to be done (Andia and Abate 2016; Taniguchi et al. 2014).

When the optimal vascularization and innervation of tendons decline, pathological features can occur. Diabetes and vasculopathies, being related to peripheral vasculo-nervous impairment, have been epidemiologically associated with tendinopathy (Abate et al. 2013a, b; Ackermann 2013).

Obesity has multiple and demonstrated harmful effects on tendons (Wearing et al. 2013; Wise et al. 2012). A significant increase in weight-bearing exponentially intensifies tendon stress. Furthermore, obese patients present systemic factors with a significant relevance in the pathogenesis of tendon tears (Ackermann and Hart 2016). Adipocytes produce factors such as chemerin and leptin that affect mesenchymal cells function, thus tissue turnover.

Additional damage to the tendon structure of collagen fibers is guaranteed by high AGEs (advanced glycation end products) derived from glucose catabolism (David et al. 2014; Franceschi et al. 2014; Abduljabbar et al. 2016). Abate et al. recently described how these metabolites develop stable covalent cross-links within tendon fibers (2013a).

11.2.2 Extrinsic Factors

11.2.2.1 Trauma and Overload Injuries

According to different loading and different anatomical regions, tendons are variously involved in overloads or trauma. Stressful situations can disclose subclinical compromised tendons due to aging, anatomical abnormalities, or comorbidities (Maffulli et al. 2005).

Direct trauma described as injuries resulting from direct impact can cause tendon ruptures. Nevertheless, more often an indirect trauma, such as an eccentric loading on muscle levers, leads to the tear.

The most often ruptured ones are the Achilles tendons, the quadriceps tendons, the rotator cuff tendons, and the biceps tendons (Paavola et al. 2005).

The pathophysiology of overuse injuries associates recurrent overloading to tendinosis/tendinitis which can proceed to micro-injuries and ultimately to a complete rupture (Kannus and Józsa 1991). Typically observed in sport and working environments, overuse injuries are a more complex field involving numerous aspects, organized by Paavola et al. in intrinsic and extrinsic factors (2005).

Intrinsic factors are muscular imbalance, muscular weakness, malalignments, limb length discrepancy, and lack of elasticity.

Extrinsic factors are training errors (distance, intensity, hill work, technique, fatigue), playing fields (consistency and irregularity), difficult environmental conditions, footwear, and equipment.

Since physical activity is practiced by people of all ages nowadays, the prevention of excessively stressful events is mandatory. In middle-aged and older patients, these events can lead to definitive rupture.

11.2.2.2 Drugs, Alcohol, and Smoking

Mainly four classes of drugs can cause tendon degeneration: in particular glucocorticoids and quinolones are better studied, while aromatase inhibitors and statins still need deeper evaluations (Kirchgesner et al. 2014).

Corticosteroids, often used as anti-inflammatory drugs in musculoskeletal disorders, have catabolic features on tendon homeostasis resulting in inhibition of new collagen and proteoglycan formation (Scutt et al. 2006). Preclinical and clinical studies have shown how glucocorticoid injections affect the biology of tendons reducing cellular turnover and, eventually, the energy to failure of the tissue (Scutt et al. 2006; Dean et al. 2014a, b; Hossain et al. 2008).

Quinolones are broad-spectrum antibiotic drugs and have toxic effects on tendons. The pathological relation between fluoroquinolones and tendon ruptures has been studied and proved by van der Linden et al. in the IMS Health database (2002). Their findings show that rupture events are rare but existing and also indicate that corticosteroid association can enhance tendon tears. These unfortunate accidents usually occur in Achilles tendon (van der Linden et al. 2002; Hori et al. 2012).

Passaretti et al. recently underlined and described the existing association between tendon failures and alcohol consumption (2016). Particularly, massive rotator cuff tears were related to high alcohol intake which is a risk factor for tendon injuries in both sexes (Passaretti et al. 2016).

The literature reported the effects of smoking cigarettes on rotator cuff degeneration and tears (Bishop et al. 2015); chronic inflammation could explain these effects on tendon homeostasis (Galatz et al. 2006).

11.3 Factors Affecting Tendon Healing

There are distinct stages of tendon pathology, from mild tendinopathy to complete tendon ruptures. In all these clinical conditions, tendon healing is a multifactorial process involving different actors who play various roles. Blood-derived cells, tissue-derived cells, and neurovascular and inflammatory mediators concur to regulate the three phases of tissue regeneration: inflammatory, reparative, and remodeling.

The medical approach to the injury can be either surgical or conservative according to the entity and the location of the trauma. The integrity of blood vessels is as essential as the close contact of tendon stumps. Surgeons should not be traumatic on bloody supplying structures while performing surgeries. Once these conditions are satisfied, the physiological processes can start.

The postoperative role of the physician is to guide patients through optimal rehabilitation without inhibiting tendon healing.

In addition to the intrinsic and extrinsic factors, there are further considerations that need to be evaluated while dealing with tendon healing.

11.3.1 Biomechanical Factors

The balance of loading stimuli during the healing of torn tendons is a matter of discussion in the field of musculoskeletal disease. The mechanobiology of tendon regeneration processes is well described by Killian et al. (2012). They described how postoperative rehabilitation can space from a total immobilization to passive motion to, eventually, overuse and from an environment leading to a catabolic state to another one leading to further micro-damages, respectively.

Several studies have shown how biological disuse of tendon can enhance the deterioration processes (Dideriksen et al. 2016; Killian et al. 2012; Bring et al. 2007). Preclinical animal models compare a healthy limb to the immobilized contralateral (Bring et al. 2009). Immobilization has been achieved by denervation, botulinum injection, or long-term immobilization with cast. These studies evince the biological reasons of tendon weakening after disuse. Metabolic activity and primary gene response decrease. In addition, the expression of sensory neuropeptide receptors guiding neuronal plasticity declines.

The adopted rehabilitation strategies are related to the nature and function of the tendon and to the type of surgical intervention.

11.3.1.1 Immobilization

Disuse has negative effects on tendon healing, but certain conditions require an initial healing time before any stress (Killian et al. 2012). Many authors, describing the rehabilitation process after rotator cuff repair, suggest a period of immobilization (Osborne et al. 2016). This allows the reinforcement of the tendon-to-bone junction after the surgical procedure. The initial protected osseointegration of anchors guarantees the stability for the following stresses (Thomson et al. 2016). Other authors however suggest that an early low-grade loading can stimulate the osseointegration (Schwartz and Thomopoulos 2013). According to how meticulous and controlled is the postoperative management of patient, an accurate choice of rehabilitation protocol can be made. The risk of overuse and consequently rupturing the repaired tendon need to be considered.

11.3.1.2 Passive Motion

When a laceration of long flexor tendons of the hand occurs, one of the main concerns is the reduced range of motion. This may result from peritendinous adhesions and scarring processes. An early and controlled passive motion is therefore required (Howell and Peck 2013).

11.3.1.3 Early Loading

In order to guarantee a correct biological healing, regardless of other factors such as peritendinous adhesions or osseointegration of materials, a certain loading is necessary to ensure a better outcome (Killian et al. 2012). Both basic science and clinical studies support the theory that early and progressive loading enhances healing processes in the postoperative rehabilitation protocol of Achilles tendon repair (Schepull and Aspenberg 2013; Majewski et al. 2008; Valkering et al. 2016; Kjaer 2014). Gene response and the nerve plasticity are enhanced, resulting in well structurally and biologically organized healed tendons (Bring et al. 2007; Eliasson et al. 2013). Greve et al. even described the use of intermittent pneumatic compression and its function of the regenerating tendon tissue (2012).

11.3.2 Nonsteroidal Anti-inflammatory Drugs (NSAIDs)

The inflammatory phase is the *conditio sine qua non* of a correct tendon regeneration after ruptures. Nonsteroidal anti-inflammatory drugs (NSAIDs) used in the first days after the trauma reduce the inflammatory phase and consequently interfere with the optimal callus formation and increase the healing period and recurrences. However, it is possible to preserve and improve tendon healing if the NSAIDs are administered after the inflammatory phase, guaranteeing a thinner tendon with better mechanical proprieties and tensile resistance. The inflammatory phase lasts for 5–7 days after the acute injury (Kjaer 2014; Virchenko 2004; Hammerman et al. 2015).

In the pathology of flexor tendons of the hand, where excessive fibrosis and adherences are worrisome and motion is early requested, NSAIDs are used to decrease the inflammatory phase and prevent flexion-extension deficits (Rouhani et al. 2013; Tan et al. 2010).

Conclusion

The pathophysiology of tendon tears is complex and multifactorial. It involves numerous intrinsic and extrinsic factors, irreversible ones and others that can be modified; in particular, a compromised vascularization and aging play an important key role. In addition, different pathologies, such as HP, gout, obesity, diabetes, and vasculopathies, have been demonstrated to interfere with the homeostasis of tendons.

Once tendon tears, the healing process starts and can be affected by biomechanical and pharmacological factors. The rehabilitation protocols must be adjusted taking into account the specific tendon nature and function, the type of treatment (surgical or conservative), and all the factors that affect the tendon healing.

References

Abate M, Schiavone C, Salini V, Andia I (2013a) Management of limited joint mobility in diabetic patients. Diabetes Metab Syndr Obes 6:197–207

Abate M, Schiavone C, Salini V, Andia I (2013b) Occurrence of tendon pathologies in metabolic disorders. Rheumatology 52:599–608

Abduljabbar FH, Aljurayyan A, Ghalimah B, Lincoln L (2016) Bilateral simultaneous quadriceps tendon rupture in a 24-year-old obese patient: a case report and review of the literature. Case Rep Orthop 2016:4713137

Ackermann PW (2013) Neuronal regulation of tendon homoeostasis. Int J Exp Pathol 94:271–286

Ackermann PW, Hart DA (2016) General overview and summary of concepts regarding tendon disease topics addressed related to metabolic disorders. Adv Exp Med Biol 920:293–298

Andia I, Abate M (2016) Hyperuricemia in tendons. Adv Exp Med Biol 920:123–132

Arverud ED, Persson-lindell O, Labruto F, Edman G, Ackermann PW (2016) Microcirculation in healing and healthy Achilles tendon assessed with invasive laser doppler flowmetry. Muscles Ligaments Tendons J 6(1):90–96

Aström M, Westlin N (1994) Blood flow in the human Achilles tendon assessed by laser Doppler flowmetry. J Orthop Res 12:246–252

Benjamin M, Kaiser E, Milz S (2008) Structure-function relationships in tendons: a review. J Anat 212:211–228

Bishop JY, Santiago-Torres JE, Rimmke N, Flanigan DC (2015) Smoking predisposes to rotator cuff pathology and shoulder dysfunction: a systematic review. Arthroscopy 31:1598–1605

Bring DKI, Kreicbergs A, Renstrom PAFH, Ackermann PW (2007) Physical activity modulates nerve plasticity and stimulates repair after achilles tendon rupture. J Orthop Res 25:164–172

Bring DKI et al (2009) Joint immobilization reduces the expression of sensory neuropeptide receptors and impairs healing after tendon rupture in a rat model. J Orthop Res 27:274–280

David MA et al (2014) Tendon repair is compromised in a high fat diet-induced mouse model of obesity and type 2 diabetes. PLoS One 9:e91234

Dean BJF et al (2014a) The risks and benefits of glucocorticoid treatment for tendinopathy: a systematic review of the effects of local glucocorticoid on tendon. Semin Arthritis Rheum 43:570–576

Dean BJF, Franklin SL, Murphy RJ, Javaid MK, Carr AJ (2014b) Glucocorticoids induce specific ion-channel-mediated toxicity in human rotator cuff tendon: a mechanism underpinning the ultimately deleterious effect of steroid injection in tendinopathy? Br J Sports Med 48:1620–1626

Dideriksen K et al (2016) Skeletal muscle adaptation to immobilization and subsequent retraining in elderly men: no effect of anti-inflammatory medication. Exp Gerontol 82:8–18

Eliasson P, Andersson T, Hammerman M, Aspenberg P (2013) Primary gene response to mechanical loading in healing rat Achilles tendons. J Appl Physiol 114:1519–1526

Franceschi F et al (2014) Obesity as a risk factor for tendinopathy: a systematic review. Int J Endocrinol 2014:670262

Franchi M, Trirè A, Quaranta M, Orsini E, Ottani V (2007) Collagen structure of tendon relates to function. ScientificWorldJournal 7:404–420. doi:10.1100/tsw.2007.92

Galatz LM et al (2006) Nicotine delays tendon-to-bone healing in a rat shoulder model. J Bone Joint Surg Am 88:2027–2034

Gao M-F, Yang H-L, Shi W-D (2013) Simultaneous bilateral quadriceps tendon rupture in a patient with hyperparathyroidism undergoing long-term haemodialysis: a case report and literature review. J Int Med Res 41:1378–1383

Gotoh M, Higuchi F, Suzuki R, Yamanaka K (2003) Progression from calcifying tendinitis to rotator cuff tear. Skelet Radiol 32:86–89

Greve K et al (2012) Metabolic activity in early tendon repair can be enhanced by intermittent pneumatic compression. Scand J Med Sci Sports 22:e55–e63. doi:10.1111/j.1600-0838.2012.01475.x

Hammerman M, Blomgran P, Ramstedt S, Aspenberg P (2015) COX-2 inhibition impairs mechanical stimulation of early tendon healing in rats by reducing the response to microdamage. J Appl Physiol 119:534–540

Hori K, Yamakawa K, Yoshida N, Ohnishi K, Kawakami J (2012) Detection of fluoroquinolone-induced tendon disorders using a hospital database in Japan. Pharmacoepidemiol Drug Saf 21:886–889

Hossain MA, Park J, Choi SH, Kim G (2008) Dexamethasone induces apoptosis in proliferative canine tendon cells and chondrocytes. Vet Comp Orthop Traumatol 21:337–342

Howell JW, Peck F (2013) Rehabilitation of flexor and extensor tendon injuries in the hand: current updates. Injury 44:397–402

Hsu HC et al (1994) Calcific tendinitis and rotator cuff tearing: a clinical and radiographic study. J Shoulder Elb Surg 3:159–164

Kannus P, Józsa L (1991) Histopathological changes preceding spontaneous rupture of a tendon: a controlled study of 891 patients. J Bone Joint Surg Am 73:1507–1525

Killian ML, Cavinatto L, Galatz LM, Thomopoulos S (2012) The role of mechanobiology in tendon healing. J Shoulder Elb Surg 21:228–237

Kirchgesner T et al (2014) Drug-induced tendinopathy: from physiology to clinical applications. Joint Bone Spine 81:485–492

Kjaer M (2014) Throw away the anti-inflammatories and start loading your damaged tendons. Aspetar Sports Med J 3:390–393

Knobloch K (2008) The role of tendon microcirculation in Achilles and patellar tendinopathy. J Orthop Surg Res 3:18

Kubo K, Kanehisa H, Kawakami Y, Fukanaga T (2001) Growth changes in the elastic properties of human tendon structures. Int J Sports Med 22:138–143

Ling SC, Chen CF, Wan RX (1990) A study on the vascular supply of the supraspinatus tendon. Surg Radiol Anat 12:161–165

Maffulli N, Renstrom P, Leadbetter W (2005) Tendon Injuries: basic science and clinical medicine. Springer-Verlag, London. doi:10.1017/CBO9781107415324.004

Majewski M, Schaeren S, Kohlhaas U, Ochsner PE (2008) Postoperative rehabilitation after percutaneous Achilles tendon repair: early functional therapy versus cast immobilization. Disabil Rehabil 30:1726–1732

Nakagawa Y (1996) Age-related changes in biomechanical properties of the Achilles tendon in rabbits. Eur J Appl Physiol Occup Physiol 73:7–10

Nickisch F (2009) Anatomy of the achilles tendon. In: The Achilles tendon: treatment and rehabilitation. Springer-Verlag, New York, pp 3–16. doi:10.1007/978-0-387-79205-7_1

Osborne JD, Gowda AL, Wiater B, Wiater JM (2016) Rotator cuff rehabilitation: current theories and practice. Phys Sportsmed 44:85–92

Paavola M, Kannus P, Järvinen M (2005) Tendon injuries: basic science and clinical medicine. Springer-Verlag, London, pp 32–39. doi:10.1007/1-84628-050-8_5

Pappu R, Jabbour SA, Regianto AM, Reginato AJ (2016) Musculoskeletal manifestations of primary hyperparathyroidism. Clin Rheumatol 35:3081–3087

Passaretti D, Candela V, Venditto T, Giannicola G, Gumina S (2016) Association between alcohol consumption and rotator cuff tear. Acta Orthop 87:165–168

Rouhani A, Tabrizi A, Ghavidel E (2013) Effects of nonsteroidal anti-inflammatory drugs on flexor tendon rehabilitation after repair. Arch Bone Jt Surg 1:28–30

Schepull T, Aspenberg P (2013) Early controlled tension improves the material properties of healing human achilles tendons after ruptures: a randomized trial. Am J Sports Med 41:2550–2557

Schwartz A, Thomopoulos S (2013) Structural interfaces and attachments in biology, pp 229–257. isbn:978-1-4614-3317-0

Scutt N, Rolf CG, Scutt A (2006) Glucocorticoids inhibit tenocyte proliferation and tendon progenitor cell recruitment. J Orthop Res 24:173–182

Sharma P, Maffulli N (2005) Tendon injury and tendinopathy: healing and repair. J Bone Joint Surg Am 87:187–202

Tan V et al (2010) Effects of nonsteroidal anti-inflammatory drugs on flexor tendon adhesion. J Hand Surg Am 35:941–947

Taniguchi Y, Matsumoto T, Tsugita M, Fujimoto S, Terada Y (2014) Spondylodiscitis and Achilles tendonitis due to gout. Mod Rheumatol 24:1026–1027

Thomson S, Jukes C, Lewis J (2016) Rehabilitation following surgical repair of the rotator cuff: a systematic review. Physiotherapy 102:20–28

Tuite DJ, Renstrom PA, O'Brien M (1997) The aging tendon. Scand J Med Sci Sports 7:72–77

Uhthoff HK, Sano H (1997) Pathology of failure of the rotator cuff tendon. Orthop Clin N Am 28:31–41

Valkering KP et al (2016) Functional weight-bearing mobilization after Achilles tendon rupture enhances early healing response: a single-blinded randomized controlled trial. Knee Surg Sports Traumatol Arthrosc. doi:10.1007/s00167-016-4270-3

van der Linden PD, Sturkenboom MCJM, Herings RMC, Leufkens HGM, Stricker BHC (2002) Fluoroquinolones and risk of Achilles tendon disorders: case-control study. BMJ 324:1306–1307

Virchenko O (2004) Parecoxib impairs early tendon repair but improves later remodeling. Am J Sports Med 32:1743–1747

Waugh CM, Blazevich AJ, Fath F, Korff T (2012) Age-related changes in mechanical properties of the Achilles tendon. J Anat 220:144–155

Wearing SC, Hooper SL, Grigg NL, Nolan G, Smeathers JE (2013) Overweight and obesity alters the cumulative transverse strain in the Achilles tendon immediately following exercise. J Bodyw Mov Ther 17:316–321

Wise BL, Peloquin C, Choi H, Lane NE, Zhang Y (2012) Impact of age, sex, obesity, and steroid use on quinolone-associated tendon disorders. Am J Med 125:1228.e23–1228.e28

Growth Factor Therapy for Tendon Regeneration

12

R. Cugat, E. Alentorn-Geli, J.M. Boffa, X. Cuscó, M. Garcia-Balletbo, P. Laiz, E. Mauri, and M. Rius

Contents

R. Cugat, M.D., Ph.D. (✉) • J.M. Boffa • X. Cuscó
E. Mauri • M. Rius
Fundación García-Cugat, Barcelona, Spain

Artroscopia GC, Orthopaedic Surgery and Traumatology, Hospital Quirón Barcelona, Barcelona, Spain

Mutualidad de Futbolistas, Real Federación Española de Fútbol, Delegación Cataluña, Barcelona, Spain
e-mail: ramon.cugat@sportrauma.com

E. Alentorn-Geli • M. Garcia-Balletbo • P. Laiz
Fundación García-Cugat, Barcelona, Spain

Artroscopia GC, Orthopaedic Surgery and Traumatology, Hospital Quirón Barcelona, Barcelona, Spain

12.1 Introduction: Epidemiology of the Tendon Injuries

Injury incidence rate of the tendons is a slightly studied topic. In the population of federated football players at Mutualitat Catalana de Futbolistes which belongs to the RFEF, the rate of tendon injuries is low, as Table 12.1 shows. The most common of the tendon injuries are affect the lower extremity, because of the overuse of them in this sport, even though all the tendons can suffer a pathology (Fig. 12.1).

The most common of the tendon injuries are:

- Patellar tendinopathy (Fig. 12.2)
- Enthesopathy of the adductor longus (Fig. 12.2)
- Hamstring tendinopathy

Table 12.1 Numer of tendon injuries compared to the total of injuries treated in the Mutualitat Catalana de Futbolistes which belongs to the Real Federación Española de Fútbol (RFEF)

Season	Affiliates	Number of injuries	Number of tendon injuries
2014–2015	151.263	25.730	73 (0.28%) tendon ruptures 781 (3.04%) tendinosis

G.L. Canata et al. (eds.), *Muscle and Tendon Injuries*, DOI 10.1007/978-3-662-54184-5_12

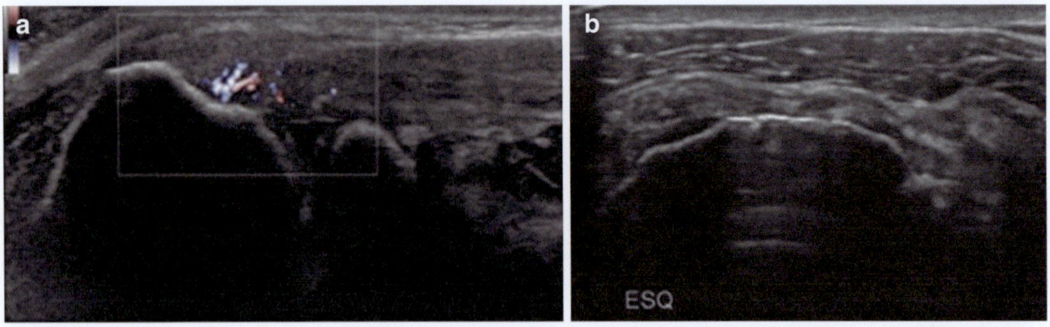

Fig. 12.1 Upper extremity injuries. (**a**) Epicondylitis in the elbow with eco-Doppler study. (**b**) Supraspinatus rupture

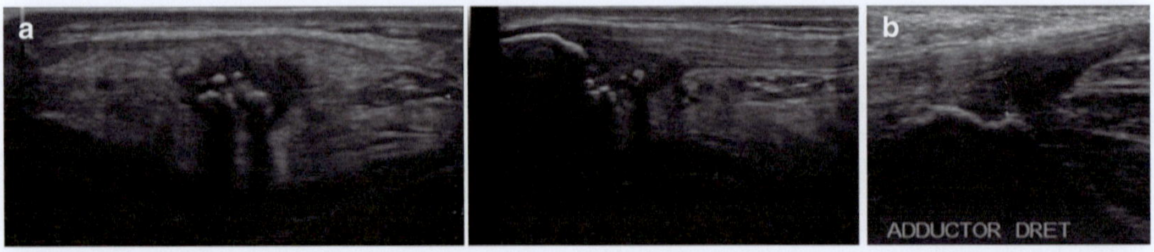

Fig. 12.2 Common injuries. (**a**) Patellar tendinopathy. Longitudinal and transversal study. (**b**) Adductor longus enthesopathy

The use of biologic therapies in tendon injuries is the present and the future in treating these injuries. The goal of these therapies is to restore the tissue with the same and indistinguishable properties from the original one. Likewise, the crux of the matter is not to repair but to regenerate, reconstruct and restore the functionality.

12.1.1 Anatomy and Histology

Tendons are fibrous connective tissue composed of collagen fibre bundles that connect muscle to bone and act as contractile force transmitters enabling skeletal movement. All these are covered by the *peritendon*.

There are anatomical sites where the tendon slides can suffer a wear disease. These sites are the bony furrows, the landmarks, where the tendon frequently has a *tendon sheath*.

In the bone soil furrows, the roof consists of a *fibrous sheath* that converts the canal in a tunnel or fibro-osseous duct and the tendon slides protected by the *synovial sheath* that has a *parietal membrane* and other *tendon membrane* that are separated by a virtual *synovial cavity* with *synovial fluid* inside. In the parietal tendon membrane and tendon membrane reflection areas, a non-ended cavity is formed. All this can be surrounded by a fascia coating thickening that also protects the tendons and is called retinaculum.

The vascularity of the tendon almost always comes from its deep side, where the mesotendon is placed, or can also come through links or vessels that come from the bone insertion.

And the last anatomical detail of the tendons is the *synovial bursa*, which is in places where it can be rubbed with other muscles or osteoligamentous structures. The bursae contain synovial fluid as a cushion to facilitate the sliding (Llusá et al. 2006).

12.1.2 Biomechanics of the Tendon

Tendons have viscoelastic behaviour; they do not act as rigid links between muscles and bones. The viscoelasticity is given by the collagen and the water and by the interaction between the collagen and the proteoglycans (Wang et al. 2012).

The mechanical proprieties of the tendon have traditionally been studied stretching an isolated tendon to failure (Butler et al. 1978). There, a force-elongation curve is obtained with four different regions. Region I is associated with non-damaging forces; in region II, the already aligned forces are stretched and at the end point some fibres start to break. Further elongation brings into region III, where fibre failure occurs unpredictably; when further elongation occurs, it brings the tendon into region IV where there is a complete failure (Maganaris et al. 2008). Different types of tendons differ in their mechanical proprieties due to their different functions.

The key to tendons' tensile strength is collagen. For about 70–80% of the dry weight, tendon is collagen type I, and in minor amounts there are collagen types III, V, IX, X, XI and XII, which also have important functions.

The tendon acts as a spring, stretching when there is a tensile force, accumulating part of this energy and liberating it when it regains its original shape. What makes it act in this way is the plasticity given by the periodic wave pattern of the collagen fibres, named the crimp pattern. When the tensile force is higher than 2%, the fibres lose its pattern, and until 4% the tendon can regain its periodic wave pattern. With a tensile force is from 4 to 8%, the fibres start to brake, and they are unable to regain completely their pattern (Maffulli 1999; Doral et al. 2010).

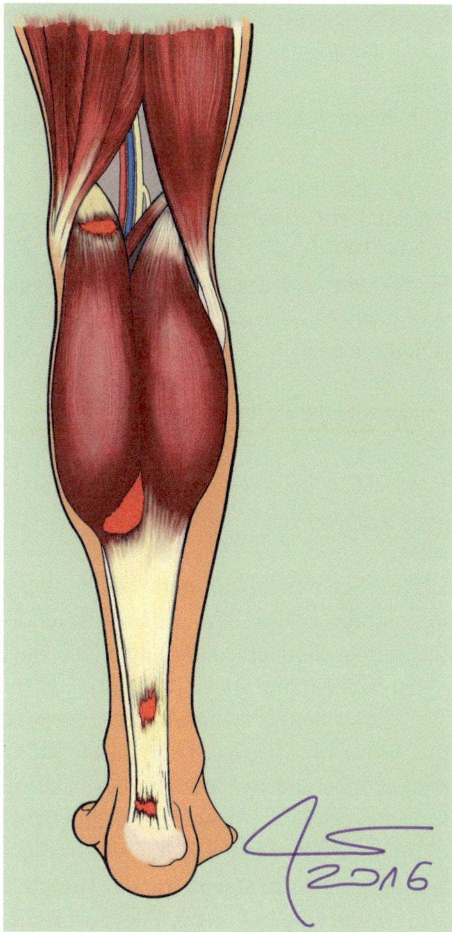

Fig. 12.3 Anatomical location of tendon injuries

12.1.3 Aetiology

The tendon injuries are often chronic, and the causes are an overload, a degenerative process or a rupture, but also it could be acute injury.

Repetitive movements both in work activity (cleaning glass, craftwork cutting, etc.) and sports activity (swimming, launching, etc.) are the cause of many of these injuries.

12.1.4 Injury Classification (Fig. 12.3)

According to the anatomical location:

1. Tendon insertion or tenoperiosteal area. These are *tendinopathy insertion* or *enthesitis* and *avulsions*.
2. Tendinous body: *swelling*, *tendinosis (degeneration)* and *partial* or *complete rupture*.
3. Musculotendinous junction: *sprains*.
4. Paratenon: *peritendinitis* and *tenosynovitis*.

12.1.5 Diagnosis

Diagnosis is performed by clinical examination and complementary studies.

Clinical Examination: Signs and Symptoms

- Pain during sports activities and in normal life. More acute when doing forced movements.
- Pain when palpating the insertion of the tendon or the tendinous body, when there is a tendinosis or an enthesitis.

- Strength decreased with or without pain when doing contraction against resistance of the injury.
- Pain when passive stretching of the injured tendon.
- Crepitation in tenosynovitis.
- "Hatchet strike defect" in complete ruptures (Cugat 1993).
- Specific test: to evaluate the rupture or injury of some tendons, such as Thompson manoeuvre in Achilles tendon.

Complementary Studies

- X-rays: Calcifications, bony protrusions and bone avulsion can be observed.
- MRI
- ULTRASOUND: Ultrasound is an imaging technique very useful to evaluate the tendons. It is a great complementary tool to the conventional radiography for an exhaustive diagnosis. Ultrasound is a non-invasive technique that allows us to use it as many as needed to do comparative and dynamic studies. The main uses are as follows: diagnosis, define the type of injury, locate and grade it, give a prognosis and suggest a treatment for the patient and also conduct the follow-up. The most frequent injuries of the tendons are tendinopathy, enteropathy, complete or partial ruptures, dislocations and partial dislocations. On the interventionist side, the ultrasounds are becoming more useful to conduct ultrasound-guided treatments. It provides precision to the treatments because it allows us to view the structure to intervene and have a precise control over the needle while doing the procedure.

12.1.6 Treatment

1. Surgical: Only when conservative treatment does not get satisfactory evolution and in big ruptures.
2. Conservative: Biologic therapy, physiotherapy and rehabilitation.

12.2 Biologic Therapy: Growth Factors

12.2.1 What Are Growth Factors?

Growth factors are substances, such as vitamins or hormones, which are required for the stimulation of growth in living cells and cellular differentiation. They are biochemical signals capable of modulating the cellular response, involved in a large number of biological functions among which cellular proliferation is important, though they also decisively affect cellular survival, migration, differentiation and even apoptosis.

Growth factors are synthetised as cellular mediators by a great amount of varied cell types, to diverse stimuli as an injury. It has been noticed that all types of connective tissues (bone, muscle, cartilage, synovial membrane, tendon, ligament, meniscus, skin, etc.) contain many of these signalling proteins which play a very important role in the remodelling and repair of the different types of connective tissue.

Growth factors carry out their function at very low concentration on body fluids and tissues, in the region of pico- or nanograms. Typically, they act by binding to a cellular receptor, which is specific for a second messenger where a tyrosine kinase protein acts. This causes a signalling cascade that ends up with a signal transduction inside the nucleus and the activation of one or more genes.

12.2.2 Mode of Action

The process of tissue regeneration includes a complex set of biological events controlled by the action and synergy of a cocktail of growth factors. There are three agents involved in tissue regeneration, the cellular component, a combination of multiple biological mediators that include growth factors and cytokines among others and a matrix or scaffold that gives support to the new tissue under construction.

The signalling pathways leading from the receptor binding to a biologic response are very complex.

Tyrosine kinase receptors are cell membrane molecules and have kinase activity, which means that they have the ability to phosphorylate or add phosphate groups on the cytoplasmic domain. A growth factor, the ligand, binds this receptor, which dimerises and activates the kinase activity (Hubbard 1999). After this activation, the receptor can add more phosphates to certain downstream targets or bring other molecules into the signalling complex by its phosphotyrosine residues (Lemmon and Schlessinger 2010). It could also be transmitted differently when the receptor does not have intrinsic tyrosine kinase activity. They instead recruit molecules, which have the ability to phosphorylate. These receptors have an intracellular domain with a protein kinase family (JAKs) which autophosphorylates and then recruits signal transducers and activators of transcription (STATs) (O'Shea et al. 2002) (Fig. 12.4).

TGF-β superfamily of ligands has intrinsic serine/threonine kinase activity and binds to a type II receptor, which is an active kinase. This binding recruits and phosphorylates a type I receptor, which can activate downstream targets, by activating receptor-regulating SMADs (R-SMAD). The SMAD complexes resulted from this activation and accumulate in the nucleus where they act as transcription factors regulating gene expression. Further signals are generally transmitted by MAPK pathway and the PLC second messenger system. These systems work in cascade and involve a series of phosphorylations from one molecule to another. A mitogenic signal allows Ras to swap its GDP (inactive) to GTP (active); this activates MAP3K (e.g. Raf), which activates MAP2K (e.g. MEK). This last activation results on a MAPK, which can now activate a transcription factor (e.g. MYC). PLC catalyses the hydrolysis of the phospholipid PIP_2 which results in two end products, DAG and IP_3. These two products are second messengers that control cellular processes and synthetise other important signalling molecules (Massagué 2012).

12.2.3 Growth Factors

PDGF in tendon

It is known that the platelet-derived growth factor, PDGF, plays an important role in the cicatrisation process of the tendon (Duffy et al. 1995). There are studies that talk about the PDGF high

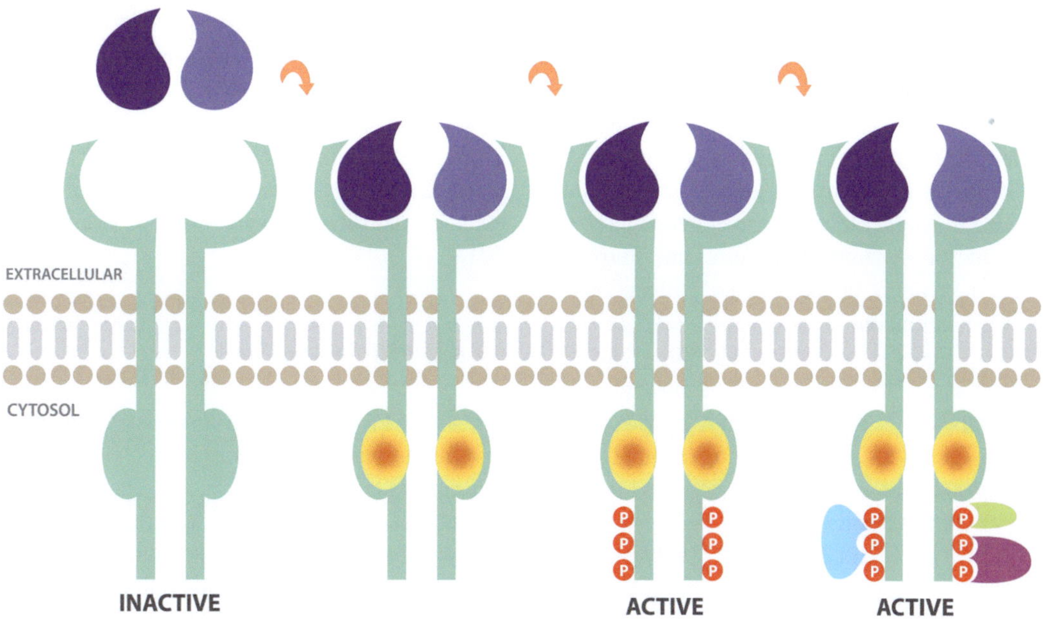

Fig. 12.4 Mechanism of action of the tyrosine kinase receptors

levels during this process, and it seems to be very important during the first part of the cicatrisation inducing other growth factors to be synthetised (Molloy et al. 2003), although there are studies that showed that PDGF is also important during the tissue remodelling process (Yoshikawa and Abrahamsson 2001).

TFG-β in tendon

TGF-β is very active during all tendinous cicatrisation phases, playing a very important role in tissue reparation stimulating extrinsic cell migration, regulating protease activity, stimulating collagen production and ending cell proliferation (Molloy et al. 2003).

As some studies show, TGF-β gene expression increases after tendon wound, and it is believed that it regulates inflammatory response (Sciore et al. 1998). Other studies have found that high TGF-β doses could have negative effects in tendon healing, e.g. fibrosis, which considerably decreases tendon mobility (Molloy et al. 2003).

IGF in tendon

In the tendon healing, the IGF stimulates fibroblast and other cell proliferation and migration to the damaged area so as to increase collagen and other extracellular matrix protein production (Molloy et al. 2003). It is also important to say that the synergy with other molecules increases its functions.

FGF in tendon

During tendon healing, FGF stimulates fibroblast proliferation in the tendon. It is proved that FGF levels are increased after a tendon injury, having the higher levels in the epitenon tenocytes and in the inflammatory cells and fibroblasts from the tendon sheath (Hsu and Chang 2004).

EGF in tendon

EGF plays an important role during the early phase of the cicatrisation. It is present in the inflammatory cells even though it is not expressed in the tenocytes of the healing area (Tsubone et al. 2004).

VEGF in tendon

VEGF is present in synovial fibroblasts and in tenocytes. It seems to play an important role in tendon angiogenesis (Hsu and Chang 2004). Its levels are insignificant in normal Achilles tendon, but they are increased after an injury. So, the increment of VEGF follows a pattern, from the outside to the injury focus (Molloy et al. 2003). This neovascularisation comes from the surface of the epitenon and provides the injury zone with extrinsic cells, nutrients and growth factors.

NGF in tendon

In human tenocytes, the presence of NGF has been shown, but there is no further information about its activity on tendinous reparation processes.

HGF in tendon

There are no studies on its activity in tendinous reparation processes.

12.3 PRP as a Medication

12.3.1 Are All PRP the Same?

Currently, there is a variety of systems for obtaining substances that contain growth factors and other elements like leukocytes, fibrin, etc. Because of this variety, the products obtained have different chemical and cellular compositions. Preclinical studies suggest that leukocytes in PRP contribute to inflammatory cytokine production in tendon healing (McCarrel et al. 2012). It also suggests that minimising leukocytes in PRP is more important than maximising platelet numbers in order to decrease inflammation and enhance matrix gene synthesis (Boswell et al. 2014).

12.3.2 PRP in Tendon

The use of PRP in tendon is increasing faster than in other tissues because from 30 to 50% of sports injuries are tendon related.

The tendon is a poorly vascularised tissue (Fenwick et al. 2002) that uses little energy and has low metabolic tax. Besides, the tendon can support high tension for a long time which means that the tissues with a high metabolic activity demand, such as cicatrisation, occur relented (Sánchez et al. 2009).

The effect of PRP in tendon tissue is similar to other tissues. The platelets, once activated, release its granule content. This content consists of important growth factors, PDGF, TGF-β, FGF, EGF, VEGF, HGF and IGF, among others, which play important roles (Molloy et al. 2003). Apart from these growth factors, this PRP therapy gives other bioactive and structural proteins, such as fibrin, fibronectin or vitronectin, which helps in intracellular adhesion and three-dimensional matrix formation (Andia et al. 2010).

12.4 Effects of PRP in Tendon Healing

12.4.1 Ultrastructural Effect

The Fernández-Sarmiento et al. study has demonstrated that PRP is associated with histological changes consistent with an accelerated and early healing process in tendon. The tendons treated with PRP showed improvements in morphometric features of fibroblast nuclei, which suggest an advanced stage of healing. After 8 weeks of treatment with PRP, the histological examination revealed a more mature organisation of collagen bundles (more packed and better oriented), lower vascular density (PRP-treated tendons exhibited faster vascular regression than tendons in the control groups) and decreased fibroblast densities than in control group tendons. The fibroblast nuclei of the tendons treated with PRP were more elongated and parallel to the tendon axis than in the control group. These findings were consistent with a more advanced stage of the healing process (Fernandez-Sarmiento et al. 2012; Fernandez-Sarmiento 2012; Domínguez et al. 2012; Fernández-Sarmiento et al. 2013).

In the II Jornadas de la Fundación Garcia Cugat in 2012, JM Dominguez and A Blanco presented "Therapy with plasma rich in growth factors in tendon ruptures" where they stated that there are obvious differences in the ultrastructure of the tendons. There are more inflammation signs in the control group at 2 and 4 weeks than in PRP group. In the PRP group, the fibroblasts have a major activity and collagen production. The collagen fibres seem to be organised better and well aligned. In the eighth week, microkeloid appeared in the control group, which could mean a loss of structure, elasticity, adhesions and recurrence of the injury. The PRP group is in a more advanced stage of cicatrisation (Figs. 12.5 and 12.6).

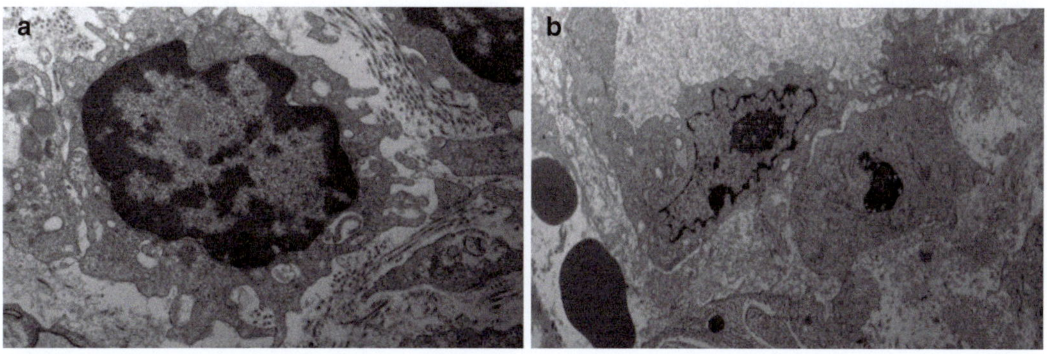

Fig. 12.5 Lymphocyte (**a**) and macrophage (**b**). Inflammation signs at 2 weeks in the control group

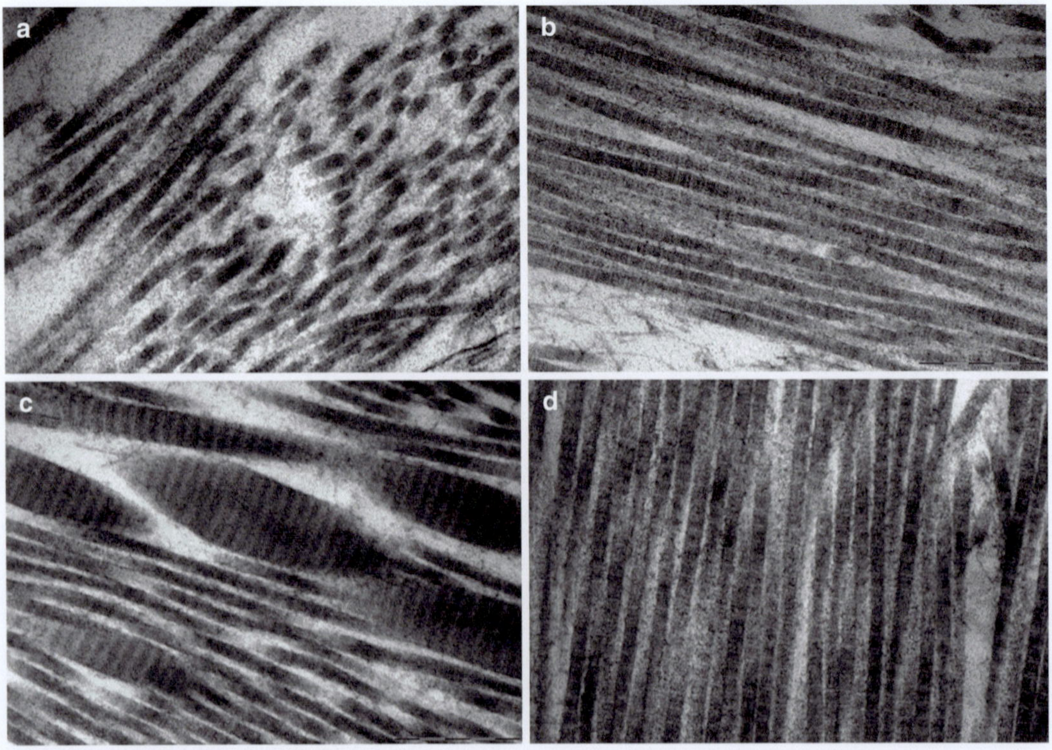

Fig. 12.6 Collagen fibre distribution. (**a**) At 4 weeks in the control group, the fibres are poorly organised. (**b**) At 4 weeks in the PRP group, mature fibres. (**c**) At 8 weeks in the control group, hypertrophic and mature fibres. (**d**) At 8 weeks in the PRP group, well-organised adult fibres

12.4.2 Biomechanical Effects

Lopez-Najera et al. study demonstrated that the application of PRP in Achilles tendon increases its repair strength at 8 weeks compared with the placebo control group, but does not modify section and tension ratios. The tension ratio progressively increases between 2 and 8 weeks compared with the ones treated with placebo (López-Nájera 2014; López-Nájera et al. 2015).

12.5 Augmentation in Surgery

In order to improve the regeneration of the tendon, the application of PRP, liquid or clot formulation, is also advised in tendinous injuries that require surgery at the end of the procedure. Also, it is advised to apply the PRP subcutaneously to improve the healing of the injured area.

In the post-surgery period, if the evolution is slower than expected, a second or third injection can be performed under ultrasound control (Fig. 12.7).

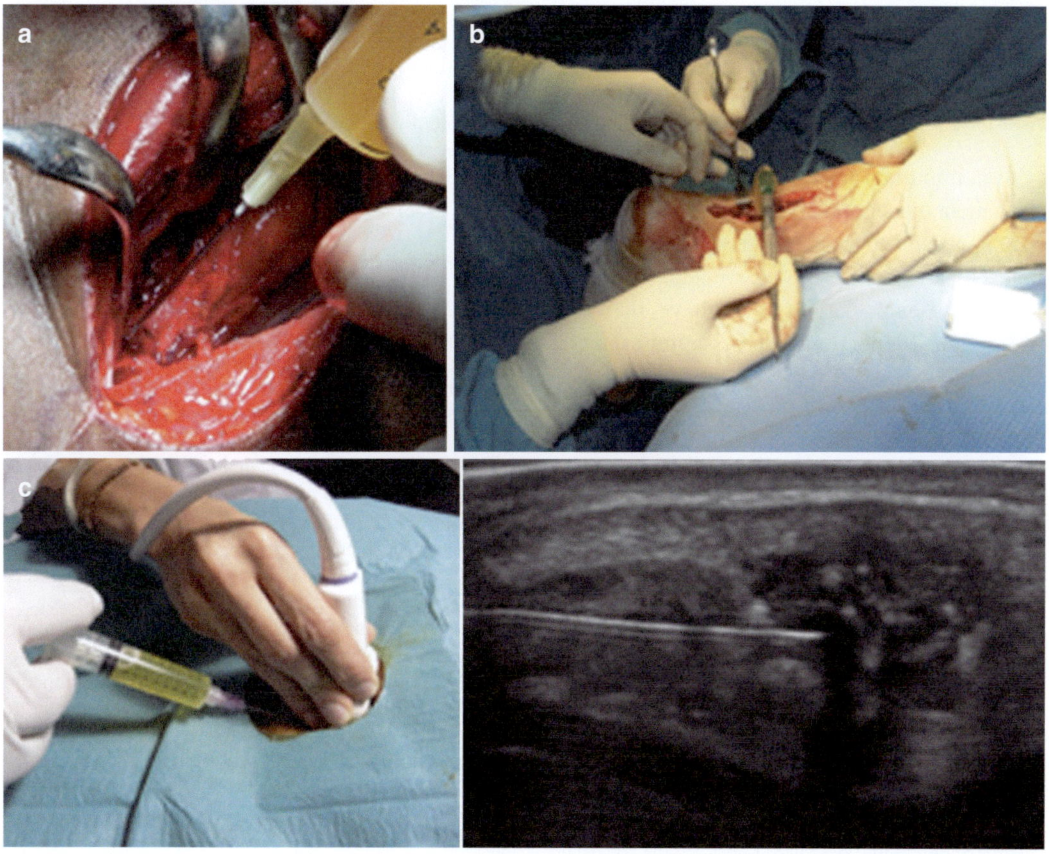

Fig. 12.7 PRP administration formula. (**a**) Liquid PRP. (**b**) Clot PRP. (**c**) Ultrasound-guided PRP injection

12.6 Physiotherapy

The role of the physiotherapy or rehabilitation is essential to recover from a tendinous injury. The rehabilitation works to diminish the pain and eliminate the problem. The main objective in this type of injuries is to eliminate the pain, regain a good range of motion and re-establish the muscle mass of the affected area.

The rehabilitation process is divided in three phases:

- First phase: the objective is to reduce the inflammation and pain.
- Second phase: the objective is to regain a good elasticity in the injured tendinous fibres. Manual exercises working with passive stretching, eccentric muscle work and cardiovascular training.

- Third phase: only will take place if the patient does not show pain. Work on gaining muscle mass through progressive strengthen exercises would be conducted.

It is important to take into consideration that the patient must not work if feeling pain, and also it is important to work progressively depending on each patient.

Finally, each patient must have their own programme depending on his injury and his characteristics.

12.7 Take-Home Message

The vast majority of tendon injuries can be solved with conservative treatment, being a minimum percentage the ones that require surgery. Biological treatments help in regenerating tissues by recovering the altered anatomy and also in recovering the decreased function within a shorter time.

Acknowledgements We thank Laura Rivilla for designing and drawing the tyrosine kinase receptor mode of action. We would also like to show our gratitude to Sue-Sonia Tizol for assistance with translation and to all football players whose images are shown in this chapter. And finally we would like to show our gratitude to Professor Dr. Alfonso Blanco for the electronic microscope images in the chapter.

References

Andia I, Sanchez M, Maffulli N (2010) Tendon healing and platelet-rich plasma therapies. Expert Opin Biol Ther 10:1415–1426. doi:10.1517/14712598.2010.514603

Boswell S, Schnabel L, Mohammed H et al (2014) Increasing platelet concentrations in leukocyte-reduced platelet-rich plasma decrease collagen gene synthesis in tendons. Am J Sports Med 42(1):42–49

Butler DL, Grood ES, Noyes FR, Zernicke RF (1978) Biomechanics of ligaments and tendons. Exerc Sport Sci Rev 6:125–181

Cugat R (1993) Patologia muscular i tendinosa del futbolista. Federació Catalana de Futbol, Barcelona

Domínguez JM, Fernández-Sarmiento J, Granados MM et al (2012) Ultrastructural study of the healing process in tenotomized achilles tendons treated with plasma rich in growth factors in sheep. Osteoarthr Cartil 20:S250–S251. doi:10.1016/j.joca.2012.02.417

Doral MN, Alam M, Bozkurt M et al (2010) Functional anatomy of the Achilles tendon. Knee Surg Sports Traumatol Arthrosc 18:638–643. doi:10.1007/s00167-010-1083-7

Duffy FJ, Seiler JG, Gelberman RH, Hergrueter CA (1995) Growth factors and canine flexor tendon healing: initial studies in uninjured and repair models. J Hand Surg Am 20:645–649. doi:10.1016/S0363-5023(05)80284-9

Fenwick SA, Hazleman BL, Riley GP (2002) The vasculature and its role in the damaged and healing tendon. Arthritis Res 4:252–260

Fernandez-Sarmiento J (2012) Evaluación de la reparación tendinosa tras la aplicación de plasma rico en factores de crecimiento en un modelo experimental de rotura del tendón de aquiles en oveja. Universidad de Córdoba, Córdoba

Fernandez-Sarmiento J, Dominguez J, Granados M, et al (2012) Histological study of the influence of plasma rich in growth factors (PRGF) in a model of tenotomized achilles tendon in sheep. KSSTA 20, Supple. issn:0942-2056.

Fernández-Sarmiento JA, Domínguez JM, Granados MM et al (2013) Histological study of the influence of plasma rich in growth factors (PRGF) on the healing of divided Achilles tendons in sheep. J Bone Joint Surg Am 95:246–255. doi:10.2106/JBJS.K.01659

Hsu C, Chang J (2004) Clinical implications of growth factors in flexor tendon wound healing. J Hand Surg Am 29:551–563. doi:10.1016/j.jhsa.2004.04.020

Hubbard SR (1999) Structural analysis of receptor tyrosine kinases. Prog Biophys Mol Biol 71:343–358

Lemmon MA, Schlessinger J (2010) Cell signaling by receptor tyrosine kinases. Cell 141:1117–1134. doi:10.1016/j.cell.2010.06.011

Llusá M, Merí A, Ruano D (2006) Manual y Atlas Fotográfico de Anatomía del Aparato Locomotor, 1st edn. Panamericana, Madrid

López-Nájera D (2014) Valoración biomecánica del efecto de la aplicación del plasma rico en plaquetas en la reparación de una lesión estándar del tendón Calcáneo Común en Ovejas. Estudio Experimental. Universidad Cardenal Herrera - CEU

López-Nájera D, Rubio-Zaragoza M, Sopena-Juncosa JJ et al (2015) Effects of plasma rich in growth factors (PRGF) on biomechanical properties of Achilles tendon repair. Knee Surg Sports Traumatol Arthrosc. doi:10.1007/s00167-015-3725-2

Maffulli N (1999) Rupture of the Achilles tendon. J Bone Joint Surg Am 81:1019–1036

Maganaris CN, Narici MV, Maffulli N (2008) Biomechanics of the Achilles tendon. Disabil Rehabil 30:1542–1547. doi:10.1080/09638280701785494

Massagué J (2012) TGFβ signalling in context. Nat Rev Mol Cell Biol 13:616–630. doi:10.1038/nrm3434

McCarrel T, Minas T, Fortier L (2012) Optimization of leukocyte concentration in platelet-rich plasma for the treatment of tendinopathy. J Bone Joint Surg Am 94(19):e143

Molloy T, Wang Y, Murrell G (2003) The roles of growth factors in tendon and ligament healing. Sports Med 33:381–394

O'Shea JJ, Gadina M, Schreiber RD (2002) Cytokine signaling in 2002: new surprises in the Jak/Stat pathway. Cell 109(Suppl):S121–S131

Sánchez M, Anitua E, Orive G et al (2009) Platelet-rich therapies in the treatment of orthopaedic sport injuries. Sports Med 39:345–354

Sciore P, Boykiw R, Hart DA (1998) Semiquantitative reverse transcription-polymerase chain reaction analysis of mRNA for growth factors and growth factor receptors from normal and healing rabbit medial collateral ligament tissue. J Orthop Res 16:429–437. doi:10.1002/jor.1100160406

Tsubone T, Moran SL, Amadio PC et al (2004) Expression of growth factors in canine flexor tendon after laceration in vivo. Ann Plast Surg 53:393–397

Wang JH-C, Guo Q, Li B (2012) Tendon biomechanics and mechanobiology—a minireview of basic concepts and recent advancements. J Hand Ther 25:133–40; quiz 141. doi:10.1016/j.jht.2011.07.004

Yoshikawa Y, Abrahamsson SO (2001) Dose-related cellular effects of platelet-derived growth factor-BB differ in various types of rabbit tendons in vitro. Acta Orthop Scand 72:287–292. doi:10.1080/00016470152846646

Biomaterials for Tendon Regeneration

13

Nuno Sevivas, Guilherme França, Nuno Oliveira, Hélder Pereira, K.W. Ng, António Salgado, and João Espregueira-Mendes

Contents

N. Sevivas (✉)
Life and Health Sciences Research Institute (ICVS), School of Medicne, University of Minho, Campus de Gualtar, 4710-057 Braga, Portugal

ICVS/3B's - PT Government Associate Laboratory, Braga/Guimarães, Portugal

Orthopaedics Department, Hospital de Braga, Braga, Portugal

Orthopaedics Department, Hospital Privado de Braga, Braga, Portugal

Clínica Espregueira-Mendes, FIFA Medical Centre of Excellence, Estádio do Dragão, Porto, Portugal
e-mail: nunosevivas@med.uminho.pt

G. França • N. Oliveira
Orthopaedics Department, Hospital de Braga, Braga, Portugal

H. Pereira
Life and Health Sciences Research Institute (ICVS), School of Medicine, University of Minho, Campus de Gualtar, 4710-057 Braga, Portugal

ICVS/3B's - PT Government Associate Laboratory, Braga/Guimarães, Portugal

3B's Research Group, Biomaterials, Biodegradables and Biomimetics, Department of Polymer Engineering, University of Minho, Headquarters of the European Institute of Excellence on Tissue Engineering and Regenerative Medicine, AvePark, Zona Industrial da Gandra, S. Cláudio do Barco, 4806-909 Caldas das Taipas, Guimarães, Portugal

Orthopaedics Department, Centro Hospitalar Póvoa de Varzim – Vila do Conde, Póvoa de Varzim, Portugal

K.W. Ng
School of Materials Science and Engineering, Nanyang Technological University, Singapore, Singapore

A. Salgado
Life and Health Sciences Research Institute (ICVS), School of Medicine, University of Minho, Campus de Gualtar, 4710-057 Braga, Portugal

ICVS/3B's - PT Government Associate Laboratory, Braga/Guimarães, Portugal

J. Espregueira-Mendes
Life and Health Sciences Research Institute (ICVS), School of Medicine, University of Minho, Campus de Gualtar, 4710-057 Braga, Portugal

ICVS/3B's - PT Government Associate Laboratory, Braga/Guimarães, Portugal

Clínica Espregueira-Mendes, FIFA Medical Centre of Excellence, Estádio do Dragão, Porto, Portugal

3B's Research Group, Biomaterials, Biodegradables and Biomimetics, Department of Polymer Engineering, University of Minho, Headquarters of the European Institute of Excellence on Tissue Engineering and Regenerative Medicine, AvePark, Zona Industrial da Gandra, S. Cláudio do Barco, 4806-909 Caldas das Taipas, Guimarães, Portugal

G.L. Canata et al. (eds.), *Muscle and Tendon Injuries*, DOI 10.1007/978-3-662-54184-5_13

13.1 Introduction

Tendons exhibit high mechanical strength, flexibility, and extensibility to perform their unique role as an active element during movement and physical exercise (Kirkendall and Garrett 1997). However, too much stress and force can be exerted on it, increasing the risk of injury, namely, at the tendon–bone interface (TBi) (Maffulli et al. 2003). Moreover, they have low metabolic rate and well-developed anaerobic mechanisms that allow them to sustain tensile loads for long periods of time. Unfortunately, this low metabolic rate also results in a slow healing after injury (Sharma and Maffulli 2005).

As a consequence the healing response is suboptimal causing scar tissue formation, which implies inferior mechanical properties (Butler et al. 2003; Khatod et al. 2003; Parchi et al. 2016; Woo et al. 1999, 2006). Physicians treat primarily tendon lesions by conservative treatment hoping that "nature" could heal the structural lesion and helping to recover or compensate function. However, when the natural healing process is not effective, surgery is needed but in this kind of lesions remains an imperfect solution. In that case, current suturing techniques do not have the expected success, often resulting in poor healing (Butler et al. 2003; Khatod et al. 2003; Laurencin and Freeman 2005; Woo et al. 2006).

Sometimes tissue transplantation is required in the surgical technique, and in that case autografting is often the preferred choice. Autografts provide a good method of replacement without the immunological response and risk of disease transmission that the allografts may carry (Hinsenkamp et al. 2012). However, there are limitations in its use related with the available quantity of autografts and also donor site morbidity concerns (Hollister 2005). As the autograft is harvested from the patient, it requires an additional procedure often resulting in pain, decreased motion, muscle atrophy, and tendonitis (Laurencin and Freeman 2005; Miller and Azar 2008; Petrigliano et al. 2006; Spindler et al. 2004; Vunjak-Novakovic et al. 2004).

The shortage of transplantable tissues and organs, as well as the donor site morbidity, has therefore boosted the birth and evolution of tissue engineering (TE) and regenerative medicine (Griffith and Naughton 2002). So, in order to overcome the existing limitations, tissue engineering has been developing new approaches combining cells, growth factors, nanoparticles, and scaffolds. The ultimate objective is to obtain a tissue that replicates the mechanical and structural properties of the native tissue.

Although TE has not progressed as successfully as anticipated since it was formalized, it still holds great potential in providing clinicians with a range of alternative solutions to repair and regenerate wounded tissues. The central dogma of TE is to use a scaffold or template as a physical and biochemical platform that mimics physiological conditions for effective wound regeneration by guiding cellular processes. Natural polymers, such as proteins and polysaccharides, are good potential materials as templates for tissue regeneration owing to their natural bioinductive abilities to improve cell–material interactions (Malafaya et al. 2007).

13.2 Tendon

Full understanding of tendon structure, behavior, and function is essential to develop and apply biomaterials as new treatment alternatives or adjuncts.

Tendon and ligament mechanical properties vary depending on their location and function, and biomaterials developed to repair these tissues must replicate those same properties in order to be successful (Hammoudi and Temenoff 2011).

Low vascularity and low cellularity associated to a rich extracellular matrix (ECM) are unique characteristics of the tendon.

13.2.1 Structure

Tendons are soft, fibrous tissues that have an organized hierarchical structure (Thorpe and Screen 2016; Wang 2006). They connect muscle to bone, and their main function is to transfer force generated from muscle to bony structures resulting in joint movement (Sharma and Maffulli 2005; Thorpe and Screen 2016).

Parallel-aligned triple-helical cross-linked collagen forms the basic component of the structure, the fibrils (10–500 nm). Various fibrils aggregate with each other and with resident tenocytes and tenoblasts to form a fiber (1–20 μm). Collagen fibers form a sinusoidal crimp structure, responsible for the early resistance to sudden tensile loads applied to tendons during muscle contraction (Khatod and Amiel 2003; Sharma and Maffulli 2005).

Fibers are surrounded by endotenon and gather in an ordered fashion to form subfascicles and fascicles (20–200 μm) that are surrounded by the epitenon. Endotenon and epitenon form a continuous fine layer of connective tissue and serve as conduits to nerves, blood, and lymphatic vessels (Hammoudi and Temenoff 2011; Sharma and Maffulli 2005; Thorpe and Screen 2016).

Tendon surface is then covered with paratenon (in regions away from joints) or synovial sheath (around joints), to facilitate movement and guarantee smooth gliding through surrounding tissues (Benjamin and Ralphs 2000; Thorpe and Screen 2016; Wang 2006). The tendon structure is represented in Fig. 13.1.

13.2.1.1 Extracellular Matrix (ECM)

As other connective tissues, tendons are mainly composed of water (55–70% total weight) (Sharma and Maffulli 2005; Thorpe and Screen

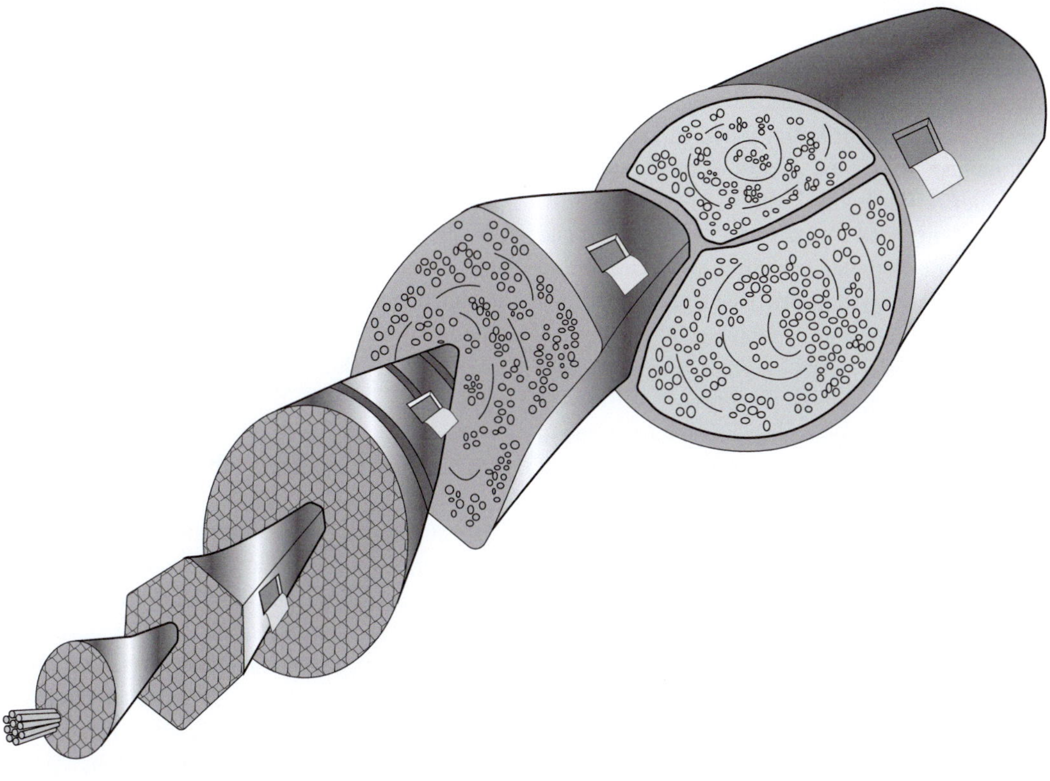

Fig. 13.1 Tendon structure (ascending order): fibrils, fibers, subfascicles, fascicles and tendon

2016). Tendon dry weight is mainly formed by ECM and cells account only for roughly 20% of total volume (Benjamin and Ralphs 2000).

The most common protein in tendons ECM is collagen, and 95% of it is **collagen type I** oriented mainly in a longitudinal fashion granting tendons high tensile strength (Hammoudi and Temenoff 2011; Thorpe and Screen 2016). **Collagen type III**, the second most common type (Thorpe and Screen 2016), is found primarily in endotenon and epitenon and, represents a less organized matrix associated with decreased strength but increased pliability. It is the main collagen type synthesized in the early phases of tendon and ligament healing (Hammoudi and Temenoff 2011; Wang 2006). **Collagen type V** can be found in the center of collagen type I fibrils and may contribute to fibrillogenesis.

Other types of collagen exist in lesser quantities (II, VI, IX, X, and XI), usually at insertion sites where they are thought to reduce stress over interface zones (Hammoudi and Temenoff 2011).

Elastin is another protein commonly found in tendons and ligaments reaching 2% of tendon dry weight (Sharma and Maffulli 2005). It usually bounds to collagen type I fibrils forming elastic fibers. They can store return energy and contribute to recover of fibril crimp structure after strain is applied to elastic fibers (Hammoudi and Temenoff 2011; Wang 2006).

Proteoglycans comprise 1–5% of tendon and ligament dry weight depending on location and function. Among their described functions, they maintain hydration of tendons, provide lubrication to the gliding fibers, improve adaptation and tensile strength, enhance compressive stiffness in fibrocartilaginous regions, and also have a role in tendon development (Hammoudi and Temenoff 2011; Thorpe and Screen 2016). The most common proteoglycan is **decorin,** making up to 80% of proteoglycan dry weight in tendons. It contributes to tendon development and is predominantly found in tensile zones, allowing tendon adaptation to tensile loads (Hammoudi and Temenoff 2011; Thorpe and Screen 2016).

Fibronectin and tenascin-C are glycoproteins found in small quantities in tendons and ligaments, and they contribute to ECM repair and mechanical stability after injury mainly by their interaction with collagen and other structural components (Hammoudi and Temenoff 2011). Moreover, Tenascin-C expression is upregulated in tendinopathy (Sharma and Maffulli 2005).

13.2.1.2 Cells

There are several types of cells present in tendons, but the majority of these cells are fibroblasts, and they are responsible for synthesizing and organizing ECM components (Benjamin and Ralphs 2000; Hammoudi and Temenoff 2011; Sharma and Maffulli 2005; Wang 2006). Fibroblasts that reside between collagen fibers, known as tenocytes, provide a complex network of cytoplasmic processes connecting adjacent cells and surrounding collagen fibers (Thorpe and Screen 2016). They are also the main cells recruited in response to injury and are able to amplify inflammatory response by secreting essential chemotactic and growth factors. Other cell types, namely, tenoblasts (tenocyte progenitor cells), chondrocytes, and synovial and vascular cells, can be found in the interfascicular space (Dyment and Galloway 2015; Sharma and Maffulli 2005).

13.2.1.3 Tendon Blood Supply

Tendon blood supply is very variable. In most of cases, tendons are supplied by intrinsic vessels (myotendinous and osteotendinous junctions) and extrinsic vessels that penetrate synovial sheath or paratenon and course deeper into the tendon through epitenon and endotenon (Sharma and Maffulli 2005).

13.2.2 Tendon–Bone interface (TBi)

TBi is a highly organized structure where two different tissues connect allowing the transmission of force produced by the muscle to the bone and resulting in movement. Briefly, it is composed of a gradual interface between tendon and bone which is composed of four zones: a dense tendon zone, non-mineralized fibrocartilage, mineralized fibrocartilage, and bone (Benjamin and Ralphs 1998).

Moreover, the tendon is composed of a highly organized collagenous extracellular matrix and parallel collagen fibers that are oriented along the long axis of the tendon. Some specialized fibroblasts (tenocytes) are distributed in parallel rows between the collagen fibers, and a few vascular structures are evident. Then, the dense collagen fibers of the tendon gradually intermesh with fibrocartilage, and the latter becomes progressively mineralized and continues into the adjacent cortical bone. There is also a distinct transition line between the mineralized and the non-mineralized fibrocartilage known as tidemark. The tidemark is a relative straight line, which indicates the production of a flat surface during the mineralization process. A histological photograph is provided showing the histological characteristics of TBi (Fig. 13.2).

13.3 Injury, Healing, and Repair

The tendon healing process after injury or surgical repair is usually predictable with three overlapping stages—(1) inflammation, (2) proliferation/matrix production, and (3) remodeling (Hope and Saxby 2007; Sharma and Maffulli 2005). In this process, the recruitment and activation of intrinsic tenocytes peaks in the proliferation phase where they are recruited from the paratenon, endotenon, and epitenon, migrate to the wound site, and begin proliferating (Garner et al. 1989; Yang et al. 2013a). All sources of tenocytes are important in synthesizing an extracellular matrix and in establishing an internal neovascular network (James et al. 2008).

In the tendon healing process and more specifically in the inflammatory phase, various kinds of cells, including fibroblasts/tenocytes,

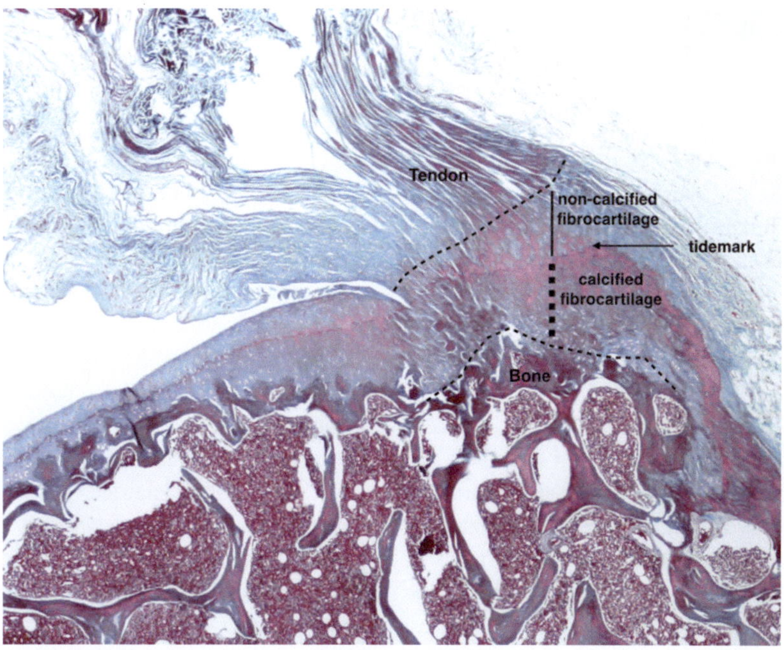

Fig. 13.2 TBi histology. The normal histology of the intact TBi is composed of four consecutive zones: a dense tendon zone, non-mineralized fibrocartilage, mineralized fibrocartilage, and bone. The tendon collagen fibers are typically oriented along the long axis of the tendon and the fibrocartilage zone becomes progressively mineralized toward the bone border. There is also a tidemark, a well-defined transition line between the non-mineralized and mineralized fibrocartilage, which indicates the production of a flat surface during the mineralization process. (Mason's Trichrome, original magnification 40×)

platelets, and MSCs, enter the wounded area, and cellular interactions play a crucial role in the healing process (Woo et al. 1999). In particular, BMSCs contribute to the process of tendon healing (Young et al. 1998). However, in the contribution of MSCs to the healing process, it is still unclear as to whether the effects are obtained by differentiation of MSCs themselves into tenocytes at the injury site (Smith and Webbon 2005) or instead they act enhancing the local biological behaviors via cell–cell contact or by the regulative effect supplying immunomodulatory and trophic factors or whether a combination of all these mechanisms occurs (Chong et al. 2009; Lange-Consiglio et al. 2013; Yagi et al. 2010).

It is currently defended that one of the possible mechanisms of the biological effects of MSCs is from paracrine factors releasing from these cells (known as "secretome") which can control regenerative mechanisms and improve the ability to control inflammation (Lange-Consiglio et al. 2013; Sevivas et al. 2016). In fact, it has been shown that the secretome of MSCs regulates cellular functions such as proliferation, differentiation, communication, and migration (Carvalho et al. 2011; Makridakis et al. 2013; Salgado and Gimble 2013; Salgado et al. 2015; Teixeira et al. 2013, 2015). Finally, from the clinical application point of view, trophic factors produced by stem cells in the form have shown to have reparative effects in spontaneous horse tendon injuries (Lange-Consiglio et al. 2013).

However, the tendon natural healing process occurs by reactive scar formation and does not achieve to obtain a tissue with the same characteristics of native tendon. Actually, even surgical repair fails in to regenerate the characteristics of tendon or TBi, resulting in a fibrous healing tissue that leads to inferior biomechanical properties, thereby increasing the likelihood of recurrence of the tear (Carpenter et al. 1998; Kovacevic and Rodeo 2008; Lui 2015; Rodeo et al. 2007). For example, in rotator cuff's TBi healing, instead of four zones, a three-layer fibrovascular construct is formed that has significantly less fibrocartilage than normal (Huegel et al. 2015), and specifically, the zone of mineralized fibrocartilage does not reform (Gerber et al. 1999).

13.4 Scaffolds and Biomaterials

TE using biomaterials is the focus of intense investigation worldwide and will probably be one of the treatments of choice for tendon and ligament injuries. It involves the use of cells, biomaterials, growth factors, or their combinations with the aim of directing a more sophisticated healing response to promote tissue repair.

TE strategies with cells require an adequate scaffold that could contain them and where cells can adhere, interact with specific growth factors and cytokines, proliferate, differentiate, and produce extracellular matrix for the success of cell therapy procedures (Krampera et al. 2006). Moreover, it provides mechanical support and may have biological properties that may favorably influence tendon-to-bone healing (Ladermann et al. 2015). Tissue regeneration through TE techniques can be achieved by culturing isolated cells on 3D scaffolds to develop biological substitutes, and for that it is important to increase the number of isolated cells (Shimode et al. 2007). Cell adhesion to the scaffold depends on the interaction that is established in between the scaffold microstructure and the cell surface receptors denominated integrins (Mora et al. 2015).

More recently, it has been used scaffolds made of biodegradable synthetic materials, which, by providing nonpermanent support to cells, can serve as temporary matrices for tissue regeneration, progressively disappearing as the new tissue is formed (Lorbach et al. 2015). Furthermore, the development of 3D electrospun scaffolds which through their close structural resemblance to ECM provide morphological cues encouraging cell growth, the application of functional tissue engineering (FTE) in scaffold design to obtain scaffolds with adequate mechanical properties and the development of fabrication techniques and coating technologies that facilitate the integration of bioactive molecules (e.g., growth factors) with scaffolds (Breidenbach et al. 2014; Hakimi et al. 2012).

13.4.1 Basic Considerations and Scaffold Design

Depending on the type of the biomaterial used, scaffolds are divided in **synthetic**, **natural**, or **composite**. There are several requirements, which should be met when designing scaffolds for tendon TE. The material should be biocompatible, promoting new tissue formation without immunological response. Sufficient void space is an important requirement in order to allow adequate nutrient delivery to the seeded or infiltrated cell population (Hollister 2005; Petrigliano et al. 2006). In fact this void space quantified as scaffold porosity is determinant for cellular proliferation and ECM formation, which enables the scaffold integration with host tissue (Hollister 2005; Laurencin and Freeman 2005; Vunjak-Novakovic et al. 2004). The goal is to achieve the same mechanical properties (e.g., elastic modulus, toughness, and ultimate strength) as the host tissue to restore normal physiologic function and prevent stress shielding of the newly formed tissue (Laurencin and Freeman 2005; Vunjak-Novakovic et al. 2004; Woo et al. 1999, 2006).

Moreover, biodegradability is an important feature. When implanting a scaffold, it is expected that this will provide the conditions for new tissue formation at the same rate of its own degradation that occurs (Doroski et al. 2007; Laurencin and Freeman 2005; Vunjak-Novakovic et al. 2004). Synthetic scaffolds offer the advantage of being able to be tuned to have a wider variety of mechanical properties and degradation characteristics through different fabrication and processing techniques. Despite these advantages, their degradation and wear products may cause an unwanted host immune response or toxicity. Natural scaffolds do not carry these risks and are readily degraded. The most popular current technique for production of nanofibrous scaffolds is electrospinning because it is a continuous, scalable process, which allows production of fibers ranging from nanometers to microns in either a random or aligned fashion (Fig. 13.3).

13.4.2 Synthetic Scaffolds

Synthetic polymers allow precise control over molecular weight, degradation time, hydrophobicity, and other attributes, yet they may not

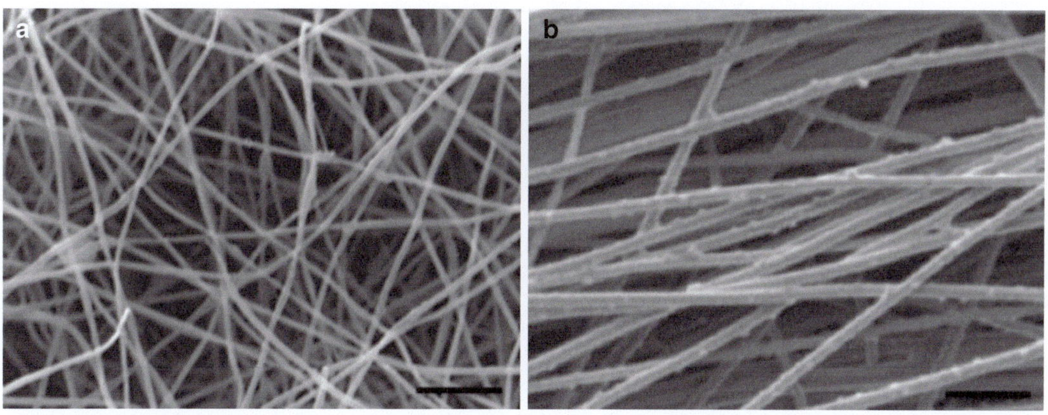

Fig. 13.3 Scanning electron microscopic images of (**a**) randomly oriented and (**b**) aligned keratin fibers fabricated by electrospinning. Scale bars represent 5 μm

interact with cells in a desired manner (Langer and Vacanti 1993).

First-generation synthetic scaffolds were inert materials, which failed to simulate the biomechanical properties of native tendon. They also did not behave as expected concerning creep, permanent deformation, stress shielding, abrasive wear and degradation, axial splitting, and extensibility (Petrigliano et al. 2006; Vunjak-Novakovic et al. 2004). Unlike the previous generation, new biomaterials have high initial strength and are designed to gradually transfer the load to the newly formed tissue, while the degradation process is progressing and the new tissue matures.

Poly(urethane) is a very heterogeneous and versatile group of polymers in what concerns their physical and mechanical properties. Depending on the fabrication process, these scaffolds can have different porosities and tunable degradation characteristics (Webb et al. 2006). These scaffolds seeded with fibroblasts have shown increased cell proliferation, matrix accumulation, and elastic modulus after a cyclic strain regimen (Webb et al. 2006). However, poly(urethanes) may release toxic degradation products and are unable to maintain similar mechanical properties to the native tendon upon degradation (Guelcher 2008).

Poly(esters) when used for tendon regeneration as scaffolds are produced in a fibrous form that is posteriorly processed to form higher ordered structures such as sheets (Deng et al. 2009; Wang et al. 2008), woven or knitted meshes (Heckmann et al. 2008), and braids (Freeman et al. 2007, 2009). PLLA, PGA, and PLGA are the most commonly used poly(esters) for tendon tissue engineering. The large interfiber pores have been shown to allow significant collagen deposition both in vitro and in vivo in a rabbit model for ACL reconstruction (Freeman et al. 2007, 2009; Van Eijk et al. 2008).

These materials have a wide range of degradation profiles and mechanical properties. However, a material that retains these properties during the replacement process by new tissue remains to be found (Vieira et al. 2009).

13.4.3 Natural Scaffolds

Also natural scaffolds have evolved during time. Initially, porous scaffolds composed of randomly oriented collagen type I fibers were used. These scaffolds without cells had suboptimal mechanical properties (Torres et al. 2000). In order to overcome this limitation, other approaches were tried. Gels composed of aligned collagen fibers seeded with MSCs and submitted to mechanical stimulation had showed significantly better mechanical properties (Altman et al. 2002; Shearn et al. 2007). MSC-seeded porous collagen sponges which generate aligned collagen fibers under cyclic strain have demonstrated increased ECM gene expression and protein deposition (Juncosa-Melvin et al. 2007). The main drawbacks of collagen matrices are the need for processing the collagen derived from animal tissue in order to remove foreign antigens and potential donor pathogens to reduce immunogenicity. These processes reduce the mechanical strength and collagen also undergoes fast in vivo degradation (Liao et al. 2008; Vieira et al. 2009).

Fibrin matrix cross-linked with thrombin and containing bone marrow stromal cells showed initially promising results, but as with collagen matrices, they are still unable to achieve the ideal mechanical properties (Liao et al. 2008; Vieira et al. 2009).

From the natural scaffolds discussed here, silk represents the strongest, being also biocompatible, promoting cell adhesion, proliferation, and ECM deposition (Vunjak-Novakovic et al. 2004). Its degradation occurs at a relative slow rate in vivo, and when its fibers are arranged in a wire rope, it achieves similar mechanical properties to those of native ligament or tendon (Chen et al. 2003, 2006; Moreau et al. 2008). However, silk presents some concerns about the adequate removal of contaminating proteins and potential immunogenicity since it is not a human native protein (Vieira et al. 2009).

13.4.4 Composite Scaffolds

Composite scaffolds are the result of the association of natural and synthetic materials in an attempt to use the positive aspects of each material in synergy. There are several studies in which fibrous scaffolds were combined with hydrogels to allow homogeneous cell seeding within the fibrous scaffold, promote the alignment of cells and ECM in the gel, reinforce the gel scaffold, and allow delivery of nutrients and growth factors through the gel (Fan et al. 2008; Hayami et al. 2010).

Some groups have been developing composite materials in order to replicate tendon interfaces. A stratified scaffold using three distinct continuous phases was produced using knitted meshes and sintered microspheres. Each phase was designed to reproduce a specific region of the tissue. This scaffold supported cell proliferation, migration, and production of ECM, maintaining distinct cellular regions and phase-specific ECM in vitro (Spalazzi et al. 2008).

Other approaches have been exploring the incorporation of ceramics with different fabrication technics to achieve graded mineral deposition (Paxton et al. 2008).

Human hair keratin offers great possibilities for tissue regeneration and repair applications because of its abundance, bioactive properties, and potential as a reliable autologous material (Rouse and Van Dyke 2010). Among existing biomaterials, fibrous matrices produced by electrospinning technique are widely used because they can mimic the nanoscale structure and complexity of the ECM and are controllable in fiber diameter and alignment (Khorshidi et al. 2016). It has been previously reported success in electrospinning randomly oriented keratin fibers by blending human hair keratin with a small amount of poly(ethylene oxide) (PEO) and showed that these are compliant for fibroblast attachment and proliferation (Sow et al. 2013).

Despite these scaffolds have an enormous potential, they are still in a premature phase of development. Their use in large scale for tendon regeneration in humans is still far from being a reality.

13.5 Tissue Engineering Strategies

The possible application of several cell types used in conjunction with biomaterials in order to improve tendon regeneration has been vastly studied. Biomaterials might be used in order to facilitate integration and recruitment of these cells from host tissue or in alternative cells can be seeded in biomaterials prior to implantation. The most promising cells for tendon regeneration are tenocytes, dermal fibroblasts, mesenchymal stem cells (MSCs), and tendon-derived stem cells (TDSCs).

13.5.1 Tenocytes

Once tenocytes are the predominant cell type found in native tendon, it is logical to integrate them in biomaterials matrices in order to try replicating native tendon. In fact, these cells are responsible for producing and maintaining the ECM which provides mechanical strength (Benjamin and Ralphs 2000). Tenocytes not only are readily incorporated into most scaffolds where they adhere and proliferate (Guelcher et al. 2008; Wang et al. 2008) but also native cells can undergo migration and infiltration into implanted scaffolds (Freeman et al. 2009). A considerable flaw in this process is the need for autogenous cells in order to avoid host immune response. These cells need to be harvested from the patient's tendons, which may lead to significant donor site morbidity.

13.5.2 Dermal Fibroblasts

Dermal fibroblasts represent a good alternative in order to overcome the difficulties and complications associated to tendon fibroblast harvesting. These cells can be obtained through a simple skin biopsy (Cornwell et al. 2004, 2007). Concerning basic behavioral characteristics, these cells adhere and proliferate in a similar way and appear to synthesize many of the same ECM components (Deng et al. 2009). Not being derived from the same tissue for which they are being applied remains the question if at long term the behavior will be similar to that of native tendon.

13.5.3 Mesenchymal Stromal Cells

Mesenchymal stromal cells are multipotent cells that can differentiate in several mesenchymal pathways. This characteristic turns these cells in a very interesting option in the field of tendon TE, with the advantage of being easy to harvest by minimally invasive needle aspiration. Also since evidence suggests MSC might be immune privileged, allogenic MSC might be used (Pittenger et al. 1999). The challenge in vivo is to achieve their maintenance and differentiation, which can be facilitated by growth factors that might be combined or delivered sequentially (Moreau et al. 2008). Human embryonic stem cells can be differentiated in MSC constituting a new source of MSC (Chen et al. 2009). However, they often cause ectopic bone formation in healed tendons which can compromise its function.

13.5.4 Tendon-Derived Stem Cells (TDSCs)

TDSCs have recently gained interest because they have the ability to promote tendon healing with no increased risk of ectopic chondro-ossification (Lui et al. 2014; Yang et al. 2013b).

13.5.5 Nanoparticles

Nanotechnology includes all techniques, which use, manipulate, or study matter between 4 and 400 atoms. Below 100 nm classic laws of Physics do not apply, which allow materials, based or manipulated with nanoparticles, to have novel properties, like size and strength beyond conventional limits (Parchi et al. 2016). These particles have vast application in tendon regeneration. They can be exploited in the manufacture of scaffolds, as carrier in gene therapy or using their anti-inflammatory properties.

Several particles have been developed and studied in order to be used in gene therapy and avoid their side effects and possible complications (Raffa et al. 2011). In an experiment to prevent peritendinous adhesion, miRNAs reducing expression of TGF-b1 were inserted into a plasmid and then were loaded into PEI-poly(lactic-co-glycolic acid) (PLGA) nanoparticles. The transfection of miRNA by PLGA nanoparticles successfully resulted in TGF-b1 inhibition, consequently inducing tendon repair, although the repaired tendon had lower strength than the control group. Due to these results, the authors concluded that pure inhibition of TGF-1b had deleterious effects, not achieving the desired healing effect (Zhou et al. 2013). The same authors hypothesized that better results could be obtained by combining TGF-1b miRNA plasmid with other growth factor's miRNAs, to be delivered simultaneously.

One of the most used and studied nanoparticles for tendon TE is silver nanoparticle (AgNP). Its ability to inhibit ATP synthesis in microorganisms, denature DNA, and block the respiratory chain made Ag be recognized as an antimicrobial agent (Morones et al. 2005). As demonstrated by in vitro experiments, AgNPs promote proliferation of primary tenocytes, as well as the production of ECM components (Kwan et al. 2014). Also in vivo these NPs have proven advantages as shown by a higher tensile modulus of tendons treated with AgNPs. Nonetheless, the tensile modulus was still significantly lower than that of a normal tendon (Kwan et al. 2014). Its antiphlogistic effect is also not negligible, reducing scar tissue formation and adhesions (Kwan et al. 2014). Other NPs have been studied as possible options for tendon regeneration although with less consistent results. A recent trend is to use these particles to enhance natural polymer matrices (Deeken et al. 2011).

13.6 Conclusion and Future Trends

Given its high frequency, low quality of tissue repair, and less than optimal clinical recovery, it is not surprising that new and innovative therapeutical strategies have become more appealing to treat tendon pathology.

The use of biomaterials, usually integrating a TE strategy, aiming to obtain a morphologically and functionally tendon similar to the original tissue is under research. Currently, its clinical use is already available but not so widespread as initially thought. However, the continuous evolution of the biomaterials and the possibility to blend it with cells and growth factors will probably allow us to regenerate tendon tissue and improve clinical outcomes when treating tendon pathology.

References

Altman G, Horan R, Martin I et al (2002) Cell differentiation by mechanical stress. FASEB J 16:270–272

Benjamin M, Ralphs JR (1998) Fibrocartilage in tendons and ligaments—an adaptation to compressive load. J Anat 193(Pt 4):481–494

Benjamin M, Ralphs J (2000) The cell and developmental biology of tendons and ligaments. Int Rev Cytol 196:85–130

Breidenbach AP, Gilday SD, Lalley AL et al (2014) Functional tissue engineering of tendon: establishing biological success criteria for improving tendon repair. J Biomech 47:1941–1948

Butler DL, Dressler M, Awad H (2003) Functional tissue engineering: assessment of function in tendon and ligament repair. In: Functional tissue engineering. Springer, New York, pp 213–226

Carpenter JE, Thomopoulos S, Flanagan CL et al (1998) Rotator cuff defect healing: a biomechanical and histologic analysis in an animal model. J Shoulder Elb Surg 7:599–605

Carvalho MM, Teixeira FG, Reis RL et al (2011) Mesenchymal stem cells in the umbilical cord: phenotypic characterization, secretome and applications in central nervous system regenerative medicine. Curr Stem Cell Res Ther 6:221–228

Chen J, Altman GH, Karageorgiou V et al (2003) Human bone marrow stromal cell and ligament fibroblast responses on RGD-modified silk fibers. J Biomed Mater Res A 67:559–570

Chen J, Horan RL, Bramono D et al (2006) Monitoring mesenchymal stromal cell developmental stage to apply on-time mechanical stimulation for ligament tissue engineering. Tissue Eng 12:3085–3095

Chen X, Song XH, Yin Z et al (2009) Stepwise differentiation of human embryonic stem cells promotes tendon regeneration by secreting fetal tendon matrix and differentiation factors. Stem Cells 27:1276–1287

Chong AK, Chang J, Go JC (2009) Mesenchymal stem cells and tendon healing. Front Biosci (Landmark Ed) 14:4598–4605

Cornwell KG, Downing BR, Pins GD (2004) Characterizing fibroblast migration on discrete collagen threads for applications in tissue regeneration. J Biomed Mater Res A 71:55–62

Cornwell KG, Lei P, Andreadis ST et al (2007) Crosslinking of discrete self-assembled collagen threads: effects on mechanical strength and cell–matrix interactions. J Biomed Mater Res A 80:362–371

Deeken CR, Cozad MJ, Bachman SL et al (2011) Characterization of bionanocomposite scaffolds comprised of amine-functionalized single-walled carbon nanotubes crosslinked to an acellular porcine tendon. J Biomed Mater Res A 96:584–594

Deng D, Liu W, Xu F et al (2009) Engineering human neo-tendon tissue in vitro with human dermal fibroblasts under static mechanical strain. Biomaterials 30:6724–6730

Doroski DM, Brink KS, Temenoff JS (2007) Techniques for biological characterization of tissue-engineered tendon and ligament. Biomaterials 28:187–202

Dyment NA, Galloway JL (2015) Regenerative biology of tendon: mechanisms for renewal and repair. Curr Mol Biol Rep 1:124–131

Fan H, Liu H, Toh SL et al (2008) Enhanced differentiation of mesenchymal stem cells co-cultured with ligament fibroblasts on gelatin/silk fibroin hybrid scaffold. Biomaterials 29:1017–1027

Freeman JW, Woods MD, Laurencin CT (2007) Tissue engineering of the anterior cruciate ligament using a braid–twist scaffold design. J Biomech 40: 2029–2036

Freeman JW, Woods MD, Cromer DA et al (2009) Tissue engineering of the anterior cruciate ligament: the viscoelastic behavior and cell viability of a novel braid–twist scaffold. J Biomater Sci Polym Ed 20:1709–1728

Garner WL, Mcdonald JA, Koo M et al (1989) Identification of the collagen-producing cells in healing flexor tendons. Plast Reconstr Surg 83:875–879

Gerber C, Schneeberger AG, Perren SM et al (1999) Experimental rotator cuff repair. A preliminary study. J Bone Joint Surg Am 81:1281–1290

Griffith LG, Naughton G (2002) Tissue engineering--current challenges and expanding opportunities. Science 295:1009–1014

Guelcher SA (2008) Biodegradable polyurethanes: synthesis and applications in regenerative medicine. Tissue Eng Part B Rev 14:3–17

Guelcher SA, Srinivasan A, Dumas JE et al (2008) Synthesis, mechanical properties, biocompatibility, and biodegradation of polyurethane networks from lysine polyisocyanates. Biomaterials 29:1762–1775

Hakimi O, Murphy R, Stachewicz U et al (2012) An electrospun polydioxanone patch for the localisation of biological therapies during tendon repair. Eur Cell Mater 24:344–357; discussion 357

Hammoudi TM, Temenoff JS (2011) Biomaterials for regeneration of tendons and ligaments. In: Burdick JA, Mauck RL (eds) Biomaterials for tissue engineering applications: a review of the past and future trends. Springer Vienna, Vienna, pp 307–341

Hayami JW, Surrao DC, Waldman SD et al (2010) Design and characterization of a biodegradable composite scaffold for ligament tissue engineering. J Biomed Mater Res A 92:1407–1420

Heckmann L, Fiedler J, Mattes T et al (2008) Interactive effects of growth factors and three-dimensional scaffolds on multipotent mesenchymal stromal cells. Biotechnol Appl Biochem 49:185–194

Hinsenkamp M, Muylle L, Eastlund T et al (2012) Adverse reactions and events related to musculoskeletal allografts: reviewed by the World Health Organisation Project NOTIFY. Int Orthop 36:633–641

Hollister SJ (2005) Porous scaffold design for tissue engineering. Nat Mater 4:518–524

Hope M, Saxby TS (2007) Tendon healing. Foot Ankle Clin 12:553–567

Huegel J, Williams AA, Soslowsky LJ (2015) Rotator cuff biology and biomechanics: a review of normal and pathological conditions. Curr Rheumatol Rep 17:476

James R, Kesturu G, Balian G et al (2008) Tendon: biology, biomechanics, repair, growth factors, and evolving treatment options. J Hand Surg Am 33:102–112

Juncosa-Melvin N, Matlin KS, Holdcraft RW et al (2007) Mechanical stimulation increases collagen type I and collagen type III gene expression of stem cell-collagen sponge constructs for patellar tendon repair. Tissue Eng 13:1219–1226

Khatod M, Amiel D (2003) Ligament biochemistry and physiology. In: Pedowitz R, O'Connor JJ, Akeson WH (eds) Daniel's knee injuries. Lippincott Williams and Wilkins, Philadelphia, pp 31–42

Khatod M, Akeson W, Amiel D (2003) Ligament injury and repair. In: Pedowitz RA, O'Connor JJ, Akeson WH (eds) Daniel's knee injuries. Lippincott Williams and Wilkins, Philadelphia, pp 185–201

Khorshidi S, Solouk A, Mirzadeh H et al (2016) A review of key challenges of electrospun scaffolds for tissue-engineering applications. J Tissue Eng Regen Med 10:715–738

Kirkendall DT, Garrett WE (1997) Function and biomechanics of tendons. Scand J Med Sci Sports 7:62–66

Kovacevic D, Rodeo SA (2008) Biological augmentation of rotator cuff tendon repair. Clin Orthop Relat Res 466:622–633

Krampera M, Pizzolo G, Aprili G et al (2006) Mesenchymal stem cells for bone, cartilage, tendon and skeletal muscle repair. Bone 39:678–683

Kwan KH, Yeung KW, Liu X et al (2014) Silver nanoparticles alter proteoglycan expression in the promotion of tendon repair. Nanomedicine 10:1375–1383

Ladermann A, Denard PJ, Collin P (2015) Massive rotator cuff tears: definition and treatment. Int Orthop 39:2403–2414

Lange-Consiglio A, Rossi D, Tassan S et al (2013) Conditioned medium from horse amniotic membrane-derived multipotent progenitor cells: immunomodulatory activity in vitro and first clinical application in tendon and ligament injuries in vivo. Stem Cells Dev 22:3015–3024

Langer R, Vacanti JP (1993) Tissue engineering. Science 260:920–926

Laurencin CT, Freeman JW (2005) Ligament tissue engineering: an evolutionary materials science approach. Biomaterials 26:7530–7536

Liao S, Chan CK, Ramakrishna S (2008) Stem cells and biomimetic materials strategies for tissue engineering. Mater Sci Eng C 28:1189–1202

Lorbach O, Baums MH, Kostuj T et al (2015) Advances in biology and mechanics of rotator cuff repair. Knee Surg Sports Traumatol Arthrosc 23:530–541

Lui PP (2015) Stem cell technology for tendon regeneration: current status, challenges, and future research directions. Stem Cells Cloning 7:163–174

Lui PP, Kong SK, Lau PM et al (2014) Allogeneic tendon-derived stem cells promote tendon healing and suppress immunoreactions in hosts: in vivo model. Tissue Eng Part A 20:2998–3009

Maffulli N, Wong J, Almekinders LC (2003) Types and epidemiology of tendinopathy. Clin Sports Med 22:675–692

Makridakis M, Roubelakis MG, Vlahou A (2013) Stem cells: insights into the secretome. Biochim Biophys Acta 1834:2380–2384

Malafaya PB, Silva GA, Reis RL (2007) Natural–origin polymers as carriers and scaffolds for biomolecules and cell delivery in tissue engineering applications. Adv Drug Deliv Rev 59:207–233

Miller R, Azar F (2008) Knee injuries. In: Canale S, Beaty J (eds) Campbell's operative orthopaedics. Mosby Elsevier, Philadelphia, pp 2346–2575

Mora MV, Iban MAR, Heredia JD et al (2015) Stem cell therapy in the management of shoulder rotator cuff disorders. World J Stem Cells 7:691–699

Moreau JE, Bramono DS, Horan RL et al (2008) Sequential biochemical and mechanical stimulation in the development of tissue-engineered ligaments. Tissue Eng A 14:1161–1172

Morones JR, Elechiguerra JL, Camacho A et al (2005) The bactericidal effect of silver nanoparticles. Nanotechnology 16:2346

Parchi PD, Vittorio O, Andreani L et al (2016) Nanoparticles for tendon healing and regeneration: literature review. Front Aging Neurosci 8

Paxton JZ, Donnelly K, Keatch RP et al (2008) Engineering the bone–ligament interface using polyethylene glycol diacrylate incorporated with hydroxyapatite. Tissue Eng A 15:1201–1209

Petrigliano FA, Mcallister DR, Wu BM (2006) Tissue engineering for anterior cruciate ligament reconstruction: a review of current strategies. Arthroscopy 22:441–451

Pittenger MF, Mackay AM, Beck SC et al (1999) Multilineage potential of adult human mesenchymal stem cells. Science 284:143–147

Raffa V, Gherardini L, Vittorio O et al (2011) Carbon nanotube-mediated wireless cell permeabilization: drug and gene uptake. Nanomedicine 6:1709–1718

Rodeo SA, Potter HG, Kawamura S et al (2007) Biologic augmentation of rotator cuff tendon-healing with use of a mixture of osteoinductive growth factors. J Bone Joint Surg Am 89:2485–2497

Rouse JG, Van Dyke ME (2010) A review of keratin-based biomaterials for biomedical applications. Materials 3:999

Salgado AJ, Gimble JM (2013) Secretome of mesenchymal stem/stromal cells in regenerative medicine. Biochimie 95:2195

Salgado AJ, Sousa JC, Costa BM et al (2015) Mesenchymal stem cells secretome as a modulator of the neurogenic niche: basic insights and therapeutic opportunities. Front Cell Neurosci 9:249

Sevivas N, Teixeira FG, Portugal R, Araujo L, Carrico LF, Ferreira N et al (2016) Mesenchymal stem cell secretome: A potential tool for the prevention of muscle degenerative changes associated with chronic rotator cuff tears. Am J Sports Med. doi:10.1177/0363546516657827

Sharma P, Maffulli N (2005) Tendon injury and tendinopathy: healing and repair. J Bone Joint Surg Am 87:187–202

Shearn JT, Juncosa-Melvin N, Boivin GP et al (2007) Mechanical stimulation of tendon tissue engineered constructs: effects on construct stiffness, repair biomechanics, and their correlation. J Biomech Eng 129:848–854

Shimode K, Iwasaki N, Majima T et al (2007) Bone marrow stromal cells act as feeder cells for tendon fibroblasts through soluble factors. Tissue Eng 13:333–341

Smith RK, Webbon PM (2005) Harnessing the stem cell for the treatment of tendon injuries: heralding a new dawn? Br J Sports Med 39:582–584

Sow WT, Lui YS, Ng KW (2013) Electrospun human keratin matrices as templates for tissue regeneration. Nanomedicine 8:531–541

Spalazzi JP, Dagher E, Doty SB et al (2008) In vivo evaluation of a multiphased scaffold designed for orthopaedic interface tissue engineering and soft tissue-to-bone integration. J Biomed Mater Res A 86:1–12

Spindler KP, Kuhn JE, Freedman KB et al (2004) Anterior cruciate ligament reconstruction autograft choice: bone-tendon-bone versus hamstring does it really matter? A systematic review. Am J Sports Med 32:1986–1995

Teixeira FG, Carvalho MM, Sousa N et al (2013) Mesenchymal stem cells secretome: a new paradigm for central nervous system regeneration? Cell Mol Life Sci 70:3871–3882

Teixeira FG, Carvalho MM, Neves-Carvalho A et al (2015) Secretome of mesenchymal progenitors from the umbilical cord acts as modulator of neural/glial proliferation and differentiation. Stem Cell Rev 11:288–297

Thorpe CT, Screen HR (2016) Tendon structure and composition. Adv Exp Med Biol 920:3–10

Torres DS, Freyman TM, Yannas IV et al (2000) Tendon cell contraction of collagen–GAG matrices in vitro: effect of cross-linking. Biomaterials 21:1607–1619

Van Eijk F, Saris DB, Creemers LB et al (2008) The effect of timing of mechanical stimulation on proliferation and differentiation of goat bone marrow stem cells cultured on braided PLGA scaffolds. Tissue Eng A 14:1425–1433

Vieira A, Guedes R, Marques A (2009) Development of ligament tissue biodegradable devices: a review. J Biomech 42:2421–2430

Vunjak-Novakovic G, Altman G, Horan R et al (2004) Tissue engineering of ligaments. Annu Rev Biomed Eng 6:131–156

Wang JH (2006) Mechanobiology of tendon. J Biomech 39:1563–1582

Wang B, Liu W, Zhang Y et al (2008) Engineering of extensor tendon complex by an ex vivo approach. Biomaterials 29:2954–2961

Webb K, Hitchcock RW, Smeal RM et al (2006) Cyclic strain increases fibroblast proliferation, matrix accumulation, and elastic modulus of fibroblast-seeded polyurethane constructs. J Biomech 39:1136–1144

Woo SL, Hildebrand K, Watanabe N et al (1999) Tissue engineering of ligament and tendon healing. Clin Orthop Relat Res 367:S312–S323

Woo SL-Y, Abramowitch SD, Kilger R et al (2006) Biomechanics of knee ligaments: injury, healing, and repair. J Biomech 39:1–20

Yagi H, Soto-Gutierrez A, Parekkadan B et al (2010) Mesenchymal stem cells: mechanisms of immunomodulation and homing. Cell Transplant 19:667–679

Yang G, Rothrauff BB, Tuan RS (2013a) Tendon and ligament regeneration and repair: clinical relevance and developmental paradigm. Birth Defects Res C Embryo Today 99:203–222

Yang Y, Zhang J, Qian Y et al (2013b) Superparamagnetic iron oxide is suitable to label tendon stem cells and track them in vivo with MR imaging. Ann Biomed Eng 41:2109–2119

Young RG, Butler DL, Weber W et al (1998) Use of mesenchymal stem cells in a collagen matrix for Achilles tendon repair. J Orthop Res 16:406–413

Zhou Y, Zhang L, Zhao W et al (2013) Nanoparticle-mediated delivery of TGF-β1 miRNA plasmid for preventing flexor tendon adhesion formation. Biomaterials 34:8269–8278

New Strategies for Muscular Repair and Regeneration

14

M. Cianforlini, V. Coppa, M. Grassi, and A. Gigante

Contents

M. Cianforlini • V. Coppa • M. Grassi • A. Gigante (✉)
Department of Clinical and Molecular Sciences, School of Medicine, Università Politecnica delle Marche, Via Tronto 10/60126, Ancona, Italy
e-mail: a.gigante@univpm.it

14.1 Introduction

Skeletal muscle injuries can stem from a variety of events, including direct, such as muscle lacerations and contusions, and indirect trauma, such as strains, and also degenerative diseases, such as muscular dystrophies (Huard et al. 2002).

Many classifications are used for muscle injuries, which sometimes causes limitations to the comprehensive study of muscle injuries and discrepancies in the uniformity for their categorization and description. In human sport clinics, the diagnosis of muscle injury is adequate in most cases, but imaging modalities such as ultrasonography, computed tomography (CT), or magnetic resonance imaging (MRI) are important to differentiate between structural lesions and functional disorders and to determine the extent of the injury.

A minor muscle injury can regenerate completely and spontaneously, whereas after severe injuries, muscle healing is incomplete, often resulting in the formation of fibrotic tissue that compromises muscle function. Despite the frequent occurrence and the presence of a body of data on the pathophysiology of muscle injuries, none of the treatment strategies adopted to date have been shown to be really effective in strictly controlled trials. Most current muscle injury treatments are based on limited experimental and clinical data and/or were only empirically tested.

G.L. Canata et al. (eds.), *Muscle and Tendon Injuries*, DOI 10.1007/978-3-662-54184-5_14

14.2 Physiopathology and Muscle Healing Process

The pathogenic process consists in consequent phases:

- Degeneration and necrosis
- Inflammation and cellular response
- Regeneration and repair
- Remodeling and fibrosis

14.2.1 Degeneration and Necrosis

The initial phase is characterized by rupture and necrosis of the myofibers. The gap created is filled with a hematoma. Late elimination of the hematoma is known to delay skeletal muscle regeneration (Beiner et al. 1999) and to promote fibrosis interfering with functional recovery.

14.2.2 Inflammation and Cellular Response

Neutrophils are the first inflammatory cells infiltrating the lesion. A large number of pro-inflammatory molecules such as cytokines (TNF-α, IL-6), chemokines (CCL17, CCL2), and growth factors (FGF, HGF, IGF-I, VEGF, TGF-β1) are secreted by neutrophils in order to create a chemo-attractive microenvironment for other inflammatory cells such as monocytes and macrophages (Tidball 1995; Toumi and Best 2003). Two types of macrophages are identified during muscle regeneration (McLennan 1996). Macrophages, infiltrating injured muscle, are key players of the healing process (Zhao et al. 2016), able to participate in the muscle regeneration process or to favor fibrosis (Munoz-Canoves and Serrano 2015).

Finally, the arrival in the damage tissue of the T lymphocytes plays an important role in the local vascularization through adhesion molecule secretion, product of growth factors (GFs), and cytokines. With the intervention of the T lymphocytes, the inflammatory response undergoes an acceleration.

14.2.3 Regeneration and Repair

Phagocytosis of damaged tissue is followed by myofibers regeneration, leading to satellite cell activation. Muscle regeneration usually starts during the first 4–5 days after injury, peaks at 2 weeks, and then gradually diminishes 3–4 weeks after injury. It is a multiple-step process including activation/proliferation of satellite cells (SCs), repair and maturation of damaged muscle fibers, and connective tissue formation. A fine balance between these mechanisms is essential for a full recovery of the contractile muscle function. Muscle fibers are postmitotic cells, which do not have the capacity to divide. Following an injury, damaged muscle fibers cannot be repaired without the presence of adult muscle stem cells (Relaix and Zammit 2012; Sambasivan et al. 2011). SCs are skeletal muscle stem cell located between the plasma membrane of myofibers and the basal lamina. Their regenerative capabilities are essential to repair skeletal muscle after injury (Hurme and Kalimo 1992; Lipton and Schultz 1979; Dumont et al. 2015). In adult muscles, SCs are found in a quiescent state and represent, depending on species, age, muscle location, and muscle type, around 5–10% of skeletal muscle cells (Rocheteau et al. 2015).

After injury, SCs become activated, proliferate, and give rise to myogenic precursor cells, known as myoblasts. After entering the differentiation process, myoblasts form new myotubes or fuse with damaged myofibers and ultimately mature in functional myofibers. Following activation, SCs proliferate and generate a population of myoblasts that can either differentiate to repair damaged fibers or, for a small proportion, self-renew to maintain the SC pool for possible future demands of muscle regeneration (Collins 2006; Dhawan and Rando 2005).

14.2.4 Remodeling and Fibrosis

The last phase is characterized by maturation of regenerated myofibers with recovery of muscle functional capacity and also fibrosis and scar tissue formation. The presence of fibrin and fibronectin into the injury site initiates the formation of an extracellular matrix that is rapidly invaded by fibroblasts (Darby et al. 2016; Desmouliere and Gabbiani 1995). Fibrogenic cytokines such as transforming growth factor-β1 (TGF-β1) participate to excessive fibroblast/myofibroblast proliferation and to an increase in type I/III collagens and laminin and fibronectin production (Lehto et al. 1985). In its initial phase, the fibrotic response is beneficial, stabilizing the tissue and acting as a scaffold for myofiber regeneration. Many growth factors are involved in the development of fibrosis, such as connective tissue growth factor (CTGF), platelet-derived growth factor (PDGF), or myostatin. TGF-β1, by stimulating fibroblasts/myofibroblasts to produce extracellular proteins such as fibronectin and type I/III collagen, has been identified as the key element in this process (Mann et al. 2011). Although fibroblasts are the major collagen-producing cells in skeletal muscle, TGF-β1 has also an effect directly on myoblasts causing their conversion to myofibroblasts.

The phases of muscle healing are almost the same in all muscle injuries (Fig. 14.1) but the functional recovery changes. Usually the healing process leads to muscle regeneration with a different scar tissue area. In the best of case the healing provides to complete resorption of the hematoma, in the almost complete regeneration of muscle damage tissue and so in a complete functional recovery that means the athlete is able to produce the same pre-injury muscle work (Huard et al. 2002). Late elimination of the hematoma is known to delay skeletal muscle regeneration, to improve fibrosis, and to reduce biomechanical properties of the healing muscle that have a negative influence on the functional recovery of the athlete. Furthermore, in rare case of major muscle injuries, some complications like myositis ossificans, cystic degeneration, heterotopic ossifications, and liquid flapper may occur.

14.3 Treatment

Most muscle injuries respond well to conservative treatment. The main indication to surgery, depending on the sport activity and the muscle group involved, is a subtotal or complete lesion of the muscle belly or an avulsion of the tendon.

The treatment strategy should be rapid and based on a correct clinical examination and instrumental diagnosis. The main objectives of the treatment are to reduce recurrence rates particularly in elite athletes, where decisions regarding return to play and player availability have significant financial or strategic consequences for the player and the team, and to minimize the absence from sport.

The pain is the first symptom and should be treated because it generates a state of muscular contraction or analgesic attitude that often affects the healing process.

PRICE (protection, rest, ice, compression, and elevation) has been central to acute soft tissue injury management for many years.

POLICE, a new acronym, which represents protection, optimal loading, ice compression, and elevation, is not simply a formula but a reminder to clinicians to think differently and seek out new and innovative strategies for safe and effective loading in acute soft tissue injury management. Optimal loading is an umbrella term for any mechanotherapy intervention and includes a wide range of manual techniques currently available; indeed, the term may include manual techniques such as massage refined to maximize the mechano-effect (Bleakley et al. 2012).

After 24–48 h from the injury, it is possible to know the lesion severity and to make decisions for recovery program. The treatment should be based on natural evolution: in the first 24–48 h, the edema and hematoma promote the fibroblast organization, and they realize the connective neoformation between 7th and 15th days.

Therefore, it is important to consider this process, because the treatment affects the scar, depending on the supplied stimuli.

The new tissue is composed of collagen maturation and it is breakable and sensible to mechanical stress. Tensile stresses allow an increase of the elasticity up to a maximum of 20%, while a load of 10–12 kg per mm^2 leads to the breakdown of the collagen fibers (Sallay et al. 1996).

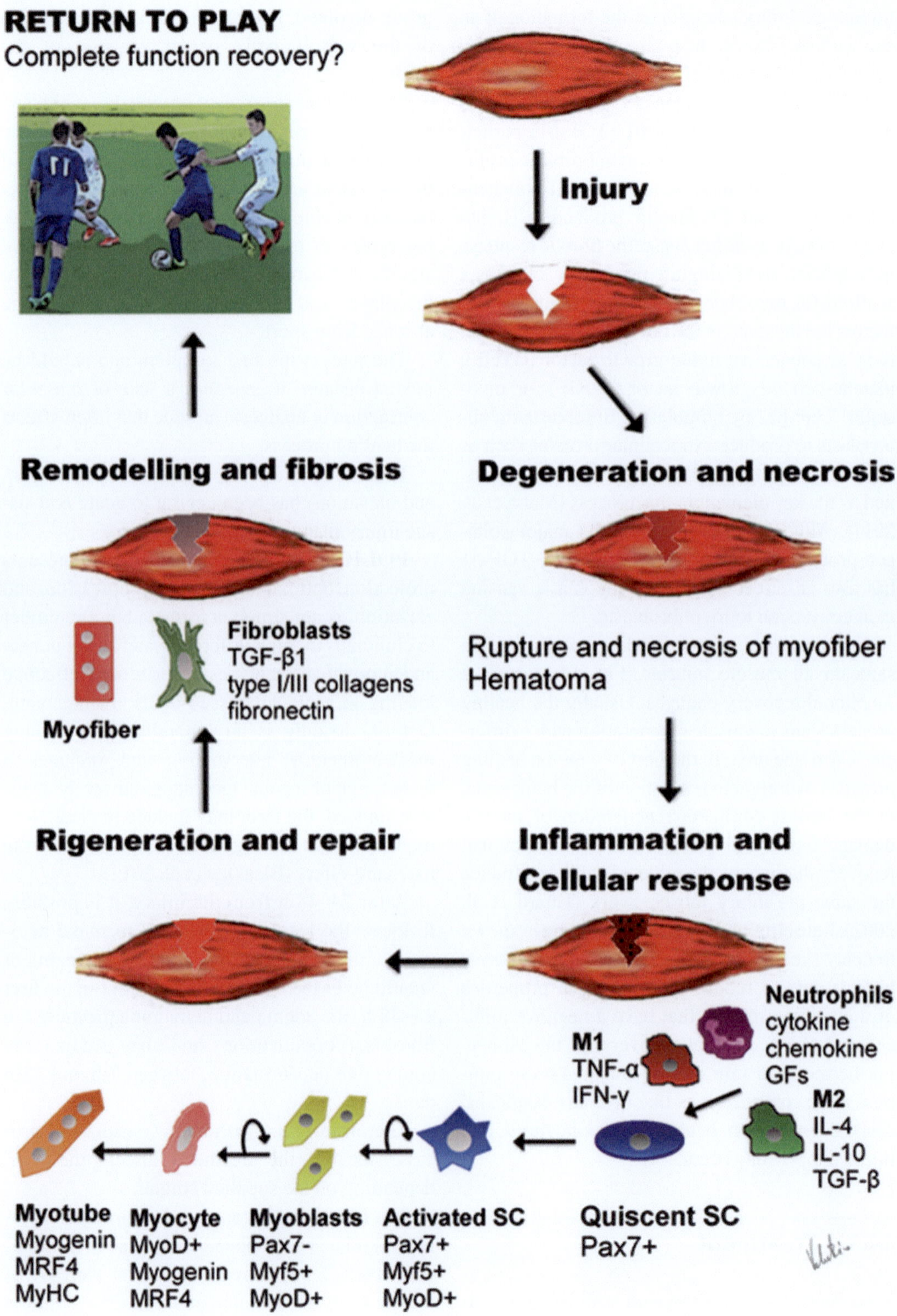

Fig. 14.1 The phases of muscle healing are almost the same in all muscle injuries after indirect trauma, but the functional recovery changes, and it is almost always incomplete for the presence of fibrotic tissue

Fisiochinesiterapic treatment in this phase should respect the healing process. The prevention of adhesions is by massage therapy initially distant from the outbreak and then, depending on the evolution, even in the scar but not earlier than 10–15 days (Järvinen et al. 2007). We should try to obtain an elastic scar in the muscle and a solid scar in the transmission structures (tendons and apparatus myoentesico) or in stabilization structures (ligaments, capsule, bands).

About **NSAIDs** some disputes exist on administration time. Some authors recommend using these drugs from the start and to suspend them after 3–5 days. Other authors indicate that the use of anti-inflammatory interferes with chemotaxis cell; with an inhibition of regenerative response, necessary for the formation of new muscle cells; and with pain that is an important parameter to the management of the first phases. These studies suggest to postpone the administration of anti-inflammatory on the 2nd or 4th day following the accident. It is considered more appropriate to use anti-inflammatory drugs from 3rd to 6th day and suspend them after the injury.

Mechanical stimulation may offer a simple and effective approach to enhance skeletal muscle regeneration. Muscle stretching can be passive or active assisted. There is no evidence that passive stretching is superior to an active protocol in terms of stretching and muscle elasticity. Mechanical forces are as important biological regulators as chemicals and genes and underline the immense potential of developing mechanotherapies to treat muscle damage (Cezar et al. 2016). Concentric and eccentric muscle contraction exercises can be started when the isometric contraction can be performed without pain. A recent study also demonstrated that a treatment based on ultrasound-guided intra-tissue percutaneous electrolysis (EPI technique) enhances the treatment of muscle injuries (Abat et al. 2015). Altogether, these results suggest that mechanical stimulation should be considered as a possible therapy to improve muscle regeneration and repair.

Kinesiotaping (neuromuscular bandage) has been introduced in recent decades. The rationale is to reduce tension on the lesion site by lifting the skin from the subcutaneous and deep tissue: the probable analgesic effect on the drainage process of these materials should get better the edema and swelling.

After scar formation and joint stability gained, we will begin on specific recovery that aims to rebuild muscle tropism, the motor pattern, and muscular strength. This stage use for the muscular tropism isometric exercises without loads and isotonic exercises (concentric and eccentric) with variable loads (from 2 to 5 kg). The sessions are to be divided in the day to avoid muscle overstress.

The different muscle contraction used in therapy must comply with the real operating conditions in athletic performance, so that the recovery of sports is as fast as possible. These treatments allow the athlete recovering quickly, while the athlete field observation in the post-treatment phases can confirm the healing and allow return to play (Gigante et al. 2014).

14.4 New Strategies for Muscular Repair and Regeneration

14.4.1 Growth Factors

Growth factors (GFs) are biologically active molecules, synthetized by the injured tissue or by other cell types into the inflammatory site, which are released in the extracellular space and modulate the regenerative response. They play a variety of roles in the different stages of muscle regeneration (Table 14.1).

Hepatocyte growth factor (HGF), fibroblast growth factor (FGF), and platelet-derived growth factor (PDGF) are of interest because of their capacity to stimulate satellite cells (Sheehan et al. 2000).

Insulin-like growth factor-1 (IGF-I) appears to be of particular importance for the muscle regeneration process. IGF-I stimulates myoblast proliferation and differentiation (Engert et al. 1996) and is implicated in the regulation of muscle growth (Schiaffino and Mammucari 2011). IGF-I improved muscle healing, and histology of the injected muscle revealed fibrosis within the

Table 14.1 Growth factor roles during the phases of muscle healing after a trauma

Growth factors	Physiological effects	Potential benefit	Main role
IGF-1	– Promotes myoblast proliferation and differentiation in vitro – Hypertrophic effect essential for muscle growth during development and regeneration – Existence of a muscle specific isoform (m IGF-1)	– Serial injections of IGF-1 improve muscle healing in vivo (Menetrey et al. 2000) – Chemotactic for fibroblasts, increase collagen production, and fibrosis development	– Central role in muscle regeneration and hypertrophy
VEGF	– Promotes angiogenesis in the healing process – Promotes myoblast migration, proliferation, and survival	– VEGF administration improves muscle regeneration (Deasy et al. 2009)	– Creates a neo-capillary network that improves the migration of satellite cell
HGF	– Promotes myoblast proliferation and inhibits myoblast differentiation (Anderson 2016) – A second set of HGF production is crucial for inflammation resolution after injury (Proto et al. 2015)	– Injection of HGF into injured muscle increased myoblast numbers but blocked the regeneration process (Miller et al. 2000)	– Activates satellite cells in the early phase of regeneration
TGF-β1	– Key regulator of the balance between muscle fibrosis and muscle regeneration – Inhibits satellite cell proliferation and differentiation in vitro	– Anti fibrotic therapy by blocking overexpression of TGF-β1 improves muscle regeneration	– Pro-fibrotic factor
FGF	– FGF-6 and FGF-2 promote satellite cell proliferation but inhibit myogenic differentiation	– Anti fibrotic therapy by blocking overexpression of TGF-β1 improves muscle regeneration (Hwang et al. 2016)	– Stimulates fibroblast proliferation

lacerated site, despite high level of IGF-I production (Lee et al. 2000). However, the efficacy of direct injection of recombinant proteins is limited by the high concentration of the factor typically required to elicit a measurable effect. This is mainly due to the bloodstream rapid clearance of these molecules and their relatively short biological half-lives.

Vascular endothelial growth factor (VEGF) has a potent angiogenic effect and is expressed in high concentration in healing flexor tendons 7–10 days following repair in animal models (Würgler-Hauri et al. 2007). Increased vascularity may improve tendon healing and contribute positively to the repair process. By targeting simultaneously angiogenesis and myogenesis, it was shown that combined delivery of VEGF and IGF-I enhances muscle regenerative process (Borselli et al. 2010).

In this direction, the use of platelet-rich plasma (PRP) is considered as a possible alternative approach based on the ability of autologous growth factors to improve skeletal muscle regeneration (Hamid et al. 2014; Hammond et al. 2009). Approximately 70% of the stored factors are secreted within the first 10 min following activation, and within the first hour almost 100% have been secreted. The degranulation of the α-granules results in the release of PDGF, TGF-β, insulin-like growth factor (IGF), and vascular endothelial growth factor (VEGF), with a host of other growth factors as well. These are native growth factors in their biologically determined ratios. These platelet growth factors enhance DNA synthesis, chemotaxis, and angiogenesis, increase collagen deposition, and stimulate synthesis of extracellular matrix.

Experimental studies on animal models showed that IGF-1, bFGF, and nerve growth factor (NGF) are potent stimulators of myoblast proliferation and fusion. Hammond et al. showed the capability of PRP to promote and accelerate myogenesis in an experimental study investigating the biomechanical and biochemical effects in rat muscle injuries (2009).

In a previous experimental study in a rat model of muscle injury, the effects of a platelet-rich fibrin matrix (PRFM) in the regeneration of damaged muscle tissue were histologically and immunohistochemically evaluated. This morphological study showed that the use of PRFM could improve muscle regeneration and long-term vascularization, suggesting that autologous PRFM may be a suitable and useful tool in the clinical treatment of muscle injuries (Gigante et al. 2012).

A side effect of the use of PRP and/or related products (e.g., PRFM) may be the occurrence of fibrosis. Visser et al. demonstrated that, in vitro, PRFM contains a significantly higher concentration of TGF-β1 compared with whole blood concentrate of similar volume. TGF-β1 has the ability to significantly increase connective cell proliferation over time, thus generating fibrotic tissue. Indeed, in an in vivo study, no increase in fibrotic tissue formation was observed during PRFM treatment in comparison with controls, suggesting that in vivo the amount of TGF-β released by PRFM might be not sufficient for this occurrence (Visser et al. 2010; Gigante et al. 2012).

Furthermore, it has been demonstrated a correlation between the concentration of growth factors and muscle regeneration. In order to closely simulate a clinical approach, Cianforlini et al. injected two different concentrations of PRP intramuscularly 24 h after the surgical trauma and evaluated, by means of histological and immunohistochemical analyses, the dose-dependent effects. Histological results confirmed the effectiveness of PRP in muscle healing and showed that the increase in PRP concentrations (i.e., GFs) in damaged muscle tissue accelerates the tissue regeneration process as well as neovascularization. Immunohistochemical data further strengthened this hypothesis detecting MyoD and myogenin-positive cells, located both inside the basal lamina of the fiber and in the interstitial spaces in the muscle sacrificed at three days and in a dose-dependent manner. It is well known that MyoD and myogenin play a key regulatory role in the processes of plasticity, adaptation, and regeneration in adult muscle. At last no significant side effects related to a higher dose of GFs were detected (Cianforlini et al. 2015).

About the efficacy of GH and IGF-1, Cianforlini et al. wanted to verify the role of GH by means of a single systemic administration in the treatment of acute muscle injury in an experimental model, verifying a possible correlation between the concentration of GH administered and tissue regeneration and fibrosis.

The action of GH is found to be ubiquitous, being increased the amount of muscle tissue and also of the endomisial and perimisiali connective tissue, with a consequent presence of exuberant scar tissue, directly proportional to the concentration of the administered GH. These are only preliminary data, but muscle regeneration and fibrosis could be both dependent from GH concentration, with an effect that would not be positive from a functional point of view, being present abundant scar tissue.

Considered as safe products, autologous PRP injections are increasingly used in patients with sports-related injuries (Engebretsen et al. 2010). Nevertheless, a recent randomized clinical trial shows no significant positive effects of PRP injections, as compared with placebo injections, in patients with muscle injuries, up to one year after injections (Reurink et al. 2014, 2015).

By recent findings, some scientific works combine PRP with Losartan (an angiotensin II type 1 receptor antagonist) (Terada et al. 2013) or PRP with the use of TGF-β1 neutralizing antibodies (Li et al. 2016). These strategies are a promising alternative to promote muscle regeneration while significantly reducing fibrosis.

14.4.2 Stem Cells

Transplantation of satellite cell-derived myoblasts has long been explored as a promising approach for treatment of skeletal muscle disorders. After an initial demonstration that normal myoblasts can restore dystrophin expression in mdx mice (Partridge et al. 1989), clinical trials, in which allogeneic normal human myoblasts were injected intramuscularly several times in dystrophic young boys muscles, have not been successful (Law et al. 1990; Mendell et al. 1995). Even recently, despite clear improvement in methodologies that enhance the success of myoblast transplantation in Duchenne patients (Skuk et al. 2007), outcomes of clinical trials are still disappointing. These experiments have raised concerns about the limited migratory and proliferative capacities of human myoblasts, as well as their limited life span in vivo. It led to the investigations of other muscle stem cell sources that could overcome these limitations and outperform the success of muscle cell transplantation. Among all these non-satellite myogenic stem cells, human mesangioblasts, human myogenic-endothelial cells, and human muscle-derived CD133+ have shown myogenic potentials in vitro and in vivo (Sampaolesi et al. 2006; Meng et al. 2014). The use of myogenic progenitor cells for improving muscle healing may become an interesting therapeutic alternative (Tedesco and Cossu 2012).

The functional recovery of muscle in a young rat model of contusion injuries is significantly improved with the combined use of Losartan and muscle-derived stem cells (Kobayashi et al. 2016). New perspectives are provided by the combination of stem cells with anti-fibrotic therapies.

14.4.3 Anti-fibrotic Agents

Considering the important role of TGF-β1 in the fibrotic cascade, the neutralization of TGF-β1 expression in injured skeletal muscle should inhibit the formation of scar tissue.

Indeed, the use of anti-fibrotic agents (decorin, relaxin, antibody against TGF-β1, AII antagonist, interferon gamma) that inactivate TGF-β1 signaling pathways reduces muscle fibrosis and, consequently, improves muscle healing, leading to a near complete recovery of lacerated muscle (Fukushima et al. 2001; Li et al. 2007).

The expression of myogenesis factor increased in mice skeletal muscles of the CCl4 + losartan group compared to the corresponding levels in the control group. It could be hypothesize that systemically elevated TGF-β1 as a result of CCl4-induced liver injury causes skeletal muscle injury, while losartan promotes muscle repair from injury via blockade of TGF-β1 signaling (Hwang et al. 2016).

Losartan, an angiotensin II receptor antagonist, neutralizes the effect of TGF-β1 and reduces fibrosis, making it the treatment of choice, since it already has FDA approval to be used clinically (Park et al. 2012; Terada et al. 2013). Suramin, also approved by the FDA, blocks TGF-β1 pathway and reduces muscle fibrosis in experimental model (Chan et al. 2003; Taniguti et al. 2011).

Also studies on the rotator cuff repair suggest the benefit effect of Licofelone (inhibitor of 5-LOX, COX-1, COX-2) on tendon healing, muscle fibrosis, and lipid accumulation (Oak et al. 2014).

In a mouse laceration model, the area of fibrosis decreased when γINF was injected at either 1 or 2 weeks after injury. More importantly, it found to improve muscle function in terms of both fast-twitch and tetanic strength. Demonstrating that γINF is a potent anti-fibrosis agent that can improve muscle healing after laceration injury (Foster et al. 2003).

14.4.4 Scaffolds

Appropriately configured materials have the ability to modulate different stages of the healing response by inducing a shift from a process of inflammation and scar tissue formation to one of constructive remodeling and functional tissue restoration. The events that facilitate such a dramatic change during the biomaterial-host interaction are complex and necessarily involve both the immune system and mechanisms of stem cell recruitment, growth, and differentiation. The biological scaffolds derived from animal ECM after a decellularization process that consists in the removal of cells associated antigens, preserving the ultrastructure and composition of the ECM.

When properly manufactured, the scaffold material increases the migration and cell survival of myogenic precursor cells (Boldrin et al. 2007). Controlling the microenvironment of injected myogenic cells using biological scaffolds enhances muscle regeneration (Borselli et al. 2011). Ideally, using an appropriate extracellular matrix (ECM) composition and stiffness, scaffolds should best replicate the in vivo milieu and mechanical microenvironment (Gilbert et al. 2010; Engler et al. 2006).

With enzymatic and chemical decellularization process, we can isolate skeletal muscle ECM; this shows to contain growth factors, glycosaminoglycans, and basement membrane structural proteins. Myogenic cells survive and proliferate on muscle ECM scaffolds in vitro, and when implanted in a rat abdominal wall injury model in vivo shows to induce a constructive remodeling response associate with scaffold degradation and myogenesis in the implant area (Wolf et al. 2012).

The Food and Drug Administration has not established standards for tissue decellularization. As a result, commercially available ECM-derived scaffolds contain different amounts of cell-associated antigenic material.

A recent study demonstrated that an acellular scaffold composed of urinary bladder porcine ECM can promote formation of new muscle tissue in mice and in humans after a volumetric muscle loss. Further more encouraging histological results, three of five patients also show a functional improvement of muscle injuries (Sicari et al. 2014).

A combination of stem cells, biomaterial-based scaffolds, and growth factors may provide a therapeutic option to improve regeneration of injured skeletal muscles (Jeon and Elisseeff 2016).

Conclusions

Skeletal muscle injuries are very frequently present in sports medicine and sport traumatology. Despite their clinical importance, the optimal rehabilitation strategies for the treatment of these injuries are not well defined. The healing process required the presence of different cell populations, up- and downregulation of various gene expressions, and participation of multiple growth factors. Scientific research so far has focused on individual elements; nowadays strategies based on the match and combination of stem cells, growth factors, and biological scaffolds have already shown promising results in animal models. A better understanding of the cellular and molecular pathways as well as a better definition of the interactions (cell-cell and cell-matrix) that are essential for effective muscle regeneration should contribute to the development of new therapies in athletes.

References

Abat F, Valles SL, Gelber PE, Polidori F, Jorda A, Garcia-Herreros S, Monllau JC, Sanchez-Ibanez JM (2015) An experimental study of muscular injury repair in a mouse model of notexin-induced lesion with EPI(R) technique. BMC Sports Sci Med Rehabil 7:7. doi:10.1186/s13102-015-0002-0

Anderson JE (2016) Hepatocyte growth factor and satellite cell activation. Adv Exp Med Biol 900:1–25. doi:10.1007/978-3-319-27511-6_1

Beiner JM, Jokl P, Cholewicki J, Panjabi MM (1999) The effect of anabolic steroids and corticosteroids on healing of muscle contusion injury. Am J Sports Med 27(1):2–9

Bleakley C M, Glasgow P, MacAuley DC (2012) PRICE needs updating, should we call the POLICE? Br J Sports Med 46:220–221. doi:10.1136/bjsports-2011-090297. Originally published online September 7, 2011

Boldrin L, Elvassore N, Malerba A, Flaibani M, Cimetta E, Piccoli M, Baroni MD, Gazzola MV, Messina C, Gamba P, Vitiello L, de Coppi P (2007) Satellite cells delivered by micro-patterned scaffolds: a new strategy for cell transplantation in muscle diseases. Tissue Eng 13(2):253–262

Borselli C, Storrie H, Benesch-Lee F, Shvartsman D, Cezar C, Lichtman JW, Vandenburgh HH, Mooney DJ (2010) Functional muscle regeneration with combined delivery of angiogenesis and myogenesis factors. Proc Natl Acad Sci U S A 107(8):3287–3292. doi:10.1073/pnas.0903875106

Borselli C, Cezar CA, Shvartsman D, Vandenburgh HH, Mooney DJ (2011) The role of multifunctional delivery scaffold in the ability of cultured myoblasts to promote muscle regeneration. Biomaterials 32(34):8905–8914. doi:10.1016/j.biomaterials.2011.08.019

Cezar CA, Roche ET, Vandenburgh HH, Duda GN, Walsh CJ, Mooney DJ (2016) Biologic-free mechanically induced muscle regeneration. Proc Natl Acad Sci U S A 113(6):1534–1539. doi:10.1073/pnas.1517517113

Chan YS, Li Y, Foster W, Horaguchi T, Somogyi G, Fu FH, Huard J (2003) Antifibrotic effects of suramin in injured skeletal muscle after laceration. J Appl Physiol 95(2):771–780. doi:10.1152/japplphysiol.00915.2002

Cianforlini M, Mattioli-Belmonte M, Manzotti S, Chiurazzi E, Piani M, Orlando F, Provinciali M, Gigante A (2015) Effect of platelet rich plasma concentration on skeletal muscle regeneration: an experimental study. J Biol Regul Homeost Agents 29(4 Suppl):47–55

Collins CA (2006) Satellite cell self-renewal. Curr Opin Pharmacol 6(3):301–306

Darby IA, Zakuan N, Billet F, Desmouliere A (2016) The myofibroblast, a key cell in normal and pathological tissue repair. Cell Mol Life Sci 73(6):1145–1157. doi:10.1007/s00018-015-2110-0

Deasy BM, Feduska JM, Payne TR, Li Y, Ambrosio F, Huard J (2009) Effect of VEGF on the regenerative capacity of muscle stem cells in dystrophic skeletal muscle. Mol Ther 17(10):1788–1798. doi:10.1038/mt.2009.136

Desmouliere A, Gabbiani G (1995) Myofibroblast differentiation during fibrosis. Exp Nephrol 3(2):134–139

Dhawan J, Rando TA (2005) Stem cells in postnatal myogenesis: molecular mechanisms of satellite cell quiescence, activation and replenishment. Trends Cell Biol 15(12):666–673

Dumont NA, Bentzinger CF, Sincennes MC, Rudnicki MA (2015) Satellite cells and skeletal muscle regeneration. Compr Physiol 5(3):1027–1059. doi:10.1002/cphy.c140068

Engebretsen L, Steffen K, Alsousou J, Anitua E, Bachl N, Devilee R, Everts P, Hamilton B, Huard J, Jenoure P, Kelberine F, Kon E, Maffulli N, Matheson G, Mei-Dan O, Menetrey J, Philippon M, Randelli P, Schamasch P, Schwellnus M, Vernec A, Verrall G (2010) IOC consensus paper on the use of platelet-rich plasma in sports medicine. Br J Sports Med 44(15):1072–1081. doi:10.1136/bjsm.2010.079822

Engert JC, Berglund EB, Rosenthal N (1996) Proliferation precedes differentiation in IGF-I-stimulated myogenesis. J Cell Biol 135(2):431–440

Engler AJ, Sen S, Sweeney HL, Discher DE (2006) Matrix elasticity directs stem cell lineage specification. Cell 126(4):677–689. doi:10.1016/j.cell.2006.06.044

Foster W, Li Y, Usas A, Somogyi G, Huard J (2003) Gamma interferon as an antifibrosis agent in skeletal muscle. J Orthop Res 21(5):798–804

Fukushima K, Badlani N, Usas A, Riano F, Fu F, Huard J (2001) The use of an antifibrosis agent to improve muscle recovery after laceration. Am J Sports Med 29(4):394–402

Gigante A, Del Torto M, Manzotti S et al (2012) Platelet rich fibrin matrix effects on skeletal muscle lesions: an experimental study. J Biol Regul Homeost Agents 26:475–484

Gigante A, Cianforlini M, Manzotti S, Ulisse S (2014) The effects of growth factors on skeletal muscle lesions. Joints 1(4):180–186

Gilbert PM, Havenstrite KL, Magnusson KE, Sacco A, Leonardi NA, Kraft P, Nguyen NK, Thrun S, Lutolf MP, Blau HM (2010) Substrate elasticity regulates skeletal muscle stem cell self-renewal in culture. Science 329(5995):1078–1081. doi:10.1126/science.1191035

Hamid MS, Yusof A, Ali MRM (2014) Platelet-rich plasma (PRP) for acute muscle injury: a systematic review. PLoS One 9(2):e90538. doi:10.1371/journal.pone.0090538

Hammond JW, Hinton RY, Curl LA, Muriel JM, Lovering RM (2009) Use of autologous platelet-rich plasma to treat muscle strain injuries. Am J Sports Med 37(6):1135–1142. doi:10.1177/0363546508330974

Huard J, Li Y, Fu FH (2002) Muscle injuries and repair: current trends in research. J Bone Joint Surg Am 84-A(5):822–832

Hurme T, Kalimo H (1992) Activation of myogenic precursor cells after muscle injury. Med Sci Sports Exerc 24(2):197–205

Hwang OK, Park JK, Lee EJ, Lee EM, Kim AY, Jeong KS (2016) Therapeutic effect of losartan, an angiotensin II type 1 receptor antagonist, on CCl4-induced skeletal muscle injury. Int J Mol Sci 17(2):227

Järvinen TA, Järvinen TL, Kääriäinen M et al (2007) Muscle injuries: optimising recovery. Best Pract Res Clin Rheumatol 21(2):317–331. pmid:17512485

Jeon OH, Elisseeff J (2016) Orthopedic tissue regeneration: cells, scaffolds, and small molecules. Drug Deliv Transl Res 6(2):105–120. doi:10.1007/s13346-015-0266-7

Kobayashi M, Ota S, Terada S, Kawakami Y, Otsuka T, Fu FH, Huard J (2016) The combined use of losartan and muscle-derived stem cells significantly improves the functional recovery of muscle in a young mouse model of contusion injuries. Am J Sports Med 44(12):3252–3261. doi:10.1177/0363546516656823

Law PK, Bertorini TE, Goodwin TG, Chen M, Fang QW, Li HJ, Kirby DS, Florendo JA, Herrod HG, Golden GS (1990) Dystrophin production induced by myoblast transfer therapy in Duchenne muscular dystrophy. Lancet 336(8707):114–115

Lee C, Fukushima K, Usas A, Xin L, Pelinkovic D, Martinek V, Huard J (2000) Biological intervention based on cell and gene therapy to improve muscle healing after laceration. J Musculoskelet Res 4(4):256–277

Lehto M, Sims TJ, Bailey AJ (1985) Skeletal muscle injury–molecular changes in the collagen during healing. Res Exp Med 185(2):95–106

Li Y, Li J, Zhu J, Sun B, Branca M, Tang Y, Foster W, Xiao X, Huard J (2007) Decorin gene transfer promotes muscle cell differentiation and muscle regeneration. Mol Ther 15(9):1616–1622. doi:10.1038/sj.mt.6300250

Li H, Hicks JJ, Wang L, Oyster N, Philippon MJ, Hurwitz S et al (2016) Customized platelet-rich plasma with transforming growth factor β1 neutralization antibody to reduce fibrosis in skeletal muscle. Biomaterials 87:147–156

Lipton BH, Schultz E (1979) Developmental fate of skeletal muscle satellite cells. Science 205(4412): 1292–1294

Mann CJ, Perdiguero E, Kharraz Y, Aguilar S, Pessina P, Serrano AL, Munoz-Canoves P (2011) Aberrant repair and fibrosis development in skeletal muscle. Skelet Muscle 1(1):21. doi:10.1186/2044-5040-1-21

McLennan IS (1996) Degenerating and regenerating skeletal muscles contain several subpopulations of macrophages with distinct spatial and temporal distributions. J Anat 188(Pt 1):17–28

Mendell JR, Kissel JT, Amato AA, King W, Signore L, Prior TW, Sahenk Z, Benson S, McAndrew PE, Rice R, Nagaraja H, Stephens R, Lantry L, Morris GE, Burghes AH (1995) Myoblast transfer in the treatment of Duchenne's muscular dystrophy. N Engl J Med 333(13):832–838

Menetrey J, Kasemkijwattana C, Day CS, Bosch P, Vogt M, Fu FH, Moreland MS, Huard J (2000) Growth factors improve muscle healing in vivo. J Bone Joint Surg [Br] 82-B:131–137. pmid:10697329

Meng J, Chun S, Asfahani R, Lochmuller H, Muntoni F, Morgan J (2014) Human skeletal muscle-derived CD133(+) cells form functional satellite cells after intramuscular transplantation in immunodeficient host mice. Mol Ther 22(5):1008–1017. doi:10.1038/mt.2014.26

Miller KJ, Thaloor D, Matteson S, Pavlath GK (2000) Hepatocyte growth factor affects satellite cell activation and differentiation in regenerating skeletal muscle. Am J Physiol Cell Physiol 278(1):C174–C181

Munoz-Canoves P, Serrano AL (2015) Macrophages decide between regeneration and fibrosis in muscle. Trends Endocrinol Metab 26(9):449–450. doi:10.1016/j.tem.2015.07.005

Oak NR, Gumucio JP, Flood MD, Saripalli AL, Davis ME, Harning JA et al (2014) Inhibition of 5-LOX, COX-1, and COX-2 increases tendon healing and reduces muscle fibrosis and lipid accumulation after rotator cuff repair. Am J Sports Med 42(12):2860–2868

Park JK, Ki MR, Lee EM, Kim AY, You SY, Han SY, Lee EJ, Hong IH, Kwon SH, Kim SJ, Rando TA, Jeong KS (2012) Losartan improves adipose tissue-derived stem cell niche by inhibiting transforming growth factor-beta and fibrosis in skeletal muscle injury. Cell Transplant 21(11):2407–2424. doi:10.3727/096368912X637055

Partridge TA, Morgan JE, Coulton GR, Hoffman EP, Kunkel LM (1989) Conversion of mdx myofibres from dystrophin-negative to -positive by injection of normal myoblasts. Nature 337(6203):176–179

Proto JD, Tang Y, Lu A, Chen WC, Stahl E, Poddar M, Beckman SA, Robbins PD, Nidernhofer LJ, Imbrogno K, Hannigan T, Mars WM, Wang B, Huard J (2015) NF-kappaB inhibition reveals a novel role for HGF during skeletal muscle repair. Cell Death Dis 6:e1730. doi:10.1038/cddis.2015.66

Relaix F, Zammit PS (2012) Satellite cells are essential for skeletal muscle regeneration: the cell on the edge returns centre stage. Development 139(16):2845–2856. doi:10.1242/dev.069088

Reurink G, Goudswaard GJ, Moen MH, Weir A, Verhaar JA, Bierma-Zeinstra SM, Maas M, Tol JL, Dutch Hamstring Injection Therapy Study I (2014) Platelet-rich plasma injections in acute muscle injury. N Engl J Med 370(26):2546–2547. doi:10.1056/NEJMc1402340

Reurink G, Goudswaard GJ, Moen MH, Weir A, Verhaar JA, Bierma-Zeinstra SM, Maas M, Tol JL, Dutch HITsI (2015) Rationale, secondary outcome scores and 1-year follow-up of a randomised trial of platelet-rich plasma injections in acute hamstring muscle injury: the Dutch Hamstring Injection Therapy study. Br J Sports Med 49(18):1206–1212. doi:10.1136/bjsports-2014-094250

Rocheteau P, Vinet M, Chretien F (2015) Dormancy and quiescence of skeletal muscle stem cells. Results Probl Cell Differ 56:215–235. doi:10.1007/978-3-662-44608-9_10

Sallay PI, Friedman RL, Coogan PG, Garrett WE (1996) Hamstring muscle injuries among water skiers: functional outcome and prevention. Am J Sports Med 24:130–136

Sambasivan R, Yao R, Kissenpfennig A, Van Wittenberghe L, Paldi A, Gayraud-Morel B, Guenou H, Malissen B, Tajbakhsh S, Galy A (2011) Pax7-expressing satellite cells are indispensable for adult skeletal muscle regeneration. Development 138(17):3647–3656. doi:10.1242/dev.067587

Sampaolesi M, Blot S, D'Antona G, Granger N, Tonlorenzi R, Innocenzi A, Mognol P, Thibaud JL, Galvez BG, Barthelemy I, Perani L, Mantero S, Guttinger M, Pansarasa O, Rinaldi C, De Angelis MGC, Torrente Y, Bordignon C, Bottinelli R, Cossu G (2006) Mesoangioblast stem cells ameliorate muscle function in dystrophic dogs. Nature 444(7119):574–579

Schiaffino S, Mammucari C (2011) Regulation of skeletal muscle growth by the IGF1-Akt/PKB pathway: insights from genetic models. Skelet Muscle 1(1):4. doi:10.1186/2044-5040-1-4

Sheehan SM, Tatsumi R, Temm-Grove CJ, Allen RE (2000) HGF is an autocrine growth factor for skeletal muscle satellite cells in vitro. Muscle Nerve 23(2):239–245

Sicari BM, Rubin JP, Dearth CL, Wolf MT, Ambrosio F, Boninger M et al (2014) An acellular biologic scaffold promotes skeletal muscle formation in mice and humans with volumetric muscle loss. Sci Transl Med 6(234):234ra58–234ra58

Skuk D, Goulet M, Roy B, Piette V, Cote CH, Chapdelaine P, Hogrel JY, Paradis M, Bouchard JP, Sylvain M, Lachance JG, Tremblay JP (2007) First test of a "high-density injection" protocol for myogenic cell transplantation throughout large volumes of muscles in a Duchenne muscular dystrophy patient: eighteen months follow-up. Neuromuscul Disord 17(1):38–46. doi:10.1016/j.nmd.2006.10.003

Taniguti AP, Pertille A, Matsumura CY, Santo Neto H, Marques MJ (2011) Prevention of muscle fibrosis and myonecrosis in mdx mice by suramin, a TGF-beta1 blocker. Muscle Nerve 43(1):82–87. doi:10.1002/mus.21869

Tedesco FS, Cossu G (2012) Stem cell therapies for muscle disorders. Curr Opin Neurol 25(5):597–603. doi:10.1097/WCO.0b013e328357f288

Terada S, Ota S, Kobayashi M, Kobayashi T, Mifune Y, Takayama K, Witt M, Vadala G, Oyster N, Otsuka T, Fu FH, Huard J (2013) Use of an antifibrotic agent improves the effect of platelet-rich plasma on muscle healing after injury. J Bone Joint Surg Am 95(11):980–988. doi:10.2106/JBJS.L.00266

Tidball JG (1995) Inflammatory cell response to acute muscle injury. Med Sci Sports Exerc 27(7):1022–1032

Toumi H, Best TM (2003) The inflammatory response: friend or enemy for muscle injury? Br J Sports Med 37(4):284–286

Visser LC, Arnoczky SP, Caballero O et al (2010) Platelet-rich fibrin constructs elute higher concentrations of transforming growth factor-β1 and increase tendon cell proliferation over time when compared to blood clots: a comparative in vitro analysis. Vet Surg 39:811–817

Wolf MT, Daly KA, Reing JE, Badylak SF (2012) Biologic scaffold composed of skeletal muscle extracellular matrix. Biomaterials 33(10):2916–2925

Würgler-Hauri CC et al (2007) Temporal expression of 8 growth factors in tendon-to-bone healing in a rat supraspinatus model. J Shoulder Elb Surg 16(5):S198–S203

Zhao W, Lu H, Wang X, Ransohoff RM, Zhou L (2016) CX3CR1 deficiency delays acute skeletal muscle injury repair by impairing macrophage functions. FASEB J 30(1):380–393. doi:10.1096/fj.14-270090

Conservative Treatments for Tendinopathy

15

F. Tencone, S. Della Villa, and A. Giannini

Contents

F. Tencone (✉) • S. Della Villa • A. Giannini
Isokinetic Medical Group, Bologna, Italy
e-mail: : f.tencone@isokinetic.com

15.1 Exercises Therapy

15.1.1 Introduction: The Importance of Loading Program in Tendinopathy

In 1998 Alfredson et al. published a key paper that changed the way we look at tendons (1998). The authors prospectively studied the effect of heavy-load eccentric calf muscle training in 15 recreational athletes who had the diagnosis of chronic Achilles tendinosis with a long duration of symptoms despite conventional nonsurgical treatment. At week 0, all patients had Achilles tendon pain not allowing running activity, and there was significantly lower eccentric and concentric calf muscle strength on the injured compared with the non-injured side. After the 12-week training period, all 15 patients were back at their preinjury levels with full running activity. There was a significant decrease in pain during activity. A comparison group of 15 recreational athletes with the same diagnosis and a long duration of symptoms had been treated conventionally. No one of the control group improved, and all patients were ultimately treated surgically.

However, despite the first encouraging results, subsequent studies have failed to reproduce the same outcome. In fact, most authors reported successfully returning 60% (Silbernagel et al. 2001; Roos et al. 2004) of participants back to sport, which contrasts with the 100% reported to have

G.L. Canata et al. (eds.), *Muscle and Tendon Injuries*, DOI 10.1007/978-3-662-54184-5_15

returned to sport in Alfredson's original paper. It was proposed that the lower success rates observed can be due to a poorer response to isolated eccentric exercises in nonathletic and female individuals when compared with athletic subjects (Maffulli and Longo 2008). A recent systematic review confirmed the success of eccentric exercises (Sussmilch-Leitch et al. 2012) even if the mechanism by which the effect is achieved remains unclear. However there is no evidence that eccentric regime is more effective than other loading programs (Malliaras et al. 2013).

Biologic tissues have the unique capacity to adapt over time increasing load tolerance and energy absorption. In tendons, changes in stiffness seem to be attributed more to adaptations of the material rather than to morphological properties. We don't know for sure if a program regime is better than other in optimizing this response. Type I collagen response to high load in normal tendon peaks at around 3 days after intense exercise (Langberg et al. 2000). Interestingly this response appears to be greater in pathological tendons than normal tendons (Kjaer et al. 2005). However, the majority of the tendon is composed not of cells but of extracellular matrix (ECM), which is a passive structure. The tendon ECM is a viscoelastic material, which means that slower loading regimes can yield greater strains than faster loading regimes, as the tendon has more time to creep (Pearson et al. 2007). This viscoelastic behavior depends on the amount of time the tendon is under load and is therefore unaffected by the mode of muscle contraction (eccentric or concentric). Slow loading may therefore produce particularly strong cell stimuli that can be beneficial to the tendon if the strain is sufficient. Taken together, all these data from in vitro and normal or pathological tendon studies suggest that loading magnitude plays the key role in contrast to muscle contraction type (Couppé et al. 2015) since contraction is slow enough.

Most of the tendinopathic area is located on the deep surface of tendons at, or close to, the bone–tendon junction. It's not possible that this is due to tensile overload because there is less elongation in this region than in the superficial portion of the tendon. The joint side of the tendon is exposed, in fact, to less tensile load (stress shielded) but may be subjected to high compressive loads against the bone (Cook and Purdam 2012). For example, with proximal hamstring tendinopathy, the tendon is thought to be compressed against the ischial tuberosity when the hip is flexed, such as during sitting. The tendon insertion and the "enthesis organ" are well engineered to absorb most functional loads and will adapt over time to higher levels of load. However, these tissues are slow to adapt to high loads and slow to resolve after insult. Reducing compressive loads in insertional tendinopathies therefore can provide an important unloading strategy for the "sensitized" tendon and must be tailored based on site of compression (Goom et al. 2016).

15.1.2 Not All Tendons Are Created Equal

Basically tendons serve to transfer tension from their respective muscle to their bony attachment. Tendons that are common sites of tendinopathy have large different morphology, so that no single characteristic emerges as key factors common to the development of tendon pain. From a clinical point of view, the differences between different sites of tendinopathy are huge. Patients with supraspinatus tendinopathy frequently report pain during night (Terabayashi et al. 2014), while Achilles tendinopathy is generally more severe at the first step in the morning. Achilles and patellar tendinopathies occur most commonly in people participating in sporting and physical activity (Järvinen 1992). Rotator cuff tear is, instead, extremely common even in normal population (Minagawa et al. 2013), and asymptomatic tear is twice as common as symptomatic tear.

Lower limb tendons have a precise biomechanical role: energy storage and release. In fact, they behave similar to a spring reducing the energy cost of human movements and to a source of power amplification for many high-powered movements (Roberts 2002). There is some evidence that this may be true even for upper limb tendons; however the muscle tendons more involved seem to be pectoral major or subscapularis, while most of rotator cuff tears are located in the supraspinatus (Roach et al. 2013). Energy storage seems not to be a key factor for upper limb tendons. Conversely upper limbs are mainly involved in reaching and pointing, movements that require a precise adjustment of muscle activity to achieve the necessary precision.

Unlike the single-joint movement, the dynamics of multi-joint movement is complex. Take the case of flexing your elbow with your arm in the horizontal plane. If your central nervous system (CNS) simply activates the biceps muscle, the elbow will flex, but its motion will impose a torque, called an interaction torque, on your shoulder. If you do not want that torque to move your upper limb while you move your lower arm around the elbow, you need to activate shoulder muscles in advance to negate interaction force. The same is true for elbow muscle. The more you need to be precise, the more muscle activation control needs to be fine adjusted. This behaviour can be different for lower limb activity, such as walking and running, that appears to be more "automatic" (Narita et al. 2002).

A recent systematic review shows that in people with tendinopathy sensory and motor system are altered bilaterally even in unilateral tendinopathy (Heales et al. 2014). This implies a potential central nervous system involvement. Interestingly among 20 studies included, there are only two studies on lower limb tendinopathy. Greater error in detection of movement was found in affected elbows of participants with lateral epicondylalgia (LE) (Juul-Kristensen et al. 2008). Consistently patients with LE have impairments in reaction time and speed of movement with reaching task (Pienimäki et al. 1997). Motor deficit may also be present in sites distant to the original site of pathology (Alizadehkhaiyat et al. 2007). All these motor control alterations may have a deepest impact where more precise muscle activation is needed, such as in reaching.

Exercises aimed to improve proprioception showed to be no more effective to improve pain compared to traditional treatments in shoulder tendinopathy (Dilek et al. 2016). Exercises to improve "stability," advocated for low back pain in the recent past, are currently reviewed for lack of any positive evidence to support their use (Wang et al. 2012). Data from low back pain studies also report hypo-activity or hyperactivity depending on the muscle and tasks investigated (Hungerford et al. 2003). Based on what we have already shown, all these data are not surprising. Proprioception is only a part of motor control and probably not the more involved in tendon pathology. Generalized muscle contraction for stability is not a good solution in movement.

To achieve correct stabilization, you have to predict the force your arm is going to experience and produce muscle contraction of the right intensity at the right time: no more, no less. In practice, this means that your CNS is "implicitly" adapted to the physical world (or, from a computational neuroscience prospective, that CNS has acquired an *internal model of dynamics*). This type of knowledge is, fortunately, implicit and has to remain so. Rather than focus on how to change motor control, it seems logic to reduce, in the short term, the need for stability, reducing the load in the tendon. There is moderate evidence for the immediate effect of several manual therapy techniques on pain and strength (Vicenzino et al. 2001). For example, in "lateral elbow mobilization with movement," a lateral humeroulnar accessory glide is applied while the patients, suffering from tennis elbow, perform their painful action (Coombes et al. 2015). For rotator cuff related shoulder pain, Lewis has proposed a method of assessment called Shoulder Symptom Modification Procedure (SSMP) (2009). The SSMP systematically investigates the effect of modifying thoracic posture, three planes of scapular posture, and humeral head position in terms of shoulder symptoms. In this process, external forces are applied to joint and painful movement tested. If this reduces or alleviates symptoms, the technique(s) founds to be beneficial during the assessment process forms part of the treatment (Lewis 2016). The common features for these proposed treatments for shoulder and elbow are that external force is applied to joint and so it may increase the articular stability changing motor command.

Predicting force is not a unique feature of the upper limb, and energy storage is not only an exclusive feature of lower limb. Rather, the relative importance of the two functions may vary between anatomical sites and be based on the prevalent activity. That has to be taken in account when we think at the rehabilitation program. We can't approach, for example, in the same way a rotator cuff tendinopathy of a professional swimmer and of a housewife.

15.1.3 Pain and Psychological Variables

Like other chronic pain conditions, in tendinopathy, there is discrepancy between tissue damage seen on clinical imaging and clinical presentation, which creates confusion for both patients and clinicians. Contradictory evidence exists on the substances responsible for pain generation, the source of these substances, and the pathways of transmission to the central nervous system.

The relationship between tendon pain and mechanical load, together with the mechano-responsiveness of tenocytes and lack of sensory innervation of the deep tendon tissue, may implicate paracrine signaling by the tendon cells. Researchers suggest that abnormal tendon cells produce signaling proteins and receptors for epinephrine, acetylcholine, glutamate, substance P, tumor necrosis factor α (TNFα), and other neuropeptides. Upregulation of these substances can produce a local response driving vascular and tenocyte responses and may also cause a neural response and provoke pain. Increases in receptors for nociceptive substances have been reported such as N-methyl-D-aspartate (NMDA) (Alfredson et al. 2001) and neurokinin-1 (NK-1) receptors (substance P) (Ljung et al. 1999).

These nociceptive signals are assessed by the CNS, but pain will not emerge until the input to the brain has been evaluated, albeit at an unconscious level. Allodynia and primary hyperalgesia are attributed to sensitization of the primary nociceptor and relate to the area of usual pain. Secondary hyperalgesia is attributed to sensitization of nociceptive neurons within the central nervous system (CNS). Tenderness and evoked pain that spread, in a non-dermatomal, non-peripheral nerve distribution, is best explained by central sensitization (Woolf and Salter 2000). The rule of central sensitization in tendinopathy is debated in literature. Plinsinga et al. (unpublished data) found no evidence of central sensitization but a reduction in lower limb loading pain threshold and an increase in pain on pain onset. This data suggest predominantly peripheral mechanisms. Conversely, there are evidences of central sensitization in tennis elbow and in rotator cuff related shoulder pain (Lim et al. 2012; Coombes et al. 2008, 2012; Gwilym et al. 2011). Again it seems that there is important difference in proportion of central involvement between the upper and lower limb.

Nociceptor signals are not the only input evaluated by the brain. Previous experiences, cultural factor, expectation of consequence, and beliefs all together contribute the implicit perception of threat to body tissues. This means that pain can be conceptualized as the conscious correlate of the implicit perception of threat to body tissues. Fear of pain develops as a result of a cognitive interpretation of pain as threatening (pain catastrophizing), and this fear affects attention processes (hypervigilance) and leads to avoidance behaviors, followed by disability, disuse, and depression. In the absence of fear-avoidance beliefs about pain, individuals are more likely to confront pain problems head-on and become more engaged in active coping to improve daily function (see Linton and Shaw (2011) for a review). In their multicenter longitudinal cohort study, Chester et al. (2016) found that in shoulder pain, psychological factors were consistently associated with patient-rated outcome, whereas clinical examination findings associated with a specific structural diagnosis were not. Mallows et al. (2016) conducted a systematic review of psychological variables in tendinopathy. While they found that there is moderate evidence that links catastrophizing and distress with LE, and moderate evidence that kinesiophobia and catastrophizing are associated with rotator cuff tendinopathy, limited evidence suggests that patellar tendinopathy is not associated with anxiety or depression and kinesiophobia may be linked with suboptimal outcomes in Achilles tendinopathy. Again literature seems to suggest that psychological factors may have different impact between the upper and lower limb.

15.1.4 To a Comprehensive Model of Tendinopathy

Recently, Coombes et al. (2008) proposed an integrative model for treating LE: they propose that LE can be conceptualized as comprising three interrelated components: (a) local tendon pathology, (b) changes in the pain system, and (c) impairment in the motor system. In their model, the authors recognized that not all LE patients have the same clinical presentation, then through comprehensive evaluation, different proportions of tendon pathology, pain system dysfunction, and motor system impairments can be used to define subgroups of LE. The healthcare practitioners should identify the relative expression of local pathology, pain, and motor system dysfunction in individual patients, so that treatment strategies may be better matched to the clinical presentation. However, this model can't be apparently generalized to other tendinopathy sites. There are different ways through which tendinopathy may produce nociception. Based on Cook et al. (n.d.), "continuum" model pain in tendon can fall into two categories: (1) reactive tendon with a first presentation of tendon pain following acute overload and (2) reactive-on-late disrepair/degenerative tendon pathology. A painful reactive or reactive-on-degenerative tendon may increase expression of nociceptive substances and their receptors, stimulating the peripheral nerve, and be interpreted as pain (Fig. 15.1). Since the degenerative portions of the tendon appear mechanically silent and structurally unable to transmit tensile load, the pain-free

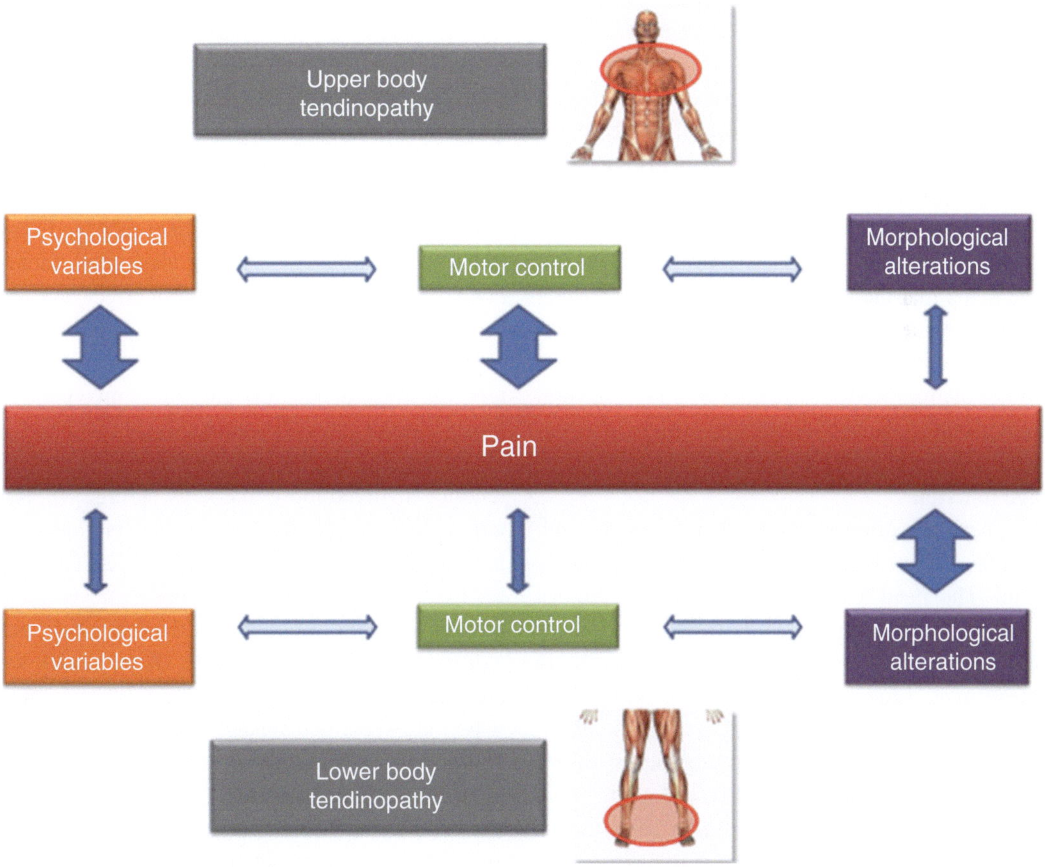

Fig. 15.1 Different burden (width of *dark blue arrows*) of various components on pain, based on upper or lower location of tendinopathy

tendon may contain substantial matrix and cell abnormalities, but limited nociceptive substance production, signaling ability, or receptor activation, which is in summary an insufficient nociceptive stimulus. This may explain, in parts, the low correlation between symptoms and alteration in traditional imaging exams.

Morphological alteration seems to produce different centralization of pain between tendinopathy sites, despite always being a chronic disease. This can be due to different impact on motor control between different sites. The presence of pain leads to inhibition or delayed activation of specific muscles or muscle groups that perform key synergistic functions. This produces alterations in the patterns of motor activity and recruitment during functional movement (Hungerford et al. 2003; Hodges and Moseley 2003). Interesting alteration in motor pattern activity is present even in expectation of pain (Tucker et al. 2012). This type of alteration exists also in lower limb tendinopathy (Chang and Kulig 2015) although may have a deepest impact where more precise control is needed. Proprioceptive representation of the painful body part in primary sensory cortex changes when pain persists (Flor et al. 1997). This may have implications for motor control because these representations are the maps that the brain uses to plan and execute movement. It is known that experimental disruption of cortical proprioceptive maps disrupts motor planning (McCormick et al. 2007). Several minor motor planning alterations may be less relevant where tendon have mostly an energy storage function.

There are different theoretical ways through which motor activity alteration may produce pain. The need to modify feed-forward control may permanently increase contribution from synergistic muscles and reduce the variability in movement. Movement variability is thought to minimize load accumulation in a specific region and to be protective for tendon morphology alteration (Stergiou and Decker 2011). Another possible mechanism is that exaggerated muscle contraction, beyond the needed for movement stability, due, for example, to error in the internal calculation of tendon load (Rio et al. 2014), significantly increases load on tendon (Maganaris and Paul 2002).

Exaggerated muscle contraction, limiting the movement of the involved area (Lund et al. 1991), can be helpful but can become detrimental if the other factors (psychological variable and morphological alteration) are relevant. Fear of pain develops as a result of a cognitive interpretation of pain as threatening (pain catastrophizing), and this fear affects attention processes (hypervigilance) and leads to altered motor behaviors, followed by tissue sensitization and then pain. Both negative affectivity (a tendency to see the cup as "half empty" rather than "half full") and threatening types of illness information can help to fuel catastrophic thoughts about pain. In absence of fear-avoidance beliefs about pain, individuals are more likely to confront pain problems head-on and become more engaged in active coping to improve daily function. If pain is framed as solely a biomedical problem, problem-solving efforts inevitably will be based on strategies to remove or reduce pain. When multiple attempts to get rid of pain fail, worries are further reinforced, and patients are stuck in an endless loop of increasing worries and failed problem-solving attempts to alleviate pain (Linton and Shaw 2011). From these descriptions, it will be clear how motor control may have an enhancement effect on relationship between pain and psychological variables. It will then not be surprising that tendinopathy in anatomical sites involved in more precise tasks is more likely to have a psychological components when compared to tendons involved more in energy storage. We are not auguring that there are some tendons that have a purely energy storage function and are not involved in joint stability, rather same tendons are more related to one aspect than the other and a different clinical presentation. In the model, we are proposing the three different components which are separated for the sake of explanation. They are, in fact, in closed correlation between them. The relative contribution from these different factors and their interactions with each other are variable, fluctuating, and unique to each individual. It is not impossible to have a patient with Achilles tendinopathy and depression and kinesiophobia; it is only less probable. Therefore also in tendinopathy, there is a need of a multidimensional clinical-reasoning approach to patient examination. This enables the clinician to recognize the relative burden and dominance of the various factors that are unique to each patient's presentation.

15.1.5 Rehabilitation Program

15.1.5.1 Phase 1: Reduce Pain (The Load Management)

Although loads appear to be the key factor, different tendons may respond differently based on their pathological state. Cook et al. (Forsdyke et al. 2016) have proposed a model of tendon pathology that can be useful to guide clinical approach. Based on this model, tendon pain presentations fall into two categories: reactive tendon with a first presentation of tendon pain following acute overload or reactive-on-late disrepair/degenerative tendon pathology. Since reactivity to load seems to be the key factor, the most important intervention in this stage is load management. This means reducing both tensile and compressive load on the tendon. Complete rest from tensile loads for a tendinopathy is contraindicated as it can decrease mechanical strength of the tendon (Reeves 2006). It's reasonable than to modify load with the goal of reducing pain. This means, in particular, reducing high-load energy storage activities that may be aggravating the pain. Volume and frequency of the highest-intensity activities, such as maximal jumping or throwing, may need to be reduced eventually in consultation with both the athlete and coach. For example, a reduction in an athlete's training load may diminish symptoms to a level that allows an athlete to continue competing. Simple training changes can reduce compressive load while maintaining tensile loads. One effective way to do this is to reduce loads in the outer muscle range, as compression of the tendon against the bone proximal to the enthesis is increased with longer muscle lengths. For upper limbs, an effective way is applying external force to joint. It is important to consider the 24-h pain behavior when implementing and progressing rehabilitation programs for tendinopathy.

Pain monitoring is a good way to control training load. A slight increase in tendon discomfort or pain is acceptable as a result of the rehabilitation program, but only for a limited period of time. Normally an increase in pain by 2–3 points on the visual analogue scale the day after taking part in rehabilitation exercises is normal, as long as it subsides within 24 h (Kountouris and Cook 2007). Any pain increase that lasts longer than 24 h should be viewed as a contraindication to progress the rehabilitation program, and appropriate adjustments should be made. The Victorian Institute of Sport Assessment (VISA) (Robinson et al. 2001) questionnaires are a series of specific validated pain and function outcome measures that can also be used to assess severity of symptoms as well as to monitor outcomes in different tendons (such as hamstring, Achilles, and patellar tendon). VISA is a 100-point scale, with higher scores representing better function and less pain. However, because of the large domain of sporting function in the VISA scores, they are not sensitive to change over a short period, and at last, 4 weeks are required between each submission. In patellar tendinopathy, Malliaras et al. (2015) suggest to measure pain response using a "pain-provocation test," such as single-leg decline squat. If the pain score on the load test (e.g., one repetition of the single-leg decline squat test at the same depth) has returned to baseline within 24 h of the activity or rehabilitation session, the load has been tolerated. If the pain is worse, load tolerance has been exceeded. The test is to be administered daily, at the same time of day, throughout the entire rehabilitation process. This approach can be extended to other tendinopathies such as LE using, for example, pain-free grip test, which is a reliable, valid, and sensitive measure (Stratford and Levy 1994). Littlewood et al. (2014) used a someway similar approach for rotator cuff related shoulder pain. However caution has to be taken in reactive shoulder and especially when psychological factors are associated (Lewis et al. 2015). Pain education may be crucial in this phase. Patient has to understand that pain is not equal to damage (Moseley 2007).

Finally clinicians have to be aware of appearance of new symptoms during the course of treatment or of symptoms that expand to sites outside and remote from the first site of presentation. This, in fact, may represent a possible sign of central sensitization (Nijs et al. 2010).

Subjecting tendons to tensile, moderate isometric loads while protecting against compression may improve recovery. Isometric also seems to be able to reduce pain through central modulation. Rio et al. (2015) show that a single resistance training bout of isometric contractions, in patients with patellar tendinopathy, reduced tendon pain immediately for at least 45 min post-intervention. The reduction in pain seems paralleled by a reduction in cortical inhibition. However, another study conducted by O'Neil et al. (unpublished data) shows that the above mentioned pain reduction does not seem to appear in patients with Achilles tendinopathy. Even if other researches are needed, isometric contractions with high load (up to 80% of maximum voluntary contraction) can be used as initial strategy if a reduction of pain is obtained. The isometric work must be composed of 5 repetitions lasting 45–60 seconds each, with a 2 minutes rest interval between the series to allow recovery. These loads can be repeated several times a day. A good prognostic sign after isometric work is an immediate reduction of pain in pain-provocation test after exercise. Even isometric must be designed in a way that compression at enthesis, in insertional tendinopathy, is not increased.

There is not a clear boundary between Phase 1 and Phase 2. Exercises that involve distant site from the original site of pathology should be introduced as soon as tolerated while maintaining Phase 1 exercises.

15.1.5.2 Phase 2: Recover Flexibility (Look at Distant Sites)

Little is known about range of motion (ROM) among patients with tendinopathy. Chimenti et al. (2016) found that during stair ascent patients with insertional Achilles tendinopathy used greater end-range dorsiflexion, less plantar flexion and lower peak ankle plantar flexor power than the control group 2016. These data seem to show that there is not restriction in ROM or isometric plantar flexor strength; altered ankle biomechanics during stair ascent were linked with greater symptom severity and likely contribute to decreased function. Conversely other authors found that patients with patellar tendinopathy showed decreased ankle dorsiflexion range of motion (Malliaras et al. 2006). Witvrouw et al. (2001) looked for risk factors for development of patellar tendinosis. They found that the only determining factor was hamstring and quadriceps reduced flexibility. From all this, albeit not conclusive data, we can hypothesis that reduced range of motion and flexibility in site of tendinopathy is not the crucial part. However altered flexibility in distal sites from the actually painful may be partial relevant because it can create biomechanical alteration.

Different tendinopathies may have different biomechanical alterations in different sports activities. People suffering ultrasuond abnormalities at their patellar tendons showed different landing patterns compared to controls (Edwards et al. 2010). Paradoxically better jumping ability has been shown to be a risk factor for developing patellar tendinopathy (Visnes et al. 2013). This may be due to a better ability to use elastic energy of tendon for force production. An altered "energy flow" from the trunk to the hand has been shown to be correlated with injury risk (Martin et al. 2014). It's difficult to find general principles that can guide functional assessment for all the tendons; however "minimum jerk" is a common feature especially of upper arms movement (Flash and Hogan 1985). Physically "jerk" is defined as the time derivative of acceleration or as the third time derivative of location. In practice, it means that if your CNS has to move your hand or some other end effector smoothly from one point to another, it should minimize the rate of changes of acceleration. If during functional assessment rapid change of acceleration is observed, this may be signs of alteration. If other flexibility, coordination, or strength deficit elsewhere in the limb are found, specific exercises can also be initiated during this initial phase. Sports with markedly different use profiles (such as baseball pitchers) may surprisingly demonstrate bilateral pathology implicating systemic or nervous system involvement in tendinopathy (Rio et al. 2016). For these reasons it is important to do a bilateral assessment and start rehabilitation as needed.

If an alteration in "kinetic chain" range of motion is found, it should be corrected with exercises that do not load the original site of pathology. Meanwhile, it is important to continue Phase 1 exercises. Finally general exercises aimed to maintain general fitness, without load altered tendon, have to be included.

15.1.5.3 Phase 3: Recover Strength (The Muscle–Tendon Specific Function)

Isotonic loads can be introduced when they can be performed with pain less than 3/10 on a numeric pain rating scale. If range of motion is restricted, for example, in the shoulder, it has to be progressed as resistance training. It is useful in the first steps of this phase to avoid compression on tendon and to maintain, if required, an external force to joint. As the symptoms improve, progression may be made by performing movement using a less stable base such as physioball and reducing external load. Then patients can switch to short lever (i.e., elbow bent for shoulder) initially without, then with, increasing weights and resistances (Lewis 2016).

In a randomized control trial, Beyer et al. found that both traditional eccentric and heavy slow resistance training (HSR) achieved equally good results in patients with Achilles tendinopathy, but that the latter tends to be associated with greater patient satisfaction after 12 weeks (2015). Kongsgaard et al. found similar results in patellar tendinopathy (2009). In HSR training three to four sets were performed progressing from an initial load based on 15 repetition maximum (15RM) to 6RM performed every second day. Different methods have been proposed to estimate RM (Niewiadomski et al. 2008). A simple way is to consider that 80% of 1RM is more or less equal to 8RM: the maximal weight that can be lifted eight times. Initially for the aim of be specific and to reduce motor control task, it's better to use single-joint specific exercises, avoiding multi-joint exercises and, for the lower limb, using only one leg. It's important, especially for energy storage tendons, to achieve heavy load (6RM) because they are associated with tendon adaptation. The clinicians have to consider both short-term and long-term reaction to load. In the short term, there will be a net loss of collagen production for 24–36 h post-exercise; for these reasons is mandatory to adequate rest days between strength sessions (Magnusson et al. 2010). In the day off isometric exercises for pain can be continued.

When heavy loads are reached (6RM), eccentric training can be introduced. Achilles tendon load and stretch are identical during the concentric and eccentric components of the traditional heel rise/drop exercise (Chaudhry et al. 2015). Muscles can produce greater maximal force eccentrically than concentrically (Enoka 1996). This can produce higher strain on tendon; however this potential is rarely utilized in practice because rehabilitation exercises seldom approach to concentric 1 RM (Malliaras et al. 2015). It's important that eccentric trainings have to be performed using significant progressive overload. Formally, the patients have to use an overload that, to be raised, need contralateral help in concentric phase. Eccentric phase has to be well performed with "minimum jerk." There are other theoretical techniques showing eccentric training useful in tendinopathy (see O'Neil et al. for a review (2015)). There is also some evidence that eccentric training may be helpful also in the upper limb (Camargo et al. n.d., 2014). We suggest to perform eccentric training only in the final steps of this phase to prepare patient to more demanding activity. Phase 3 exercises should be continued throughout rehabilitation and to return to sport.

15.1.5.4 Phase 4: Recover Coordination (The Kinetic Chain Function)

The purpose of Phase 4 is to introduce more functional tasks: during this rehabilitation period the differences between tendons increase. According to the hypothesis already presented the functional task of lower limbs is to store and release energy, whereas upper limbs have to predict forces. As already described this distinction depends also from the patient activities. Upper limbs multi-joint coordination exercises have to be firstly introduced as closed chain exercises, such as push-up or modified push-up. Progression is performed using less stable base and/or open chain. For example, to treat a shoulder tendinopathy we can introduce external rotation exercises with unsupported abduction/flexion, with progressive increase of elastic resistance or free weight loads as tolerated. (Lewis et al. 2015).

Treat movement dysfunction may be extremely tricky. It is difficult to find an optimal coordination for most of the human movement, if not impossible nowadays. Imposing a "correct" way to move is complicated and may be even detrimental especially when variability is needed (Stergiou and Decker 2011). Giving learners instructions that refer to the coordination of their body movements—as is typically done in teaching motor skills—has not been shown to be optimal for learning (Wulf et al. 1998) and may reduce variability. Most of the motor learning happens without any formal instructions. A 1-year-old child normally walks easily even if he's not able to understand a single word. His brain has an "internal model of dynamics" that is well adapted to physical forces such as interactional torque and is able to predict it. This is called unsupervised motor learning. Reinforcement learning (RL) is learning by interacting with an environment. It means learning from the consequences of one's actions, rather than from being explicitly taught and selecting actions on the basis of past experiences (exploitation) and also by new choices (exploration), which is essentially trial-and-error learning. There are good evidences that the CNS uses some forms of RL (Graybiel 2005; Tanaka et al. 2004). According to the constrained action hypothesis (CAH), an internal focus is associated with "conscious" control processes interfering with automatic control processes (Wulf et al. 2001). Learning from error implies that we need to reduce error in the long run. In movements such as hitting a nail with a hammer, minimalizing errors means that the center of the hammer must get as close as possible to the center of the nail. This achieves reducing variability at the end effector. Then it is generally mandatory to increase "good variability" (Wu and Latash 2014) elsewhere (Todorov and Jordan 2002). For this reason, conscious control, for example, of shoulder may reduce variability in shoulder movement that may be detrimental for tendon and function. So during this phase of rehabilitation, exercises have to be focused to end effector (external focusing) trying to forget as much as possible the painful tendon.

During the landing phase of a vertical jump, peak patellar tendon forces have been estimated to be 5.17 ± 0.86 body weight, with a loading rate of 38.06 ± 11.55 body weight per second (Janssen et al. 2013). In contrast, bilateral leg press (which is not an energy storage loading exercise) performed with a resistance equal to three times the body weight exerts a patellar tendon force equivalent to 5.2 body weight and a loading rate estimated at around 2 body weight per second (Reeves et al. 2003). The major change through these activities is rate of loading of the tendon, which should be progressed gradually through relevant energy storage activities for patients. Initially, simple weight-bearing exercises, such as single-leg squats, step downs, or lunges, can be performed at a speed appropriate for the patient's functional level. The speed of the exercise is progressively increased until the patient becomes proficient to perform the exercise as fast as athletic or functional activities.

After satisfactory completion of simple faster movements, more demanding exercises, such as hopping, skipping, or jumping squats, can be added to improve the kinetic chain function. Progression is guided by pain experienced in provocation test 24 h after exercise. A helpful habit is to use a training diary on which the athlete keeps the level of pain during activity and during the next day (especially morning stiffness). Exercises that implement energy storage can be very demanding for tendons; for this reason, it is better to perform this type of exercise every third day, in consideration of collagen turnover (Cook and Purdam 2012). It's important to continue Phase 1, Phase 2, and Phase 3 exercises in the days off, with a progressive and careful load increase. Malliaras et al. (2015) suggest that the volume is progressed before the intensity. Especially in athletes, the purpose of Phase 4 is to build power. Power is a function of strength (force) and speed (velocity) of movement and is important in most sporting activities. Power has to be at least as in the contralateral limb. We advise to use a functional test that mimics sport-specific demands of the subject such as maximal vertical hop height. If pain rises during Phase 4, it is important to return to Phase 1 exercises and progress as soon as the pain has returned to normal.

15.1.5.5 Phase 5: Return to Sport (Sport-Specific Exercises)

In these return-to-sports phase, specific exercises are introduced. This part of the rehabilitation program must be carefully planned in consultation with the athlete and their coach so that it involves sessions of gradually increasing intensity and volume with appropriate rest periods. For the most of the sports, jogging is a base activity and needs to be introduced at this stage of the rehabilitation program. Running retraining seems to be a promising way to reduce pain moving the load from the pathological structure. The aim of running retraining is to identify the theoretical mechanics contributing to tissue overload and then facilitate the desired changes (for a complete review, see Barton et al. (2016)). For example, increasing step rate may reduce soleus muscle force during stance and be helpful in Achilles tendinopathy (Lenhart et al. 2014).

It's also important to introduce load monitoring. The rating of perceived exertion (RPE) (Ritchie 2012) has been used by clinicians, coaches, and researchers as a simple tool to monitor and adjust exercise intensity (Saw et al. 2015). Silbernagel et al. (2015) proposed to subdivide activities' intensity based on pain (assessed with numeric pain rating scale) and RPE in three different groups. Mild activities can be performed every day, moderate activities every two days, while high-level activities require 3 days of recovery. When the athlete can jog without increasing their pain, more demanding sport-specific exercises including sprinting, jumping/landing, acceleration, and change of direction activities are added. Similar interval training has been developed for overhead athletes (Axe et al. 2009). Reduced energy transfer to the shoulder would potentially result in higher requirements at the shoulder itself, potentially leading to early fatigue of the rotator cuff muscles. Thus it is important to assess that any potentially biomechanical alterations are resolved.

This final phase may be the most critically one. It's not infrequent that pain may rise again when athlete returns to normal activity. Mild pain, that do not limit sports activity, may remain (van der Plas et al. 2012). Recurrence of symptoms is not infrequent, and the athlete may be more susceptible to change of intensity of activity. Excessive and rapid increases in training loads are likely responsible for a large proportion of non-contact, soft-tissue injuries. The training intensity used during rehabilitation is usually lower than the normal training. So athletes can't simply return to normal training but have to shift from rehabilitation exercises to sport-specific activities for monitoring load. We recommend, for this propose, to use the "acute/chronic workload ratio" as proposed by Blanch and Gabbett (2016). It is important to consider tendinopathy as a treatable pathology but not always a curable one. This change of vision is to be sheared with athletes and coaches. When athletes may return to play, they are not "healed" and need special attentions. As a maintenance program, once athletes have returned to sport, it's helpful to use Phase 2 strengthening exercises at least twice per week.

Rehabilitation phase	Functional impairment	Exercise type	Duration
Phase 1	Load and pain management	Reduce loading	Weeks 2–3
Phase 2	Recover flexibility	Correct biomechanical alteration	Weeks 3–4
Phase 3	Muscle–tendon function	Single-joint strengthening	Weeks 3–8
Phase 4	Kinetic chain function	Multi-joint strengthening and flexibility	Weeks 8–14
Phase 5	Sport-specific exercises and return to sport	Shifting from rehabilitation to normal training	Months 3–6

15.2 Nonsteroidal Anti-inflammatory Drugs

Oral nonsteroidal anti-inflammatory drugs (NSAIDs) have been used extensively for decades to treat pain associated with tendon overuse. In their systematic review, Bret et al. (Andres and Murrell 2008) identified 37 randomized clinical trials or systematic reviews that evaluate NSAIDs in the treatment of tendinopathy, but only 17 studies were placebo controlled. Boudreault et al. (2014) recently evaluated the effectiveness of NSAIDs in rotator cuff tendinopathy. Their meta-analysis reveals that there is low-to-moderate grade evidence that NSAIDs are effective in reducing short-term pain without an improvement in function. Interestingly, in terms of pain and function, oral anti-inflammatory drugs in the short term are as effective as corticosteroid injections. Scott et al. (2011) found no randomized control trails that evaluated the effect of NSAIDs on symptoms lasting longer than 3 months. A trial, which included patients with chronic Achilles tendinopathy of less than 6 months, found identical treatment outcomes in subject randomly assigned to receive piroxicam or placebo tablets (Aström and Westlin 1992). Finally, a recent Cochrane review (Pattanittum et al. 2013) concludes that "*there remains limited evidence from which to draw firm conclusions about the benefits or harms of topical or oral NSAIDs in treating lateral elbow pain*." Overall, the evidence suggests both oral and local NSAIDS are effective in relieving the pain associated with tendinopathy in the short term (7–14 days). Oral and local NSAIDs appear effective in the treatment of acute shoulder bursitis/tendonitis. It may be due to the involvement of the "enthesis organ" (Kehl et al. 2016) in tendinopathy. Not surprisingly, the patients who presented with a longer duration and greater severity of symptoms were more likely to have a poor response to both corticosteroid injection and/or oral NSAIDs. However, recent research shows that NSAIDs may have a possible negative consequences on the long-term healing process (Su and O'Connor 2013). In addition, long-term NSAIDs use increases the risk of gastrointestinal, cardiovascular, and renal complications associated with these medications. Overall, a short course of NSAIDs appears a reasonable option for the treatment of acute pain associated with tendon overuse. In all cases, if chosen, NSAID treatments should always be kept as short as possible.

15.3 Physical Therapy Modalities

There are a wide variety of modalities available to the physical therapist, and it is difficult to predict which technique or group of techniques a given therapist will utilize. Low-level laser treatment (LLLT) has been studied extensively with mixed results. Overall some studies showed improvement treating tendinopathy with LLLT compared to placebo (Bjordal et al. 2006; England et al. 1989), but many showed no difference (Basford et al. 2000; Bingöl et al. 2005). A recent systematic review assessed LLLT in tendinopathy and found there that low-level laser treatment is more effective than placebo in treating tendinopathy (Nogueira and Júnior 2015). Other physical therapy modalities have not been studied extensively but have similar conflicting results in the literature. A recent systematic review found that patients with persistent plantar fasciitis may benefit from therapeutic ultrasound (Yu et al. 2016). Pooled data from trials evaluating the treatment of lateral epicondylitis with ultrasound compared to controls showed the estimated difference in success rate to be 15% (van der Windt et al. 1999). Some benefits with therapeutic ultrasound used in the treatment of lateral epicondylitis and calcific tendonitis of the supraspinatus are reported (Philadelphia Panel 2001).

Iontophoresis and phonophoresis involve using ionizing current or ultrasound to deliver medications locally. Corticosteroids and NSAIDS are commonly used with these modalities. There are only few controlled studies in literature, and most reported no improvement compared to controls (Runeson and Haker 2002). Transverse friction massage has also been used to treat tendinopathy, but, to our knowledge, no studies showed a benefit of deep friction massage over other physical therapy modalities (Stasinopoulos and Stasinopoulos 2004). A recent Cochrane review found no sufficient evidence to determine the effects of deep transverse friction on pain, improvement in grip strength, and functional status for patients with lateral elbow tendinitis (Loew et al. 2014). Hyperthermia has also been used in the treatment of tendinopathy. This modality involves using deep-heating machines that combine a superficial cooling system with a microwave-powered heating system. This can increase the temperature of target tissues approximately 4 °C without damaging the skin. Presumably this increased temperature results in increased blood flow and subsequent healing to the damaged area. One randomized clinical trial has been recently published evaluating hyperthermia compared to therapeutic ultrasound in the treatment of tendinopathy. This trial report improvements in pain and patient satisfaction in the hyperthermia group compared to the ultrasound group (Giombini et al. 2006).

In summary, there is currently little and conflicting evidence available to support the use of most physical therapy modalities including LLLT, iontophoresis, phonophoresis, therapeutic ultrasound, or deep friction massage. Further research with higher-powered studies would be useful to determine the most effective physical therapy regime for the treatment of tendinopathies.

15.4 Corticosteroid

Corticosteroid injections have been a mainstay in the treatment of tendinopathy. Despite their widespread use, there is some controversy as to their usefulness and safety in this setting. Several studies report good short-term pain control (≤6 weeks) with corticosteroid injections in patients with lateral epicondylitis and shoulder impingement (Smidt et al. 2002a; Verhaar et al. 1996). The long-term efficacy of corticosteroid injections for tendinopathy has not been demonstrated. Corticosteroid injections for lateral epicondylitis do not provide any long-term benefit (6–12 months) compared with placebo, NSAIDs, or physical therapy in randomized, controlled studies (Smidt et al. 2002b). A recent study by Coombes et al. (2013) shows that the use of corticosteroid may be even detrimental in a long time. In this study, the authors find that among patients with chronic unilateral lateral epicondylalgia, the use of corticosteroid injection with respect to placebo injection resulted in worse clinical outcomes after 1 year, and even physiotherapy is able to reverse this outcome.

Mixed results have been published also regarding the long-term benefits of sub-acromial corticosteroid injections for rotator cuff tendinopathy. An extensive systematic review evaluating the efficacy of corticosteroid injections in the treatment of rotator cuff disease recently reported little or no evidence to support the use of corticosteroid injections for these patients (Koester et al. 2007).

Analyzing the effectiveness of corticosteroid injections in the medium-term treatment of tendinopathy, there is a question of safety with using these medications in this setting (Kleinman and Gross 1983). Several cases of Achilles tendon rupture have been reported after corticosteroid injections. More recently, Gill et al. (2004) described a series of 83 injections in the Achilles region without serious complication. The key point is they injected the steroid under fluoroscopic guidance around the tendon but not within the substance of the tendon. Of note, only 40% of the patients in this series reported improvement after the procedure at the 2-year follow-up.

In summary, corticosteroid injections have been used for decades in the treatment of tendinopathy. There is strong evidence that they relieve pain in the short term up to 6 weeks, but there is no evidence that they provide any benefit in the long term (beyond 6 months) for the treatment of chronic tendinopathy, and some evidence that their use can even be detrimental. There are also some reports that show that they can be detrimental in long terms. Even if it seems that the risks associated with corticosteroid injections can be minimized by injecting under image guidance to ensure the injection is paratendinous rather than intratendinous, the authors do not advice the use of steroid in tendinopathy.

15.5 Glyceryl Trinitrate Patches

Nitric oxide (NO) is a soluble molecule produced by a family of enzymes called nitric oxide synthases (NOS). In large doses, NO can be toxic, but in smaller physiological doses, it acts as a cellular messenger and appears to play a role in blood pressure, memory, and host defense. NO appears to play a role in tendon healing after injury. In a rat Achilles tendon healing model (Murrell et al. 1997), inhibition of NOS resulted in a decreased cross-sectional area and load to failure of the healing tendon. NO was delivered transcutaneously to the area of painful tendinopathy using commercially available glyceryl trinitrate (GTN) patches. Patients generally place the patch directly over the area of greatest tenderness/pain, and they are instructed to change the patch every 24 h. The patches were worn for more or less 6 months.

There are some randomized, controlled, double-blind clinical studies designed to determine whether the topical administration of NO would enhance tendon healing in humans. Again there are mixed results. Despite the first clinical data were hopeful (Paoloni et al. 2003, 2005, 2009), subsequent studies do not support these treatments (Steunebrink et al. 2013; Cumpston et al. 2009). A Cochrane systematic review found some evidence only from one study with high risk of bias on the effectiveness of topical glyceryl trinitrate for rotator cuff disease in acute phase (less than 7 days duration) but that there is insufficient evidence to be certain about their longer-term effects (Cumpston et al. 2009).

There is some question whether nitric oxide simply has an analgesic effect or a healing effect in the treatment of tendinopathy. The most commonly described side effect seen with this treatment modality is headache. The headaches can be severe enough to cause cessation of treatment. Based on these evidences, the authors recommend GTN in tendinopathy only when other treatments have failed.

Acknowledgments The authors would like to thank Dr. Franco Cento for the extended review.

References

Alfredson H, Pietilä T, Jonsson P et al (1988) Heavy-load eccentric calf muscle training for the treatment of chronic Achilles tendinosis. Am J Sports Med 26:360–366

Alfredson H, Forsgren S, Thorsen K et al (2001) In vivo microdialysis and immunohistochemical analyses of tendon tissue demonstrated high amounts of free glutamate and glutamate NMDAR1 receptors, but no signs of inflammation, in Jumper's knee. J Orthop Res 19:881–886. doi:10.1016/S0736-0266(01)00016-X

Alizadehkhaiyat O, Fisher AC, Kemp GJ et al (2007) Upper limb muscle imbalance in tennis elbow: a functional and electromyographic assessment. J Orthop Res 25:1651–1657. doi:10.1002/jor.20458

Andres BM, Murrell GAC (2008) Treatment of tendinopathy: what works, what does not, and what is on the horizon. Clin Orthop Relat Res 466:1539–1554. doi:10.1007/s11999-008-0260-1

Aström M, Westlin N (1992) No effect of piroxicam on achilles tendinopathy. A randomized study of 70 patients. Acta Orthop Scand 63:631–634

Axe M, Hurd W, Snyder-Mackler L (2009) Data-based interval throwing programs for baseball players. Sports Health 1:145–153. doi:10.1177/1941738108331198

Barton CJ, Bonanno DR, Carr J et al (2016) Running retraining to treat lower limb injuries: a mixed-methods study of current evidence synthesised with expert opinion. Br J Sports Med 50:513–526. doi:10.1136/bjsports-2015-095278

Basford JR, Sheffield CG, Cieslak KR (2000) Laser therapy: a randomized, controlled trial of the effects of low intensity Nd:YAG laser irradiation on lateral epicondylitis. Arch Phys Med Rehabil 81:1504–1510. doi:10.1053/apmr.2000.17812

Beyer R, Kongsgaard M, Hougs Kjær B et al (2015) Heavy slow resistance versus eccentric training as treatment for Achilles tendinopathy: a randomized controlled trial. Am J Sports Med 43:1704–1711. doi:10.1177/0363546515584760

Bingöl Ü, Altan L, Yurtkuran M (2005) Low-power laser treatment for shoulder pain. Photomed Laser Surg 23:459–464. doi:10.1089/pho.2005.23.459

Bjordal JM, Lopes-Martins RAB, Iversen VV (2006) A randomised, placebo controlled trial of low level laser therapy for activated Achilles tendinitis with microdialysis measurement of peritendinous prostaglandin E_2 concentrations. Br J Sports Med 40:76–80. doi:10.1136/bjsm.2005.020842

Blanch P, Gabbett TJ (2016) Has the athlete trained enough to return to play safely? The acute:chronic workload ratio permits clinicians to quantify a player's risk of subsequent injury. Br J Sports Med 50:471–475. doi:10.1136/bjsports-2015-095445

Boudreault J, Desmeules F, Roy J-S et al (2014) The efficacy of oral non-steroidal anti-inflammatory drugs for rotator cuff tendinopathy: a systematic review and meta-analysis. J Rehabil Med 46:294–306. doi:10.2340/16501977-1800

Camargo PR, Alburquerque-Sendín F, Salvini TF (2014) Eccentric training as a new approach for rotator cuff tendinopathy: review and perspectives. Published Online First. doi:10.5312/wjo.v5.i5.634

Camargo PR, Avila MA, Alburquerque-Sendín F et al Eccentric training for shoulder abductors improves pain, function and isokinetic performance in subjects with shoulder impingement syndrome—a case series. Rev Bras Fisioter 16:74–83

Chang Y-J, Kulig K (2015) The neuromechanical adaptations to Achilles tendinosis. J Physiol 593:3373–3387. doi:10.1113/JP270220

Chaudhry S, Morrissey D, Woledge RC et al (2015) Eccentric and concentric loading of the triceps surae: an in vivo study of dynamic muscle and tendon biomechanical parameters. J Appl Biomech 31:69–78. doi:10.1123/jab.213-0284

Chester R, Jerosch-Herold C, Lewis J et al (2016) Psychological factors are associated with the outcome of physiotherapy for people with shoulder pain: a multicentre longitudinal cohort study. Br J Sports Med. doi:10.1136/bjsports-2016-096084

Chimenti RL, Forenza A, Previte E et al (2016) Forefoot and rearfoot contributions to the lunge position in individuals with and without insertional Achilles tendinopathy. Clin Biomech 36:40–45. doi:10.1016/j.clinbiomech.2016.05.007

Cook JL, Purdam C (2012) Is compressive load a factor in the development of tendinopathy? Br J Sports Med 46:163–168. doi:10.1136/bjsports-2011-090414

Cook JL, Rio E, Purdam CR et al Revisiting the continuum model of tendon pathology: what is its merit in clinical practice and research? Br J Sports Med. doi:10.1136/bjsports-2015-095422

Coombes BK, Bisset L, Vicenzino B et al (2008) A new integrative model of lateral epicondylalgia. Published Online First. doi:10.1136/bjsm.2008.052738

Coombes BK, Bisset L, Vicenzino B (2012) Thermal hyperalgesia distinguishes those with severe pain and disability in unilateral lateral epicondylalgia. Clin J Pain 28:595–601. doi:10.1097/AJP.0b013e31823dd333

Coombes BK, Bisset L, Brooks P et al (2013) Effect of corticosteroid injection, physiotherapy, or both on clinical outcomes in patients with unilateral lateral epicondylalgia: a randomized controlled trial. JAMA 309:461–469. doi:10.1001/jama.2013.129

Coombes BK, Bisset L, Vicenzino B (2015) Management of lateral elbow tendinopathy-one size does not fit all. J Orthop Sports Phys Ther 45:1–38. doi:10.2519/jospt.2015.5841

Couppé C, Svensson RB, Silbernagel KG et al (2015) Eccentric or concentric exercises for the treatment of tendinopathies? J Orthop Sport Phys Ther 45:1–25. doi:10.2519/jospt.2015.5910

Cumpston M, Johnston RV, Wengier L et al (2009) Topical glyceryl trinitrate for rotator cuff disease. In: Buchbinder R (ed) Cochrane database of systematic reviews. John Wiley & Sons, Ltd., Chichester, UK . doi:10.1002/14651858.CD006355.pub2CD006355

Dilek B, Gulbahar S, Gundogdu M et al (2016) Efficacy of proprioceptive exercises in patients with subacromial impingement syndrome. Am J Phys Med Rehabil 95:169–182. doi:10.1097/PHM.0000000000000327

Edwards S, Steele JR, McGhee DE et al (2010) Landing strategies of athletes with an asymptomatic patellar tendon abnormality. Med Sci Sports Exerc 42:2072–2080. doi:10.1249/MSS.0b013e3181e0550b

England S, Farrell AJ, Coppock JS et al (1989) Low power laser therapy of shoulder tendonitis. Scand J Rheumatol 18:427–431

Enoka RM (1996) Eccentric contractions require unique activation strategies by the nervous system. J Appl Physiol 81

Flash T, Hogan N (1985) The coordination of arm movements: an experimentally confirmed mathematical model. J Neurosci 5:1688–1703. PMID: 4020415

Flor H, Braun C, Elbert T et al (1997) Extensive reorganization of primary somatosensory cortex in chronic back pain patients. Neurosci Lett 224:5–8

Forsdyke D, Smith A, Jones M et al (2016) Psychosocial factors associated with outcomes of sports injury rehabilitation in competitive athletes: a mixed studies systematic review. Br J Sports Med 50(9):537–544. doi:10.1136/bjsports-2015-094850

Gill SS, Gelbke MK, Mattson SL et al (2004) Fluoroscopically guided low-volume peritendinous corticosteroid injection for Achilles tendinopathy. A safety study. J Bone Joint Surg Am 86–A:802–806

Giombini A, Di Cesare A, Safran MR et al (2006) Short-term effectiveness of hyperthermia for supraspinatus tendinopathy in athletes: a short-term randomized controlled study. Am J Sports Med 34:1247–1253. doi:10.1177/0363546506287827

Goom TSH, Malliaras P, Reiman MP et al (2016) Proximal hamstring tendinopathy: clinical aspects of assessment and management. J Orthop Sports Phys Ther 46:483–493. doi:10.2519/jospt.2016.5986

Graybiel AM (2005) The basal ganglia: learning new tricks and loving it. Curr Opin Neurobiol 15:638–644. doi:10.1016/j.conb.2005.10.006

Gwilym SE, Oag HCL, Tracey I et al (2011) Evidence that central sensitisation is present in patients with shoulder impingement syndrome and influences the outcome after surgery. Bone Joint J 93:498–502. doi:10.1302/0301-620X.93B4.25054

Heales LJ, Lim ECW, Hodges PW et al (2014) Sensory and motor deficits exist on the non-injured side of patients with unilateral tendon pain and disability—implications for central nervous system involvement: a systematic review with meta-analysis. Br J Sports Med 48:1400–1406. doi:10.1136/bjsports-2013-092535

Hodges PW, Moseley GL (2003) Pain and motor control of the lumbopelvic region: effect and possible mechanisms. J Electromyogr Kinesiol 13:361–370. doi:10.1016/S1050-6411(03)00042-7

Hungerford B, Gilleard W, Hodges P (2003) Evidence of altered lumbopelvic muscle recruitment in the presence of sacroiliac joint pain. Spine (Phila Pa 1976) 28:1593–1600

Janssen I, Steele JR, Munro BJ et al (2013) Predicting the patellar tendon force generated when landing from a jump. Med Sci Sports Exerc 45:927–934. doi:10.1249/MSS.0b013e31827f0314

Järvinen M (1992) Epidemiology of tendon injuries in sports. Clin Sports Med 11:493–504

Juul-Kristensen B, Lund H, Hansen K et al (2008) Poorer elbow proprioception in patients with lateral epicondylitis than in healthy controls: a cross-sectional study. J Shoulder Elb Surg 17:S72–S81. doi:10.1016/j.jse.2007.07.003

Kehl AS, Corr M, Weisman MH (2016) Review: enthesitis: new insights into pathogenesis, diagnostic modalities, and treatment. Arthritis Rheumatol 68:312–322. doi:10.1002/art.39458

Kjaer M, Langberg H, Miller BF et al (2005) Metabolic activity and collagen turnover in human tendon in response to physical activity. J Musculoskelet Neuronal Interact 5:41–52

Kleinman M, Gross AE (1983) Achilles tendon rupture following steroid injection. Report of three cases. J Bone Joint Surg Am 65:1345–1347

Koester MC, Dunn WR, Kuhn JE et al (2007) The efficacy of subacromial corticosteroid injection in the treatment of rotator cuff disease: a systematic review. J Am Acad Orthop Surg 15:3–11

Kongsgaard M, Kovanen V, Aagaard P et al (2009) Corticosteroid injections, eccentric decline squat training and heavy slow resistance training in patellar tendinopathy. Scand J Med Sci Sports 19:790–802. doi:10.1111/j.1600-0838.2009.00949.x

Kountouris A, Cook J (2007) Rehabilitation of Achilles and patellar tendinopathies. Best Pract Res Clin Rheumatol 21:295–316. doi:10.1016/j.berh.2006.12.003

Langberg H, Skovgaard D, Asp S et al (2000) Time pattern of exercise-induced changes in type I collagen turnover after prolonged endurance exercise in humans. Calcif Tissue Int 67(1):41–44. doi:10.1007/s00223001094

Lenhart RL, Thelen DG, Wille CM et al (2014) Increasing running step rate reduces patellofemoral joint forces. Med Sci Sports Exerc 46:557–564. doi:10.1249/MSS.0b013e3182a78c3a

Lewis JS (2009) Rotator cuff tendinopathy/subacromial impingement syndrome: is it time for a new method of assessment? Br J Sports Med 43:259–264. doi:10.1136/bjsm.2008.052183

Lewis J (2016) Masterclass rotator cuff related shoulder pain: assessment, management and uncertainties. Published Online First. doi:10.1016/j.math.2016.03.009

Lewis J, McCreesh K, Roy J-S et al (2015) Rotator cuff tendinopathy: navigating the diagnosis-management conundrum. J Orthop Sport Phys Ther 45:923–937. doi:10.2519/jospt.2015.5941

Lim ECW, Sterling M, Pedler A et al (2012) Evidence of spinal cord hyperexcitability as measured with nociceptive flexion reflex (NFR) threshold in chronic lateral epicondylalgia with or without a positive neurodynamic test. J Pain 13:676–684. doi:10.1016/j.jpain.2012.04.005

Linton SJ, Shaw WS (2011) Impact of psychological factors in the experience of pain. Phys Ther 91

Littlewood C, Malliaras P, Mawson S et al (2014) Self-managed loaded exercise versus usual physiotherapy treatment for rotator cuff tendinopathy: a pilot randomised controlled trial. Physiotherapy 100:54–60. doi:10.1016/j.physio.2013.06.001

Ljung B-O, Forsgren S, Fridén J (1999) Substance P and calcitonin gene-related peptide expression at the extensor carpi radialis brevis muscle origin: implications for the etiology of tennis elbow. J Orthop Res 17:554–559. doi:10.1002/jor.1100170414

Loew LM, Brosseau L, Tugwell P et al (2014) Deep transverse friction massage for treating lateral elbow or lateral knee tendinitis. In: Brosseau L (ed) Cochrane database of systematic reviews. John Wiley & Sons, Ltd., Chichester, UK . doi:10.1002/14651858.CD003528.pub2CD003528

Lund JP, Donga R, Widmer CG et al (1991) The pain-adaptation model: a discussion of the relationship between chronic musculoskeletal pain and motor activity. Can J Physiol Pharmacol 69:683–694

Maffulli N, Longo UG (2008) How do eccentric exercises work in tendinopathy? Rheumatology 47:1444–1445. doi:10.1093/rheumatology/ken337

Maganaris CN, Paul JP (2002) Tensile properties of the in vivo human gastrocnemius tendon. J Biomech 35:1639–1646

Magnusson SP, Langberg H, Kjaer M (2010) The pathogenesis of tendinopathy: balancing the response to loading. Nat Rev Rheumatol 6:262–268. doi:10.1038/nrrheum.2010.43

Malliaras P, Cook JL, Kent P (2006) Reduced ankle dorsiflexion range may increase the risk of patellar tendon injury among volleyball players. J Sci Med Sport 9:304–309. doi:10.1016/j.jsams.2006.03.015

Malliaras P, Barton CJ, Reeves ND et al (2013) Achilles and patellar tendinopathy loading programmes: a systematic review comparing clinical outcomes and identifying potential mechanisms for effectiveness. Sports Med 43:267–286. doi:10.1007/s40279-013-0019-z

Malliaras P, Cook J, Purdam C et al (2015) Patellar tendinopathy: clinical diagnosis, load management, and advice for challenging case presentations. J Orthop Sport Phys Ther 45:887–898. doi:10.2519/jospt.2015.5987

Mallows A, Debenham J, Walker T et al (2016) Association of psychological variables and outcome in tendinopathy: a systematic review. Br J Sports Med 43:255–266. doi:10.1136/bjsports-2016-096154

Martin C, Bideau B, Bideau N et al (2014) Energy flow analysis during the tennis serve: comparison between

injured and noninjured tennis players. Am J Sports Med 42:2751–2760. doi:10.1177/0363546514547173
McCormick K, Zalucki N, Hudson ML et al (2007) Faulty proprioceptive information disrupts motor imagery: an experimental study. Aust J Physiother 53:41–45. doi:10.1016/S0004-9514(07)70060-0
Minagawa H, Yamamoto N, Abe H et al (2013) Prevalence of symptomatic and asymptomatic rotator cuff tears in the general population: from mass-screening in one village. J Orthop 10:8–12. doi:10.1016/j.jor.2013.01.008
Moseley GL (2007) Reconceptualising pain according to modern pain science. Phys Ther Rev 12:169–178. doi:10.1179/108331907X223010
Murrell GAC, Szabo C, Hannafin JA et al (1997) Modulation of tendon healing by nitric oxide. Inflamm Res 46:19–27. doi:10.1007/s000110050027
Narita K, Murata T, Honda K et al (2002) Subthalamic locomotor region is involved in running activity originating in the rat ventromedial hypothalamus. Behav Brain Res 134:275–281
Niewiadomski W, Laskowska D, Gąsiorowska A et al (2008) Determination and prediction of one repetition maximum (1RM): safety considerations. J Hum Kinet 19:109–120. doi:10.2478/v10078-008-0008-8
Nijs J, Van Houdenhove B, Oostendorp RAB (2010) Recognition of central sensitization in patients with musculoskeletal pain: application of pain neurophysiology in manual therapy practice. Man Ther 15:135–141. doi:10.1016/j.math.2009.12.001
Nogueira AC Jr, Júnior MJ (2015) The effects of laser treatment in tendinopathy: a systematic review. Acta Ortop Bras 23:47–49. doi:10.1590/1413-78522015230100513
O'Neill S, Watson PJ, Barry S (2015) Why are eccentric exercises effective for Achilles tendinopathy? Int J Sports Phys Ther 10:552–562
Paoloni JA, Appleyard RC, Nelson J et al (2003) Topical nitric oxide application in the treatment of chronic extensor tendinosis at the elbow: a randomized, double-blinded, placebo-controlled clinical trial. Am J Sports Med 31:915–920
Paoloni JA, Appleyard RC, Nelson J et al (2005) Topical glyceryl trinitrate application in the treatment of chronic supraspinatus tendinopathy: a randomized, double-blinded, placebo-controlled clinical trial. Am J Sports Med 33:806–813. doi:10.1177/0363546504270998
Paoloni JA, Murrell GAC, Burch RM et al (2009) Randomised, double-blind, placebo-controlled clinical trial of a new topical glyceryl trinitrate patch for chronic lateral epicondylosis. Br J Sports Med 43:299–302. doi:10.1136/bjsm.2008.053108
Pattanittum P, Turner T, Green S et al (2013) Non-steroidal anti-inflammatory drugs (NSAIDs) for treating lateral elbow pain in adults. Cochrane Database Syst Rev 5:CD003686. doi:10.1002/14651858.CD003686.pub2
Pearson SJ, Burgess K, Onambele GNL (2007) Creep and the in vivo assessment of human patellar tendon mechanical properties. Clin Biomech 22(6):712–717. doi:10.1016/j.clinbiomech.2007.02.006
Philadelphia Panel (2001) Philadelphia Panel evidence-based clinical practice guidelines on selected rehabilitation interventions for shoulder pain. Phys Ther 81:1719–1730
Pienimäki TT, Kauranen K, Vanharanta H (1997) Bilaterally decreased motor performance of arms in patients with chronic tennis elbow. Arch Phys Med Rehabil 78:1092–1095
Reeves ND (2006) Adaptation of the tendon to mechanical usage. J Musculoskelet Neuronal Interact 6:174–180
Reeves ND, Maganaris CN, Narici MV (2003) Effect of strength training on human patella tendon mechanical properties of older individuals. J Physiol 548:971–981. doi:10.1113/jphysiol.2002.035576
Rio E, Moseley L, Purdam C et al (2014) The pain of tendinopathy: physiological or pathophysiological? Sports Med 44:9–23. doi:10.1007/s40279-013-0096-z
Rio E, Kidgell D, Purdam C et al (2015) Isometric exercise induces analgesia and reduces inhibition in patellar tendinopathy. Br J Sports Med 49:1277–1283. doi:10.1136/bjsports-2014-094386
Rio E, Kidgell D, Moseley GL et al (2016) Tendon neuroplastic training: changing the way we think about tendon rehabilitation: a narrative review. Br J Sports Med 50:209–215. doi:10.1136/bjsports-2015-095215
Ritchie C (2012) Rating of perceived exertion (RPE). J Physiother 58:62. doi:10.1016/S1836-9553(12)70078-4
Roach NT, Venkadesan M, Rainbow MJ et al (2013) Elastic energy storage in the shoulder and the evolution of high-speed throwing in Homo. Nature 498:483–486. doi:10.1038/nature12267
Roberts TJ (2002) The integrated function of muscles and tendons during locomotion. Comp Biochem Physiol A Mol Integr Physiol 133:1087–1099
Robinson JM, Cook JL, Purdam C et al (2001) The VISA-A questionnaire: a valid and reliable index of the clinical severity of Achilles tendinopathy. Br J Sports Med 35:335–341. doi:10.1136/BJSM.35.5.335
Roos EM, Engström M, Lagerquist A et al (2004) Clinical improvement after 6 weeks of eccentric exercise in patients with mid-portion Achilles tendinopathy—a randomized trial with 1-year follow-up. Scand J Med Sci Sports 14:286–295. doi:10.1111/j.1600-0838.2004.378.x
Runeson L, Haker E (2002) Iontophoresis with cortisone in the treatment of lateral epicondylalgia (tennis elbow)—a double-blind study. Scand J Med Sci Sports 12:136–142. doi:10.1034/j.1600-0838.2002.02142.x
Saw AE, Main LC, Gastin PB et al (2015) Monitoring the athlete training response: subjective self-reported measures trump commonly used objective measures: a systematic review. Br J Sports Med 12:32–65. doi:10.1136/bjsports-2015-094758
Scott A, Huisman E, Khan K (2011) Conservative treatment of chronic Achilles tendinopathy. CMAJ 183:1159–1165. doi:10.1503/cmaj.101680
Silbernagel KG (2015) A proposed return-to-sport program for patients with midportion Achilles tendinopa-

thy: rationale and implementation. J Orthop Sport Phys Ther 45. doi:10.2519/jospt.2015.5885

Silbernagel KG, Thomeé R, Thomeé P et al (2001) Eccentric overload training for patients with chronic Achilles tendon pain—a randomised controlled study with reliability testing of the evaluation methods. Scand J Med Sci Sports 11:197–206

Smidt N, van der Windt DA, Assendelft WJ et al (2002a) Corticosteroid injections, physiotherapy, or a wait-and-see policy for lateral epicondylitis: a randomised controlled trial. Lancet 359:657–662. doi:10.1016/S0140-6736(02)07811-X

Smidt N, Assendelft WJJ, van der Windt DAWM et al (2002b) Corticosteroid injections for lateral epicondylitis: a systematic review. Pain 96:23–40

Stasinopoulos D, Stasinopoulos I (2004) Comparison of effects of exercise programme, pulsed ultrasound and transverse friction in the treatment of chronic patellar tendinopathy. Clin Rehabil 18:347–352. http://www.ncbi.nlm.nih.gov/pubmed/15180116. Accessed 5 Dec 2016

Stergiou N, Decker LM (2011) Human movement variability, nonlinear dynamics, and pathology: is there a connection? Hum Mov Sci 30:869–888. doi:10.1016/j.humov.2011.06.002

Steunebrink M, Zwerver J, Brandsema R et al (2013) Topical glyceryl trinitrate treatment of chronic patellar tendinopathy: a randomised, double-blind, placebo-controlled clinical trial. Br J Sports Med 47:34–39. doi:10.1136/bjsports-2012-091115

Stratford PW, Levy DRMD (1994) Assessing valid change over time in patients with lateral epicondylitis at the elbow. Clin J Sport Med 4:88–91

Su B, O'Connor JP (2013) NSAID therapy effects on healing of bone, tendon, and the enthesis. J Appl Physiol 115

Sussmilch-Leitch SP, Collins NJ, Bialocerkowski AE et al (2012) Physical therapies for Achilles tendinopathy: systematic review and meta-analysis. J Foot Ankle Res 5:1. doi:10.1186/1757-1146-5-15

Tanaka SC, Doya K, Okada G et al (2004) Prediction of immediate and future rewards differentially recruits cortico-basal ganglia loops. Nat Neurosci 7:887–893. doi:10.1038/nn1279

Terabayashi N, Watanabe T, Matsumoto K et al (2014) Increased blood flow in the anterior humeral circumflex artery correlates with night pain in patients with rotator cuff tear. J Orthop Sci 19:744–749. doi:10.1007/s00776-014-0604-5

Todorov E, Jordan MI (2002) Optimal feedback control as a theory of motor coordination. Published Online First. doi:10.1038/nn963

Tucker K, Larsson A-K, Oknelid S et al (2012) Similar alteration of motor unit recruitment strategies during the anticipation and experience of pain. Pain 153:636–643. doi:10.1016/j.pain.2011.11.024

van der Plas A, de Jonge S, de Vos RJ et al (2012) A 5-year follow-up study of Alfredson's heel-drop exercise programme in chronic midportion Achilles tendinopathy. Br J Sports Med 46:214–218. doi:10.1136/bjsports-2011-090035

van der Windt DA, van der Heijden GJ, van den Berg SG et al (1999) Ultrasound therapy for musculoskeletal disorders: a systematic review. Pain 81:257–271

Verhaar JA, Walenkamp GH, van Mameren H et al (1996) Local corticosteroid injection versus Cyriax-type physiotherapy for tennis elbow. J Bone Joint Surg Br 78:128–132

Vicenzino B, Paungmali A, Buratowski S et al (2001) Specific manipulative therapy treatment for chronic lateral epicondylalgia produces uniquely characteristic hypoalgesia. Man Ther 6:205–212. doi:10.1054/math.2001.0411

Visnes H, Aandahl HÅ, Bahr R (2013) Jumper's knee paradox—jumping ability is a risk factor for developing jumper's knee: a 5-year prospective study. Br J Sports Med 47:503–507. doi:10.1136/bjsports-2012-091385

Wang X-Q, Zheng J-J, Yu Z-W et al (2012) A meta-analysis of core stability exercise versus general exercise for chronic low back pain. PLoS One 7:e52082. doi:10.1371/journal.pone.0052082

Witvrouw E, Bellemans J, Lysens R et al (2001) Intrinsic risk factors for the development of patellar tendinitis in an athletic population. A two-year prospective study. Am J Sports Med 29:190–195

Woolf CJ, Salter MW (2000) Neuronal plasticity: increasing the gain in pain. Science 288:1765–1769

Wu Y-H, Latash ML (2014) The effects of practice on coordination. Exerc Sport Sci Rev 42:37–42. doi:10.1249/JES.0000000000000002

Wulf G, Höß M, Prinz W (1998) Instructions for motor learning: differential effects of internal versus external focus of attention. J Mot Behav 30:169–179. doi:10.1080/00222899809601334

Wulf G, McNevin N, Shea CH (2001) The automaticity of complex motor skill learning as a function of attentional focus. Q J Exp Psychol A 54:1143–1154. doi:10.1080/713756012

Yu H, Randhawa K, Côté P et al (2016) The effectiveness of physical agents for lower-limb soft tissue injuries: a systematic review. J Orthop Sport Phys Ther 46:523–554. doi:10.2519/jospt.2016.6521

Use of Nutraceuticals for Tendinopathies

16

Marco Antônio Percope de Andrade,
Guilherme Moreira de Abreu-e-Silva,
and Túlio Vinícius Oliveira de Campos

Contents

M.A.P. de Andrade, M.D., Ms.C., Ph.D. (✉)
Orthopaedic Department, Universidade Federal de Minas Gerais, Belo Horizonte, Brazil

Departamento de Aparelho Locomotor, Universidade Federal de Minas Gerais, Av. Prof. Alfredo Balena, 110, Santa Efigênia, CEP: 30130-100, Belo Horizonte, MG, Brazil
e-mail: marcoapercope@gmail.com

G.M. de Abreu-e-Silva, M.D., Ms.C., Ph.D.
T.V.O. de Campos, M.D., Ms.C.
Orthopaedic Department, Universidade Federal de Minas Gerais, Belo Horizonte, Brazil

16.1 Introduction

The importance of tendinopathies in the clinical scenario has increased recently. It may be attributed to the increase of sport activities, life expectancy, and other factors such as environment, diet, systemic diseases, and some drug therapies (e.g., fluoroquinolones). In fact, not only athletes but also the general population suffer from inflammatory or degenerative tendon conditions which may be attributed to the quality of tendon tissue and mechanical overuse (Fusini et al. 2016).

Recently, basic and clinical researches have advocated the prescription of oral medication aiming to modulate pathways which determine tendon structure and resistance.

The term "nutraceutical" was coined from "nutrition" and "pharmaceutical" in 1989 by DeFelice and was originally defined as "a food that provides health benefits, including the prevention and/or treatment of a disease". In general, nutraceuticals have late onset of action and should be devoid of adverse effects. They are not under rigorous control and licensing processes as drugs and do not require robust clinical support to be sold as treatment alternatives (Percope de Andrade et al. 2015).

Oral supplements of glucosamine and chondroitin sulfate, vitamin C, hydrolyzed type 1 collagen, L-arginine alpha-ketoglutarate, curcumin, boswellic acid, methylsulfonylmethane, and bromelain increase the concentration of beneficial

G.L. Canata et al. (eds.), *Muscle and Tendon Injuries*, DOI 10.1007/978-3-662-54184-5_16

compounds in tendon and may help to preserve, or even repair, the damaged structures.

The aim of the present chapter is to review the basic and clinical data that support the use of nutraceuticals in the management of tendon disease.

16.2 Basic Science

16.2.1 Glucosamine and Condroitin Sulfate

Lippiello demonstrated that bovine tenocytes were stimulated by the addition of a combination of glucosamine and chondroitin sulfate to the culture medium. That pair of substances increased collagen synthesis by 22% in tenocytes. After 48 h exposure, epitenon and tenocyte cells presented a greater production of radiolabeled hydroxyl-proline (Lippiello 2006).

Tenotomized rats treated with oral glucosamine and chondroitin supplements showed more organized collagen bundles and less inflammation than controls fed with placebo. After eight weeks, rats fed with glucosamine and chondroitin had greater tendon strength in biomechanical tests (Ozer et al. 2011).

Topical application of chondroitin has beneficial effects in rabbit's tendon characteristics by preventing the degenerative cascade of proteases and inflammation on tendon structure induced by collagenase (Oryan et al. 2008).

16.2.2 Vitamin C

Vitamin C is a critical element in the synthesis of procollagen chains. It acts as coenzyme of proline hydroxylase. In fact, it is a cofactor of hydroxylation (Fusini et al. 2016).

Experimental research shows that tenocytes cultured in a medium without ascorbate synthesized collagen at only a third of the normal level. Addition of ascorbate to avian tendon cells increased procollagen translation by six times (Kao et al. 1976).

Vitamin C alone is not able to increase collagen synthesis and secretion. In fact, tenocytes treated with ascorbate maintained a large pool of procollagen despite changes in translation or secretion rate. These results are compatible with a possible feedback mechanism between the levels of internal procollagen pool and the rates of collagen synthesis and secretion (Schwarz et al. 1981).

Ascorbic acid may act as an antioxidant agent. Vitamin C increased reduced glutathione tissue quantity two weeks after injury, in comparison to a group treated with saline. The treatment with ascorbate also improved the gliding resistance of tendons and reduced the fibrotic scar at the site of injury (Hung et al. 2013).

A study with 42 healthy female Wistar albino rats proved that high-dose vitamin C supplementation every 2 days may have stimulating effects on healing of a full-thickness Achilles tendon rupture (Omeroglu et al. 2009).

16.2.3 Hydrolyzed Type 1 Collagen

The role of collagen 1 on tenocyte or tenoblast culture is unknown.

Investigation of the effects of collagen peptide ingestion on rabbit's tendon extracellular matrix demonstrates that hydrolyzed type 1 collagen peptides affect the size of collagen fibrils and composition of glycosaminoglycans in Achilles tendon. The ingestion of type 1 collagen increased the amount of dermatan sulfate and lowered the percentage of hyaluronic acid. The rise of this biochemical component would enhance the mechanical properties of Achilles tendon (Minaguchi et al. 2005).

16.2.4 L-Arginine Alfa-Ketoglutarate

L-arginine is an essential amino acid required by the enzymatic family of nitric oxide synthase (NOS) to produce nitric oxide (NO) which is a crucial factor in tendon healing process.

In a rat model, uninjured tendons did not present NOS activity. After surgical tenotomy, NOS enzyme increased its activity reaching a maximum after 7 days, with reduction near baseline levels at day 14 (Murrell 2007a).

Inhibition of NOS activity with oral administration of an analogue of L-arginine-N ω-nitro-L-arginine methyl ester (L-NAME) resulted in significant reduction of cross-sectional area and failure load of injured Achilles tendons (Murrell et al. 1997).

In animal models, the addition of competitive NOS inhibitors impaired tendon healing, while the addition of NO enhanced tendon healing (Murrell 2007b).

The levels of transforming growth factor (TGF) β undergo a change during physiological repair process. At the beginning they rise, and after about 3 weeks, they gradually decrease to slowly reach control levels. Conversely, if L-NAME is given at injury time, the macrophage infiltrates continue to express high level of TGF-β. Following an injury, iNOS activity increases during the acute phase of inflammation, and then gradually tends to normalize. Treatment of injured tendon with L-NAME, however, inhibits iNOS activity. L-NAME-treated rats showed increased adhesion of peritoneal macrophages to epitenon monolayers in vitro. In addition, the treatment of acute tendon injury with NO inhibitor causes a long-lasting and wide accumulation of many inflammatory cells in the subcutaneous tissue, muscle, and tendon as a response of chronic inflammation. Thus, the formation of NO is a key event for tendon healing process because its inhibition increases the level of TGF-β and development of fibrosis and chronic inflammation (Darmani et al. 2004).

16.2.5 Curcumin

Curcumin is an antioxidant extracted from *Curcuma longa* which has a potential role in prevention of oxidative stress damage. Increased vascularization is a very common finding in tendinopathy. Curcumin inhibits the formation of new blood vessels in a mouse model (Arbiser et al. 1998).

Long-term oral administration of curcumin decreased cross-linking of collagen and restored its original characteristics (Pari and Murugan 2007; Sajithlal et al. 1998).

Curcumin targets NF-κB signaling pathway by inhibiting inflammation and apoptosis induced by IL-1β in vitro. Curcumin achieves its anti-inflammatory effects by downregulation of matrix metalloproteinase-1, metalloproteinase-9, and metalloproteinase-13, cyclooxygenase-2, inhibition of caspase-3, and Bax pathway leading to apoptosis. It also stimulates cell survival by promoting Bcl-2 pathway (Buhrmann et al. 2011).

Oral administration of curcumin (100 mg/kg of body weight) has been tested to manage patellar tendon injury in Sprague-Dawley rats. Histological examination revealed deposition of well-organized collagen fibers and improvement of tendon biomechanical properties (Jiang et al. 2016).

16.2.6 Boswellic Acid

Boswellic acid (BA), extracted from *Boswellia serrata*, is considered an active treatment for chronic inflammatory diseases. Although BA is often used in combination with other nutraceuticals, we could not find articles describing the effects of BA on tenocytes.

16.2.7 Methylsulfonylmethane (MSM)

Methylsulfonylmethane (MSM) is an oral supplement recommended to treat conditions such as pain, inflammation, allergies, arthritis, and parasitic and bacterial infections.

This sulfur-containing compound is found in a variety of human food like vegetables, grains, fruits, and beverages. It is a natural substance with efficacious analgesic and anti-inflammatory properties used in the management of osteoarthritis.

There is no study concerning the use of MSM on tenocytes (Magnuson et al. 2007).

16.2.8 Bromelain

Bromelain is an ensemble of proteases derived from pineapple stem with some therapeutic effects in inflammatory diseases. In vitro, experiments have shown that bromelain was able to remove several essential cell surface molecules for leukocyte trafficking (Aiyegbusi et al. 2010).

Aiyegbusi et al. observed that the flesh and bark extract of pineapple plant, which contains the enzyme bromelain, promoted murine tenoblast proliferation. Inversely, leaves and core extracts reduced tenocytes population.

The effects of fresh pineapple juice and commercial bromelain on tenocyte proliferation were studied by Aiyegbusi. They observed that tenocyte population of bromelain group had significantly increased in comparison to control and fresh pineapple juice groups. Pineapple juice, however, significantly lowered the MDA level compared with both the control and bromelain-treated group.

16.3 Clinical Evidence

The management of tendinopathies with oral supplements is relatively new. Current clinical studies often test combination of substances and compare the results of medication to physical activity interventions or other treatments.

A clinical study, comparing the effects of glucosamine or indomethacin administration in the management of Achilles peritendinitis, showed that glucosamine had a better overall therapeutic effect on 2/3 of the patients compared to 1/3 of the patients treated with indomethacin (Sundqvist et al. 1987).

Oral supplementation of hydrolyzed type 1 collagen, arginine L-alpha-ketoglutarate, MSM, and bromelain has a potential role in tendon healing and lowering pain related to tendinopathy.

Also, it has been demonstrated that these agents may act in human arthroscopic rotator cuff tear repair. Nutraceutical supplementation for 3 months after rotator cuff repair lowered postoperative shoulder pain and led to a slight improvement in repair integrity. Otherwise, it was not possible to find any objective functional improvement (Gumina et al. 2012).

Notarnicola et al. showed that extracorporeal shockwave therapy results would be boosted by administration of dietary supplements containing L-arginine-α-ketoglutarate, Vinitrox™ (a polyphenolic compound), MSM, bromelain, type 1 collagen, and vitamin C. The effects of nutraceutical supplementation and extracorporeal shockwave therapy were studied in patients with insertional Achilles tendinopathy. The combined treatment lead to a lower level of pain and better results at Ankle-Hindfoot scale and Roles and Maudsley score than isolated extracorporeal shockwave therapy (Notarnicola et al. 2012).

The dietary supplement TENDOACTIVE™ (Bioiberica S.A., Palafolls, Spain) composed by mucopolisaccharides, type 1 collagen, and vitamin C has been tested to manage different tendinopathies (Achilles, patellar, and common extensor tendons). The overall results suggest improvement of symptoms and healing of injured tendons (Arquer et al. 2014; Shakibaei et al. 2011).

Merolla et al. assessed the analgesic effect of a dietary compound named TENDISULFUR® (Laborest SpA, Nerviano, Italy) in patients with a full-thickness supraspinatus tendon rupture treated arthroscopically. This oral supplement contains glucosamine and chondroitin sulfate, vitamin C, type 1 collagen, L-arginine-α-ketoglutarate, Boswellic acid, curcumin, and MSM. Patients were randomly assigned to dietary supplement or placebo for 2 months. After 1 week, treatment group showed significantly lower level of VAS, night pain, and pain after activity. Constant-Murley score and simple shoulder test (SST) did not differ between the two groups. The authors concluded that TENDISULFUR® alleviated short and partially mid-term pain but did not affect long-term pain (Merolla et al. 2015).

The majority of clinical studies investigating nutraceuticals' use in tendinopathy treatment have methodological limitations. They have methodological pitfalls as absence of estimation of number of patients to treat, low values in power, error, and outcome assessment. Furthermore, sample size calculation has rarely been performed, and it is not clear who evaluated the patients during the study (the treating physician or an independent investigator).

16.4 Take-Home Message

- Tendinopathy is a common and difficult to manage disorder. The risk of recurrence is high and a "gold standard" therapy is still not available.
- Nutraceuticals emerge as candidates to reduce symptoms attributed to tendinopathies, prevent tendon rupture, and improve recovery from trauma or surgery.
- Ethical and economic issues impair the trustworthy of the best scientific evidence.
- There is a myriad of preclinical studies supporting the use of nutraceuticals supplementation to improve outcomes while approaching tendinopathies.
- Despite the reliable evidence from preclinical studies, clinical studies are scant and biased.

References

Aiyegbusi AI, Duru FI, Awelimobor D, Noronha CC, Okanlawon AO (2010) The role of aqueous extract of pineapple fruit parts on the healing of acute crush tendon injury. Nig Q J Hosp Med 20:223–227

Arbiser JL, Klauber N, Rohan R, van Leeuwen R, Huang MT, Fisher C (1998) Curcumin is an in vivo inhibitor of angiogenesis. Mol Med 4:376–383

Arquer A, García M, Laucirica JA (2014) Eficacia y seguridad de un tratamiento oral a base de mucopolisacáridos, colágeno tipo i y vitamina C en pacientes con tendinopatías. Apunts. Medicina de l'Esport 49:31–36

Buhrmann C, Mobasheri A, Busch F (2011) Curcumin modulates nuclear factor kappaB (NF-kappaB)-mediated inflammation in human tenocytes in vitro: role of the phosphatidylinositol 3-kinase/Akt pathway. J Biol Chem 286:28556–28566

Darmani H, Crossan J, McLellan SD, Meek D, Adam C (2004) Expression of nitric oxide synthase and transforming growth factor-beta in crush-injured tendon and synovium. Mediat Inflamm 13:299–305

Fusini F et al (2016) Nutraceutical supplement in the management of tendinopathies: a systematic review. Muscles Ligaments Tendons J 6(1):48–57

Gumina S, Passaretti D, Gurzi MD, Candela V (2012) Arginine L-alpha-ketoglutarate, methylsulfonylmethane, hydrolyzed type I collagen and bromelain in rotator cuff tear repair: a prospective randomized study. Curr Med Res Opin 28:1767–1774

Hung LK, Fu SC, Lee YW, Mok TY, Chan KM (2013) Local vitamin-C injection reduced tendon adhesion in a chicken model of flexor digitorum profundus tendon injury. J Bone Joint Surg Am 95:e41

Jiang D, Gao P, Lin H, Geng H (2016) Curcumin improves tendon healing in rats: a histological, biochemical, and functional evaluation. Connect Tissue Res 57:20–27

Kao WW, Flaks JG, Prockop DJ (1976) Primary and secondary effects of ascorbate on procollagen synthesis and protein synthesis by primary cultures of tendon fibroblasts. Arch Biochem Biophys 173:638–648

Lippiello L (2006) Collagen synthesis in tenocytes, ligament cells and chondrocytes exposed to a combination of glucosamine HCl and chondroitin sulfate. Evid Based Complement Alternat Med 4(2):219–224

Magnuson BA, Appleton J, Ames GB (2007) Pharmacokinetics and distribution of [35S]methylsulfonylmethane following oral administration to rats. J Agric Food Chem 55:1033–1038

Merolla G, Dellabiancia F, Ingardia A, Paladini P, Porcellini G (2015) Co-analgesic therapy for arthroscopic supraspinatus tendon repair pain using a dietary supplement containing *Boswellia serrata* and *Curcuma longa*: a prospective randomized placebo-controlled study. Musculoskelet Surg 99:43–52

Minaguchi J, Koyama Y, Meguri N et al (2005) Effects of ingestion of collagen peptide on collagen fibrils and glycosaminoglycans in Achilles tendon. J Nutr Sci Vitaminol 51:169–174

Moraes JR, Facco GG, Moraes FR, Filho JRE, Miyazato LG, Beretta DC (2009) Effects of glycosaminoglycan polysulphate on the organisation of collagen fibres in experimentally induced tendonitis in horses. Vet Rec 165:203–205

Murrell GA (2007a) Using nitric oxide to treat tendinopathy. Br J Sports Med 41:227–231

Murrell GA (2007b) Oxygen free radicals and tendon healing. J Shoulder Elbow Surg 16:208–214

Murrell GA, Szabo C, Hannafin JA (1997) Modulation of tendon healing by nitric oxide. Inflamm Res 46:19–27

Notarnicola A, Pesce V, Vicenti G, Tafuri S, Forcignano M, Moretti B (2012) SWAAT study: extracorporeal shock wave therapy and arginine supplementation and other nutraceuticals for insertional Achilles tendinopathy. Adv Ther 29:799–814

Omeroglu S, Peker T, Turkozkan N, Omeroglu H (2009) High-dose vitamin C supplementation accelerates the Achilles tendon healing in healthy rats. Arch Orthop Trauma Surg 129:281–286

Oryan A, Goodship AE, Silver IA (2008) Response of a collagenase-induced tendon injury to treatment with a polysulphated glycosaminoglycan (Adequan). Connect Tissue Res 49:351–360

Ozer H, Taskesen A, Kul O, Selek HY, Turanli S, Kose K (2011) Effect of glucosamine chondroitin sulphate on repaired tenotomized rat Achilles tendons. Jt Dis Relat Surg 22:100–106

Pari L, Murugan P (2007) Influence of tetrahydrocurcumin on tail tendon collagen contents and its properties in rats with streptozotocin-nicotinamide-induced type 2 diabetes. Fundam Clin Pharmacol 21:665–671

Percope de Andrade MA, Campos TV, Abreu-E-Silva GM (2015) Supplementary methods in the nonsurgical treatment of osteoarthritis. Arthroscopy 31(4): 785–792

Sajithlal GB, Chithra P, Chandrakasan G (1998) Effect of curcumin on the advanced glycation and cross-linking of collagen in diabetic rats. Biochem Pharmacol 56:1607–1614

Schwarz RI, Mandell RB, Bissell MJ (1981) Ascorbate induction of collagen synthesis as a means for elucidating a mechanism of quantitative control of tissue-specific function. Mol Cell Biol 1:843–853

Shakibaei M, Buhrmann C, Mobasheri A (2011) Anti-inflammatory and anti-catabolic effects of TENDOACTIVE® on human tenocytes in vitro. Histol Histopathol 26:1173–1185

Sundqvist H, Forsskahl B, Kvist M (1987) A promising novel therapy for Achilles peritendinitis: double-blind comparison of glycosaminoglycan polysulfate and high-dose indomethacin. Int J Sports Med 8:298–303

Surgical Treatment of Acute and Chronic Muscle Injuries

17

F. Benazzo, M. Bargagliotti, A. Combi, and G. Zanon

Contents

F. Benazzo (✉) • M. Bargagliotti • G. Zanon
Department of Orthopedics and Traumatology, University of Pavia, IRCCS Policlinico San Matteo, P.le Golgi 19, 27100 Pavia, Italy
e-mail: fbenazzo@unipv.it; f.benazzo@smatteo.pv.it; marcobarga@libero.it

A. Combi
Department of Orthopedics and Traumatology, AO Santa Croca e Carle, via Michele Coppino 26, 12010 Cuneo, Italy

17.1 Introduction

Muscle injuries (MI) can stem from a variety of events, including direct (i.e., muscle contusions) and indirect trauma (i.e., muscle strains) (Crisco et al. 1994; Garrett 1990; Huard et al. 2002).

The professional and recreational activities are one of the most common causes; therefore, there is a strict connection with the modern sports traumatology. They represented 48% of all injuries during track and field competition in a recent International Association of Athletics Federations (IAAF) study and more than 31% of all injuries in professional soccer players (Ekstrand et al. 2011; Hägglund et al. 2005).

Thigh muscle damage presents the most common injury in track and field athletes (16%) like soccer player, rugby (10.4%), basketball (17.7%), and American football (46%/22% practice/games) (Alonso et al. 2009; Malliaropoulos et al. 2010; Lopez et al. 2012; Borowski et al. 2008; Feeley et al. 2008).

The relevance of this problem is even more obvious if the frequency is compared to anterior cruciate ligament ruptures, which occur in the same squad statistically only 0.4 times per season (Walden et al. 2011).

There is no consensus when a surgical approach should be implemented because a lot of authors often apply an experience-based medicine especially in the serious situations. Despite this, fortunately most of muscle injuries can be treated conservatively, as skeletal muscles have a

G.L. Canata et al. (eds.), *Muscle and Tendon Injuries*, DOI 10.1007/978-3-662-54184-5_17

high endogenous capacity for repair. In literature a lot of studies and reviews well describe good/excellent results using conservative treatments, mainly in nonprofessional populations, and consist of rest, nonsteroidal anti-inflammatory drugs (NSAIDs), physical therapy, and an exercise program. Steroid and PRP injection has also been proposed as a treatment to decrease the symptoms and promote the muscle repair (Cacchio et al. 2011; Mason et al. 2012; Levine et al. 2000; Zanon et al. 2016; Heiderscheit et al. 2010).

Surgical treatment is dictated by the clinical and imaging (ultrasonography, MRI, or CT scan) presentation of the injury and can be individually tailored to the patient's functional needs (Ekstrand et al. 2011; Boutin et al. 2002; Askling et al. 2007).

A judicious interpretation of all these elements is the key to obtain a suitable approach. However, there are many classification systems with different terminologies that make the accurate decision for a better treatment a difficult task (Mueller-Wohlfahrt et al. 2013).

In literature several studies with a long-term and mid-term follow-up reported good/excellent results using the surgical approach, despite that this management is potentially subjected to intra- and postoperative complications (severe postoperative hematoma, thrombosis, myositis ossificans, and infections) (Ramos et al. 2015).

17.2 Definition and Classification of the Muscle Injuries

The muscle injuries present a heterogeneous group of muscle disorders, which have traditionally been difficult to categorize. This is an important keypoint because it is closely connected with a specific damage-related treatment, especially concerning a surgical approach (Armfield et al. 2006).

Today, it is well established in the international experience that muscles often involved in damages are the biarticular muscles or those with a more complex architecture (e.g., adductor longus, hamstring, etc.) used to undergo eccentric contraction and contain primarily fast-twitch type 2 muscle fibers (Jarvinen et al. 2005; Anderson et al. 2001; Noonan and Garrett 1999).

This is a typical situation occurring during jumping and running sports, with accelerations and sudden decelerations like in football players, sprinters, and basketball players. In football/soccer, for example, in the 92% the four major muscle groups of the lower limbs are involved: hamstrings 37%, adductors 23%, quadriceps 19%, and calf muscles 13%. As much as 96% of all muscle injuries in football/soccer occur in noncontact situations, whereas contusions are more frequently encountered in contact sports, like rugby, American football, and ice hockey (Ekstrand et al. 2011; Lopez et al. 2012).

Defining injuries as acute or chronic is clinically relevant in many cases, where these terms have implications regarding the anatomic pathologic abnormalities and especially the tissue quality, which sometimes may necessitate a surgical approach. The current literature varies greatly in defining the terms acute and chronic damage (Flint et al. 2014).

We define "chronic" the muscle injuries when the problem persists for more than 4 months from the first traumatic event, and it was not allowed a complete healing process (Murray and Lowe 2009). Therefore, in these situations it is reported that a higher rate of recurrent damage of the same muscle caused longer period of absence from the field than the initial injury.

Different classification systems are then published regarding the grading and the amount of tissue damage (Bryan 2009).

Some of them use only a physical examination approach, others considering the image data (using ultrasound or MRI) and more recent are the mixed-classifications. O'Donoghue devised one of the more widely used clinical MI grading systems in 1962 (1962).

This system uses a classification that is based on injury severity and the objective functional loss. Takebayashi et al. (1995) proposed in 1995 an ultrasound-based three-grade classification system ranging from a grade 1 injury with less than 50% of the muscle involved, grade 2 presenting a partial tear with more than 50% of the muscle involved, and up to grade 3 with a complete tear. Peetrons in 2002 (2002) has recommended a similar grading. The current most widely used classification is an MRI-based graduation defining four grades: grade 0 with no pathological findings, grade 1 with a muscle edema only but without tissue damage, grade 2 as partial muscle tear, and grade 3 with a complete muscle tear

(Stoller 2007). The limitations of the previous grading systems are a lack of prognostic information for the clinician such as length of muscle tear on MRI, MRI "negative" injuries, distance from the origin, cross-sectional area of edema, and involvement of the tendon (Connell et al. 2004; Ekstrand et al. 2012; Cross et al. 2004; Gibbs et al. 2004; Slavotinek 2010; Cohen et al. 2011).

Recently, the Munich Consensus has proposed in 2013 an alternative muscle grading system mixing clinical and image data. The Munich grading system classifies injuries as either "functional" (fatigue-induced, delayed-onset muscle soreness (DOMS), spine-related neuromuscular dysfunction, or muscle-related neuromuscular dysfunction) or "structural" muscle pathology, where the "structural" classes are further divided into three essential grades of muscle injury: minor, moderate, and complete (Mueller-Wohlfahrt et al. 2013; Meyer and Prior 2000).

The British Athletics Muscle Injury Classification proposes another "mixed" grading system (2014) for hamstring injuries, based on the available evidence which should provide a sound diagnostic base for therapeutic decision-making and prognostication. Injuries are graded 0–4 based on MRI features, with grades 1–4 including an additional suffix "a," "b," or "c" if the injury is "myofascial," "musculotendinous," or "intratendinous" (Pollock et al. 2014).

This classification system can provide a reproducible diagnostic framework for enhanced clinical management of muscle injury but not provide reliable information on player readiness to return to play (Reurink et al. 2014).

17.3 Surgical Treatment Options: The Decision-Making Approach for the Most Frequent Muscle Injuries

17.3.1 Acute Muscle Insertional Injuries

One of the most important indications for a surgical treatment of acute muscle injuries are the insertional detachment from the bone origin. Sometimes, they occur with a direct avulsion of a little piece of the bone, particularly in young patients. The muscle's tendons or the miotendinous junctions are always involved. These situations often follow a violent or explosive muscular contraction against a fixed resistance, sudden deceleration, or stretching of the involved muscle or as a result of a direct trauma (Almekinders 1991; Kujala et al. 1997).

In these situations there is a partial or complete loss of the muscular preload length, and their function and contraction properties are compromised. The management is to reinsert the muscles in the correct anatomical footprint, using simple stiches (resorbable or not resorbable wires) or devices like screws, anchors, or cortical buttons (Caekebeke et al. 2016).

Very often, the long strong biarticular muscles or those with a more complex architecture are involved. For example, the 80% cases of proximal hamstring injuries are represented by an avulsion of the tendons from the ischial tuberosity, but it represents only the 20% of all hamstring pathologies (De Smet and Best 2000; Hallen and Ekstrand 2014; Cohen and Bradley 2007) (Fig. 17.1).

Quadriceps disinsertions from the patella are instead an uncommon problem with an incidence of 1.37/100,000 patients per year, affecting predominantly middle-aged males (male/female [4.2:1]; mean age, 51.1 years) and even more rare is the proximal complete avulsion from the anterosuperior iliac spine (Clayton and Court-Brown 2008).

Concerning the distal biceps avulsions and/or ruptures, they are relatively rare with an incidence rate of about 1.2–2.5 per 100,000 (Safran and Graham 2002; Kelly et al. 2015).

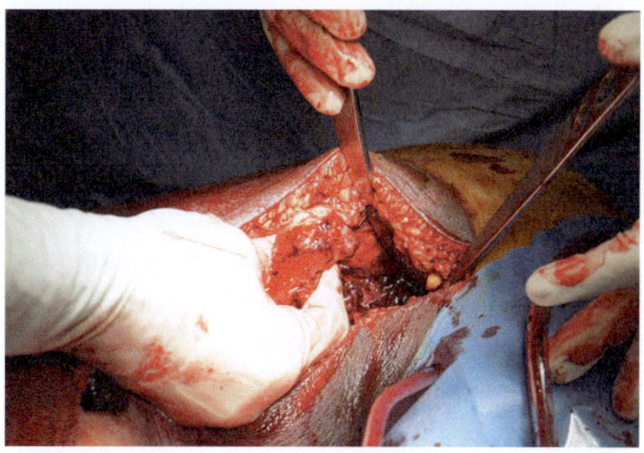

Fig. 17.1 Complete avulsion of the proximal hamstrings' tendon from the ischial tuberosity in a 40-years-old female

The pathogenetic causes are different: studies support eccentric overload as the most common mechanism of injury. High-energy contact trauma is also reported in the quadriceps disinsertions, while the most common mechanism by which distal biceps, pectoralis major, and hamstring avulsions occur is a fall on the outstretched hand or a final phase of a jump. Degeneration, inflammation, hypovascularization, or friction of the tendon is known to contribute to the possibility of rupture (Devereaux and ElMaraghy 2013; Belli et al. 2001; Weiss et al. 2000; LaPrade et al. 2015).

Also medications can predispose to muscle avulsion such as anabolic steroids, statins, locally injected corticosteroids, prolonged use of systemic corticosteroids, and antibiotics (e.g., fluoroquinolones) (Celic et al. 2012; David et al. 1995; Liow and Tavares 1995). Not so rare is then the involvement, caused by the same injured mechanisms, of other anatomical structures during a muscles avulsion. For example, there is a strict relation between distal hamstring disinsertion (i.e., distal origin of the semimembranosus) and other tears like the anterior cruciate ligament (ACL), menisci, and/or the posterior cruciate ligament (PCL) (Khoshnoodi et al. 2014; Vanek 1994). Khoshnoodi et al. reported, for example, a case of an isolated semimembranosus insertional avulsion with a PCL tear, medial meniscal tear, and capsular rupture in a 26-year-old football player (Khoshnoodi et al. 2014). According to the literature, the surgical treatment is recommended in case of complete disinsertion, especially in young active sportsmen, and generally if the retraction from the bone is greater than 2 cm (i.e., hamstring injuries) (Fig. 17.2). One of the most important aspects in these situations is the early identification and a well-timed surgical treatment. The results of previous studies regarding the timing of surgery are conflicting: today, the common consensus is that patients with acute repairs have better outcomes when compared with chronic surgical treatment, due to an easier and faster postoperative recovery (Sallay et al. 2008; Sarimo et al. 2008). The literature suggests also that the early surgical reattachment gives the athletes a greater chance of returning to their pre-injury level of sport, especially for the lower limb muscle avulsions (Harris et al. 2011; Kurosawa et al. 1996). Ten patients presenting with complete proximal hamstring tendon tears were confirmed on MRI. All patients underwent surgical exploration and repair of the torn tendons with the aim of returning to normal activities and sports. All patients were semi-professional or professional athletes and presented within five weeks of their injury (average 12 days, range 4–35 days).An excellent outcome was found in terms of return to normal activities and sports. Early surgical repair and physiotherapy has been noted to be associ- ated with a good outcome and enables an early return to high level sports after complete tear of the proximal hamstring tendons (Konan and Haddad 2010). Lempainen et al. showed, with a case series of 18 operatively treated distal hamstring muscle tears in athletes, excellent results in 13 cases. Fourteen of the 18 patients were able to return to their former level of sport after an average of 4 months (range 2–6 months) (Lempainen et al. n.d.). O'Shea et al. demonstrated in 27 patients after quadriceps reinsertion (average 17 days between injury and surgery) excellent clinical outcomes over a period of seven years, and they were all able to return to pre-injury levels of activity (2002). In a review that evaluated 18 studies, including 286 operative and 14 nonoperative cases, Harris JD et al. concluded that surgical repair of complete proximal hamstring ruptures improved clinical outcomes than a conservative treatment (2011). Also Sallay

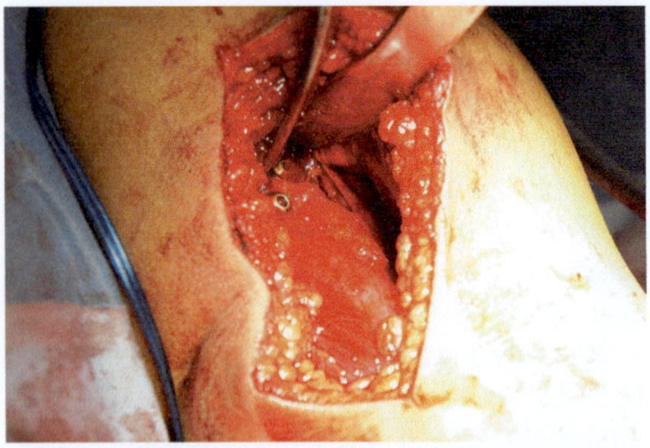

Fig. 17.2 Reinsertion and fixation of the bone fragment of the ischial tuberosity after the complete proximal hamstrings' tendon avulsion using metal screws in a young 17-year-old football player

et al. with a retrospectively reviewed 25 cases surgical repaired over a 12-year period using bone anchors reported good results: in 92% cases no pain and in 98% no differences with the isokinetic test comparing the injured limb with the uninvolved one. In that study all the patients had an avulsion from the bone of all the three tendons (2008). But other papers have shown a low rate of return to pre-injury activity levels. For example, Konrath et al. found that 51% of patients who underwent a quadriceps reinsertion were unable to return to their pre-injury activity level. In this study, although 79% of players were described as recovering fully from their injury, only 50% of all injured players returned to play in regular-season NFL games (1998). Several series and descriptions are available in the literature about different surgical techniques, and good/excellent results are reported by the authors (Mica et al. 2009; Sarimo et al. 2008; Chakravarthy et al. 2005; LaPrade et al. 2015; Branch and Anz 2015; Boublik et al. 2013; Petilon et al. 2005). The fixation of the tendons usually is performed using an open surgical approach in order to have a better anatomical exposure and an easier technique. Different devices can be used due to an anatomical reconstruction and to obtain a stronger suture of the tendons to the bone (Gidwani et al. 2004; Wooton et al. 1990; West et al. 2008). In this way, some authors have proposed reinforcements of the damaged tissue using, for example, autograft, allograft, or synthetic mesh augmentation (Sarimo et al. 2008; West et al. 2008; Ding et al. 2016; Morrey et al. 2016). Recently, mini-invasive techniques such as a percutaneous fixation of the muscle's avulsion (Watts et al. 2014) or an endoscopic approach allowing a safe approach to the area of injury were also showed. The benefit of it is to reduce the morbidities associated with an open approach (Guanche 2015; Bhatia 2016). Concluding, the management of muscle avulsions must be focused at first time in a correct diagnosis and at second in the reconstruction/reinsertion thinking about the dimension of the damage, the quality of the muscle origin, and the type of patients. In order of this reason, according with the literature, we remember some useful tips for a correct management of these situations, due to simplifying of the surgical procedure and reducing the operative time:

- Use the most simple surgical approach considering our surgical skills.
- Identify and protect the vascular and nervous complex.
- Identify and mobilize the muscle's origin.
- Clean and remove completely the hematoma, fibrotic, and soft tissue.
- Denude the bone from the periosteum to enhance healing of the muscle insertion.
- Suture the insertional origin of the muscle reducing any tension of the tissue (i.e., flexion of the knee if proximal hamstring reinsertion).
- Protect the surgical gesture and the healing process employing an immobilization with a cast or plaster for some days (7–15) after surgery.

17.3.2 Acute Muscle Belly Injuries

Direct muscle contusions are one of the most common causes of discontinuity of muscle bellies.

More rarely the cause depends on a violent contraction or forceful stretching of the muscle or an uncoordinated force acting on the tightly contracted muscle (Praemer et al. 1992; Zarins and Ciullo 1983).

The surgical treatment of acute damage is therefore necessary in the grade III–IV (total) muscle tissue injuries (Almekinders 1991; Kujala et al. 1997).

In these situations there is a subtotal or complete loss of the contractile muscle capacity (caused from the interruption of the muscle fibers) compromising its function. The regenerative capacity of the injured skeletal muscle is limited, and therefore suturing the transected muscle may help the tissue heal and prevent complications. Some authors have reported good/excellent results after repair, but unfortunately it does not prevent the formation of scar tissue (Chien et al. 1991; Gilcreest 1933). Aarimaa et al. showed, in an experimental study, that volumetric muscle loss greater than 50% cannot be biologically repaired and, consequently, result in a residual important loss of function (2004).

Repair of muscle belly lacerations is technically demanding because the sutures pull out, and the likelihood of clinical failure is high. Thereby, a complete MI like a laceration can bring about permanent functional disability and muscle weakness (Julien and Mudgal 2011). Different suture techniques have been described in literature, but still the best suture is debated: today the therapeutic management is unclear with no definite guidelines. This is caused by the great heterogeneity of the muscle belly lesions and of patients. Many features are already identified: dimension and extension of the lesion, quality and kind of the damage tissue, type of suture, and time between injury and surgery (Jarvinen and Lehto 1993). For example, the role of epimysium (the connective tissue sheath around a muscle) is not well defined in surgical repair. Furthermore, the epimysium-based repair has been reported to be important for superior stitching of forearm muscle belly lacerations (Botte et al. 1987). As for the hand surgeons, where the epitendinous repair has become a common practice because of its biomechanical strength, different authors found similar advantages in epimysial-based repair in muscle bellies. The incorporation of the epimysium improves surgical repair because incorporation of fibrous portions of the muscle improves tension bearing and may permit a better sliding (Heckman and Levine 1978).

Heterogeneous outcomes are also reported using different types of sutures. Chien et al., for example, showed better results with the modified Kessler suture (with 5–0 Mersilene) than either simple suturing with 2–0 Dexon or simple suturing with a tendon graft (1991). Contrary to Chien, Kragh J.F. Jr. et al. had shown that the better method of repair for suturing muscle is the use of combination stitches and not only the same type (2005).

In this paper the authors tested Kessler stitches and the combination of Mason-Allen and perimeter stitches. Individual stitches were placed in the muscle belly of quadriceps femoris from a pig cadaver and were tensioned mechanically. The maximum loads and strains were measured and failure modes recorded. The mean load and strain for the Kessler stitches were significantly less than those for combination stitches. Despite these considerations, it is a common consensus that immediate repair strength is important because healing is better when motion is started 5 days after repair, and this is useful to prevent hard anelastic scar (Jarvinen and Lehto 1993).

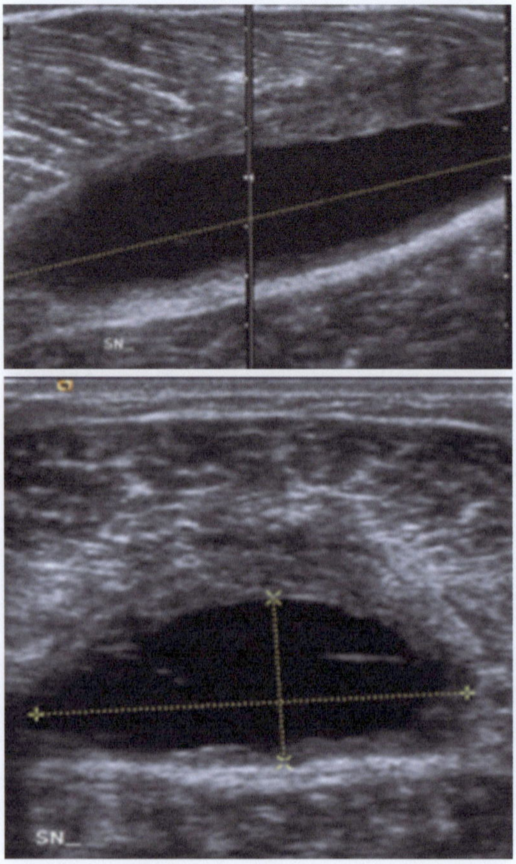

Fig. 17.3 Intramuscular *rectus femoris* III grade lesion hematoma in 26-year-old sportsman

During an acute muscle injury, another important indication for a surgical approach is also when a large intramuscular hematoma is associated with the tissue damage (Fig. 17.3) (Almekinders 1991; Kujala et al. 1997).

In some situations, especially after a direct trauma, a localized bleeding can form a hematoma associated with the tissue damage. There are two types of hematoma: intramuscular and intermuscular. The prognosis for intermuscular hematomas is better, but the persistence of swelling after 48–72 h increases pain intensity, extension of tenderness, prolonged restricted limb range of motion, and pain. In few of these cases, the hematoma becomes so large as to generate a compartment syndrome giving compression of vessels and nerves with a reduction of the distal pulses or paresthesia (Botte et al. 1987; Heckman and Levine 1978; Kragh et al. 2005; McQueen et al. 2000).

It is crucial to identify these situations adopting a mini-invasive surgical approach to remove the hematoma aimed to prevent a complete invasive fasciotomies.

17.3.3 Chronic Muscles Injuries

The surgical management of chronic muscle injuries is today unclear, and no definite guidelines are yet published. Very often the persistence of discomfort and pain are the symptoms most frequently reported by the patients for a long time (duration > 4–6 months) after an acute damage, and the loss of function with worsening performances sometimes may require in these situations a remote surgical treatment (Hope and McQueen 2004; Ramdass et al. 2007; Erturan et al. 2013). Several studies showed a closed correlation between acute muscle injuries and chronic ones: Murray and Lowe have demonstrated that a previous hamstring damage displays the greatest risk factor with two to six times elevated re-injury rates (2009).

In literature, there is discrepancy of the results about the surgical treatment of chronic muscle injuries, as there is no common consensus because authors often apply an experience-based medicine. Two are then the most important correlated difficulties occurring during the surgical approach in these situations, and often they are the cause of poor outcome: the quality of the residual tissue and the retraction of the previous scar. Regarding the first complication, in literature different strategies in order to reinforce the peri-lesional *cloth*, especially if the injury takes place in the extremities of the muscle tissue (miotendinous/tendinous side), are described. Some papers reported good results using the autografts, allografts, and also muscular transpositions. Lempainen et al., for example, proposed surgical reconstruction technique for complete chronic proximal hamstring rupture by use of fascia lata autograft augmentation in five cases with good results at 12 months follow-up. The authors suggest this technique when the primary repair has failed or in chronic injuries where there is a large defect with loss of healthy tissue (Lempainen et al. 2007).

Sarimo et al. reported, for example, on 41 proximal hamstring ruptures, of which 19 patients had surgical repair with greater than 3 months' delay. The risk for a poor outcome was 28 times greater for those with a delay in treatment. The authors found also a strict correlation between outcomes and quality of the peri-lesional residual muscular tissue (Sarimo et al. 2008).

In a cohort study, about 72 patients comparing the functional outcomes and return to sports after acute, chronic repair, and allograft reconstruction for proximal hamstring ruptures, the authors showed that surgery after 6 weeks from the injury had poorer outcomes for return to sports (70.2% cases versus 80.3%) and a trend toward inferior outcomes compared with the acute repair (Rust et al. 2014).

The retraction and the scarring pose are another significant dilemma for the surgeon, very often directly related to the severity of the soft tissue damage. Therefore, the surgical management should be considered if, after an adequate postoperative rehabilitation and stretching protocols, the patient complains of persistence of pain and stiffness after a previously injured muscle. In these chronic cases, the scar tissue formation and adhesions restricting the articular range of motion should be suspected, and surgical fibrinolysis and revision of the scar tissue can be considered. In literature several authors proposed, in addition of this procedure, also the use of autograft or allograft augmentation in order to resolve the muscular retraction of the scar. Murray and Lowe published a case report of a cyclist with a 6-year-old chronic proximal hamstring rupture treated with Achilles allograft reconstruction with a reinforcement of the footprint using suture anchors (2009).

Rust et al. proposed allograft reconstruction for chronic hamstring injuries with greater than 5–6 cm of scar retraction (2014).

Darlis and Widmer recommended the use of an allograft/autograft when anatomic repair of the distal biceps cannot be achieved by native tendon beyond 70–90 flexion (Darlis and Sotereanos 2006; Widmer and Tashjian 2010).

But the harvesting autograft may cause donor site morbidity and additional operating time to harvest and requires prepping and draping of the lower extremity. Allograft increases cost and carries a small but inherent risk of disease transmission (Robertson et al. 2006).

Another strategy to treat and resolve the muscular scar retraction after a wrong healing of an acute muscular complete tear is the musculotendinous surgical release. In the beginning this technique was introduced like a viable solution for the treatment of spastic hemiplegia in the cerebral palsy of the childhood. In these situations, due to a congenital damage of the central nervous system, children have a permanent hypertonia of the lower limbs generating a joint dysfunction by a fixed muscle contraction. Several authors proposed different surgical techniques: one of the most used is the transverse Vulpius recession of the gastroc-soleus, as to reduct the contraction of the calf in order to restore the proper functioning of affected limb (Tinney et al. 2015).

Today, the musculotendinous surgical release is also a useful trick very popular especially between the shoulder surgeons: the retraction is one of the most important limiting factors for successful surgical repair of the cuff (Meyer et al. 2012).

In literature this technique is also proposed like an excellent treatment in chronic miotendinous junction pathology, due to reducing the pain and discomfort of the tendinopathy. For example, several surgical techniques (arthroscopic, mini-open, and percutaneous) are described for the treatment of the chronic lateral epicondylitis (Grewal et al. 2009).

Concluding, the surgical treatment is required also in case of complications that occurred after acute muscle injuries. One example is the myositis ossificans (MO) (Fig. 17.4). Generally, it is related to trauma from a single blow or repeated episodes of microtraumas, and it can be diagnosed and monitored by serial X-rays, being radiologically evident 3–6 weeks after injury (Parikh et al. 2002; Renstrom 2003). The most common reported sites of MO are in the thigh and arm muscles: quadriceps femoris, brachialis, and the adductor. In the majority of cases, it is asymptomatic and can be managed with nonoperative treatments with spontaneous resolution monitored by imaging exams. If MO progress to permanently limit range of motion and function with pain or when the lesion is vulnerable to a repeated trauma causing disability, surgical intervention to remove persistent calcium deposits can be pointed out. Surgery should not be attempted until 4–6 months after trauma to allow for complete maturation of the process (De Maeseneer et al. 1997; Ben Hamida et al. 2004).

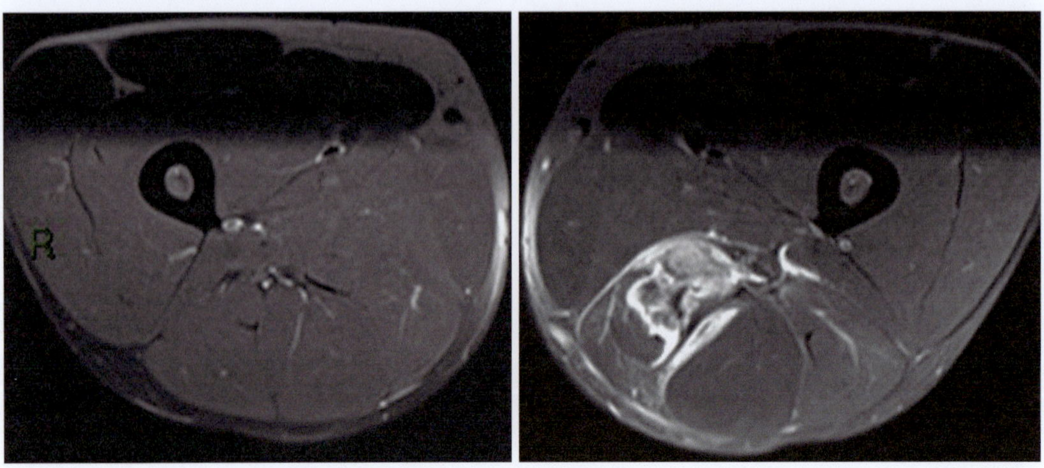

Fig. 17.4 Sagittal T2-weighted magnetic resonance imaging scan of a myositis ossificans of the 29-year-old professional soccer player

References

Aarimaa V, Kaariainen M, Vaittinen S et al (2004) Restoration of myofiber continuity after transection injury in the rat soleus. Neuromuscul Disord 14:421–428

Almekinders LC (1991) Results of surgical repair versus splinting of experimentally transected muscle. J Orthop Trauma 5:173–176

Alonso JM, Junge A, Renstrom P et al (2009) Sports injuries surveillance during the 2007 IAAF World Athletics Championships. Clin J Sport Med 19:26–32

Anderson K, Strickland SM, Warren R (2001) Hip and groin injuries in athletes. Am J Sports Med 29:521–533

Armfield DR, Kim DH, Towers JD et al (2006) Sports-related muscle injury in the lower extremity. Clin Sports Med 25:803–842

Askling CM, Tengvar M, Saartok T et al (2007) Acute first-time hamstring strains during high-speed running: a longitudinal study including clinical and magnetic resonance imaging findings. Am J Sports Med 35:197–206

Belli P, Costantini M, Mirk P, Leone A, Pastore G, Marano P (2001) Sonographic diagnosis of distal biceps tendon rupture: a prospective study of 25 cases. J Ultrasound Med 20(6):587–595

Ben Hamida KS, Hajri R, Kedadi H, Bouhaouala H, Salah MH, Mestiri A et al (2004) Myositis ossificans circumscripta of the knee improved by alendronate. Joint Bone Spine 71(2):144–146

Bhatia DN (2016) Endoscopic repair of acute and chronic retracted distal biceps ruptures. J Hand Surg Am 41(12):e501–e507. pii:S0363-5023(16)30630-X

Borowski LA, Yard EE, Fields SK et al (2008) The epidemiology of US high school basketball injuries, 2005–2007. Am J Sports Med 36:2328–2335

Botte MJ, Gelberman RH, Smith DG et al (1987) Repair of severe muscle belly lacerations using a tendon graft. J Hand Surg Am 12(3):406–412

Boublik M, Schlegel TF, Koonce RC, Genuario GW, Kinkartz JD (2013) Quadriceps tendon injuries in National Football League players. Am J Sports Med 41:1841

Boutin RD et al (2002) MR imaging of sports-related muscle injuries. Radiol Clin N Am 40:333

Branch EA, Anz AW (2015) Distal insertions of the biceps femoris: a quantitative analysis. Orthop J Sports Med 3(9):2325967115602255

Bryan DJ (2009) Gastrocnemius vs. soleus strain: how to differentiate and deal with calf muscle injuries. Curr Rev Muscoskelet Med 2:74–77

Cacchio A, Rompe JD, Furia JP, Susi P, Santili V, Paulis F (2011) Shockwave therapy for the treatment of chronic proximal hamstring tendinopathy in professional athletes. Am J Sports Med 39:146–153

Caekebeke P, Vermeersch N, Duerinckx J, van Riet R (2016) Radiological and clinical evaluation of the transosseous cortical button technique in distal biceps tendon repair. J Hand Surg Am 41(12):e447–e452. pii:S0363-5023(16)30504-4

Celic EC, Ozbaydar M, Ofluoglu D, Demircay E (2012) Simultaneous and spontaneous bilateral quadriceps tendons rupture. Am J Phys Med Rehabil 91(7):631–634

Chakravarthy J, Ramisetty N, Pimpalnerkar A et al (2005) Surgical repair of complete proximal hamstring tendon ruptures in water skiers and bull riders: a report of four cases and review of the literature. Br J Sports Med 39:569–572

Chien SH, Chen SK, Lin SY, Chen SS, Wu HS (1991) Repair method and healing of skeletal muscle injury. Gaoxiong Yi Xue Ke Xue Za Zhi 7:481–488

Clayton RA, Court-Brown CM (2008) The epidemiology of musculoskeletal tendinous and ligamentous injuries. Injury 39:1338–1344

Cohen S, Bradley J (2007) Acute proximal hamstring rupture. J Am Acad Orthop Surg 15(6):350–355

Cohen SB, Towers JD, Zoga A et al (2011) Hamstring injuries in professional football players: magnetic resonance imaging correlation with return to play. Sports Health 3:423–430

Connell DA, Schneider-Kolsky ME, Hoving JL et al (2004) Longitudinal study comparing sonographic and MRI assessments of acute and healing hamstring injuries. AJR Am J Roentgenol 183:975–984

Crisco JJ, Jokl P, Heinen GT, Connell MD, Panjabi MM (1994) A muscle contusion injury model. Biomechanics, physiology, and histology. Am J Sports Med 22(5):702–710

Cross TM, Gibbs N, Houang MT et al (2004) Acute quadriceps muscle strains: magnetic resonance imaging features and prognosis. Am J Sports Med 32:710–719

Darlis NA, Sotereanos DG (2006) Distal biceps tendon reconstruction in chronic ruptures. J Shoulder Elb Surg 15:614–619

David HG, Green JT, Grant AJ, Wilson CA (1995) Simultaneous bilateral quadriceps rupture: a common complication of anabolic steroid abuse. J Bone Joint Surg Br 77(1):159–160

De Maeseneer M, Jaovisidha S, Lenchik L, Vaughan LM, Russack V, Sartoris DJ et al (1997) Myositis ossificans of the foot. J Foot Ankle Surg 36(4):290–293

De Smet AA, Best TM (2000) MR imaging of the distribution and location of acute hamstring injuries in athletes. AJR Am J Roentgenol 174(2):393–399

Devereaux MW, ElMaraghy AW (2013) Improving the rapid and reliable diagnosis of complete distal biceps tendon rupture: a nuanced approach to the clinical examination. Am J Sports Med 41(9):1998–2004

Ding DY, Ryan WE, Strauss EJ, Jazrawi LM (2016) Chronic distal biceps repair with an Achilles allograft. Arthrosc Tech 5(3):e525–e529

Ekstrand J, Hägglund M, Waldén M (2011) Epidemiology of muscle injuries in professional football (soccer). Am J Sports Med 39:1226–1232

Ekstrand J, Healy JC, Waldén M et al (2012) Hamstring muscle injuries in professional football: the correlation of MRI findings with return to play. Br J Sports Med 46:112–117

Erturan G, Davies N, Williams H, Deo S (2013) Bilateral simultaneous traumatic upper arm compartment syn-

dromes associated with anabolic steroids. J Emerg Med 44(1):89–91
Feeley BT, Kennelly S, Barnes RP et al (2008) Epidemiology of National Football League training camp injuries from 1998 to 2007. Am J Sports Med 36:1597–1603
Flint JH, Wade AM, Jeffrey Rue JF, Rue JP (2014) Defining the terms acute and chronic in orthopaedic sports injuries: a systematic review. Am J Sports Med 42:235
Garrett WE Jr (1990) Muscle strain injuries: clinical and basic aspects. Med Sci Sports Exerc 22(4):436–443
Gibbs NJ, Cross TM, Cameron M et al (2004) The accuracy of MRI in predicting recovery and recurrence of acute grade one hamstring muscle strains within the same season in Australian Rules football players. J Sci Med Sport 7:248–258
Gidwani S, Jagiello J, Bircher M (2004) Avulsion fracture of the ischial tuberosity in adolescents: an easily missed diagnosis. BMJ 239:99–100
Gilcreest EL (1933) The common syndrome of rupture, dislocation and elongation of the long head of the biceps brachii. Surg Gynecol Obstet 58:322–339
Grewal R, MacDermid JC, Shah P, King GJ (2009) Functional outcome of arthroscopic extensor carpi radialis brevis tendon release in chronic lateral epicondylitis. J Hand Surg Am 34(5):849–857
Guanche CA (2015) Hamstring injuries. J Hip Preserv Surg 2(2):116–122
Hägglund M, Waldén M, Ekstrand J (2005) Injury incidence and distribution in elite football—a prospective study of the Danish and the swedish top divisions. Scand J Med Sci Sports 15:21–28
Hallen A, Ekstrand J (2014) Return to play following muscle injuries in professional footballers. J Sports Sci 32(13):1229–1236
Harris JD, Griesser MJ, Best TM, Ellis TJ (2011) Treatment of proximal hamstring rupture-a systematic review. Int J Sports Med 32:490–495
Heckman JD, Levine MI (1978) Traumatic closed transection of the biceps brachii in the military parachutist. J Bone Joint Surg Am 60:369–372
Heiderscheit BC, Sherry MA, Silder A, Chumanov ES, Thelen DG (2010) Hamstring strain injuries: recommendations for diagnosis, rehabilitation, and injury prevention. J Orthop Sports Phys Ther 40(2):67–81
Hope MJ, McQueen MM (2004) Acute compartment syndrome in the absence of fracture. J Orthop Trauma 4:220–224
Huard J, Li Y, Fu FH (2002) Muscle injuries and repair: current trends in research. J Bone Joint Surg Am 84(5):822–832
Jarvinen MJ, Lehto MU (1993) The effects of early mobilisation and immobilisation on the healing process following muscle injuries. Sports Med 15:78–89
Jarvinen TA, Jarvinen TL, Kaariainen M et al (2005) Muscle injuries: biology and treatment. Am J Sports Med 33:745–764
Julien TP, Mudgal CS (2011) Anchor suture technique for muscle belly repair. Tech Hand Up Extrem Surg 15:257
Kelly MP, Perkinson SG, Ablove RH, Tueting JL (2015) Distal biceps tendon ruptures: an epidemiological analysis using a large population database. Am J Sports Med 43(8):2012–2017
Khoshnoodi P, Tehranzadeh AD, Dunn JM, Tehranzadeh J (2014) Semimembranosus tendon avulsion fracture of the posteromedial tibial plateau associated with posterior cruciate ligament tear and capsular rupture. Skelet Radiol 43(2):239–242
Konan S, Haddad F (2010) Successful return to high level sports following early surgical repair of complete tears of the proximal hamstring tendons. Int Orthop 34(1):119–123
Konrath GA, Chen D, Lock T et al (1998) Outcomes following repair of quadriceps tendon ruptures. J Orthop Trauma 12(4):273–279
Kragh JF, Svoboda SJ, Wenke JC, Ward JA, Walters T (2005) Suturing of lacerations of skeletal muscle. J Bone Joint Surg (Br) 87-B:1303–1305
Kujala UM, Orava S, Järvinen M (1997) Hamstring injuries: current trends in treatment and prevention. Sports Med 23:397–404
Kurosawa H, Nakasita K, Nakasita H, Sasaki S, Takeda S (1996) Complete avulsion of the hamstring tendons from the ischial tuberosity. A report of two cases sustained in Judo. Br J Sports Med 30:72–74
LaPrade F, Wijdicks CA et al (2015) Structural properties of the intact proximal hamstring origin and evaluation of varying avulsion repair techniques: an in vitro biomechanical analysis. Am J Sports Med 43:721
Lempainen L, Sarim J, Orava S (2007) Recurrent and chronic complete ruptures of the proximal origin of the hamstring muscles repaired with fascia lata autograft augmentation. Arthroscopy 23(4):441.e1–441.e5
Lempainen L, Sarimo J, Mattila K, Heikkila J, Orava S Distal tears of the hamstring muscles: review of the literature
Levine WN, Bergfeld JA, Tesssendorf W, Moorman CT III (2000) Intra-muscular corticosteroid injection for hamstring injuries. A 13-year experience in the National Football League. Am J Sports Med 28:297–300
Liow RY, Tavares S (1995) Bilateral rupture of the quadriceps tendon associated with anabolic steroids. Br J Sports Med 29(2):77–79
Lopez V Jr, Galano GJ, Black CM et al (2012) Profile of an American amateur rugby union sevens series. Am J Sports Med 40:179–184
Malliaropoulos N, Papacostas E, Kiritsi O et al (2010) Posterior thigh muscle injuries in elite track and field athletes. Am J Sports Med 38:1813–1819
Mason DL, Dickens V, Vail A (2012) Rehabilitation for hamstring injuries. Cochrane Database Syst Rev 12:CD004575
McQueen MM, Gaston P, Court-Brown CM (2000) Acute compartment syndrome. Who is at risk? J Bone Joint Surg (Br) 82(2):200–203
Meyer RA, Prior BM (2000) Functional magnetic resonance imaging of muscle. Exerc Sport Sci Rev 28:89–92
Meyer DC, Farshad M, Amacker NA, Gerber C, Wieser K (2012) Quantitative analysis of muscle and tendon retraction in chronic rotator cuff tears. Am J Sports Med 40:606

Mica L, Schwaller A, Stoupis C et al (2009) Avulsion of the hamstring muscle group: a follow-up of 6 adult non-athletes with early operative treatment: a brief report. World J Surg 33:1605–1610

Morrey MC, Barlow JD, Abdel MP, Hanssen AD (2016) Synthetic mesh augmentation of acute and subacute quadriceps tendon repair. Orthopedics 39(1):e9–13

Mueller-Wohlfahrt HW, Haensel L, Mithoefer K, Ekstrand J, English B, McNally S et al (2013) Terminology and classification of muscle injuries in sport: the Munich consensus statement. Br J Sports Med 47:342–350

Murray PJ, Lowe WR (2009) Achilles allograft reconstruction of a chronic complete proximal hamstring rupture. Knee Surg Sports Traumatol Arthrosc 17:1360–1363

Noonan TJ, Garrett WE Jr (1999) Muscle strain injury: diagnosis and treatment. J Am Acad Orthop Surg 7:262–269

O'Donoghue DO (1962) Treatment of injuries to athletes. WB Saunders, Philadelphia

O'Shea K, Kenny P, Donovan J, Condon F, McElwain JP (2002) Outcomes following quadriceps tendon ruptures. Injury 33:257–260

Parikh J, Hyare H, Saifuddin A (2002) The imaging features of posttraumatic myositis ossificans, with emphasis on MRI. Clin Radiol 57:1058–1066

Peetrons P (2002) Ultrasound of muscles. Eur Radiol 12:35–43

Petilon J, Carr DR, Sekiya JK, Unger DV (2005) Pectoralis major muscle injuries: evaluation and management. J Am Acad Orthop Surg 13(1):59–68

Pollock N, James SLJ, Lee JC, Chakraverty R (2014) British athletics muscle injury classification: a new grading system. Br J Sports Med 48:1347–1351

Praemer A, Furner S, Rice DP (1992) Musculoskeletal conditions in the United States. Park Ridge, Illinois, American Academy of Orthopaedic Surgeons

Ramdass MJ, Singh G, Andrews B (2007) Simvastatin-induced bilateral leg compartment syndrome and myonecrosis associated with hypothyroidism. Postgrad Med J 83(977):152–153

Ramos LA, de Carvalho RT, Abdalla RJ, Ingham SJM (2015) Surgical treatment for muscle injuries. Curr Rev Muscoskelet Med 8:188–192

Renstrom P (2003) Muscle injuries. In: Ekstrand J, Karlsson J, Hodson A (eds) Football medicine. Martin Dunitz, London, pp 217–228

Reurink G, Goudswaard GJ, Tol JL et al (2014) MRI observations at return to play of clinically recovered hamstring injuries. Br J Sports Med 48:1370–1376

Robertson A, Nutton RW, Keating JF (2006) Current trends in the use of tendon allografts in orthopaedic surgery. J Bone Joint Surg Br 88:988–992

Rust DA, Giveans MR, Stone RM, Samuelson KS, Larson CM (2014) Functional outcomes and return to sports after acute repair, chronic repair, and allograft reconstruction for proximal hamstring ruptures. Am J Sports Med 42:1377

Safran MR, Graham SM (2002) Distal biceps tendon ruptures: incidence, demographics, and the effect of smoking. Clin Orthop Relat Res 404:275–283

Sallay PI, Friedman RL, Coogan PG et al (2008) Subjective and functional outcomes following surgical repair of complete ruptures of the proximal hamstring complex. Orthopedics 31:1092–1096

Sarimo J, Lempainen L, Mattila K et al (2008) Complete proximal hamstring avulsions: a series of 41 patients with operative treatment. Am J Sports Med 36:1110–1115

Slavotinek J (2010) Muscle injury: the role of imaging in prognostic assignment and monitoring of muscle repair. Semin Musculoskelet Radiol 14:194–200

Stoller DW (2007) MRI in orthopaedics and sports medicine, 3rd edn. Wolters Kluwer/Lippincott, Philadelphia

Takebayashi S, Takasawa H, Banzai Y et al (1995) Sonographic findings in muscle strain injury: clinical and MR imaging correlation. J Ultrasound Med 14:899–905

Tinney A, Thomason P, Sangeux M, Khot A, Graham HK (2015) The transverse Vulpius gastrocsoleus recession for equinus gait in children with cerebral palsy. Bone Joint J 97-B(4):564–571

Vanek J (1994) Posteromedial fracture of the tibial plateau is not an avulsion injury. A case report and experimental study. JBJS 76(2):290–292

Walden M, Hagglund M, Magnusson H et al (2011) Anterior cruciate ligament injury in elite football: a prospective three-cohort study. Knee Surg Sports Traumatol Arthrosc 19:11–19

Watts CD, Hartzler RU, Cross WW (2014) Open reduction and percutaneous fixation of a rare hamstring avulsion fracture. BMJ Case Rep. doi:10.1136/bcr-2014-205256

Weiss C, Mittelmeier M, Gruber G (2000) Do we need MR images for diagnosing tendon ruptures of the distal biceps brachii? The value of ultrasonographic imaging. Ultraschall Med 21(6):284–286

West JL, Keene JS, Kaplan LD (2008) Early motion after quadriceps and patellar tendon repairs: outcomes with single-suture augmentation. Am J Sports Med 36(2):316–323

Widmer BJ, Tashjian RZ (2010) Treatment of distal biceps tendon ruptures. Am J Orthop (Belle Mead NJ) 39:288–296

Wooton JR, Cross MJ, Holt KWG (1990) Avulsion of the ischial apophysis: the case for open reduction and internal fixation. J Bone Joint Surg Am 72B:625–627

Zanon G, Combi F, Combi A, Perticarini L, Sammarchi L, Benazzo F (2016) Platelet-rich plasma in the treatment of acute hamstring injuries in professional football players. Joints 4(1):17–23

Zarins B, Ciullo JV (1983) Acute muscle and tendon injuries in athletes. Clin Sports Med 2:167–182

Rotator Cuff Tendinopathy

18

Stephanie C. Petterson, Margaret Harvey, and Kevin D. Plancher

Contents

S.C. Petterson, M.P.T., Ph.D.
Orthopaedic Foundation, Stamford, CT, USA

M. Harvey, D.O.
Plancher Orthopaedics & Sports Medicine, New York, NY, USA

K.D. Plancher, M.D. (✉)
Orthopaedic Foundation, Stamford, CT, USA

Plancher Orthopaedics & Sports Medicine, New York, NY, USA

Department of Orthopaedic Surgery, Albert Einstein College of Medicine, New York, NY, USA
e-mail: kplancher@plancherortho.com

Rotator cuff disease has been described as a progressive disorder of the rotator cuff tendons, beginning with an acute tendinitis, progressing to tendinosis with degeneration and partial-thickness tearing, and can result in full-thickness rupture (Neer 1983). The incidence of rotator cuff tendinopathy has been reported at 0.3–5.5% with an annual prevalence from 0.5 to 7.4% (Littlewood et al. 2014).

The term tendinopathy describes a painful condition that develops in or around tendons potentially due to an imbalance between pathologic responses from tendon overuse and regenerative changes, leading to impaired functional mobility (Andres and Murrell 2008a; Factor and Dale 2014). In 1983, Neer described the pathophysiology of rotator cuff disease in three stages, impingement syndrome to partial and complete rotator cuff tears (1983). More recently, Lewis suggests a continuum from reactive to disrepair and finally degenerative tendinopathy (2010). While histological evidence suggests that little or no inflammation is present, chronic changes include degeneration and disorganization of collagen fibers, increased cellularity, and tendon thickening (Fukuda et al. 1990a).

The etiology of rotator cuff tendinopathy and rotator cuff failure is likely multifactorial from a combination of intrinsic, extrinsic, and environmental factors (Seitz et al. 2011; Lewis 2010). Extrinsic factors (i.e., bony or soft tissue) cause compression of the rotator cuff tendons, while intrinsic (e.g., aging, decreased vascularity,

G.L. Canata et al. (eds.), *Muscle and Tendon Injuries*, DOI 10.1007/978-3-662-54184-5_18

altered biology, tendon overuse) mechanisms are generally associated with degeneration of the rotator cuff tendon (Seitz et al. 2011). These factors can contribute to tendon wear, fraying, and ultimately a partial- or full-thickness rotator cuff tear. An understanding of the anatomy of the rotator cuff tendons and histology of chronic tendinopathy as well as extrinsic and intrinsic causes of tendinopathy is required to fully understand how to accurately diagnose and treat rotator cuff tendinopathy.

18.1 Anatomy and Function

The rotator cuff consists of four muscles: the supraspinatus, infraspinatus, teres minor, and subscapularis. They originate on the scapula and insert into the greater and lesser tuberosities of the humerus (Busconi and Schepsis 2005). These muscles end in short, flat tendons which fuse with the fibrous capsule to form the musculotendinous cuff. The fusion occurs approximately 1.27 to 1.90 cm. from the point of insertion onto the humerus (DePalma and Brand 2008). The supraspinatus footprint is 23 × 16 mm and inserts at the articular surface from the bicipital groove to the top of the bare area (Curtis et al. 2006). The infraspinatus footprint is 29 × 19 mm and wraps around the posterior border of the supraspinatus, framing the bare area. The teres minor footprint measures 29 × 21 mm and is posterior to the infraspinatus. The subscapularis footprint is located on the lesser tuberosity, adjacent to the biceps groove, and measures 40 × 20 mm (Curtis et al. 2006). The rotator cuff plays a role in providing internal and external rotation of the glenohumeral joint, but perhaps a more critical role is in stabilizing the humeral head and preventing superior translation of the humeral head during arm elevation because of the relative location to the humeral head and via its active compression mechanism against the glenoid (Sharkey and Marder 1995).

The subacromial space, defined by the coracoacromial ligament and acromioclavicular joint superiorly, the anterior edge and undersurface of the acromion, and the humeral head inferiorly, houses the rotator cuff tendons, the long head of the biceps tendon, and the coracoacromial ligament. On average, the subacromial space, measured as the width of the space between the inferior surface of the acromion and the head of the humerus and anteroposterior radiograph, is 1–1.5 cm; however, it varies based on the acromial shape (Umer et al. 2012; Petersson and Redlund-Johnell 1984). Under normal circumstances, there is room for the tendon to travel; however, in pathologic states, there may not be sufficient room for the tendon, and "impingement" occurs.

18.2 Extrinsic Causes

Extrinsic mechanisms of rotator cuff tendinopathy often result in mechanical compression of the bursal side of the rotator cuff tendon due to narrowing of the subacromial space arising from anatomic or biomechanical factors, or a combination (Seitz et al. 2011). Subacromial impingement, first described by Watson-Jones in 1940 as impingement of the lateral acromion on the rotator cuff during the mid-arc of abduction, is the most common form of external impingement (Busconi and Schepsis 2005; Watson-Jones 1940). In his classic article in 1972, Neer coined the term "impingement syndrome," implicating the anterior acromion, the coracoacromial ligament, and the acromioclavicular joint as the root cause (1972). His theory of the rotator cuff and undersurface of the humeral head encountering the undersurface of the anterior acromion and coracoacromial ligament led to the recommendation to perform an anterior acromioplasty to manage primary impingement (Neer 1972).

Anatomic factors that may narrow the subacromial space include acromion shape and prominent osseous changes to the inferior aspect of the acromioclavicular joint or coracoacromial ligament (Farley et al. 1990; Ogawa et al. 2005). In 1986, Bigliani classified the acromion into three types based on shape: type I, flat; type II, curved; and type III, hooked (Bigiliani et al. 1986). Multiple studies have determined that there is an association between acromion shape

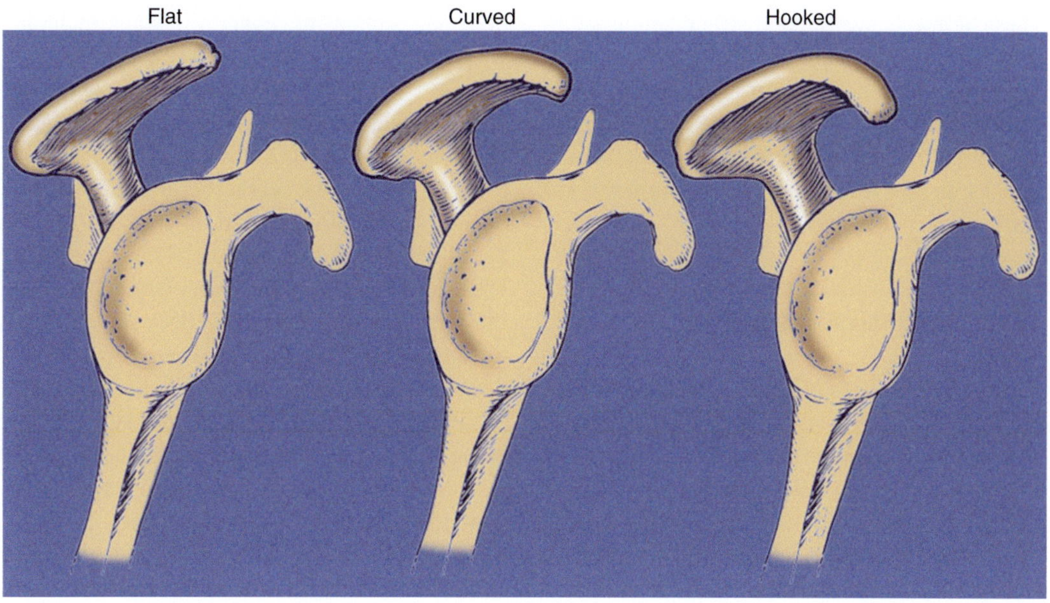

Fig. 18.1 Bigliani classification of acromial shape: type I (*flat*), type II (*curved*), and type III (*hooked*). Copyright Kevin D. Plancher, MD

and severity of rotator cuff pathology (Ogawa et al. 2005; Bigliani et al. 1991; Epstein et al. 1993). The geometry of the type II or III acromion leads to a reduction in the subacromial space and therefore a greater risk of impingement, whereas a type III acromion has also been associated with a higher incidence of rotator cuff tears (Bigliani et al. 1991; Epstein et al. 1993; Toivonen et al. 1995) (Fig. 18.1). Arthritic changes of the acromioclavicular joint have been theorized as a cause of external impingement of the rotator cuff tendons (Neer 1972, 1983; Petersson and Gentz 1983). Cuomo demonstrated that inferior spurs of the distal clavicle associated with acromioclavicular joint arthrosis correlate with the presence of rotator cuff pathology (Cuomo et al. 1998).

There is significant evidence that anatomic variants may contribute to an extrinsic mechanism of rotator cuff tendinopathy. However, the presence alone of these external factors may be insufficient to result in rotator cuff tendinopathy (Seitz et al. 2011). Soslowsky et al. found that external compression of rotator cuff tendons in rats with normal activity did not cause pathologic changes; however, when coupled with overuse activity, there was a significant effect on tendon injury (2002). Therefore, it can be theorized that extrinsic causes may be a factor in rotator cuff tendinopathy; however, there is likely an overuse component involved.

Functional range of motion of the shoulder can alter the dimensions of the subacromial space and contribute to clinical signs of secondary impingement syndrome, specifically shoulder abduction and rotation (Matthews and Fadale 1989; Graichen et al. 1999). The distance between the humerus and the acromion is reduced by almost 50% when the shoulder moves from 30° to 120° of abduction with the minimum distance between the acromion and humerus being the smallest when the arm is externally rotated 90° (DePalma and Brand 2008; Graichen et al. 1999). The supraspinatus is closest to the anteroinferior border of the acromion when the arm is in 90° of abduction and 45° of internal rotation (Graichen et al. 1999). On the contrary, while arm elevation leads to a decrease in subacromial space width, adduction muscle forces substantially increase the acromiohumeral distance and claviculohumeral distance compared to abduction muscle forces (138% at 90° relative to abduction forces).

These biomechanics support strengthening of the adductor muscles, including the latissimus dorsi, subscapularis, and teres major and minor, in both conservative and postoperative rehabilitation programs to avoid and lessen the symptoms of impingement syndrome (Hinterwimmer et al. 2003).

18.3 Intrinsic Causes

Intrinsic mechanisms originate in the tendon itself and have a multitude of causes which include natural process of aging (Tempelhof et al. 1999; Milgrom et al. 1995), microvascular blood supply (Biberthaler et al. 2003; Fukuda et al. 1990b), morphology, and mechanical properties (Michener et al. 2003). Age has been shown to have a negative influence on tendon properties including decreased collagen orientation, cellularity, compliance, elasticity, and overall tensile strength (Seitz et al. 2011). There is a decrease in total glycosaminoglycans and proteoglycans in the supraspinatus tendon with age (Riley et al. 1994).

Rotator cuff tendon vascularity may play a role in rotator cuff tendinopathy. Codman described a "critical zone" in the supraspinatus tendon approximately 1 cm from the insertion on the greater tubercle, also the most common site of rotator cuff tendon injury (Petri et al. 1987; Codman 1934). Multiple studies have confirmed this hypovascular zone of the distal 2 cm of the supraspinatus tendon, predisposing the rotator cuff tendon to injury due to poor healing potential (Biberthaler et al. 2003; Brooks et al. 1992; Fukuda et al. 1990b). However, other studies refute this concept and have demonstrated no region of avascularity in the critical zone. The role vascularity plays in rotator cuff tendinopathy therefore remains unclear (Matthews and Fadale 1989; Levy et al. 2008; Longo et al. 2008).

18.4 Diagnosis

No single test can efficiently diagnose rotator cuff tendinopathy. Diagnosis involves the combination of a thorough history, physical examination, and supporting imaging studies including x-rays and MRI. Pain, weakness, and loss of shoulder motion are common complaints (Fongemie et al. 1998). Pain is generally exacerbated by overhead activities as the rotator cuff passes through the coracoacromial arch, frequently occurs at night, and may radiate into the deltoid and scapular regions (Fongemie et al. 1998). Patients may also complain of pain and difficulty reaching behind the back such as when tucking in shirt or placing a wallet in the back pocket and even when reaching out to the side.

Several key maneuvers are essential to include in the physical examination to aid in the diagnosis of subacromial impingement syndrome. A combination of a positive Hawkins-Kennedy impingement test, painful arc of motion, and a positive infraspinatus test yields a >95% likelihood of a diagnosis of impingement, whereas, when these tests are negative, the likelihood of impingement is <24%.

The Neer impingement sign causes provocation of pain at the anterolateral edge of the acromion when the examiner passively forward flexes the arm greater than 120° with the humerus internally rotated and the scapula stabilized (Fig. 18.2). The Neer sign has a sensitivity and specificity of 72 and 60%, respectively (Hegedus et al. 2012). Hawkins and Kennedy also described an alternative impingement test which elicits symptoms when the arm is placed in 90° forward elevation and then gently internally rotated (Fig. 18.3). The Hawkins-Kennedy sign has a sensitivity and specificity of 79 and 59%, respectively (Hegedus et al. 2012). These impingement tests place the greater tuberosity, rotator cuff, or biceps tendon against the undersurface of the acromion or coracoacromial ligament causing aggravation of an inflamed bursa. A painful arc of motion between 60° and 120° of active forward elevation in the plane of the scapula is also indicative of impingement. The patient often reports pain or painful catching in the shoulder. This test has a sensitivity of 73.5% and specificity of 81.1% (Factor and Dale 2014). Lastly, the infraspinatus muscle test performed with the arm at the side and the elbow flexed to 90° elicits pain when the patient resists against an internal rotation force.

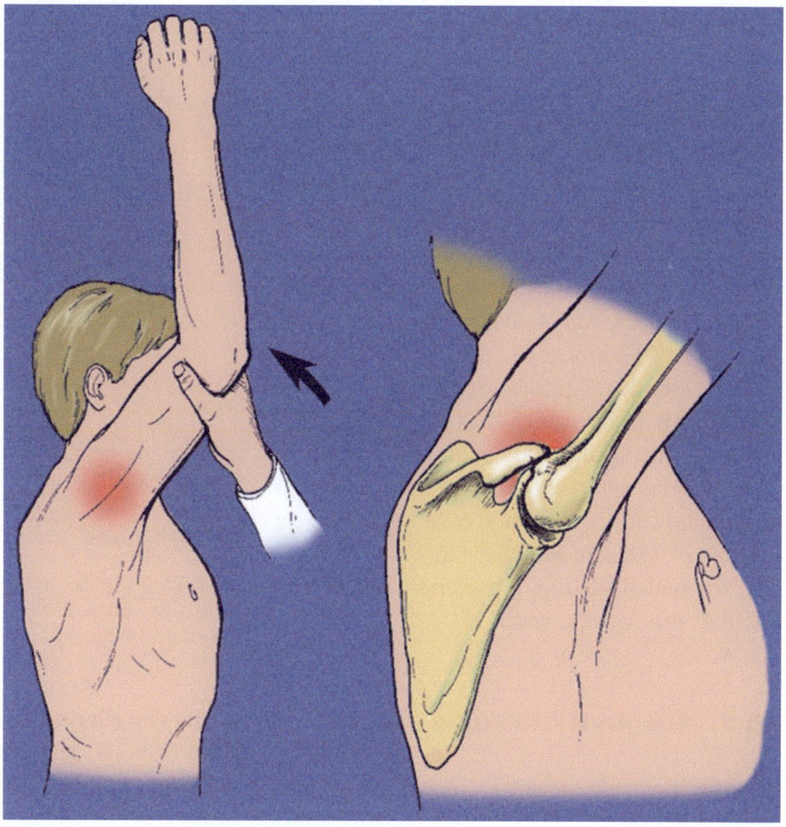

Fig. 18.2 Neer impingement sign. The examiner stabilizes the scapula and passively flexes the arm greater than 120° with the arm internally rotated. Provocation of pain at the anterolateral edge of the acromion is indicative of subacromial impingement. Copyright Kevin D. Plancher, MD

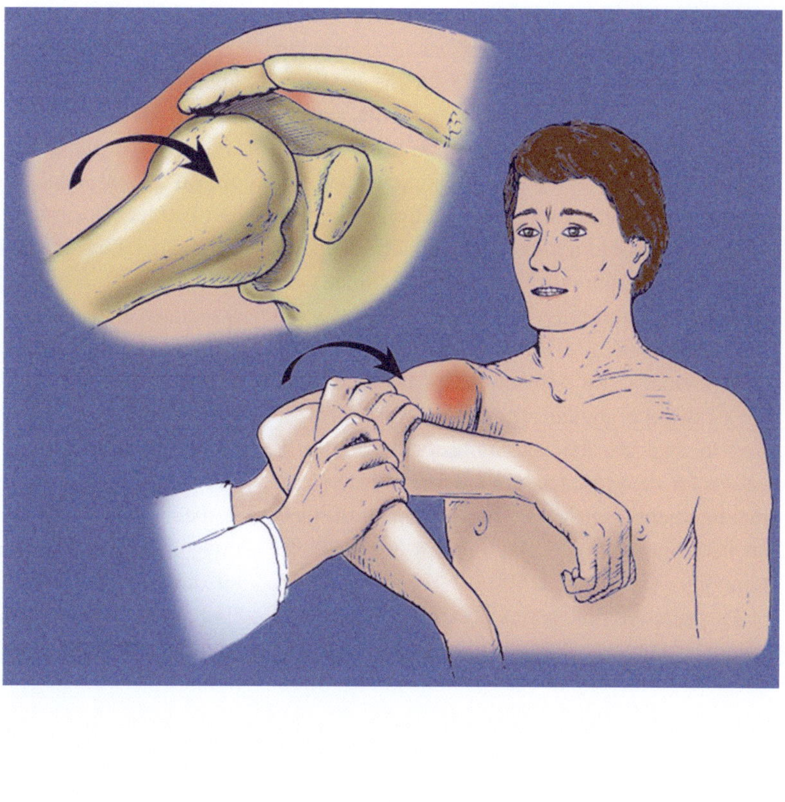

Fig. 18.3 Hawkins-Kennedy impingement test. The patient's arm is positioned in 90° of forward elevation with the elbow flexed to 90°. The examiner then gently internally rotates the arm. Provocation of pain at the anterolateral edge of the acromion is indicative of subacromial impingement. Copyright Kevin D. Plancher, MD

Many disorders of the shoulder present similar to subacromial impingement syndrome. A diagnostic lidocaine anesthetic injection into the subacromial space can improve the accuracy of the diagnosis of subacromial impingement syndrome. We inject 10 mL of 1% lidocaine using a 25-gauge, 1½ in. needle into the subacromial space through an anterior approach. Ultrasound can be used as an adjunct to guide the needle to ensure accuracy. Alternatively, the needle can be placed 1 cm inferior to the posterolateral corner of the acromion directed toward the coracoid. Provocative maneuvers should be performed following the injection to confirm the diagnosis. Alleviation of symptoms on impingement tests is highly indicative of subacromial impingement syndrome. The authors believe that a 1½ in. needle is essential if using a posterior approach to avoid a false-negative result.

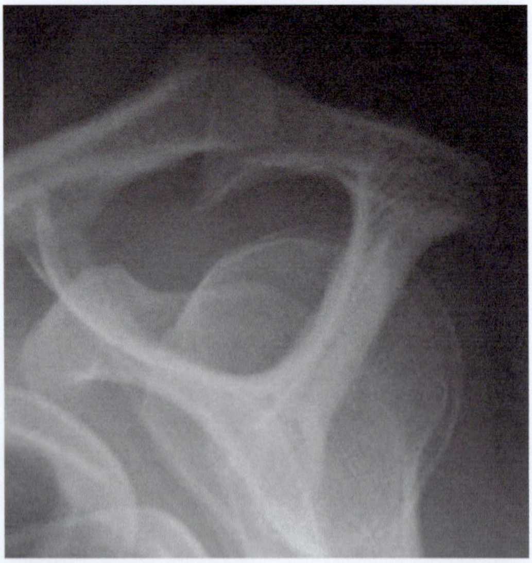

Fig. 18.4 Scapular outlet view demonstrating a type III, *hooked*, acromion. The scapular outlet view best evaluates acromial morphology

18.5 Diagnostic Imaging

The specificity of special tests on physical examination is relatively low; therefore, imaging of the shoulder should also be utilized in the diagnostic process in order to make an accurate and complete assessment of the underlying pathology (Silva et al. 2010). Radiographs can aid in evaluating acromial morphology, assessing for the presence of subacromial spurs and calcific tendinitis and for the presence of degenerative changes at the greater tuberosity, the acromioclavicular joint, or anterior acromion. A supraspinatus outlet view radiograph is best to evaluate acromial shape. The scapular outlet view, on the other hand, best evaluates the anteroinferior acromion (Fig. 18.4). This view is a true scapulolateral with the x-ray tube angled 5–10° caudally. An AP view of the shoulder with the x-ray tube angled 30° caudally can also be used to evaluate the anteroinferior acromion as well as for the presence of a calcified coracoacromial ligament (Fig. 18.5). This AP caudal tilt view has been shown to have the highest interobserver reliability (Kitay et al. 1995).

This radiographic series is extremely useful in surgical planning to determine the amount of resection necessary to establish a flat acromion. A study by Kitay et al. demonstrated that the distance from the acromial cortex to the end of the acromial spur on x-ray significantly correlated with intraoperative spur length (1995). Acromial slope measured on the supraspinatus outlet view, which was shown to have less intraobserver reliability than the caudal tilt view, significantly correlated with intraoperative acromial thickness. Therefore, the authors believe these views should be included in routine radiographic evaluation and surgical planning when presented with suspected subacromial impingement or rotator cuff involvement prior to acromioplasty.

Magnetic resonance imaging (MRI) can also be useful to evaluate soft tissue and bony pathology associated with rotator cuff pathology and assess the subacromial-subdeltoid bursa. MRI evaluation of rotator cuff tendinopathy has a reported sensitivity of 84–96% (Quinn et al. 1995; Balich et al. 1997). Tendinopathy is characterized on MRI as increased intra-substance signal on short TE sequences, not as bright as fluid on T2-weighted images (Buchbinder et al. 2008). Coronal or sagittal oblique cuts are best to evaluate subacromial spurs as well as acromion type (Fig. 18.6) Small spurs appear black (hypointensity) on T2-weighted images, whereas larger spurs appear as high signal

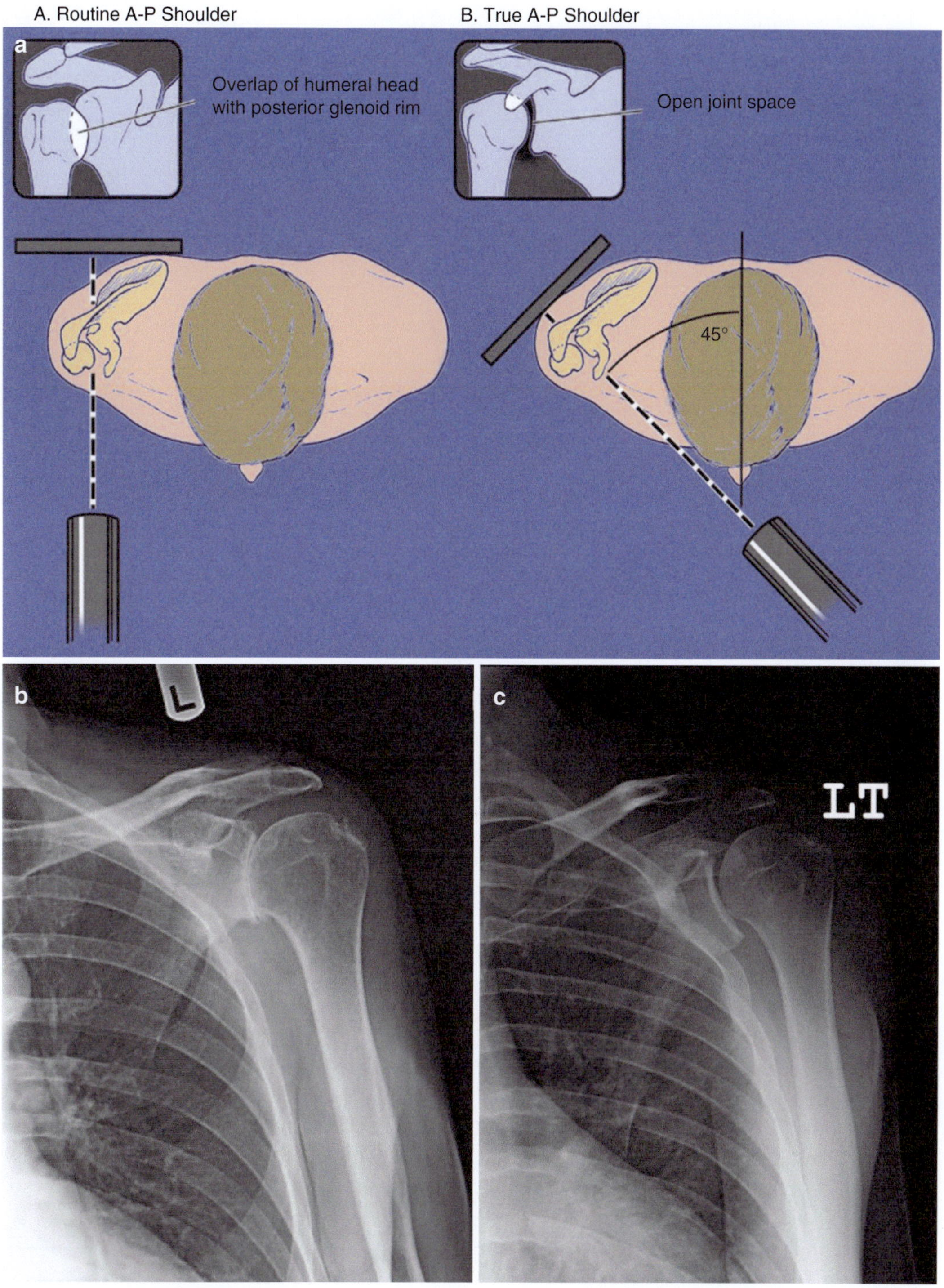

Fig. 18.5 (**a**) Artwork demonstrating the difference and correct way to obtain a true versus routine AP view of the shoulder. (**b**) Routine AP in a left shoulder. (**c**) True AP (Grashey) in a left shoulder. Copyright Kevin D. Plancher, MD

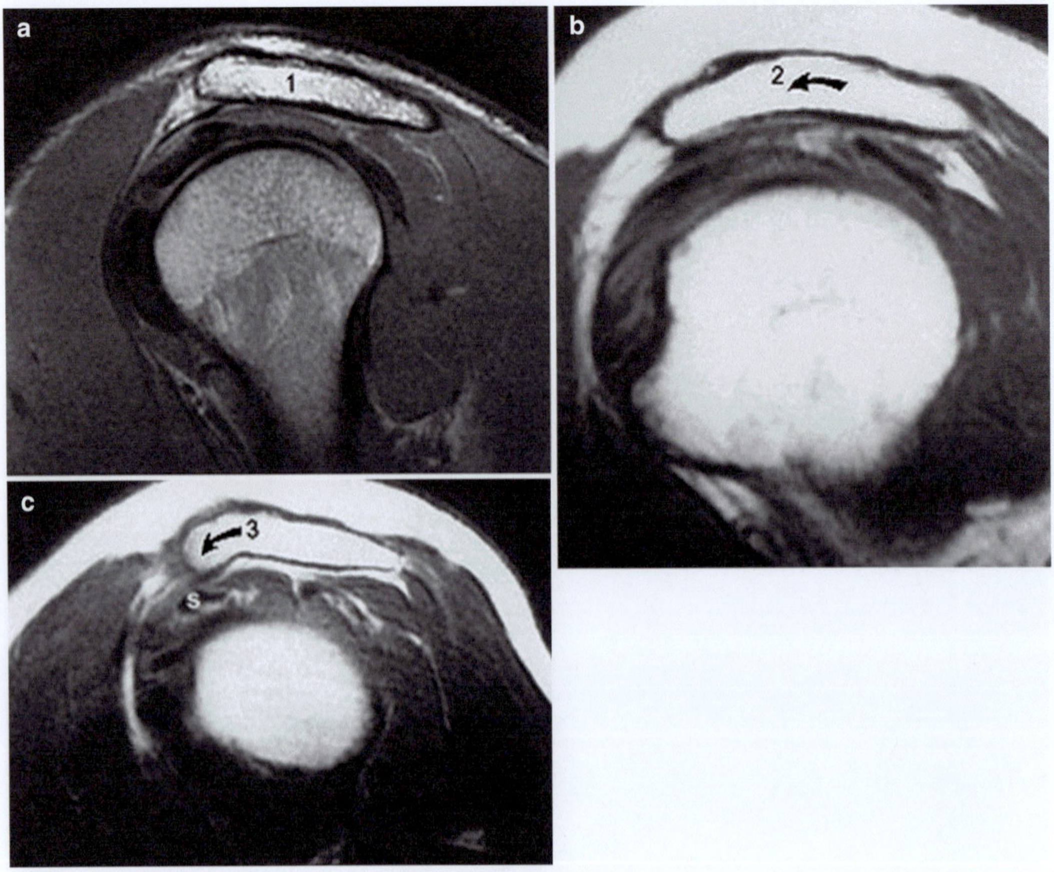

Fig. 18.6 MRI evaluation of acromial morphology. (**a**) Type I, *flat*. (b) Type II, *curved*. (c) Type III, *hooked*. Copyright Kevin D. Plancher, MD

on both T1-weighted and T2-weighted images because they contain marrow. Degenerative changes of the acromioclavicular joint can also be visualized on MRI, indicated by hypertrophy of the joint capsule as a medium signal intensity surrounding the acromioclavicular joint on pulse sequences with short repetition time (TR) and short echo time (TE). Changes in the subacromial-subdeltoid bursa and peri-bursal fat are signs of a rotator cuff tear as a complete tear allows extension of intra-articular fluid in the bursa. This is represented as high signal intensity or white within the bursa on T2-weighted images.

The use of ultrasound, computed tomography (CT), and MRI has been shown to be reliable methods for measuring acromiohumeral distance (McCreesh et al. 2013). Normal acromiohumeral distance is approximately 10.5–11 mm and is smaller in females compared to males (Cotty et al. 1988; Kim et al. 2014). The distance is also dependent on arm position and has been shown to be smallest (8.1–9.9 mm), when the arm is flexed to 90° and in neutral rotation and is largest in positions of internal rotation (range, 11.2–12.2 mm) (Kim et al. 2014). Additionally, an acromiohumeral distance less than 7 mm has been correlated with a complete rotator cuff tear (Weiner and Macnab 1970; Fehringer et al. 2008; Henseler et al. 2014).

18.6 Treatment

Oral NSAIDS are commonly utilized as the initial treatment for tendinopathy. Multiple studies have demonstrated the effectiveness of oral and local NSAIDS in the treatment of acute shoulder tendinopathy (Mena et al. 1986; Mazieres et al. 2005;

Petri et al. 1987, 2004). Patients who present with a longer duration and greater severity of symptoms are less likely to have a positive response with NSAIDS (Andres and Murrell 2008b).

Physical therapy is also a common treatment for rotator cuff tendinopathy. Physical therapy for rotator cuff tendinopathy generally focuses on rotator cuff strengthening, scapular stabilization, as well as improving the biomechanics of the shoulder. There appears to be moderate evidence that manual physical therapy may decrease pain in rotator cuff tendinopathy; however, it is unclear if it improves overall function (Bang and Deyle 2000; Desjardins-Charbonneau et al. 2015).

Corticosteroid injections, most commonly subacromial injections, have also been a mainstay of treatment for rotator cuff tendinopathy. The mechanism of action is to locally decrease inflammation and improve the ability to perform exercises and improve function (Griffin 2005). Alvarez found no improvement in symptoms with an injection of betamethasone versus Xylocaine in range of motion or improving quality of life (Alvarez et al. 2005). In contrast, multiple studies have demonstrated at least short-term improvement after a corticosteroid subacromial injection (Celik et al. 2009; Yu et al. 2006). In general, it is recommended to attempt conservative treatment of a course of NSAIDS, physical therapy, and possibly a steroid injection prior to any surgical treatment.

Orthobiologics are emerging in the treatment of tendon pathologies. Platelet-rich plasma (PRP) and stem cell injections are two methods of introducing growth factors from autologous or allogeneic sources that can be used in isolation or as adjuvant therapies to augment tendon healing. While still in their infancy, these modalities show promise in addressing the underlying pathologic processes to promote an optimal healing environment (Freitag et al. 2014; Kesikburun et al. 2013; Scapone et al. 2013; Abdulrazzak et al. 2010). These modalities can be introduced via direct injection or intraoperative application to improve the effectiveness of conservative and surgical treatments.

Surgery is typically indicated after a failed 6-month course of conservative treatment, confirmed anatomic variants or changes, in the absence or presence of a rotator cuff tear. The results of surgery for rotator cuff tendinopathy are difficult to interpret. If a surgical procedure is performed, it is generally to perform an acromioplasty, assess the rotator cuff, and debride the bursa and tendon as indicated. Favorable results have been seen in the vast majority of studies (Bengtsson et al. 2006; Nutton et al. 1997; Stephens et al. 1998). A randomized study comparing acromioplasty or supervised exercises versus placebo demonstrated improvement in both the exercise and acromioplasty group (Brox et al. 1993).

18.7 Summary

Rotator cuff tendinopathy is a common orthopedic disorder that can be difficult to treat effectively. Whether this is a result of intrinsic and extrinsic causes or a combination, the accepted treatment algorithm begins with conservative treatment. Surgery is only considered when nonoperative treatment fails in the presence of anatomic variants with or without a rotator cuff tear.

References

Abdulrazzak H, Moschidou D, Jones G, Guillot PV (2010) Biological characteristics of stem cells from foetal, cord blood and extraembryonic tissues. J R Soc Interface 7(Suppl 6):S689–S706

Alvarez CM, Litchfield R, Jackowski D, Griffin S, Kirkley A (2005) A prospective, double-blind, randomized clinical trial comparing subacromial injection of betamethasone and xylocaine to xylocaine alone in chronic rotator cuff tendinosis. Am J Sports Med 33(2):255–262

Andres BM, Murrell GA (2008a) Treatment of tendinopathy: what works, what does not, and what is on the horizon. Clin Orthop Relat Res 466(7):1539–1554

Andres BM, Murrell GA (2008b) Treatment of tendinopathy: what works, what does not, and what is on the horizon. Clin Orthop Relat Res 466(7):1539–1554

Balich SM, Sheley RC, Brown TR, Sauser DD, Quinn SF (1997) MR imaging of the rotator cuff tendon: interobserver agreement and analysis of interpretive errors. Radiology 204:191–194

Bang MD, Deyle GD (2000) Comparison of supervised exercise with and without manual physical therapy for patients with shoulder impingement syndrome. J Orthop Sports Phys Ther 30:126–137

Bengtsson M, Lunsgo K, Hermodsson Y, Nordqvist A, Abu-Zidan FM (2006) High patient satisfaction after arthroscopic subacromial decompression for shoulder

impingment: a prospective study of 50 patients. Acta Orthop 77:138–142
Biberthaler P, Wiedemann E, Nerlich A, Kettler M, Mussack T, Deckelmann S, Mutschler W (2003) Microcirculation associated with degenerative rotator cuff lesions. In vivo assessment with orthogonal polarization spectral imaging during arthroscopy of the shoulder. J Bone Joint Surg Am 85-A(3):475–480
Bigiliani BU, Morrison ES, April EW (1986) The morphology of the acromion and its relationship to rotator cuff tears. Orthop Trans 10:216
Bigliani LU, Ticker JB, Flatow EL, Soslowsky LJ, Mow VC (1991) The relationship of acromial architecture to rotator cuff disease. Clin Sports Med 10:823–838
Brooks CH, Revell WJ, Heatley FW (1992) A quantitative histological study of the vascularity of the rotator cuff tendon. J Bone Joint Surg Br 74(1):151–153
Brox JI, Staff PH, Ljunggren AE, Brevik JI (1993) Arthroscopic surgery compared with supervised exercises in patients with rotator cuff disease (stage II impingement syndrome). BMJ 307:899–903
Buchbinder R, Green S, Roud JM (2008) Corticosteroid injections for shoulder pain. Cochrane Database Syst Rev 1:CD004016
Busconi BD, Schepsis AA (2005) Sports medicine. Lippincott Williams and Wilkins, Philadelphia, PA
Celik D, Atalar AC, Buclu A, Demirhan M (2009) The contribution of subacromial injection to the conservative treatment of impingement syndrome. Acta Orthop Traumatol Turc 43(4):331–335
Codman EA (1934) The shoulder: rupture of the supraspinatus tendon and other lesion in or about the subacromial bursa. Thomas Todd, Boston
Cotty P, Proust F, Bertrand P et al (1988) Rupture of the rotator cuff. Quantification of indirect signs in standard radiology and the Leclercq maneuver. J Radiol 69(11):633–638
Cuomo F, Kummer FJ, Zuckerman JD, Lyon T, Blair B, Olsen T (1998) The influence of acromioclavicular joint morphology on rotator cuff tears. J Shoulder Elb Surg 7:555–559
Curtis A, Burbank KM, Tierney JJ, Scheller AD, Curran AR (2006) The insertional footprint of the rotator cuff: an anatomic study. Arthroscopy 22(6):603–609
DePalma AF, Brand RA (2008) Surgical anatomy of the rotator cuff and the natural history of degenerative periarthritis. Clin Orthop Relat Res 466(3):543–551
Desjardins-Charbonneau A, Jean-Sebastien R, Clermnt ED, Pierre F, MacDermid JC, Francois D (2015) The efficacy of manual therapy for rotator cuff tendinopathy: a systematic review and meta-analysis. J Orthop Sports Phys Ther 45(5):330–350
Epstein RE, Schweitzer ME, Frieman BG, Fenlin JM Jr, Mitchell DG (1993) Hooked acromion: prevalence on MR images of painful shoulders. Radiology 187:479–481
Factor D, Dale B (2014) Current concepts of rotator cuff tendinopathy. Int J Sports Phys Ther 9(2):274–288
Farley TE, Neumann CH, Steinbach LS, Peterson SA (1990) The coracoacromial arch: MR evaluation and correlation with rotator cuff pathology. Skelet Radiol 23:641–645
Fehringer EV, Rosipal CE, Rhodes DA et al (2008) The radiographic acromiohumeral interval is affected by arm and radiographic beam position. Skelet Radiol 37(6):535–539
Fongemie AE, Buss DD, Rolnick SJ (1998) Management of shoulder impingement syndrome and rotator cuff tears. Am Fam Physician 57(4):667–674
Freitag J, Lenssen R, Slimmon D, Balster S (2014) The effect of platelet-rich-plasma injections in the nonsurgical treatment of a partial rotator cuff tear. Int J Case Rep Images 5(7):524–530
Fukuda H, Hamada K, Yamanaka K (1990a) Pathology and pathogenesis of bursal-side rotator cuff tears viewed from en bloc histologic sections. Clin Orthop Relat Res 254:75–80
Fukuda H, Hamada K, Yamanaka K (1990b) Pathology and pathogenesis of bursal-side rotator cuff tears viewed from en bloc histologic sections. Clin Orthop Relat Res 254:75–80
Graichen H, Bonel H, Stammberger T, Englmeier KH, Reiser M, Eckstein F (1999) Subacromial space width changes during abduction and rotation—a 3-D MR imaging study. Surg Radiol Anat 21(1):59–64
Griffin LY (ed) (2005) Essentials of musculoskeletal care, 3rd ed, section 2 edn. American Academy of Orthopaedic Surgeons, Rosemont, IL
Hegedus EJ, Goode AP, Cook CE, Michener L, Myer CA, Myer DM, Wright AA (2012) Which physical examination tests provide clinicians with the most value when examining the shoulder? Update of a systematic review with meta-analysis of individual tests. Br J Sports Med 46(14):964–978
Henseler JF, de Witte PB, de Groot JH, van Zwet EW, Nelissen RG, Nagels J (2014) Cranial translation of the humeral head on radiographs in rotator cuff tear patients: the modified active abduction view. Med Biol Eng Comput 52(3):233–240
Hinterwimmer S, Von Eisenhart-Rothe R, Siebert M et al (2003) Influence of adducting and abducting muscle forces on the subacromial space width. Med Sci Sports Exerc 35(12):2055–2059
Kesikburun S, Kenan A, Yilmaz B, Yasar E, Yazicioglu K (2013) Platelet-rich plasma injections in the treatment of chronic rotator cuff tendinopathy. A randomized controlled trial with 1-year follow up. Am J Sports Med 41(11):2609–2616
Kim H, Kim B, Shim J, Kwon H, Jung J (2014) Comparative analysis of acromiohumeral distances according to the locations of the arms and humeral rotation. J Phys Ther Sci 26(1):97–100
Kitay GS, Iannotti JP, Williams GR, Haygood T, Kneeland BJ, Berlin J (1995) Roentgenographic assessment of acromial morphologic condition in rotator cuff impingement syndrome. J Shoulder Elb Surg 4(6):441–448
Levy O, Relwani J, Zaman T, Even T, Venkateswaran B, Copeland S (2008) Measurement of blood flow in the rotator cuff using laser Doppler flowmetry. J Bone Joint Surg Br 90(7):893–898. doi:10.1302/0301-620X.90B7.19918

Lewis JS (2010) Rotator cuff tendinopathy: a model for the continuum of pathology and related management. Br J Sports Med 44(13):918–923
Littlewood C, May S, Walters S (2014) Epidemiology of rotator cuff tendinopathy:a systematic review. Should Elb 5:256–265
Longo UG, Franceschi F, Ruzzini L, Rabitti C, Morini S, Maffulli N, Denaro V (2008) Histopathology of the supraspinatus tendon in rotator cuff tears. Am J Sports Med 36(3):533–538. Epub 2007 Nov 15
Matthews LS, Fadale PD (1989) Subacromial anatomy for the arthroscopist. Arthroscopy 5(1):36–40
Mazieres B, Rouanet S, Guillon Y, Scarsi C, Reiner V (2005) Topical ketoprofen patch in the treatment of tendinitis: a randomized, double blind, placebo controlled study. J Rheumatol 32:1563–1570
McCreesh KM, Crotty JM, Lewis JS (2015) Acromiohumeral distance measurement in rotator cuff tendinopathy: is there a reliable, clinically applicable method? A systematic review. Br J Sports Med 49(5):298–305
Mena HR, Lomen PL, Turner LF, Lamborn KR, El B (1986) Treatment of acute shoulder syndrome with flurbiprofen. Am J Med 80:141–144
Michener LA, McClure PW, Karduna AR (2003) Anatomical and biomechanical mechanisms of subacromial impingement syndrome. Clin Biomech 18(5):369–379
Milgrom C, Schaffler M, Gilbert S, van Holsbeeck M (1995) Rotator-cuff changes in asymptomatic adults. The effect of age, hand dominance and gender. J Bone Joint Surg Br 77(2):296–298
Neer CS (1972) Anterior acromioplasty for the chronic impingement syndrome in the shoulder: a preliminary report. J Bone Joint Surg Am 54(1):41–50
Neer CS (1983) Impingement lesions. Clin Orthop Relat Res 173:70–77
Nutton RW, McBirnie JM, Phillips C (1997) Treatment of chronic rotator-cuff impingement by arthroscopic subacromial decompression. J Bone Joint Surg Br 79:73–76
Ogawa K, Yoshida A, Inokuchi W, Naniwa T (2005) Acromial spur:relationship to aging and morphologic changes in the rotator cuff. J Shoulder Elb Surg 14:591–598
Petersson CJ, Gentz CF (1983) Ruptures of the supraspinatus tendon. The significance of distally pointing acromioclavicular osteophytes. Clin Orthop Relat Res:143–148
Petersson CJ, Redlund-Johnell I (1984) The subacromial space in normal shoulder radiographs. Acta Orthop Scand 55(1):57–58
Petri M, Dobrow R, Neiman R, Whiting-O'Keefe Q, Seaman WE (1987) Randomized, double-blinded, placebo-controlled study of the treatment of the painful shoulder. Arthritis Rheum 30:1040–1045
Petri M, Hufman SL, Waser G, Cui H, Snabes MC, KM V (2004) Celecoxib effectively treats patients with acute shoulder tendinitis/bursitis. J Rheumatol 31:1614–1620
Quinn SF, Sheley RC, Demlow TA, Szumowski J (1995) Rotator cuff tendon tears: evaluation with fatsuppressed MR imaging with arthroscopic correlation in 100 patients. Radiology 195:497–500
Riley GP, Harrall RL, Constant CR, Chard MD, Cawston TE, Hazleman BL (1994) Glycosaminoglycans of human rotator cuff tendons: changes with age and in chronic rotator cuff tendinitis. Ann Rheum Dis 53(6):367–376
Scapone M, Rabaago D, Snell E, Demeo P, Ruppert K et al (2013) Effectiveness of platelet-rich plasma injection for rotator cuff tendinopathy: a prospective open-label study. Global Adv Health Med 2(2):26–31
Seitz AL, McClure PW, Finucane S, Boardmann DN, Michener LA (2011) Mechanisms of rotator cuff tendinopathy: intrinsic, extrinsic or both? Clin Biomech 26:1–12
Sharkey NA, Marder RA (1995) The rotator cuff opposes the superior translation of the humeral head. Am J Sports Med 23(3):270–275
Silva RT, Hartmann LG, Laurino CF, Bilo JP (2010) Clinical and ultrasonographic correlation between scapular dyskinesia and subacromial space measurement among junior elite tennis players. Br J Sports Med 44(6):407–410
Soslowsky LJ, Thomopoulos S, Esmail A, Flanagan CL, Iannoti JP, Williamson JD III et al (2002) Rotator cuff tendinosis in an animal model: role of extrinsic and overuse factor. Ann Biomed Eng 30:1057–1063
Stephens SR, Warren RF, Payne LZ, Tl W, Altchek DW (1998) Arthroscopic acromioplasty: a 6 to 10 year follow up. Arthroscopy 14:382–388
Tempelhof S, Rupp S, Seil R (1999) Age-related prevalence of rotator cuff tears in asymptomatic shoulders. J Shoulder Elb Surg 8(4):296–299
Toivonen DA, Tuite MJ, Orwin JF (1995) Acromial structure and tears of the rotator cuff. J Shoulder Elbow Surg 4:376–383
Umer M, Qadir I, Azam M (2012) Subacromial impingement syndrome. Orthop Rev 4(2):e18
Watson-Jones R (1940) Fractures and other bone and joint injuries. Williams and Wilkins, Baltimore, MD
Weiner DS, Macnab I (1970) Superior migration of the humeral head. A radiological aid in the diagnosis of tears of the rotator cuff. J Bone Joint Surg Br 52(3):524–527
Yu CM, Chen CH, Liu HT, Dai MH, Wang IC, Wang KC (2006) Subacromial injections of corticosteroids and xylocaine for painful subacromial impingement syndrome. Chang Gung Med J 29(5):474–479

Anterosuperior Rotator Cuff Ruptures

19

Alessandro Castagna, Raffaele Garofalo, and Marco Conti

Contents

A. Castagna (✉) • R. Garofalo • M. Conti
Shoulder and Elbow Unit, Humanitas Institute IRCCS, Rozzano, Milan, Italy

Upper limb Unit, F. Miulli Hospital Acquaviva delle fonti, Bari, Italy
e-mail: alex.castagna@tin.it

19.1 Introduction

Massive rotator cuff tears have been described as lesions having a diameter more than 5 cm (Cofield 1991) or involving two or more tendons (Warner and Gerber 1997). Most part of the papers in the literature focused on the posterosuperior massive rotator cuff. This term indicated a pattern tear in which at least the supraspinatus and infraspinatus tendon are injured.

The anterosuperior rotator cuff tear was first defined by Novè-Josserand et al. in 1997 as a "full-thickness supraspinatus tear that extends anterior to its border involving the rotator interval structures and subscapularis tendon" (1997). This pattern of lesion is much less common and behaves differently from the posterior superior tear (Gerber and Krushell 1991). The incidence of anterosuperior rotator cuff tears has been reported to occur anywhere from 2 to 24% and is likely to be underreported and undertreated (Flury et al. 2006; Namdari et al. 2008). The specific feature of this lesion are related to anatomy, clinical presentation, prognosis, and treatment.

The subscapularis represents the anterior portion of rotator cuff, and it is very important to stabilize the shoulder on the coronal and on the transverse plane. The fibers of the upper part of the subscapularis tendon fuse with the most anterior fibers of supraspinatus tendon forming the anterior cable that is a very important structure to start the arm elevation and stabilize the humeral head during this motion. A recent clinical paper

G.L. Canata et al. (eds.), *Muscle and Tendon Injuries*, DOI 10.1007/978-3-662-54184-5_19

confirm this evidence and furthermore showed that a dysfunction of the entire subscapularis (upper and lower part) and supraspinatus was associated with a loss of active elevation and was a risk factor to develop a pseudoparalytic shoulder (Collin et al. 2014). Anatomic relationship with the rotator interval (superior glenohumeral ligament [SGHL], coracohumeral ligament [CCHL]), and the long head of the biceps tendon determines specific clinical implication and influences the treatment of this injury.

Furthermore, differently from other tendons, once torn, the subscapularis tendon is prone to retraction and the development of irreversible changes of the muscle. After a delay of several months or longer, repair of the retracted tendon can be difficult or impossible.

This chapter will provide an overview of anatomy, epidemiology, clinical evaluation, and imaging of anterosuperior rotator cuff lesions. Additionally, this chapter will detail our treatment and provide data regarding expected outcomes of treatment of anterosuperior rotator cuff tears.

19.2 Relevant Anatomy and Pathology

The rotator cuff is a continuous tendinous band that is intimately connected with the glenohumeral articular capsule. It can be divided into three parts: the posterior cuff with the infraspinatus tendon and the teres minor tendon, the superior cuff with the supraspinatus tendon, and the anterior cuff with the subscapularis tendon and the rotator interval. The rotator interval also includes the intra-articular portion of the tendon of the long head of the biceps (LHBT).

The subscapularis muscle originates from the anterior surface of the scapula and typically is split into the upper two thirds and lower third. The upper two thirds insert on the lesser tuberosity, the lower, muscular part wing onto the humeral metaphysis. The upper tendinous portion is what can be visualized arthroscopically. The upper portion of the subscapularis tendon interdigitates with the anterior fibers of the supraspinatus tendon and contributes together with coracohumeral ligament to form the anterior part of rotator cuff cable. The subscapularis tendon and the supraspinatus tendon are thereby intertwined for approximately 1 cm before inserting into the lesser and greater tuberosity, respectively. From the intra-articular point of view, the insertion of upper part of subscapularis is at the same level of superior glenohumeral ligament that contributes to form the medial sling of pulley system of LHBT. The supraspinatus muscle originates in the supraspinatus fossa of the scapula superior to the scapular spine. The muscle inserts via a strong tendon on the superior facet of the greater tuberosity. Many fibers of the supraspinatus tendon extend medially to form the lateral wall of the bicipital groove and merge with the subscapularis tendon.

The rotator interval is composed of the coracohumeral ligament, the superior glenohumeral ligament, the joint capsule, and expansions of the subscapularis and supraspinatus tendons. The coracohumeral ligament is the dominant structure of the rotator interval. It bridges the subscapularis and the supraspinatus tendons and ensures continuity of the rotator cuff. It is triangular, with its base at the coracoid, its apex over the bicipital groove, one side inserting mainly into the greater tuberosity, and one side inserting mainly into the lesser tuberosity. It becomes intimately associated with the glenohumeral joint capsule and covers the LHBT.

Isolated subscapularis tears are relatively uncommon and however when isolated are more commonly associated with trauma in comparison to other types of rotator cuff injuries. The trauma very often is in forced external rotation with an adducted arm (Gerber and Krushell 1991) or an abducted arm (i.e., anterior shoulder dislocation) (Deutsch et al. 1997). The rupture of the supraspinatus may preexist or may occur at the time of the injury or as a degenerative secondary development. A lesion of the subscapularis and supraspinatus can cause inflammation and distension of the ligamentous pulley and bicipital sheath, ultimately destabilizing the LHBT within its groove (Habermeyer et al. 2004). The reported prevalence of LHBT lesions associated with subscapularis tears ranged from 63 to 85% (Bartl et al. 2011).

In an anterosuperior rotator cuff tear, the subscapularis and supraspinatus tears become extended and retracted medially along the direction of tendon and muscle, resulting in involvement of the medial sling of the LHBT. Eventually, a thickened margin may form between the subscapularis and supraspinatus tendons.

The leading edge of a torn subscapularis can be difficult to identify arthroscopically because of retraction and scarring in anterosuperior rotator cuff tears. In 2003 Lo and Burkhart described the comma sign as an arthroscopic landmark to identify the torn subscapularis stump to mobilize and repair the tendon. They described the comma sign as tissue composed of the humeral attachments of the superior glenohumeral and coracohumeral ligaments that concomitantly tear and remain attached to the superolateral corner of the subscapularis. The recognition of this structure is very important to guide the repair of the anterosuperior tear (Lo and Burkhart 2003).

Different age groups often present with a different injury pattern of the anterosuperior rotator cuff tendon. A traumatic isolated subscapularis or anterosuperior rotator cuff tear has been well described in young-aged athletes. This kind of lesion can range from articular-sided partial tears with instability of LHBT to a large tears combined with pain and stiffness.

Middle-aged and elderly people, on the other hand, may present with a massive tear that is often the result of an acute extension of a prior minimally symptomatic chronic tear (acute on chronic tear), leading to instability and possible pseudoparalytic shoulder sometimes associated with an anterosuperior escape. Often, in these patients, the trauma consisted of an anterior shoulder dislocation.

Finally the anterosuperior tear could result from a progressive wear of the rotator cuff, typically in elderly people, that starts to become progressively symptomatic because of LHBT pathology or because of painful or shoulder weakness.

19.3 Clinic and Imaging

Clinical presentation for injury of the anterosuperior rotator cuff tear is extremely variable, particularly because the injury could be acute and traumatic versus degenerative; furthermore, it is also related to the tear extension.

Three types of clinical presentations could be more characteristic: chronic and progressive shoulder pain following a traumatic event, pseudoparalytic shoulder, and progressive pain, without any history of trauma, sometimes associated with shoulder stiffness. Pain is constant and aggravated by using the arm at the side or above the head. Night pain is also a common feature. The pattern of pain is not distinctly different from that of isolated supraspinatus tears particularly in cases in which only the superior one-third of the subscapularis tendon is involved. One-third of patients could present with a pseudoparalytic shoulder. Passive range of motion is preserved, but active elevation is limited to less than 90 degrees. Pseudoparalysis is typically associated with large multiple tendon rotator cuff tears. Shoulders with pain and stiffness (decrease of active and passive range of motion) are rare. Pain and stiffness are not specific for any type of lesion or severity of injury. Since the proximal LHBT derives medial stability from the subscapularis tendon insertion, biceps tendon symptoms may be present with a subscapularis tendon tear. Tenderness in the anterior region over the bicipital groove and lesser tuberosity is very common particularly in acute cases. In chronic cases, this could be confounding just because symptoms related to LHBT are commonly associated with cuff pathology.

Tucking one's shirt in the back may be particularly troublesome as this requires coupled internal rotation and extension. A long-standing massive anterosuperior rotator cuff can lead to progressive superior and anterosuperior migration of the humeral head. Usually in this condition, patients will reveal a pseudoparalytic shoulder associated with a dynamic anterosuperior escape.

Clinical examination findings include increased passive external rotation, especially in adduction, as well as loss of internal rotation strength in case of complete subscapularis tendon tear. The "Belly Press" test (or Napoleon test), where the patient attempts to apply pressure to the abdomen while maintaining a straight wrist, has been shown to be reasonably sensitive for subscapularis tears. A decrease in the ability to maintain a forward position of the elbow compared with contralateral side is also considered positive for insufficiency of subscapularis tendon. This test and lift-off test has been described by Gerber and Krushell (1991). A prerequisite to perform the lift-off test is that patient should have a minimal pain with motion and should be able to internally rotate the arm. A positive test occurs when the patient is unable to lift or maintain the hand away from the back. In the complete tear, the hand cannot be held off the back in any capacity, but in partial lesions, the hand may drop toward the back but without dropping to rest on the back. The lift-off sign is less useful in patients experiencing extreme pain with internal rotation and in patients with stiffness which prevents adequate internal rotation for the test.

The "bear-hug" test, first described by Barth et al. (2006) has been shown by Chao and Thomas et al. (2008) to be perhaps the best test for detecting upper subscapularis tendon tears. To perform this maneuver, the examiner asks the patient to place the involved side hand on the contralateral shoulder with the elbow in 45 degrees of forward flexion and the fingers extended. The patient then attempts to resist an external force by trying to pull the hand away from the shoulder in a perpendicular fashion. The test is positive when the patient is unable to move the hand on the opposite shoulder or shows weakness compared with contralateral shoulder. The bear-hug test is particularly sensitive and specific for tears of the upper subscapularis. Sometimes this test could be only painful, but this is not sensitive for a subscapularis tear. Of the tests specifically evaluating the anterosuperior rotator cuff, Jobe's empty can test and full can test is employed to evaluate supraspinatus integrity (Itoi 2013). Obviously, also the subacromial impingement test, the Neer test (1972), and the Hawkins and Kennedy (1980) could be positive. Dynamic anterosuperior subluxation of the humeral head associated with active elevation of the arm indicates a large tear of the subscapularis and supraspinatus tendons.

The patient performs resisted abduction with the examiner observing from behind. Dynamic anterior subluxation occurs during the initial degrees of abduction and may occasionally be palpated under the deltoid rather than be observed.

Pathology involving the LHBT remains an enigma to clinical diagnosis. Although most completely ruptured biceps are easily detectable on clinical examination by the ball-like deformity of the biceps muscle belly present when the arm is elevated to 90 degrees and the elbow is forcibly flexed, more subtle bicipital problems are difficult to diagnose. The palm-up test can be performed with the elbow extended and the forearm supinated. The patient is asked to elevate the arm against resistance (Speed's test). If pain is elicited along the anterior part of the biceps, the test is positive. Although other tests have been described (Yergason's test, O'Brien's test), none of these tests have been found to be very specific for bicipital lesions. On the other hand, dislocation or subluxation of LHBT cannot be reliably detected clinically. A slight clicking sound perceived by the patient and the examiner during rotation is uncommon and may or may not be caused by biceps dislocation.

About the **imaging studies**, plain radiographs (X-ray) are the initial studies required for patients with a suspected rotator cuff tear. X-ray normally is negative and does not give direct information of a rotator cuff tear. In case of long-standing massive rotator cuff tear, a superior migration of humeral head with a reduced acromiohumeral distance (normal value more than 7 mm) could be observed.

Cystic lesions or sclerosis of the lesser tuberosity suggests an anterior rotator cuff lesion. A sclerosis of the greater tuberosity indicated a lesion of the superior cuff. Anterior subluxation is often not readily identifiable using conventional radiography, although it may be suspected on axillary views.

Additional studies, however, are necessary to evaluate anterosuperior cuff including magnetic resonance imaging (MRI), MRI with intra-articular contrast injection (artro-MRI), CT arthrography (CTA), and ultrasonography (US).

The US is routinely used in some centers for inexpensive evaluation of the rotator cuff. It allows for dynamic evaluation particularly of the LHBT. However, it requires an experienced operator, and the interpretation of the results is operator dependent; furthermore, it does not have any ability to show fatty infiltration, muscle atrophy, and grade of tendon retraction. According to some authors (Edwards et al. 2005), CT scan with or

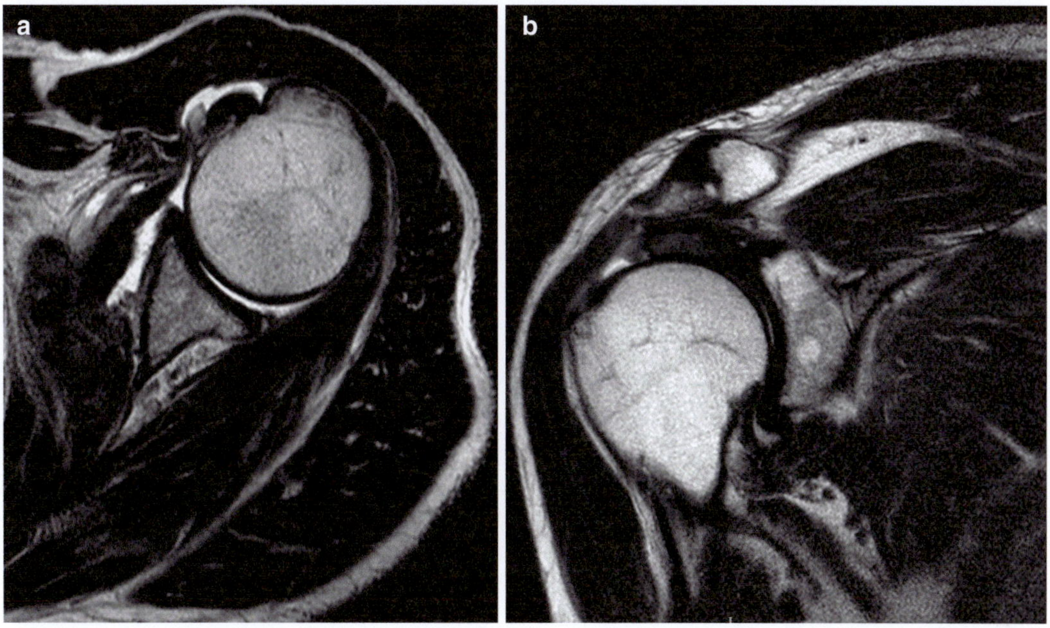

Fig. 19.1 T2-weighted MRI axial (**a**) and coronal oblique view (**b**) showing an anterosuperior rotator cuff tear. On axial view the tear of subscapularis and, on the coronal oblique view, the tear of anterior part of supraspinatus are shown

without arthrography is very useful to diagnose injury of anterosuperior rotator cuff.

Dislocation and subluxation of the long head of the biceps tendon are readily identifiable particularly with arthro-CT scan. In most centers, MRI is used to evaluate the rotator cuff because it offers excellent soft tissue visualization (Fig. 19.1). Different criteria taking in account size of tear, thinning of tendon, retraction, shape, traumatic or degenerative features, and fatty infiltration could be used to understand if the tear is reparable or not (Loew et al. 2015). The Goutallier system of staging changes in the rotator cuff muscle (grade 0, no fatty deposits; grade 1, some fatty streaking within muscle; grade 2, more muscle than fat; grade 3, fat equal to muscle; grade 4, more fat than muscle) is based on CT (Goutallier et al. 1994) and has been adapted to MRI, although MRI studies tend to overestimate the degree of fatty infiltration (Fuchs et al. 1999). Tung et al. reported that only the 31% of subscapularis tears confirmed at arthroscopy were detected at preoperative time on standard MRI (2001) (Fig. 19.5). In particular the small tears were frequently missed, whether tears involving 50% or more of the tendon insertion were more readily detected. Another study confirmed this finding, even when artro-MRI was used. In this study, subscapularis tears were identified in 40 shoulders at the time of arthroscopy, whereas a lesion was identified in only 15 shoulders in a preoperative MRI. These findings indicate that sensitivity to identify subscapularis tears does not dramatically increase even with the use of arthrography, particularly in case of smaller partial-thickness tear (Foad and Wijdicks 2012).

19.4 Treatment

Different considerations should be done before discussing the options of treatment. First of all as with the other tendons of rotator cuff, in cases with a small, degenerative tear with a well-compensated shoulder function in a low-demand patient, a conservative treatment could be attempted. No steroidal anti-inflammatory drugs, injections, and physical therapy to improve pain and function are the mainstay of this treatment. On the other hand, dysfunction of the entire subscapularis is a risk factor for pseudoparalytic shoulder. For function to be preserved in patients with anterosuperior rotator cuff tears, it may be important to avoid fatty infiltration with anterior extension into the lower subscapularis tendon (Collin et al. 2014). Without treatment, rupture of the subscapularis leads to pain, loss of function, and shoulder weakness. In the long term, dynamic anterior instability can lead to the development of glenohumeral arthrosis (Flury et al. 2006). In consequence, an acute traumatic tear of the anterosuperior rotator cuff more typically should be repaired surgically as soon as possible. Subscapularis tendon in particular is prone to retraction and early irreversible changes of the muscle. Inferior clinical results have been reported with delayed repair of subscapularis tear, and, in many cases, the subscapularis was found not repairable at the time of surgery (Mansat et al. 2003). As discussed before, the anterosuperior tear often results by a traumatic event. Often these patients coming to our attention because of pain, loss of function, and stiffness after a trauma, stiffness could be probably related to the proximity of LHBT and rotator interval. These patients could be treated with physical therapy and planned repair. During surgery a release of rotator interval should be done. Some authors believe that, given the critical role of the subscapularis in glenohumeral kinematics, even in the presence of a complete long-standing tear with a substantial fatty infiltration, an attempt to repair the subscapularis also for its tenodesis effect should be done (Denard et al. 2011; Koo and Burkhart 2012). Other authors, however, think that patients with evidence of fatty degenerated subscapularis tendon associated with a static anterior subluxation of humeral head should not undergo a repair operation.

The biomechanical rationale to repair the subscapularis becomes most important in case of an anterosuperior rotator cuff tear. The anterior part of supraspinatus and superior part of subscapularis are connected by a comma-shaped arc of tissue called the comma sign. The comma sign is very helpful to find the subscapularis tendon particularly in chronic case when the subscapularis retract medially to the glenoid. The comma sign represent the superior glenohumeral ligament and the medial segment of the coracohumeral ligament that are torn off the humerus at the upper border of the subscapularis footprint (Lo and Burkhart 2003; Visonà et al. 2015a). Repairing the upper part of subscapularis together with comma system restores a part of the anterior attachment of the rotator cable. Recently, however, some authors noted that in patients treated with arthroscopic repair of anterosuperior tears of the rotator cuff, the technique of in-continuity repair did not produce better clinical outcomes or structural integrity than the technique involving disruption of the tear margin. If the muscle in an anterosuperior rotator cuff tear is of good quality, it does not appear to matter whether the tear margin between the subscapularis and supraspinatus is preserved or disrupted (Kim et al. 2014).

For the repair of anterosuperior rotator cuff tear, arthroscopic and open technique has been described.

Open technique could be a good option in rare case of isolated traumatic tear of subscapularis tendon particularly when the lesion involves all the length of the subscapularis (tendon and muscular portion). Open surgery is also indicated for management of extra-articular lesions or tears involving the myotendineous portion (Di Schino et al. 2012).

Anterosuperior rotator cuff tear can be arthroscopically repaired with the patient in a beach chair or lateral decubitus position (Fig. 19.2). We use three or four portals to work around the shoulder: posterior, anterosuperior, and one or two subacromial portals. We use a 30° arthroscopy all the time of the procedure. Proper manipulation of the arm can be useful for visualizing the subscapularis. Bringing the arm into forward and internal rotation could be useful to examine the tendon.

In the lateral decubitus, the so-called posterior lever push in which the assistant applies a lever from anterior to posterior associated with an internal rotation could help to better visualize the tendon and the extent of the lesion.

Once the lesion is identified, we start to prepare and repair.

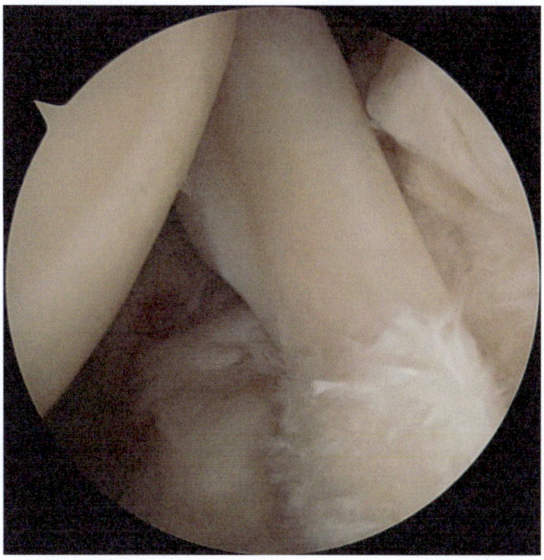

Fig. 19.2 Left shoulder observed through a posterior portal. A complete anterosuperior tear is shown. The LHBT appears in the middle

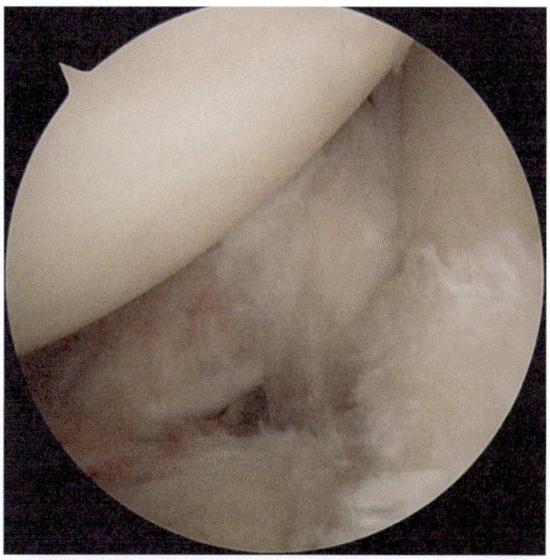

Fig. 19.3 Intra-articular view of a left shoulder. The upper part of the subscapularis tendon is grasped and the comma sign is evident. The comma sign is a combination of medial pulley, coracohumeral ligament, and interval capsule

In case of acute on chronic case and in any case with a retracted subscapularis tendon, we prefer to repair anterior part of the cuff through an intra-articular approach using the suture anchor technique with or without in-continuity repair (Fig. 19.3). This depends from pattern of tear, from grade of retraction of the subscapularis and supraspinatus tendon, and from the tissue quality. One posterior and one anterosuperior portal could be enough to treat this tear. One or two triple loaded suture anchors using a mattress stitch associated with two simple stitches could be used. Suture could be passed with different tools according to the preference of surgeon. In general one anchor per linear centimeter of torn tendon should be used. When using anchors most subscapularis tears could be repaired with a single-row technique with good results (Fig. 19.4) (Ide et al. 2007). There is a high correlation between subscapularis tear and LHBT pathology, and often the LHBT pathology should be treated and at the same time the subscapularis tendon pathology. If the LHBT is altered in the groove, a tenotomy or an associated tenodesis (subpectoral tenodesis) with a screw could be done working once the subscapularis tendon is repaired, on the anterior space of the shoulder. In case in which the LHBT is just unstable without any pathology in the groove, an associated tenodesis at the anchor used to repair the subscapularis tendon is carried out.

Whenever it is possible, in case of anterosuperior rotator cuff, we prefer to use transosseous repair. In particular this technique is done in case

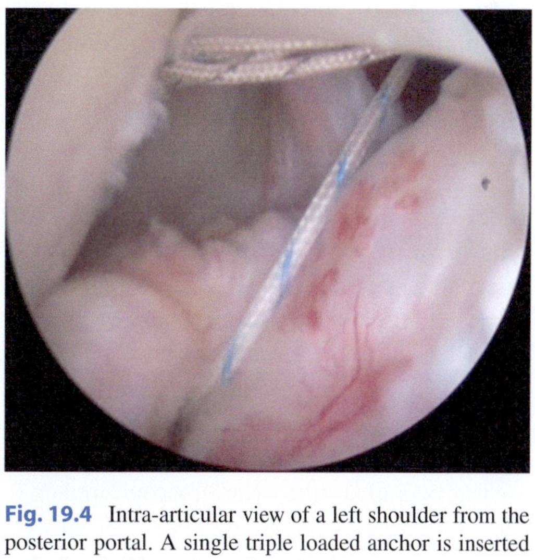

Fig. 19.4 Intra-articular view of a left shoulder from the posterior portal. A single triple loaded anchor is inserted at the level of footprint and repair of subscapularis tendon is started

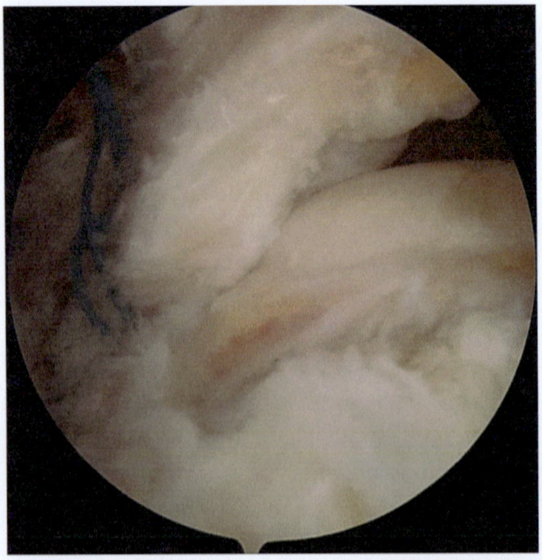

Fig. 19.5 The scope is on the posterolateral subacromial portal. A traction suture (*green*) is inserted on the upper part of the subscapularis tendon

in which the tendons are not so much retracted or stiff and the technique of in-continuity repair could be used. In this case, we start tissue mobilization during the articular phase of arthroscopy. The subscapularis is mobilized and a traction stitch is used to assist in the reduction. Then the scope is moved into subacromial space (Fig. 19.5). The space is cleaned and the superior cuff is freed from adhesions. The footprint of tendon is prepared. Different tunnels could be made, according to the size of tear, using the ArthroTunneler™ (Tornier, Edina, MN) device (Garofalo et al. 2012) We perform the repair with the scope in posterolateral portal and using as working portal the anterolateral, anterior, and posterior portals. In case of anterosuperior tear with the interval in continuity, we prefer to not disrupt the margin between the supraspinatus and subscapularis, and we pass the anterior sutures to repair the most anterosuperior part of tear altogether (Fig. 19.6). This technique of repair is more easy and fast to do. Furthermore, this allows to reapproximate the superior cuff (Fig. 19.7).

The overall results of arthroscopic repair of the anterosuperior rotator cuff tear are promising; however, early recognition and treatment of tear improve prognosis after repair (Kim et al. 2014; Bennett 2003; Visonà et al. 2015b; Schnaser et al. 2013). Younger age of patients, less degree of tissue retraction, less fatty infiltration, and the possibility to repair the subscapularis tendon lead to a better clinical result.

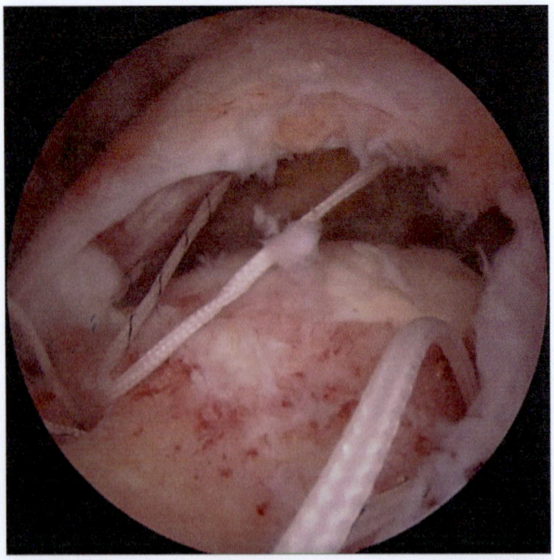

Fig. 19.6 Left shoulder: The scope is on the posterolateral portal. Different sutures are passed in bone tunnel according to the tear size. The most anterior sutures (*blue/white* and *black/white*) are passed in the anterior part of rotator cuff (repair in continuity)

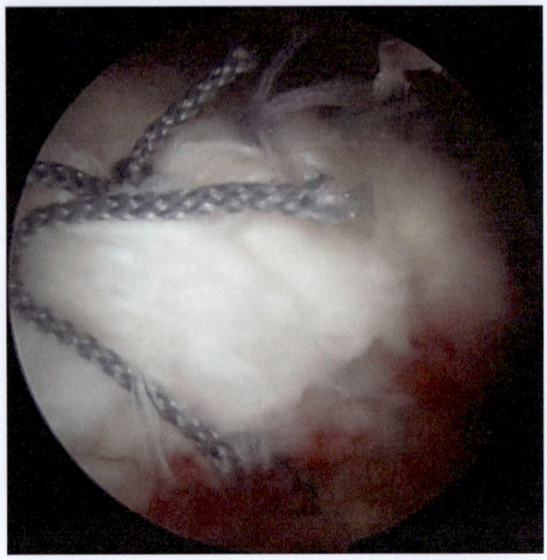

Fig. 19.7 The scope is on the posterolateral portal. Final view of massive rotator cuff repaired with six transosseous sutures

References

Barth JR, Burkhart SS, DeBeer JF (2006) The bear-hug test: a new and sensitive test for diagnosing a subscapularis tear. Arthroscopy 22(10):1076–1084

Bartl C, Salzmann GM, Seppel G et al (2011) Subscapularis function and structural integrity after arthroscopic repair of isolated subscapularis tears. Am J Sports Med 39(6):1255–1262

Bennett WF (2003) Arthroscopic repair of anterosuperior (supraspinatus/subscapularis) rotator cuff tears: a prospective cohort with 2- to 4-year follow-up. Classification of biceps subluxation/instability. Arthroscopy 19(1):21–33

Chao S, Thomas S, Yucha D, Kelly JD 4th, Driban J, Swanik K (2008) An electromiyographic assessment of the "bear hug": an examination for the evaluation of the subscapularis muscle. Arthroscopy 24(11):1265–1270

Cofield RH (1991) Tears of the rotator cuff. In: Instructional course lectures. American Academy of Orthopaedic Surgeons, Rosemont, IL, pp 258–271

Collin P, Matsumura N, Ladermann A, Denard PJ, Walch G (2014) Relationship between massive chronic rotator cuff tear pattern and loss of active shoulder range of motion. J Shoulder Elb Surg 23:1195–1202

Denard PJ, Ladermann A, Burkhart SS (2011) Arthroscopic management of subscapularis tears. Sports Med Arthrosc 19(4):333–341

Deutsch A, Altchek DW, Veltri DM, Potter HG, Warren RF (1997) Traumatic tears of the subscapularis tendon: clinical diagnosis, magnetic resonance imaging findings, and operative treatment. Am J Sports Med 25:13–22

Di Schino M, Augerau B, Nich C (2012) Does open repair of anterosuperior rotator cuff tear prevent muscular atrophy and fatty infiltration? Clin Orthop Relat Res 470:2776–2784

Edwards TB, Walch G, Novè-Josserand L, Gerber C (2005) Anterior superior rotator cuff tears. Repairable and irreparable tears. In: JJP W, Iannotti JP, Flatow EL (eds) Complex revision problems in shoulder suregry, 2nd edn. Lippincott Williams and Wilkins, Philadelphia, pp 107–128

Flury MP, John M, Goldhan J, Schwyzer HK, Simmen BR (2006) Rupture of the subscapularis tendon (isolated or in combination with supraspinatus tear): when is repair indicated? J Shoulder Elb Surg 15(6):659–664

Foad A, Wijdicks CA (2012) The accuracy of magnetic resonance imaging and magnetic resonance arthrogram versus arthroscopy in the diagnosis of subscapularis tendon injury. Arthroscopy 28(5):636–641

Fuchs B, Weishaupt D, Zanetti M, Hodler J, Gerber C (1999) Fatty degeneration of the muscles of the rotator cuff: assessment by computed tomography versus magnetic resonance imaging. J Shoulder Elb Surg 8:599–605

Garofalo R, Castagna A, Borroni M, Krishnan SG (2012) Arthroscopic transosseous (anchorless) rotator cuff repair. Knee Surg Sports Traumatol Arthrosc 20(6):1031–1035

Gerber C, Krushell RJ (1991) Isolated rupture of the tendon of the subscapularis muscle. Clinical features in 16 cases. J Bone Joint Surg Br 73:389–394

Goutallier D, Postel JM, Bernageau J, Lavau L, Voisin MC (1994) Fatty muscle degeneration in cuff ruptures. Pre- and postoperative evaluation by CT scan. Clin Orthop Relat Res 304:78–83

Habermeyer P, Magosch P, Pritsch M, Scheibel MT, Lichtenberg S (2004) Anterosuperior impingement of the shoulder as a result of pulley lesions: a prospective arthroscopic study. J Shoulder Elb Surg 13:5–12

Hawkins RJ, Kennedy JC (1980) Impingement syndrome in athletes. Am J Sports Med 8:151–158

Ide J, Tokiyoshi A, Hirose J, Mizuta H (2007) Arthroscopic repair of traumatic combined rotator cuff tears involving the subscapularis tendon. J Bone Joint Surg Am 89(11):2378–2388

Itoi E (2013) Rotator cuff tear: physical examination and conservative treatment. J Orthop Sci 18:197–204

Kim SJ, Jung M, Lee JH, Kim C, Chun YM (2014) Arthroscopic repair of anterosuperior rotator cuff tears: in-continuity technique vs. disruption of subscapularis-supraspinatus tear margin: comparison of clinical outcomes and structural integrity between the two techniques. J Bone Joint Surg Am 96(24):2056–2061

Koo SS, Burkhart SS (2012) Subscapularis tendon tears: identifying mid to distal footprint disruptions. Arthroscopy 26(8):1130–1134

Lo IK, Burkhart SS (2003) (2003). The comma sign: an arthroscopic guide to the torn subscapularis tendon. Arthroscopy 19:334–337

Loew M, Magosch P, Lichtenberg S, Haebermeyer P, Porschke F (2015) How to discriminate between acute traumatic and chronic degenerative rotator cuff lesions: an analysis of specific criteria on radiography and magnetic resonance imaging. J Shoulder Elb Surg 24(11):1685–1693

Mansat P, Frankle MA, Cofield RH (2003) Tears in the subscapularis tendon: descriptive analysis and results of surgical repair. Joint Bone Spine 70:342–347

Namdari S, Henn F, Green A (2008) Traumatic anterosuperior rotator cuff tears: the outcome of open surgical repair. J Bone Joint Surg Am 90:1906–1913

Neer CS II (1972) Anterior acromioplasty for the chronic impingement syndrome in the shoulder: a preliminary report. J Bone Joint Surg Am 54:41–50

Nove'-Josserand L, Gerber C, Walch G (1997) Lesions of the anterosuperior rotator cuff. In: Warner JJP, Iannotti JP, Gerberc C (eds) Complex and revision problems in shoulder surgey. Lippincott-Raven, Philadelphia, pp 165–176

Schnaser E, Toussaint B, Gillespie R, Lefebvre Y, Gobezie R (2013) Arthroscopic treatment of anterosuperior rotator cuff tears. Orthopedics 36(11):e1394–e1340

Tung G, Yoo D, Levine S, Brody J, Green A (2001) Subscapularis tendon tear: primary and associated signs on MRI. J Comput Assist Tomogr 25:417–424

Visonà E, Cerciello S, Godenèche A, Neyton L, Fessy MH, Novè-Josserand L (2015a) The "comma sign": ana antomical investigation (dissection of the rotator interval in 14 cadaveric shoulders). Surg Radiol Anat 37(7):793–798

Visonà E, Paladini P, Merolla G, Cerciello S, Porcellini G (2015b) Strength recovery after arthroscopic antero-superior cuff repair: analysis of a consecutive series. Musculoskelet Surg 99:S37–S42

Warner JJP, Gerber C (1997) Massive tears of the postero-superior rotator cuff. In: Warner JJP, Iannotti JP, Gerberc C (eds) Complex and revision problems in shoulder surgey. Lippincott-Raven, Philadelphia, pp 177–203

Long Head of the Biceps Tendinopathy

20

Andrew E. Apple, Michael J. O'Brien,
and Felix H. Savoie III

Contents

A.E. Apple, M.D. • M.J. O'Brien, M.D.
F.H. SavoieIII, M.D. (✉)
Department of Orthopaedic Surgery, Tulane
University School of Medicine,
New Orleans, LA, USA
e-mail: fsavoie@tulane.edu

20.1 Anatomy

The long head of the biceps (LHB) tendon originates from the superior glenoid labrum at the supraglenoid tubercle. Typically, its origin is posterior in up to 85% of shoulders (Nho et al. 2010). For approximately 35 mm, the tendon course is intra-articular until it reaches the bicipital groove, which lies between the greater and lesser tuberosities. Despite its intra-articular position, the tendon remains extrasynovial. The bicipital groove is hourglass in shape, with the widest portion at the superior aspect measuring from 9 to 12 mm wide and about 2.2 mm deep. The midportion of the groove narrows to a width of 6.2 mm and the depth slightly increases to 2.4 mm. The average length of the bicipital groove is 5 cm. Additional soft tissue restraints serve to stabilize the tendon within the bicipital groove, namely, the biceps sling, which receives contributions from the subscapularis, supraspinatus, coracohumeral ligament, and superior glenohumeral ligament. The transverse humeral ligament also contributes to the soft tissue envelope of the LHB tendon in the groove. As the tendon exits the bicipital groove, the pectoralis major tendon provides stability (Rudzki et al. 2015).

The function of the LHB tendon remains controversial, but some studies describe its role in shoulder stability in overhead throwing athletes (Longo et al. 2011). Some authors have also noted a 10% decrease in forearm supination strength and elbow flexion strength

G.L. Canata et al. (eds.), *Muscle and Tendon Injuries*, DOI 10.1007/978-3-662-54184-5_20

after spontaneous rupture of the biceps, possibly elucidating the tendon's role in those actions (Rudzki et al. 2015).

20.2 Pathology

The natural history of LHB pathology begins with either dysvascular degeneration (tendinosis) or inflammation (tendinitis), in which the tendon becomes inflamed and hyperemic as it undergoes repetitive mechanical insults. The synovial sheath that encases the tendon may also develop synovitis. As more intra-tendinous signal changes occur, the tendon is prone to partial tearing and degenerative changes (Fig. 20.1). The tendon becomes thick and fibrotic, which can lead to decreased or aberrant motion in the bicipital groove, finally resulting in spontaneous rupture of the LHB tendon (McDonald et al. 2013). Although isolated LHB tendinopathy is possible, it usually occurs concomitantly with other shoulder pathologies such as rotator cuff disease. Other entities that may be responsible for irritation of the LHB tendon

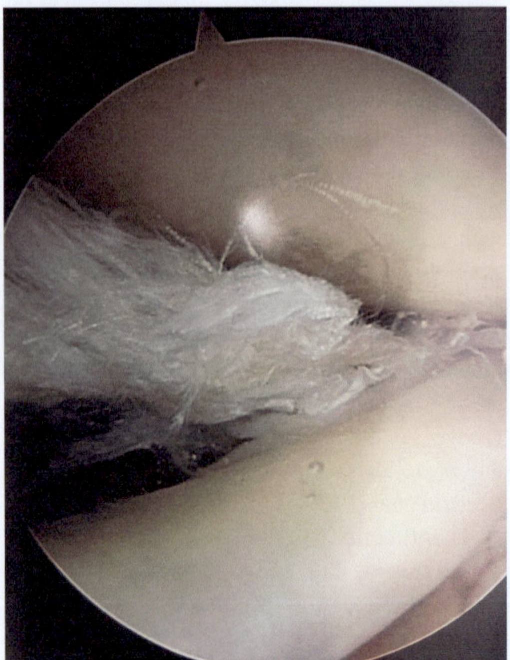

Fig. 20.1 Arthroscopic view of the biceps tendon with partial tearing and fraying

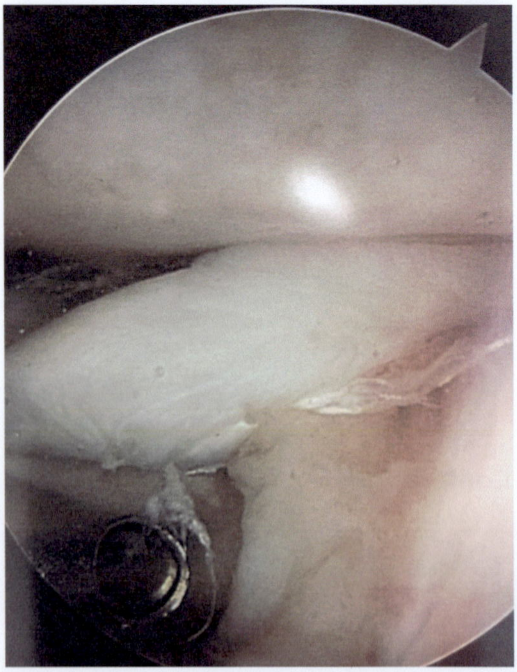

Fig. 20.2 Arthroscopic view of the biceps tendon subluxed out of the bicipital groove

include bicipital groove osteophytes and associated groove stenosis, systemic inflammatory disease, lesions of the soft tissues encompassing the biceps pulley, and superior labrum anterior to posterior (SLAP) tears. LHB tendon pathology may also be related to instability of the tendon as it traverses the bicipital groove. Instability can range from mild subluxation of the tendon to complete dislocation out of the bicipital groove (Fig. 20.2). Elser et al. (2011) found up to a 32% incidence of biceps pulley injury in a series of shoulder arthroscopies, and pulley lesions were commonly associated with SLAP tears and rotator cuff injuries.

20.3 History and Physical Exam

The typical description of LHB pathology is progressive anterior shoulder pain associated with chronic overuse syndromes. In younger patients with suspected LHB pathology, participation in overhead sports is common. A single traumatic event is also possible, during which the patient may hear an audible pop. Additional shoulder pathology can raise suspicion for LHB tendon instability. For instance, a tear of the subscapularis tendon may lead to LHB instability due to its intimate association as part of the biceps pulley.

One indication of LHB pathology is point tenderness to palpation of the tendon within the bicipital groove. The tendon can be palpated in the rotator interval, at the transverse humeral ligament, and beneath the attachment of the pectoralis major tendon insertion. We believe palpation to be the most diagnostic physical exam finding of biceps pathology. Physical exam maneuvers that elicit LHB tendon pain include Speed's test and Yergason's test. A positive Speed's test is indicated by pain with resisted forward flexion with the forearm extended and fully supinated. The Yergason test evokes pain with resisted forearm supination with the elbow flexed at 90 degrees and the arm adducted. These tests, however, may also be positive in SLAP tears, but in true SLAP lesions, there will be humeral head subluxation and a positive labral click, with the pain felt "deep," while the biceps will be less deep, more painful, and usually without a labral click. The "3-Pack" exam, coined by O'Brien, incorporates bicipital groove palpation, the throwing test, and active compression test. With high inter-rater reliability and sensitivity, the "3-Pack" exam can isolate biceps-labral complex lesions specific to three different zones: inside, junctional, and bicipital groove (Taylor et al. 2016). If the patient has sustained a spontaneous rupture of the biceps tendon, a "Popeye" sign may be evident in which an enlarged distal biceps mass is visualized (Rudzki et al. 2015) (Figs. 20.3 and 20.4).

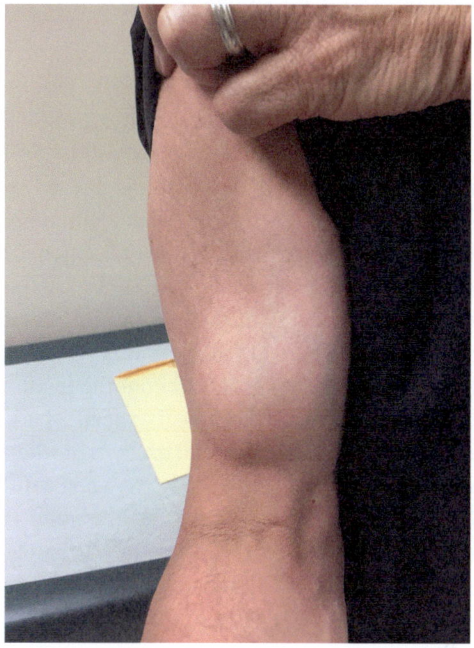

Fig. 20.3 Clinical photographs of a patient with a "Popeye" sign, which is a distal biceps mass indicative of biceps tendon rupture

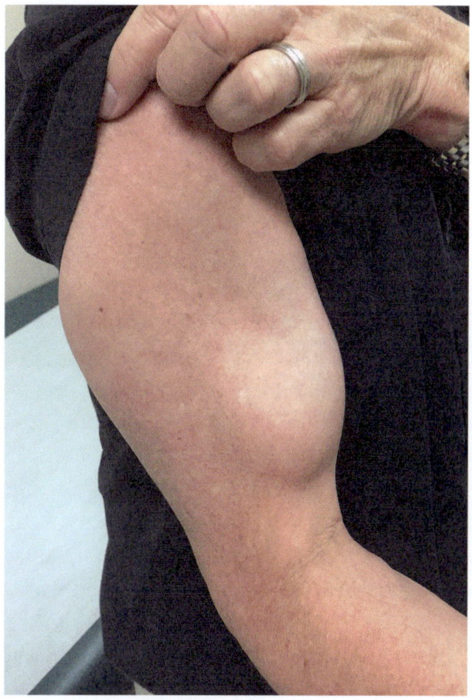

Fig. 20.4 Clinical photographs of a patient with a "Popeye" sign, which is a distal biceps mass indicative of biceps tendon rupture

Differential Diagnosis for Long Head of the Biceps Tendon Pathology:

- LHB tendinopathy/tenosynovitis
- LHB partial tear
- LHB rupture
- LHB instability (subluxation and/or dislocation)
- SLAP tear
- Acromioclavicular joint pathology
- Anterosuperior rotator cuff tear
- Subcoracoid impingement
- Subscapularis pathology

20.4 Diagnosis

Further workup of suspected LHB tendon lesions may include imaging and injections. A standard radiographic series of the shoulder will assist in identifying other potential causes of shoulder pain. Magnetic resonance imaging (MRI) is frequently utilized in the assessment of shoulder pathology. Not only can MRI assist in diagnosis of isolated LHB tendon injuries, but it can also aid in diagnosing concomitant shoulder pathology. MRI allows assessment of the tendon itself and its milieu, including its sheath, peritendinous fluid, and the bicipital groove. Further, magnetic resonance arthrography may be useful in isolated LHB tendon injuries. Ultrasound is another imaging modality of use, in particular, due to the ability for a dynamic exam. The tendon can be visualized during a subluxation event and assessed for complete rupture. If a skilled ultrasonographer is available, ultrasound can be more cost-effective. Corticosteroid injections into the biceps tendon sheath can prove to be both diagnostic and therapeutic (Nho et al. 2010).

20.5 Treatment

Non-operative management of LHB tendinopathy consists of rest, activity modifications, anti-inflammatory medications, and physical therapy. Corticosteroid injections, as mentioned above, can be administered in the subacromial space, glenohumeral joint, or directly into the tendon sheath. The glenohumeral injection may spread to the LHB tendon sheath based on their anatomic relationship (Nho et al. 2010). Hashiuchi et al. (2011) determined that LHB tendon sheath injections performed under ultrasound guidance were more accurate in their series of 30 biceps sheath injections evaluated with postinjection computed tomography. Care must be taken to inject corticosteroids into the bicipital groove and not the tendon substance, which may be detrimental to the tendon itself (Nho et al. 2010). Spontaneous complete ruptures of the LHB tendon are typically treated non-operatively with minimal consequence due to the "autotenodesis" phenomenon. Residual symptoms may include cosmetic concerns related to the "Popeye" deformity and a fatigue-related cramping of the biceps brachii muscle. The "autotenodesis" effect occurs due to the tendon's soft tissue restraints keeping it in the bicipital groove and the hourglass shape of the groove creating a bottleneck for the wide portion of the tendon as it retracts distally (Rudzki et al. 2015).

When non-operative treatment fails, the discussion of surgical management is initiated and may relate to associated shoulder pathology. Isolated LHB tendinopathy surgical indications include partial-thickness tearing or fraying greater than 25–50% of the tendon diameter and persistent subluxation or dislocation. Other relative indications for surgical management of the LHB are SLAP tears and intraoperative findings suggestive of biceps pathology at the time of surgery for other pathologies (Khazzam et al. 2012). Factors to consider in surgical decision-making include the patient's activity level, hand dominance, age, and functional expectations.

Current surgical management of the long head of the biceps tendon can be categorized as debridement, tenotomy, or tenodesis. Debridement is typically elected if less than 30% of the tendon diameter is involved (Khazzam et al. 2012). Arthroscopic tenotomy is performed utilizing the standard posterior viewing portal and working through the anterosuperior portal. Various instruments can be used to transect the tendon at its origin and the LHB tendon retracts into the bicipital groove. Some authors have described maintaining a wider portion of tendon to secure in the narrow portion of the groove or including a piece of labrum in the transection to prevent distal migration of the tendon through the bicipital groove (Rudzki et al. 2015) (Fig. 20.5). Goubier et al. (2014) described looping the free edge of biceps tendon about itself to provide substantial bicipital groove restraint. A neat tendon edge should be maintained to prevent subsequent mechanical symptoms.

Techniques for tenodesis include interference screw, suture anchor, unicortical button,

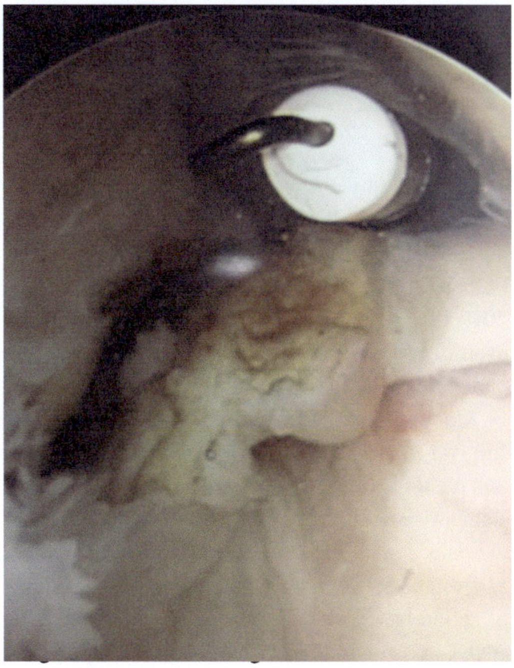

Fig. 20.5 Arthroscopic view of a biceps tenotomy, retaining a wide portion of the tendon to prevent retraction of the remaining tendon distally through the bicipital groove

tendon and then placing two suture anchors. One anchor is placed proximally, and the second anchor is placed 1–1.5 cm distal to the first. Chiang et al. (2016) compared suture anchor tenodesis with interference screw technique. Their technique for the Y-knot all-suture anchor fixation included bicortical drilling, was performed in a series of cadavers, and compared this fixation to interference screw tenodesis models with biomechanical testing. The all-suture anchor technique proved to have an equivalent ultimate failure load, but increased displacement with cyclic loading.

Button tenodesis can achieve either unicortical or bicortical fixation. Care is taken with bicortical drilling as the axillary and radial nerves are at risk. The transected LHB tendon is whipstitched and threaded through the button, which is passed through the drill hole. A tension-slide technique is used to secure the construct (Rudzki et al. 2015).

Soft tissue tenodesis is performed by suturing the LHB tendon to the overlying soft tissue roof of the bicipital groove. The percutaneous

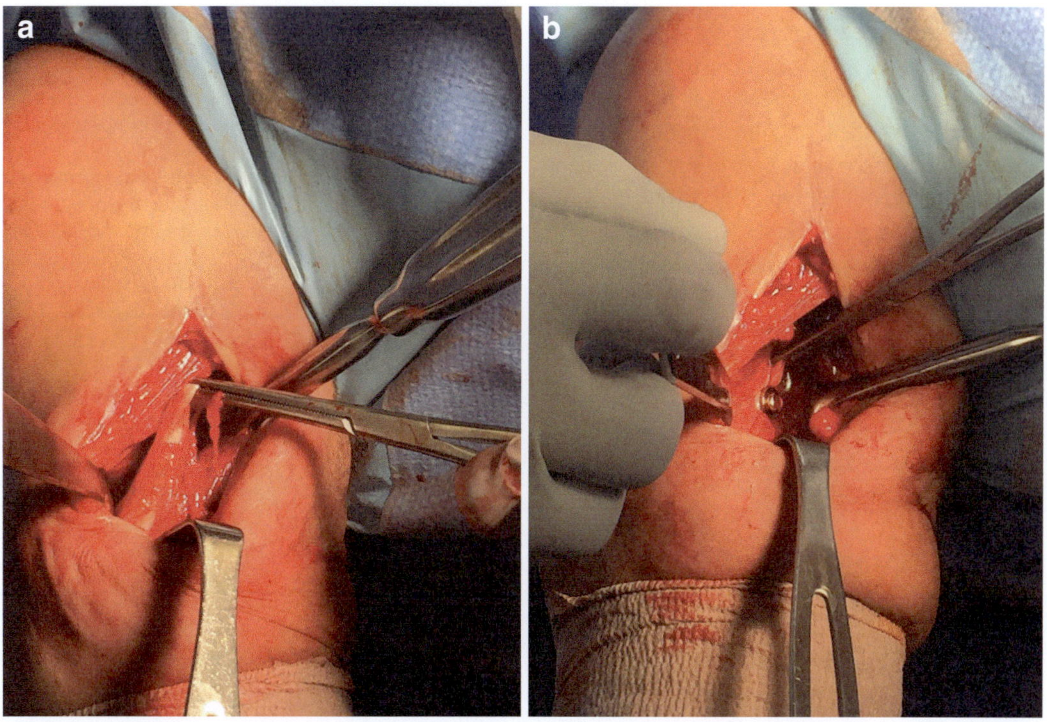

Fig. 20.6 Photographs of an open subpectoral biceps tenodesis. (**a**) Isolation of the biceps tendon. (**b**) Final construct after tenodesis with a screw and washer

intra-articular transtendon (PITT) technique described by Sekiya et al. (2003) uses a spinal needle to capture the biceps tendon via the lateral rotator interval. Sutures are shuttled through the soft tissue construct and the procedure is repeated 5–6 cm distally for dual fixation.

O'Brien has described a soft tissue tenodesis technique in which he transfers the long head to the short head to maintain the normal anatomy and course for the muscle with excellent results (Drakos et al. 2008).

Werner et al. (2014) compared arthroscopic suprapectoral tenodesis to open subpectoral tenodesis in patients with isolated superior labrum or LHB pathology. Both procedures resulted in equally excellent clinical and functional outcomes at 2 years of follow-up. Both techniques utilized interference screws for tenodesis fixation. Kolz et al. (2015) performed biomechanical studies on the LHB tendon in both the suprapectoral and subpectoral regions and found that the tendon had a higher tensile strength in the suprapectoral region. They also found that the suprapectoral region can resist higher failure loads. Based on this study, they concluded that tenodesis in the suprapectoral region may yield a stronger construct.

Postoperative care depends on the operative technique performed and any other associated pathology addressed at the time of surgery. Patients receiving tenotomy are typically placed in a sling for 1 week until pain subsides, with gradual return to activity. For tenodeses, patients are immobilized in a sling for approximately 4 weeks and begin active elbow flexion at 6–8 weeks postoperatively. This course allows for the tenodesis site to heal appropriately (Patel et al. 2016).

20.6 Discussion

In comparing LHB tenotomy with tenodesis, major differences include the formation of a "Popeye" deformity and fatigue-related cramps, both of which are more likely after tenotomy. In tenodesis, the length-tendon relationship is maintained, while tenotomized patients may exhibit a slight decrease in strength with forearm supination and elbow flexion (Patel et al. 2016). Friedman et al. (2015) evaluated patients younger than age 55 for 3 years after tenotomy or tenodesis. "Popeye" deformity and cramping were more common in the tenotomy group. However, functional and subjective outcome scores were similar after 3 years. Potential complications of LHB tenodesis may include persistent pain, tenodesis failure, and refractory tenosynovitis (Virk et al. 2016). In the case of tenodesis failure, symptoms usually remit over time, similar to if the patient had a spontaneous LHB rupture.

Many techniques have been described for the surgical treatment of long head of the biceps tendon pathology, with limited data on a clear-cut gold standard procedure. Equipped with knowledge of the risks and benefits of each technique, the patient and surgeon should arrive at an appropriate course of action based on patient expectations, functional status, cosmetic concerns, and demographics. Surgeon proficiency with each technique should also play a role in operative planning.

References

Chiang FL, Hong C, Chang C et al (2016) Biomechanical comparison of all-suture anchor fixation and interference screw technique for subpectoral biceps tenodesis. Arthroscopy 32:1247–1252

Drakos MC, Verma NN, Gulotta LV et al (2008) Arthroscopic transfer of the long head of the biceps tendon: functional outcome and clinical results. Arthroscopy 24:217–223

Elser F, Braun S, Dewing CB et al (2011) Anatomy, function, injuries, and treatment of the long head of the biceps brachii tendon. Arthroscopy 27:581–592

Friedman JL, FitzPatrick JL, Rylander LS et al (2015) Biceps tenotomy versus tenodesis in active patients younger than 55 years. Orthop J Sports Med 3:1–6

Goubier JN, Bihel T, Dubois E, Teboul F (2014) Loop biceps tenotomy: an arthroscopic technique for long head of biceps tenotomy. Arthrosc Tech 3:e427–e430

Hashiuchi T, Sakurai G, Morimoto M et al (2011) Accuracy of the biceps tendon sheath injection: ultrasound-guided or unguided injection? A randomized controlled trial. J Shoulder Elb Surg 20:1069–1073

Khazzam M, George MS, Churchill RS et al (2012) Disorders of the long head of biceps tendon. J Shoulder Elb Surg 21:136–145

Kolz CW, Suter T, Henninger HB (2015) Regional mechanical properties of the long head of the biceps tendon. Clin Biomech 30:940–945

Longo UG, Loppinni M, Marineo G et al (2011) Tendinopathy of the tendon of the long head of the biceps. Sports Med Arthrosc Rev 19:321–332
McDonald LS, Dewing CB, Shupe PG et al (2013) Disorders of the proximal and distal aspects of the biceps muscle. J Bone Joint Surg Am 95:1235–1245
Nho SJ, Strauss EJ, Lenart BA et al (2010) Long head of the biceps tendinopathy: diagnosis and management. J Am Acad Orthop Surg 18:645–656
Patel KV, Bravman J, Vidal A et al (2016) Biceps tenotomy versus tenodesis. Clin Sports Med 35:93–111
Rudzki JR, Shaffer BS (2015) Arthroscopic treatment of biceps tendinopathy. In: Wiesel SW (ed) Operative techniques in orthopaedic surgery. Lippincott Williams & Wilkins, Philadelphia, pp 55–67
Sekiya JK, Elkousy HA, Rodosky MW (2003) Arthroscopic biceps tenodesis using the percutaneous intra-articular transtendon technique. Arthroscopy 19:1137–1141
Tarleton AA, Zhou L, O'Brien MJ, Savoie FH (2015) Arthroscopic biceps tenodesis from a superior viewing portal in the shoulder. Arthrosc Tech 4:e383–e389
Taylor SA, Newman AM, Dawson C et al (2016) The "3-pack" examination is critical for comprehensive evaluation of the biceps-labrum complex and the bicipital tunnel: a prospective study. Arthroscopy 33(1):28–38. doi:10.1016/j.arthro.2016.05.015
Virk M, Nicholson GP (2016) Complications of proximal biceps tenotomy and tenodesis. Clin Sports Med 35:181–188
Werner BC, Evan CL, Holzgrefe RE et al (2014) Arthroscopic suprapectoral and open subpectoral biceps tenodesis: a comparison of minimum 2-year clinical outcomes. Am J Sports Med 42:2583–2590

Medial and Lateral Epicondylitis 21

L.A. Pederzini and F. Di Palma

Contents

L.A. Pederzini • F. Di Palma (✉)
Orthopaedic and Arthroscopic Department,
New Sassuolo Hospital, via F. Ruini, 2, 41049
Sassuolo, Modena, Italy
e-mail: gigiped@hotmail.com; felice.dipalma@libero.it

21.1 Epitrochleitis

The medial epicondylitis, or "golfer's elbow," is a painful syndrome that affects the medial compartment of the elbow often with pain irradiation to the forearm and ipsilateral wrist, caused usually by a functional overload of flexor-pronator muscles of the forearm that anatomically have a common tendon that inserts on the medial epicondyle (Plancher et al. 1996).

The common tendon is on the anteroinferior surface of the epicondyle just proximal to the anterior bundle of the medial collateral ligament.

Despite the name given to this pathology, it is not exclusive of golfers, but it is a disorder related to specific work tasks and to particular sports including golf.

Tennis players and other athletes who use repetitively the flexion-extension of the wrist and fingers can develop this painful syndrome too.

In particular, the type of racket grip and rotator effects given to the ball is responsible of a medial painful syndrome much more common now than in the past.

Sports that can frequently determine this disease are, therefore, golf, tennis, throwing sports, and weight lifting (Plancher et al. 1996).

Common daily activities requiring continuous flexion-extension movements of the elbow and wrist can cause medial epicondylitis like drawing,

G.L. Canata et al. (eds.), *Muscle and Tendon Injuries*, DOI 10.1007/978-3-662-54184-5_21

hammering, chopping wood, using a computer, cooking, and screwing.

The involved muscles are usually the flexor carpi radialis and pronator teres and less frequently palmaris longus, the flexor carpi ulnaris, and the flexor digitorum superficialis.

Repeated microtrauma causes microtears and weakening of the flexor carpi radialis or the pronator teres near their common origin on the medial epicondyle characterized by fibroblastic tendinosis with proliferation of vascular granulation tissue. The histology of the tendon becomes abnormal and can ultimately lead to avulsion of the flexor-pronator origin (Kraushaar and Nirschl 1999). The process becomes chronic with a failed healing response.

Usually it affects people over 35 years (Kraushaar and Nirschl 1999) old.

If not well treated, it can cause chronic elbow pain and joint stiffness.

Medial epicondylitis can be classified (Gabel and Morrey 1995) into three types: type I (isolated medial epicondylitis), type IIA (medial epicondylitis with minimum or medium ulnar neuropathy), and type IIB (medial epicondylitis with moderate or severe ulnar neuropathy).

21.1.1 Physical Examination

Patients typically present with chronic medial elbow pain. They may complain of weak grasp, difficulty in bending the fingers, and paresthesias in the fourth and fifth finger.

The onset can be insidious with increasing symptoms or acute.

The diagnosis of medial epicondylitis can be difficult because of the differential diagnosis including several disorders such as compression of the anterior interosseous nerve, arthritis, arthrofibrosis, cervical radiculopathy, cubital tunnel syndrome, loose bodies, medial epicondyle avulsion, osteophytes, synovitis, medial collateral ligament instability, and extension valgus overload (Dlabach and Baker 2001).

A complete history, physical examination, and additional diagnostic studies are necessary to make the correct diagnosis.

Physical examination shows tenderness at the origin of the flexor-pronator mass on the medial epicondyle increased by resisted wrist flexion and pronation.

The point of maximum tenderness is approximately 5 mm distal and anterior to the midpoint of the medial epicondyle (Dlabach and Baker 2001).

Physical examination of the ulnar nerve and valgus stress tests should be negative to confirm the diagnosis of isolated medial epicondylitis.

The ulnar collateral ligament must be examined to rule out instability or partial tear. Pain along the ulnar collateral ligament with valgus stress tested between 30° and 80° of flexion is an indication of instability.

The medial epicondylitis can occur as a secondary phenomenon with ulnar collateral ligament injury. In this case the principal cause of the disease which needs to be treated remains.

A complete neurologic examination of the cervical spine, shoulder, and wrist should be performed. Radiographic examination, including anteroposterior, lateral, and axial views, may show other causes of medial-sided pain as fractures, osteoarthritis, or ossification.

Imaging techniques such as MRI or ultrasound are performed to complete diagnosis.

Ultrasound (Lin 2012) study of the elbow is increasingly used in the absence of radiation exposure and easily accessible and reduces costs. Furthermore, it allows a dynamic assessment of the joint compared to other imaging studies.

Most of the typical pathologic findings of medial epicondylitis are usually found in the aforementioned muscles. The common tendon of flexion-pronator mass can show hypoechogenicity, loss of normal fibrillar structure, increased caliber, partial- or full-thickness tears, calcification, and hyperemia (seen with Doppler examination).

Ultrasound examination especially during valgus stress tests may be very helpful in assessing possible injury of the ulnar collateral ligament.

Young patients may develop lesions caused by valgus overuse, which, occurring on immature skeleton, may generate osteochondritis dissecans of the lateral humeral condyle and epicondyle fragmentation or injury of the ulnar collateral ligament that can be diagnosed by ultrasounds.

Electromyography and nerve conduction studies are indicated in patients with abnormal neurological findings during physical examination.

21.1.2 Treatment

The medial epicondylitis management is initially based on the nonoperative treatment.

The goal is to diminish pain and inflammation with:

- Resting from sports or from activities that cause pain
- Local cryotherapy for 15–20 min 3–4 times daily for 3 weeks
- The use of oral nonsteroidal anti-inflammatory drugs
- Stretching exercises
- Reducing the workload at the elbow while protecting the elbow with an elastic bandage and keeping wrist stiff during all activities in which weights are lifted

If this therapy is not successful in diminishing the symptoms, 1–2 injections of corticosteroids can be taken into account.

A gradual return to sports and work activities is possible when the patient does not complain of pain and starts practicing with the typical movements of his activities.

Patients with persistent symptoms after 6–12 months of nonoperative management should be considered candidate for surgical treatment (Gerard and Gabel 2001; Ciccotti 1999; Baker and Cummings 1998).

Treatments include percutaneous release (Baumgard and Schwartz 1982) and open debridement with or without common tendon detachment (Nirschl 1992; Vangsness and Jobe 1991).

The majority of surgical techniques for the medial epicondylitis are open procedures.

The procedure described by Nirschl (1992) consists of excising the pathologic tissue of the common tendon of the flexor-pronator mass leaving intact the normal tissue.

Vangsness and Jobe (1991) prefer to detach the origin of the flexion-pronator mass, remove the pathologic tissue, and reattach the origin of the flexor-pronator mass tendon.

With these procedures, the ulnar nerve is decompressed and transposed in patients with ulnar nerve symptoms.

21.1.3 Surgical Technique

Brachial plexus block or general anesthesia is usually performed for this surgery.

The patient is placed supine on the operating table. The involved extremity is exsanguinated and the tourniquet inflated.

A curved skin incision is performed just posterior to the medial epicondyle. The cutaneous nerves and the ulnar nerve are identified and protected during surgery.

The common tendon of flexor-pronator mass is exposed and the pathologic tissue identified and removed, leaving the normal tissue intact.

The ulnar collateral ligament is evaluated.

The defect can be sutured with absorbable suture or can be left free.

The ulnar nerve is transposed only in case of neurological symptoms. It is then performed hemostasis after tourniquet release. Subcutaneous and skin closure are performed.

Postoperatively, patients begin wrist and hand motion exercises immediately.

Posterior splint is used for about 7–10 days. The sutures are removed at 12–15 days, and elbow range-of-motion exercises are begun.

After about 3 weeks, strengthening exercises are started.

A longer period of immobilization is indicated in patients who undergo to ulnar collateral ligament reconstruction (Gabel and Morrey 1995; Kurvers and Verhaar 1995; Stahl and Kaufman 1997).

21.2 Lateral Epicondylitis

Lateral epicondylitis or "tennis elbow" is a degenerative tendinopathy of the extensor carpi radialis brevis (ECRB) and the common extensor tendon which is inserted on the lateral epicondyle of the elbow and affects both sportsmen and manual workers.

Epicondylitis is the most common lateral overload tendinopathy of the elbow (Jones and Savoie 1993; Field and Savoie 1998).

It is more common among athletes who practice activities for at least 2 h per week, 3–4 times more common in athletes over 40 years (Field and Savoie 1998).

There is no significant difference between male and female.

Regarding pathophysiology, it was thought that repetitive microtrauma to the common extensor origin at the lateral epicondyle produced inflammation within the common tendon of the extensor muscles. More recently, investigators of the pathoetiology of lateral epicondylitis have failed to detect signs of inflammation in patients with chronic tennis elbow and prefer the terminology "lateral tennis elbow" or "tendinosis of the elbow" to describe the condition.

The most likely hypothesis seems to be a microscopic lesion of ECRB from repeated microtrauma that causes the formation of a reparative tissue that looks like angiofibroblastic hyperplasia (Plancher et al. 1996; Baker and Jones 1999).

Subsequently, the process of micro-lesions and tissue repair leads to a tendon function failure.

The patient typically presents a recent history of functional elbow overuse with insidious onset of pain in the lateral aspect of the elbow (usually the dominant), although this condition is not always present.

21.2.1 Physical Examination

The diagnosis is essentially clinical.

The pain is exacerbated by resisted wrist dorsiflexion with the elbow extended. Swelling is not usually present. Physical examination shows tenderness over the lateral epicondyle especially just distal and anterior to the lateral epicondyle.

Elbow range of motion typically is equal to the contralateral side, but throwing athletes can have a loss of extension.

X-rays are usually normal.

The differential diagnosis should be made with the compression of the radial nerve and compressive neuropathy of the posterior interosseous nerve, intra-articular pathologies of the elbow, posterolateral impingement, posterolateral rotatory instability, osteoarthritis of the radial head, cervical radiculopathy, loose bodies, fracture of the radial head, and lateral synovial fringe.

21.2.2 Treatment

Lateral epicondylitis usually heals with conservative treatment in 90–95% of cases. Conservative treatment consists of rest, NSAIDs, injection, activity modification, strengthening exercises, laser therapy, ultrasound therapy, pulsed electromagnetic field therapy, iontophoresis, stretching, acupuncture, and shockwave therapy (Leach and Miller 1987).

More recently, therapies involving injections of blood plasma that has been enriched with platelets (PRP) have been introduced (Mishra and Pavelko 2006; Taylor et al. 2002; Edwards and Calandruccio 2003; Connel et al. 2006). As a concentrated source of autologous platelets, PRP contains several different growth factors and other cytokines that can stimulate healing of soft tissue. The platelet-rich plasma is a volume of fractionated plasma which is obtained by centrifuging the blood and the subsequent separation of platelets from other blood components. Wound-healing and tissue-repairing processes involve a complex cellular and molecular response, mediated by a wide range of growth factors and cytokines released from the plasma and intracellular granules of platelets stored within α-granules.

The PRP applied at the site of the lesion provides higher quantities of these mediators with the aim to facilitate and accelerate the healing processes, increasing local blood supply through the stimulation of new blood vessel formation.

The aim of the injection therapy with PRP is to reduce or eliminate pain and inflammation and recover the functional motion.

Some authors have shown that the injection of PRP determines the release in the pathologic tendon tissue of a series of cellular and humoral substances which leads, through a biological complex process, to a tissue healing (Mishra and Pavelko 2006; Taylor et al. 2002). The procedure according to some authors leads to a clinical improvement and also a good morphologic tendon aspect (Edwards and Calandruccio 2003).

There are a small number of patients who do not have imaging changes before and after treatment, even having a good clinical improvement studied by different scores (VAS and Nirschl scores).

The poor regenerative capacity of the tendons should perhaps be sought in their poor blood supply resulting in reduced oxygenation and nutrition of tissue, characteristic which explains the low-potential healing and consequently the difficult treatment (Connel et al. 2006).

21.2.3 Surgical Technique

Nonoperative treatment is the gold standard for this pathology.

However, from 5% to 10% (in some studies up to 25%) of these patients develop a set of symptoms that may require surgical treatment. Pain at night usually convinces the patient for a more invasive treatment. Surgical treatment should be considered in patients treated conservatively for at least 6 months.

Surgical treatment can be open, percutaneous, or arthroscopic, with success percentages that range from good to excellent from <65% to 95% of cases (Baker and Jones 1999).

They have described several open techniques, the first of which in 1955 by Bosworth (1955). Later technique improvements have been made by Coonrad and Hooper (1973), Nirschl and Pettrone (1979), Baumgard and Schwartz (1982), and Baker et al. (2000). Bosworth proposed four types of surgical procedures: the complete cutting of the common tendon insertion of the extensor muscles mass, the cutting of common tendon with the synovial fringe removal on the radial head, the complete cutting of the common tendon of the extensor muscle mass and the resection of the annular ligament, and finally vertical split of the common tendon origin of the extensor muscle mass, associated with the partial annular ligament resection and repair of the origin of the extensors with a suture above the radial head (Bosworth 1955).

Nirschl and Pettrone (1979) reported their technique in 1979. This technique is performed with an anterior approach to the epicondyle. Then the proximal insertion of the extensor carpi radialis longus (ECRL) on the distal humerus is released and retracted anteriorly in order to expose the extensor carpi radialis brevis (ECRB). At this point, the ECRB is retracted from its proximal origin in order to expose pathologic tissue. They remove all pathology found, the ECRB is released from its origin, and multiple microperforations are performed to the anterior surface of the lateral epicondyle. An anatomical repair of the ECRL and ECRB and EDC concludes the technique.

Baumgard and Schwartz (1982) described a percutaneous release in 1982. Baker reported his experience and introduced arthroscopic classification of the lateral epicondylitis. Baker's arthroscopic classification provides three types of lesions: Type I: no tear of the lateral joint capsular; Type II: longitudinal lesion to the lateral joint capsular; and Type III: complete breakage of lateral joint capsular with retraction and wide exposure of ECRB tendon insertion.

Arthroscopic treatment of lateral epicondylitis is performed with local anesthetic nerve block or general anesthesia. The involved extremity is exsanguinated and the tourniquet inflated.

The patient is in prone position.

Once good viewing of the internal surface of the ECRB and lateral joint capsular has been obtained, if these structures are intact, arthroscopic debridement of the capsule proceeds through the lateral portal. Having removed the portion of this lateral capsule, the internal surface of the ECRB can be seen. At this point, the arthroscopic release phase can begin, starting from the point of lesion and continuing proximally toward the origin of the muscular insertion at the lateral epicondyle by radio-frequency hook. Subsequently, a burr to decorticate the lateral epicondyle is used or microfractures in order to promote the repair process are performed, thanks to the bleeding thus obtained.

A local anesthetic is then injected into the lateral portal to decrease postoperative pain. After surgery, a 90° elbow posterior splint with radiocarpal joint in hyperextension is used for 15 days, starting active and passive physiokinetic therapy, progressive ROM, cryotherapy, and gradual strengthening exercises at around 4–6 weeks once complete ROM has been reached.

Return to sports at around 8–10 weeks postoperative.

Conclusions

The lateral epicondylitis is much more frequent than the medial.

Most of patients with lateral or medial epicondylitis respond to a nonoperative treatment. However, in chronic cases, surgery should be considered with failure of nonoperative treatment.

The open technique is the preferred method for the medial epicondylitis.

Referring to lateral epicondylitis, arthroscopic treatment should be the first choice with a success rate equal to the open treatment. In expert hands, this procedure is simple, safe, repeatable, and efficient. The technique preserves the insertion of the other extensor tendons. It allows for shorter, early rehabilitation if compared to other techniques. Long-term subjective and objective results are good to excellent in 75% of patients, and the return to the same level of previous sport is early and complete. Arthroscopy is less traumatic, allows treatment of associated intra-articular disorders, and allows a faster return to work or sports compared to traditional open procedure.

References

Baker CL, Cummings PD (1998) Arthroscopic management of miscellaneous elbow disorders. Oper Tech Sports Med 6:16–21

Baker CL, Jones GL (1999) Current concepts: arthroscopy of the elbow. Am J Sports Med 27:251–264

Baker CL Jr, Murphy KP, Gottlob CA, Curd DT (2000) Arthroscopic classification and treatment of lateral epicondylitis: two-year clinical results. J Shoulder Elb Surg 9:475–482. doi:10.1067/mse.2000.108533

Baumgard SH, Schwartz DR (1982) Percutaneous release of the epicondylar muscles for humeral epicondylitis. Am J Sports Med 10:233–236. doi:10.1177/036354658201000408

Bosworth DM (1955) The role of the orbicular ligament in tennis elbow. J Bone Joint Surg Am 37:527–534

Ciccotti MG (1999) Epicondylitis in the athlete. Instr Course Lect 48:375–381

Connel DA, Ali KE, Ahmad M et al (2006) Ultrasound-guided autologus blood injection for tennis elbow. Skelet Radiol 35:371–377

Coonrad RW, Hooper WR (1973) Tennis elbow: its course, natural history, conservative and surgical management. J Bone Joint Surg Am 55:1177–1182

Dlabach JA, Baker CL (2001) Lateral and medial epicondylitis in the overhead athlete. Oper Tech Orthop 11(1):46–54

Edwards SG, Calandruccio JH (2003) Autologus blood injections for refractory lateral epicondylitis. Am J Hand Surg 28(2):272–278

Field LD, Savoie FH (1998) Common elbow injuries in sport. Sports Med 26:193–205

Gabel GT, Morrey BF (1995) Operative treatment of medial epicondylitis. Influence in concomitant ulnar neuropathy at the elbow. J Bone Joint Surg Am 77:1065–1069

Gerard T, Gabel MD (2001) Management of medial epicondylitis in the throwing athlete. Oper Tech Sport Med 9(4):205–210

Jones GS, Savoie EH (1993) Arthroscopic capsular release of flexion contractures (arthrofibrosis) of the elbow. Arthroscopy 9:277

Kraushaar BS, Nirschl RP (1999) Current concepts review: tendinosis of the elbow (tennis elbow). J Bone Joint Surg Am 81:259–278

Kurvers H, Verhaar J (1995) The results of operative treatment of medial epicondylitis. J Bone Joint Surg Am 77:1374–1379

Leach RE, Miller JK (1987) Lateral and medial epicondylitis of the elbow. Clin Sports Med 6:259–273

Lin C-W (2012) Yan-Hao Chen, wen-Shiang Chen Application of Ultrasound and Ultrasound-guided intervention for evaluating elbow Joint Pathologies. J Med Ultrasound 20:87–95

Mishra A, Pavelko T (2006) Treatment of chronic elbow tendinosis with bufferede platelet-rich plasma. Am J Sports Med 10(10):1–5

Nirschl RP (1992) Elbow tendinosis/tennis elbow. Clin Sports Med 11:851–870

Nirschl RP, Pettrone F (1979) Tennis elbow: the surgical treatment of lateral epicondylitis. J Bone Joint Surg Am 61:832–841

Plancher KD, Halbrecht J, Lourie GM (1996) Medial and lateral epicondylitis in the athlete. Clin Sports Med 15:283–305

Stahl S, Kaufman T (1997) Ulnar nerve injury at the elbow after steroid injection for medial epicondylitis. J Hand Surg Br 22:69–70

Taylor MA, Norman TL, Clovis NB et al (2002) The response of the rabbit patellar tendons after autologus blood injection. Med Sci Sports Exerc 34(1):70–73

Vangsness CT, Jobe FW (1991) Surgical treatment of medial epicondylitis: results in 35 elbows. J Bone Joint Surg Br 73:409–411

Disorders of the Distal Biceps Tendon

22

Madeleine Bain, Joideep Phadnis, and Gregory Bain

Contents

M. Bain (✉)
University of Adelaide, Adelaide, SA, Australia
e-mail: madeleine.bain@student.adelaide.edu.au

J. Phadnis, MBChB, MRCS, SportsMed, FRCS
Department of Orthopaedic Surgery and Trauma, Flinders Medical Centre, Adelaide, SA, Australia

G. Bain, MBBS, FRACS, FA(Ortho)A, PhD
Department of Orthopaedic Surgery and Trauma, Flinders Medical Centre, Adelaide, SA, Australia

Department of Orthopaedic Surgery and Trauma, Flinders University, Adelaide, SA, Australia
e-mail: greg@gregbain.com.au

22.1 Background

Rupture of the distal biceps tendon is an uncommon and often overlooked injury. It is the consequence of eccentric contracture against forced extension, resulting in significant weakness of both supination and flexion (Nesterenko et al. 2010). Distal tendon ruptures make up 3–12% of all biceps injuries (D'Alessandro et al. 1993) and occur most frequently in the dominant arm of males between 40 and 60 (Ramsey 1999), with increased risk in smokers (Safran and Graham 2002) and anabolic steroid users (Visuri and Lindholm 1994).

Partial tears of the distal biceps tendon are less common than complete rupture and pose several clinical challenges. These injuries are commonly overlooked due to their subtle presentation and variable clinical examination and as yet no well-defined management pathway due to the paucity of evidence (Bain et al. 2008). Endoscopy has been shown to be a valuable diagnostic tool in partial tears that can aid in determining pathology, severity and therefore management. Chronic distal biceps tendon tears are frequently accompanied by tendon retraction, pseudotendon formation and scar tissue. However, these have had positive outcomes with grafting or fixation in extreme flexion (Morrey et al. 2014). Outcomes for open and endoscopic approaches have been positive, with satisfactory results achieved when utilising the Endobutton, suture anchors, interference screws and transosseous repairs (Bain et al. 2000; Boyd and Anderson 1961; Gregory et al. 2009; Heinzelmann et al. 2009).

G.L. Canata et al. (eds.), *Muscle and Tendon Injuries*, DOI 10.1007/978-3-662-54184-5_22

22.2 Anatomy

The biceps brachii originates and inserts as two discrete heads to provide both elbow supination and flexion. The long head of biceps courses parallel to the short head on the radial side of the upper arm, with varying amounts of interdigitating muscle fibres (Eames et al. 2007). Three zones of the distal biceps tendon have been described, (1) pre-aponeurosis at the musculotendinous junction, (2) aponeurosis at the origin of the lacertus fibrosus and (3) post-aponeurosis, where it will insert into the ulnar aspect of the radial tuberosity (Eames et al. 2007). The lacertus fibrosus is a trilayer structure and arises from primarily the long head of biceps, enveloping the proximal forearm flexor muscles to insert on the subcutaneous anterior ulna (Eames et al. 2007).

The long head passes posterior to the short head, to insert into an oval footprint more proximally and posteriorly at the radial tuberosity (Eames et al. 2007; Jarrett et al. 2012). The short head fans out over the long head and inserts distally on the radial tuberosity, where variation in the size and location of the tendon footprint can predispose to impingement against the ulna (Bain et al. 2016). The tendon footprint has a mean area of 108 mm^2, length 21 mm and width 7 mm (Athwal et al. 2007). In the fully supinated forearm, the long head is the primary supinator, as the lever arm created by the radial tuberosity generates greater rotational torque. The short head's distal attachment produces greater elbow flexion to complement the brachialis (Eames et al. 2007).

The bicipitoradial bursa is teardrop shaped and encloses the entire distal biceps tendon, closely adherent to the tendons ulnar aspect. In elbow extension, it is between the biceps tendon and brachialis muscle and in pronation between the proximal radius and biceps tendon (Fig. 22.1).

The distal biceps tendon receives dual blood supply, proximally the brachial artery and distally the recurrent radial artery. A relative hypovascular region exists adjacent to the site of tendon insertion, which may further increase its susceptibility to injury. The rupture usually occurs at the tendon insertion in an area of preexisting degeneration (Ramsey 1999).

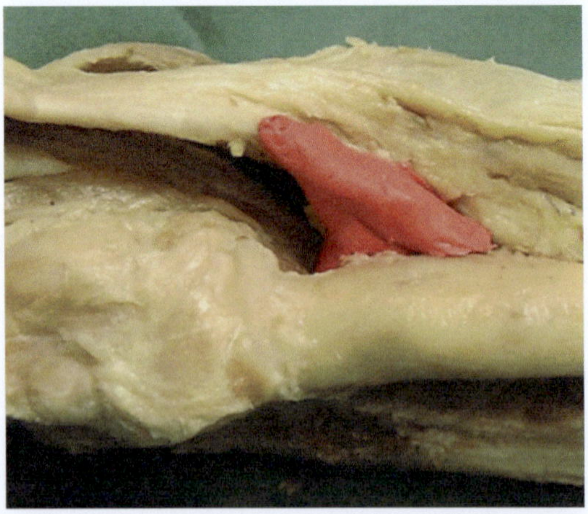

Fig. 22.1 The bicipitoradial bursa is highlighted between the distal biceps tendon and the radius (proximal, *left*; distal, *right*) (Permission granted from (Eames and Bain 2006))

22.3 Clinical Assessment

22.3.1 History

The presentation is typically of a sudden onset of pain and weakness following an eccentric load. This acute pain is felt in the antecubital fossa or, less commonly, posterolateral elbow (Bain et al. 2016; Dürr et al. 2000) and may be associated with an audible 'pop' (Ramsey 1999) and weak supination and flexion.

Chronic pain may occur in older patient with distal biceps tendonitis/tendinosis or bicipitoradial bursitis. This is typically an aching anterior elbow pain exacerbated by specific activities. In contrast to complete rupture, tendinopathy favours females, particularly those with comorbidities, such as immunosuppression, diabetes and hypothyroidism (Bain et al. 2016; Phadnis and Bain 2017).

22.3.2 Physical Examination

A distal biceps tendon acute rupture is a clinical diagnosis. It may present with ecchymosis and swelling of the antecubital fossa with a visible and palpable defect in the distal biceps muscle belly that is accentuated on active flexion (Ramsey

1999). Assessment of strength generally shows weakness of supination greater than flexion as the biceps is the primary forearm supinator, while the brachialis is able to compensate for elbow flexion.

The hook sign is a useful clinical test. It is described as positioning the elbow flexed to 90° with the forearm maximally supinated. From the lateral side, the examiner's finger is hooked beneath the distal biceps tendon in the antecubital fossa (O'Driscoll et al. 2007). In a normal patient, approximately 1 cm of the examiners finger is able to hook beneath the tendon and pull forwards, indicating an intact hook test (O'Driscoll et al. 2007). Abnormalities have been further subclassified by the senior author from the hook tests' initial interpretation; see Table 22.1. Assessment of tendon laxity and its ability to yield against resistance are used for grading. This classification is correlated with MRI findings and the pathologies in which they might appear, as described in Table 22.2. The integrity of the lacertus fibrosus is difficult to assess clinically, and it can be unclear if it remains intact in the presence of a retracted tendon (Bain et al. 2016).

Examination findings in partial tears are often subtle, making it difficult to clinically diagnose.

Table 22.1 Clinical assessment and interpretation of the hook test

Hook test finding	Grade	Features of tendon
Normal	N	Taut, unyielding and symmetric with contralateral arm
Abnormal	A1	Taut, but yielding and asymmetric with contralateral arm
Abnormal	A2	Lax and asymmetric
Abnormal	A3	Absent cord

Reproduced from Bain et al. (2016)

Table 22.2 Classification of distal biceps pathologies with clinical and radiological findings

Grade	Injury	Clinical	Hook test	MRI	Recommended management
0	Tendinosis, bursitis	Atraumatic, tender, swollen	N	Bursitis, effusion, tendinosis	Nonoperative, bursectomy, biopsy
1A	Low-grade partial tear (<50% footprint detachment)	Pain and weakness against resistance	N, A1	Bursitis, effusion, footprint irregularity	Endoscopic debridement
1B	Isolated head rupture	Weakness against resistance	A1	Isolated head avulsion	Repair isolated head
1C	High-grade partial tear (>50% footprint detachment)	Pain and weakness against resistance	A1	Incomplete footprint detachment	Complete and repair
2	Complete tendon rupture, lacertus intact	Tendon medialised by intact lacertus, marked weakness	A2	Complete footprint detachment, tendon within sheath	Repair
3	Complete tendon and lacertus rupture with retraction	Retracted muscle, marked weakness	A3	Complete footprint detachment, retracted tendon and muscle	Repair
4A	Chronic rupture	Tendon medialised by intact lacertus, marked weakness	A1, A2	Complete detachment and contracted tendon within sheath (A2). A pseudotendon may bridge the native tendon to the footprint (A1)	Repair
4B	Chronic retracted rupture	Retracted muscle, marked weakness	A3	Complete footprint detachment, retracted tendon within fibrous cocoon	Repair in flexion or use tendon graft

Reproduced from Bain et al. (2016)

We have found a number of interesting clinical examination techniques for assessment of the partial distal biceps tendon tears and bursitis. (1) Rotating the forearm, the biceps musculotendinous junction can be seen to migrate proximally and distally. (2) Pain is elicited in passive pronation. (3) Marked supination weakness in maximum flexion. (4) With the elbow in 90° of flexion and full supination, there is localised pain and tenderness over the insertion with supination against resistance. Crepitus may also be present (Bain et al. 2016), in addition to a palpable biceps tendon in the antecubital fossa (Dellaero and Mallon 2006).

22.3.3 Imaging

Plain radiographs may only identify non-specific hypertrophic bone formation over the radial tuberosity (Ramsey 1999); therefore, AP and lateral films should be sought for preoperative planning, but not diagnostic confirmation of tendon rupture.

Medial approach ultrasound views through the pronator window are shown to be valuable to visualise the ulnar facing radial tuberosity; however, it is less reliable than MRI (Smith et al. 2010).

MRI is beneficial for diagnostic confirmation in addition to classification of the tear. A FABS view (flexion 90°, abducted shoulder 90° and supination) is an easily reproducible technique to visualise the full length of the tendon in one section (Giuffrè and Moss 2004) (Fig. 22.2). Comparison of intraoperative findings and MRI revealed that complete rupture is reliably detected on MRI with sensitivity of 100% (Festa et al. 2010). Partial ruptures were detected at a sensitivity of only 59%, and those requiring surgical repair were indistinguishable from nonoperative management (Festa et al. 2010).

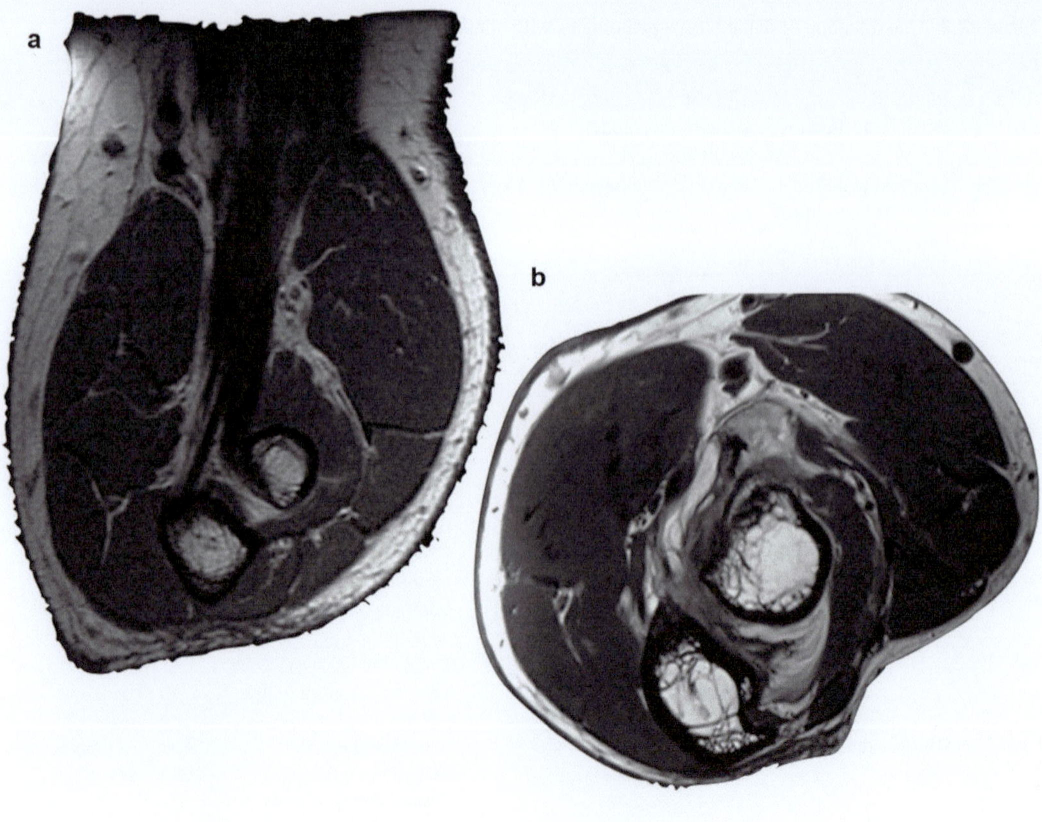

Fig. 22.2 Magnetic resonance imaging of the distal biceps tendon in the FABS position. (**a**) Partial tear of the distal biceps tendon. (**b**) Complete tear, with thickening of the proximal tendon

22.4 Classification

Various classifications exist to describe distal biceps tendon pathology. Injuries can be described relative to the degree (partial or complete), duration (acute or chronic) or anatomical zone relative to the aponeurosis described above. Biceps tendon insertion (zone 3) is the most common site of pathology and has been graded 0–4 (see Table 22.2). This grading system identifies the pathology and guides management based upon clinical and radiological findings. As there is overlap amongst grades, assessment of the hook test needs to be interpreted.

22.5 Indication for Endoscopy

The use of endoscopy in distal biceps pathology can be both diagnostic and therapeutic. Endoscopy enables visualisation of the tendon to differentiate complete from partial tears and to assess the quality of the remaining tendon. Fibrous tissue and pseudotendon that may develop in chronic injury can be identified and debrided, and the retracted residual tendon can be retrieved with this technique. Endoscopic repair is relatively contraindicated in patients with abnormal anatomy, such as following surgery or trauma to the antecubital fossa or elbow. After becoming comfortable with diagnostic endoscopy, the surgeon can progress to debridement procedures including synovectomy, surgical release of partial tears and debridement of the tuberosity (Bain et al. 2016).

22.6 Surgical Techniques

22.6.1 Two-Incision Technique

The two-incision technique was initially described by Boyd and Anderson (1961), with a modification by Bourne and Morrey (1991). A 3–4 cm transverse incision is made in the antecubital fossa. The lateral cutaneous nerve of the forearm is identified and protected, and a grasping stitch is used to secure the tendon. In maximal supination, a blunt artery forceps is advanced along the medial border of the radius through the dorsolateral aspect of the forearm. Caution should be taken to avoid disturbing the periosteum to reduce the risk of radioulnar synostosis. A second incision is made over the tip of the forceps. The forearm is then pronated to expose the radial tuberosity, while also protecting the posterior interosseous nerve by removing it from the operative field.

The radial tuberosity is burred to accept the tendon and drill holes in the margin to accept sutures from the tendon (Mazzocca et al. 2008). The sutures are passed anterior to posterior with the aid of forceps and tied firmly over the bone surface (Phadnis and Bain 2015). This technique is complicated by the formation of heterotopic ossification and radioulnar synostosis. The chance of this can be reduced by not violating the periosteum over the ulna and irrigating the wound (Mazzocca et al. 2008).

22.6.2 Single Anterior Incision: Endobutton Technique

Various techniques have been described utilising the single incision approach. Endobuttons, interference screws and suture anchors have all been used with positive outcomes (Gregory et al. 2009; Heinzelmann et al. 2009; McKee et al. 2005; Peeters et al. 2009; Sharma and MacKay 2005). A longitudinal anterior incision is made distal to the antecubital fossa. The lateral cutaneous nerve of the forearm is identified and protected. The tendon stump is grasped and debrided. A number 2 FiberWire Krackow suture is inserted, leaving the free ends exiting the distal tendon. The radial tuberosity is then exposed with 90° retractors and maximal supination and elbow extension (Bain et al. 2000). A cortical window over the footprint surface is debrided with a high-speed burr and a 4 mm drill advanced through to the reach the posterior side.

A space of 2 mm is left when the free strands from the tendon are secured to the Endobutton. This enables manipulation of the Endobutton when passed through the radial cortex. Suture

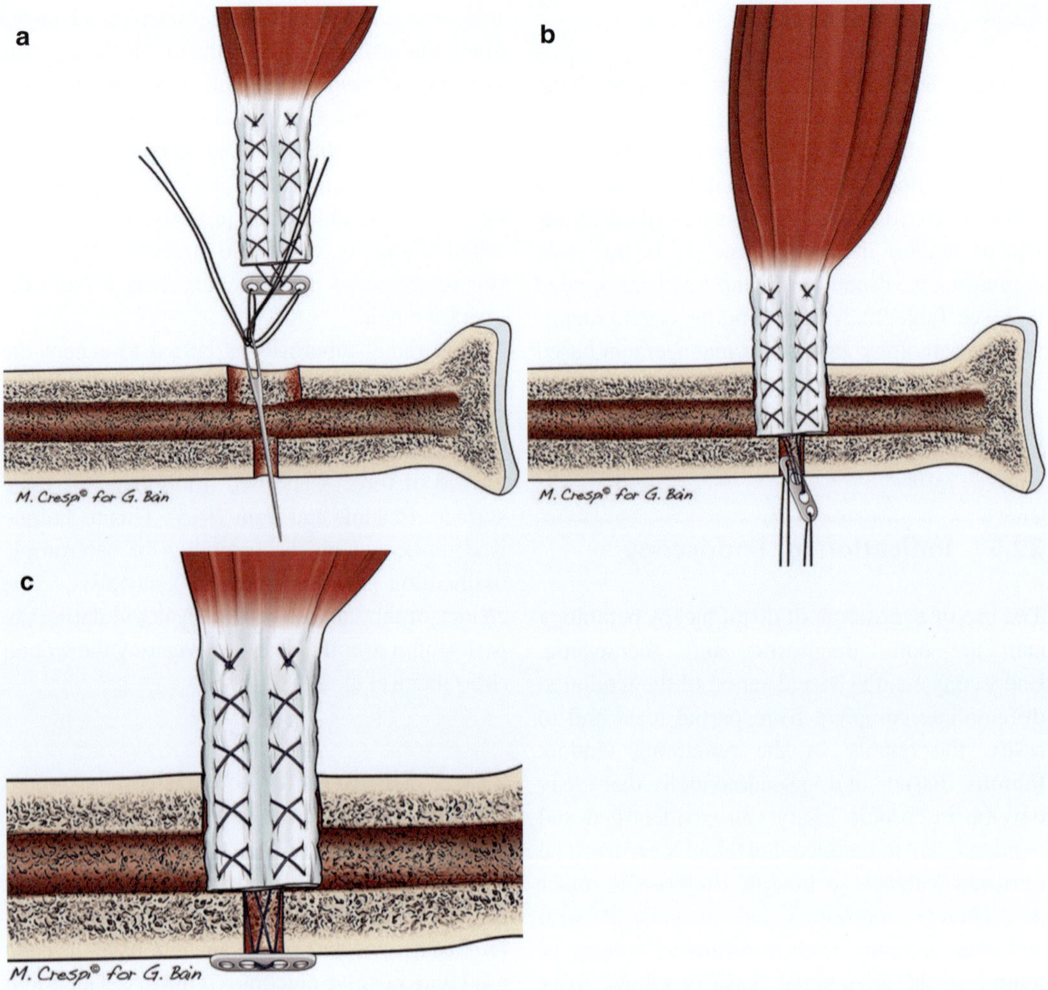

Fig. 22.3 Fixation of the tendon using the Endobutton technique. (**a**) Leading and trailing sutures thread through straight-eyed needle. (**b**) Endobutton advanced by applying tension to leading suture under fluoroscopic guidance. (**c**) Endobutton secured on the dorsal radius, and leading and trailing sutures removed

material is placed at both of the outermost holes of the Endobutton. Both sutures are threaded onto a straight needle and advanced through the drill hole (Fig. 22.3a). The needle is angled in an ulnar direction, to avoid the posterior interosseous nerve and then pierces the posterior forearm. Tension is put on the leading suture first to manipulate the Endobutton and allow it to pass through the cortex, then the trailing suture to fix it in place (Fig. 22.3b). Fluoroscopy and examining range of motion should be performed to ensure fixation before the sutures are removed (Fig. 22.3c) (Bain et al. 2000).

Due to the radial tuberosity's ulnar position, this technique does not restore the tendons' anatomical position. Currently, the author uses endoscopic-assisted Endobutton placement, discussed below, to allow the footprint repair to be achieved.

22.6.3 Endoscopic-Assisted Repair

The patient is positioned supine with the elbow flexed to 10°, thereby reducing anterior soft tissue tension (Phadnis and Bain 2015). A 2 cm

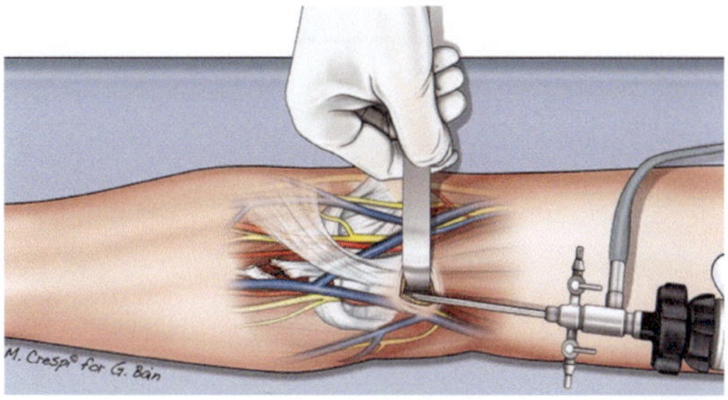

Fig. 22.4 Positioning the scope during distal biceps tendon endoscopy of the right elbow (Image provided by Dr Gregory Bain)

longitudinal incision is made over the biceps tendon, 2 cm distal to the anterior elbow crease. The lateral cutaneous nerve of the forearm is identified and protected, and the radial artery deeper in the wound is retracted or cauterised. The bicipitoradial bursa is identified, and a small transverse portal is made on the radial side at its apex. The 4-mm arthroscope is introduced; a hooded scope provides extra retraction (Fig. 22.4). Maintaining a medial position from the entry point will enable the median nerve and brachial artery to be protected. Forearm rotation will provide dynamic tendon views and assist in the identification of relevant anatomical structures. The condition of the tendon and its sheath can be assessed, while also being able to identify the radial tuberosity, the bursitis and even the pseudotendon in chronic cases (Bain et al. 2016; Phadnis and Bain 2015). In acute injuries, integrity of the tendon sheath may be maintained with the bursa still adherent to the footprint (Bain et al. 2016). Chronic injuries may appear with retraction of the tendon stump and development of a pseudotendon. This dense tissue does not contain any tendon but can mask the tendon, which is hidden inside (Phadnis and Bain 2015). An intact lacertus fibrosus may tether the residual tendon and prevent it from retracting. In order to achieve adequate tendon mobilisation, it may require release from the lacertus fibrosus.

The tendon is debrided to expose healthy tissue with a full-radius resector, without teeth or suction, in order to prevent damage to surrounding tissue. Through this same incision, an arthroscopic hook can be used to probe the insertion site. If the tear is <25% of the tendon insertion, it may be debrided. Larger tears will involve release of the remaining tendon with scissors placed into the proximal tendon bone junction (Dürr et al. 2000). With a complete tear, the natural footprint can be debrided with a chondrotome (Fig. 22.5).

The tendon stump is prepared with a Krackow whipstitch with a minimum of three throws along the length of the tendon. The four FiberWire strands exit the tendon surface on the superior aspect to avoid interference between the tendon and the bone surface (Phadnis and Bain 2015). The tuberosity is prepared with a high-speed burr, shaver, rongeur or curette as required, until superficial bleeding is visible (Fig. 22.6). A 2.5-mm drill is then used to create two oblique holes from the anterior cortex of the radius to just posterior of the footprint.

A Tuohy epidural needle is loaded with a nylon suture loop protruding by 2 cm. The needle is advanced through each hole, and the needle is grasped from the posterior radius with an angled Lahey clamp (Fig. 22.7). The clamp is slightly opened to allow the suture to be grasped and then delivered to the anterior wound. When the needle is removed, the two free ends exit the anterior surface and the loop through the posterior hole. The prepared biceps tendon is oriented so the ulnar strands from the short head are placed through the distal hole and the radial strands of the long head through the proximal. The FiberWire suture of the tendon is then thread through an Endobutton and tied firmly to the bone surface (Fig. 22.8a, b). The risk of impingement is lessened by aiming the drill away from the posterior interosseous nerve and placing the Endobutton under direct vision. Smaller burr holes also minimise the risk of proximal radius fractures. The tourniquet is released, haemostasis achieved and wound closed. The patient is discharged with a sling and can mobilise the arm, but no sport should be played for 3–6 months.

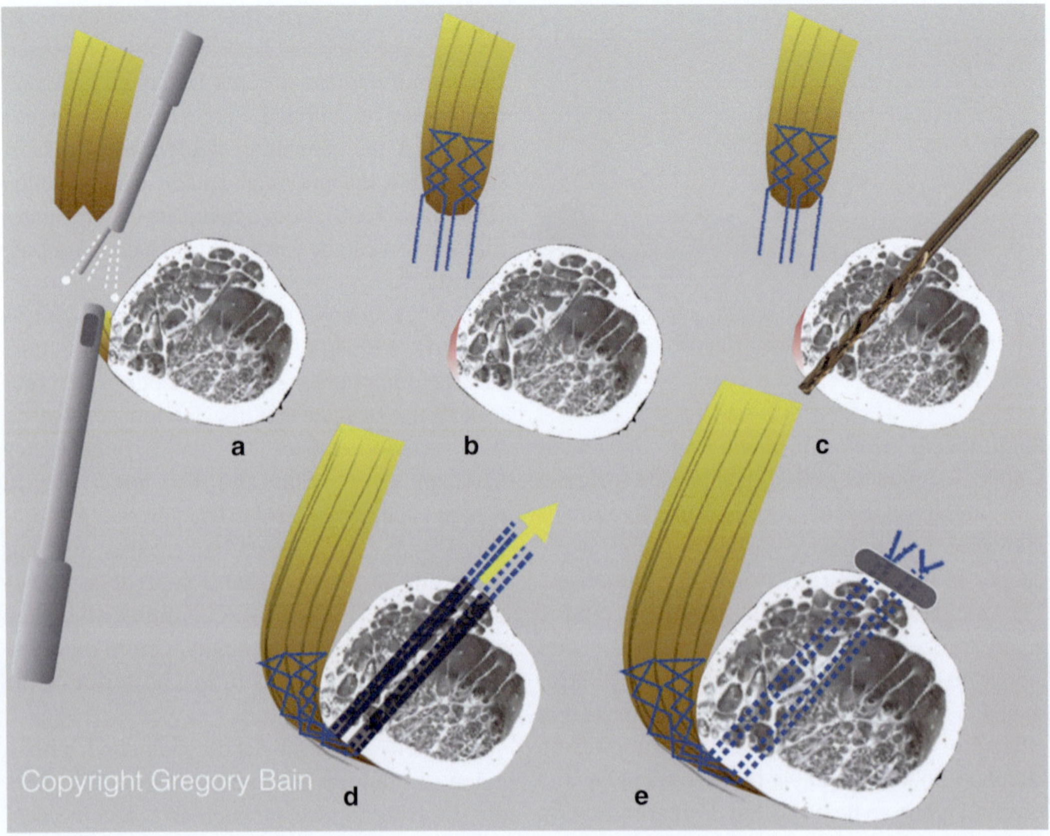

Fig. 22.5 Distal biceps tendon endoscopic-assisted repair. (**a**) Debridement of the torn tendon stump and burring of the radial tuberosity surface. (**b**) Tendon stump is prepared with a whipstitch with non-absorbable suture material. (**c**) Two oblique drill holes created from the radial anterior cortex to the dorsal ulnar surface. (**d**) Looped nylon suture material advanced through drill holes. (**e**) Sutures tied over the Endobutton, securing the tendon to the ulnar aspect of the tuberosity

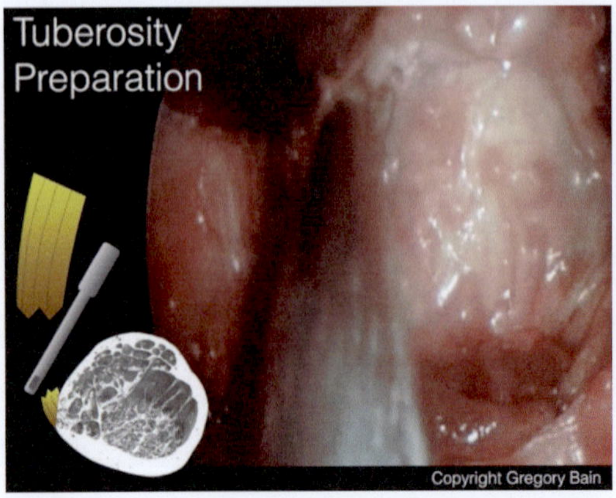

Fig. 22.6 Endoscopic-assisted debridement of the radial tuberosity

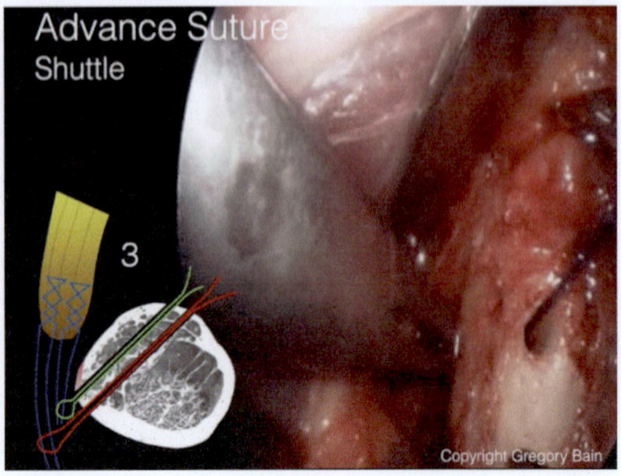

Fig. 22.7 The suture material is advanced through the oblique drill holes and grasped on the posterior aspect

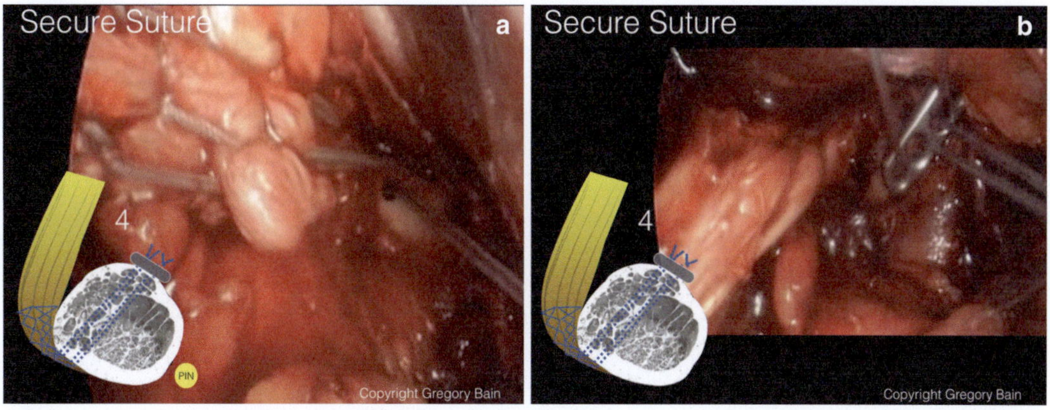

Fig. 22.8 Fixation of the distal biceps tendon to the radial tuberosity. (**a**) The suture restores the tendon to the radial tuberosity. (**b**) The Endobutton is securely fastened to the anterior radius

22.6.4 Chronic Biceps Tendon Rupture

The management of chronic biceps tendon rupture is operative if the patient has a high demand and at low surgical risk. An open approach is usually used, the tendon identified and mobilised. In severe cases, semitendinosus autograft or allograft can be used. Repairs in extreme flexion have been shown to have good outcomes, with no loss of motion compared to the contralateral side (Dillon et al. 2011; Morrey et al. 2014). Surgery in chronic cases can be complicated by neurovascular damage, significant tendon retraction and reduced tendon mobilisation, likely requiring augmentation if retracted greater than 4 cm (Dillon et al. 2011).

22.7 Outcomes

The outcome postsurgical repair of distal biceps tendon rupture is positive. Following repair, physiotherapy can be used to improve strength, and mobility should be encouraged for patients with grade 0 and 1A. Patients with grade 1B to grade 4 are advised to use a sling and mobilise as tolerated with no resisted flexion or supination for 6 weeks. In a series of 23 patients, Morrey et al. (Morrey et al. 2014) found that all patients were subjectively very satisfied or satisfied with the outcome and full return to work. Dillon et al. (Dillon et al. 2011) established that Endobutton produced no loss of motion and recovered 101% of flexion strength and 99% supination strength. Conversely, unrepaired biceps tendon rupture was found by Freeman et al. to have a 37% decrease in supination strength and a statistically insignificant 7% in elbow flexion strength. Endurance is also reduced in nonoperative management, with 47% supination deficit and 21% in flexion (Baker and Bierwagen 1985; Freeman et al. 2009).

22.8 Complications

Reported complications include infection, rerupture, pain, haematoma, neurological complications and fracture through proximal radius drill holes. Complication rates increase in revision or chronic injuries. Nerve palsies are usually transient and most commonly involve the lateral cutaneous nerve of the forearm, posterior interosseous nerve, superficial branch of the radial nerve and, infrequently, the median nerve (Gregory et al. 2009). Rare complications including heterotopic ossification and radioulnar synostosis have also been reported and are associated with the two-incision technique (Peeters et al. 2009).

References

Athwal G, Steinmann S, Rispoli D (2007) The distal biceps tendon: footprint and relevant clinical anatomy. The Journal of Hand Surgery 32(8):1225–1229

Bain G, Johnson L, Turner P (2008) Treatment of partial distal biceps tendon tears. Sports Med Arthrosc Rev 16(3):154–161

Bain G, Phadnis J, Saeed H (2016) Biceps tendon pathology. In: Pederzini L, Eygendaal D, Denti M (eds) Elbow and Sport, 1st edn. Springer, New York, pp 143–152

Bain G, Prem H, Heptinstall R, Verhellen R, Paix D (2000) Repair of distal biceps tendon rupture: a new technique using the Endobutton. J Shoulder Elb Surg 9(2):120–126

Baker B, Bierwagen D (1985) Rupture of the distal tendon of the biceps brachii. Operative versus non-operative treatment. J Bone Joint Surg 67(3):414–417

Bourne M, Morrey B (1991) Partial rupture of the distal biceps tendon. Clin Orthop Relat Res 271:143–148

Boyd H, Anderson L (1961) A method for reinsertion of the distal biceps brachii tendon. The Journal of Bone & Joint Surgery 43(7):1041–1043

D'Alessandro D, Shields C, Tibone J, Chandler R (1993) Repair of distal biceps tendon ruptures in athletes. Am J Sports Med 21(1):114–119

Dellaero D, Mallon W (2006) Surgical treatment of partial biceps tendon ruptures at the elbow. J Shoulder Elb Surg 15(2):215–217

Dillon M, Bollier M, King J (2011) Repair of acute and chronic distal biceps tendon ruptures using the Endobutton. Hand 6(1):39–46

Dürr H, Stäbler A, Pfahler M, Matzko M, Refior H (2000) Partial rupture of the distal biceps tendon. Clin Orthop Relat Res 374:195–200

Eames M, Bain G (2006) Distal biceps tendon endoscopy and anterior elbow arthroscopy portal. Tech Shoulder Elbow Surg 7(3):139–142

Eames M, Bain G, Fogg Q, Van Riet R (2007) Distal biceps tendon anatomy: a cadaveric study. J Bone Joint Surg (Am) 89:1044–1045

Festa A, Mulieri P, Newman J, Spitz D, Leslie B (2010) Effectiveness of magnetic resonance imaging in detecting partial and complete distal biceps tendon rupture. J Hand Surg 35(1):77–83

Freeman C, McCormick K, Mahoney D, Baratz M, Lubahn J (2009) Nonoperative treatment of distal biceps tendon ruptures compared with a historical control group. J Bone Joint Surg (Am) 91(10):2329–2334

Giuffrè B, Moss M (2004) Optimal positioning for MRI of the distal biceps brachii tendon: flexed abducted supinated view. Am J Roentgenol 182(4):944–946

Grégory T, Roure P, Fontés D (2009) Repair of distal biceps tendon rupture using a suture anchor: description of a new endoscopic procedure. Am J Sports Med 37(3):506–511

Heinzelmann A, Savoie F, Ramsey J, Field L, Mazzocca A (2009) A combined technique for distal biceps repair using a soft tissue button and biotenodesis interference screw. Am J Sports Med 37(5):989–994

Jarrett C, Weir D, Stuffmann E, Jain S, Miller M, Schmidt C (2012) Anatomic and biomechanical analysis of the short and long head components of the distal biceps tendon. J Shoulder Elb Surg 21(7):942–948

Mazzocca A, Spang J, Arciero R (2008) Distal biceps rupture. Orthop Clin N Am 39(2):237–249

McKee M, Hirji R, Schemitsch E, Wild L, Waddell J (2005) Patient-oriented functional outcome after repair of distal biceps tendon ruptures using a single-incision technique. J Shoulder Elb Surg 14(3):302–306

Morrey M, Abdel M, Sanchez-Sotelo J, Morrey B (2014) Primary repair of retracted distal biceps tendon ruptures in extreme flexion. J Shoulder Elb Surg 23(5):679–685

Nesterenko S, Domire Z, Morrey B, Sanchez-Sotelo J (2010) Elbow strength and endurance in patients with a ruptured distal biceps tendon. J Shoulder Elb Surg 19(2):184–189

O'Driscoll S, Goncalves L, Dietz P (2007) The hook test for distal biceps tendon avulsion. Am J Sports Med 35(11):1865–1869

Peeters T, Ching-Soon N, Jansen N, Sneyers C, Declercq G, Verstreken F (2009) Functional outcome after repair of distal biceps tendon ruptures using the Endobutton technique. J Shoulder Elb Surg 18(2):283–287

Phadnis J, Bain G (2015) Endoscopic-assisted distal biceps footprint repair. Tech Hand Up Extrem Surg 19(2):55–59

Phadnis J, Bain G (2017) Distal biceps tendinopathy. In: Ring D, Steinmann S (eds) Advanced reconstruction: elbow, 2nd edn. American Academy of Orthopaedic Surgeons, Rosemont, IL, pp 81–90

Ramsey M (1999) Distal biceps tendon injuries: diagnosis and management. J Am Acad Orthop Surg 7(3):199–207

Safran M, Graham S (2002) Distal biceps tendon ruptures: incidence, demographics and the effect of smoking. Clin Orthop Relat Res 404:275–283

Sharma S, MacKay G (2005) Endoscopic repair of distal biceps tendon using an endobutton. Arthroscopy 21(7):891–897

Smith J, Finnoff J, O'Driscoll S, Lai J (2010) Sonographic evaluation of the distal biceps tendon using a medial approach. J Ultrasound Med 29(5):861–865

Visuri T, Lindholm H (1994) Bilateral distal biceps tendon avulsions with use of anabolic steroids. Med Sci Sports Exerc 26(8):941–944

Hand and Wrist Tendinopathies

23

Margaret Woon Man Fok, Bo Liu, John White, and Gregory Bain

Contents

M.W.M. Fok (✉)
Department of Orthopaedics and Traumatology, Queen Mary Hospital, The University of Hong Kong, Pok Fu Lam, Hong Kong
e-mail: margaret_fok@yahoo.com

B. Liu
Department of Hand Surgery, Beijing Ji Shui Tan Hospital, Beijing, China
e-mail: bobliu7@hotmail.com

J. White • G. Bain
Department of Orthopaedic Surgery, Flinders University and Flinders Medical Centre, Adelaide, SA, Australia
e-mail: dr.jwhite@ashna.net; admin@gregbain.com.au

Injuries to the tendons or its associated structures of hands and wrists are common in sport activities. They are easily missed and are usually underestimated by the patients themselves. They can occur after a single traumatic injury or can be resulted from repetitive insults. Tendons can either be avulsed from bone, e.g. flexor digitorum profundus (FDP) tendon avulsion (jersey finger) and terminal finger extensor tendon avulsion (mallet finger), or subluxated from its designated route, e.g. extensor tendon subluxation or extensor carpi ulnaris (ECU) subluxation. Meanwhile, the tendon sheath can also undergo inflammation and result in stenosing tendonitis, e.g. trigger finger and de Quervain's disease.

23.1 Acute Conditions

The common hand and wrist tendinopathies that are resulted from a single traumatic event are jersey fingers, mallet fingers and extensor tendon subluxation. They are often treated as sprain and are being disregarded.

23.1.1 Flexor Digitorum Profundus (FDP) Tendon Avulsion

Flexor digitorum profundus tendon avulsion, also commonly referred as jersey finger, describes an injury which is seen in American football when a tackler grasps the jersey of another player while he pulls away. It occurs when the distal

G.L. Canata et al. (eds.), *Muscle and Tendon Injuries*, DOI 10.1007/978-3-662-54184-5_23

interphalangeal joint (DIPJ) of a finger is forcefully extended from an actively flexed position. A painful "pop" may be felt at times. The ring finger is the most commonly affected finger (Leddy and Parker 1977). It is postulated that it has the least independent movement of all fingers (Leddy and Parker 1977; Gunter 1960; Lunn and Lamb 1984).

Leddy and Parker first proposed to classify the injury into three types in 1977 based on the point of failure and the extent of the retraction of the avulsed tendon (Leddy and Parker 1977). It is later being modified to include types 4 and 5 (Fig. 23.1) (Al-Qattan 2001; Smith 1981).

Patient with jersey finger usually presents with a stiff and swollen finger with a classic description of the injury mechanism. A loss of DIPJ flexion is observed. Tenderness may be felt along the flexor tendon sheath, and a mass suggesting the location of the FDP stump can sometimes be palpated. Radiographs of the affected finger are taken to assess bone integrity of the distal phalanx. Dynamic ultrasound and MRI can also be used to confirm the diagnosis and to assess the extent of stump retraction.

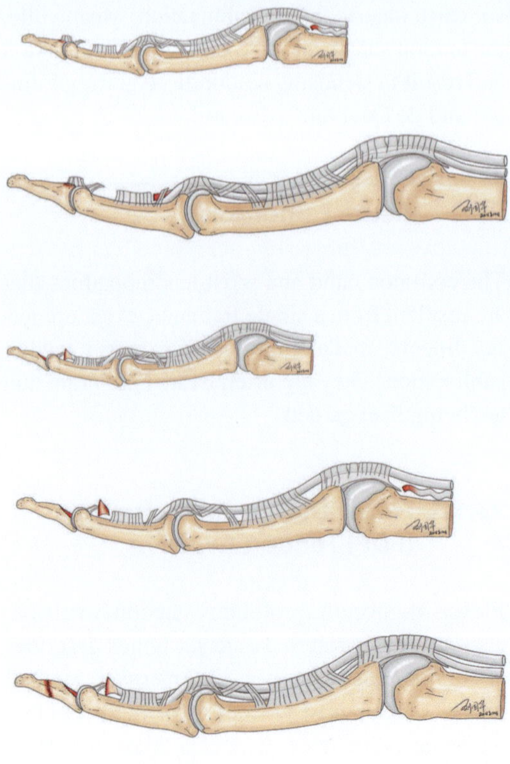

Fig. 23.1 Classification of jersey fingers Type 1 - 5 (copyright Dr. Margaret Fok)

23.1.1.1 Management

Surgical treatment is advocated for all types of jersey fingers in the acute settings. The classification system bears prognostic value. As there is a loss of nutrient supply of the tendon with the rupture of both short and long vinculum in type 1 injury, early surgery of tendon to bone repair within 10 days is advised to prevent necrosis of the tendon (Leddy and Parker 1977). Meanwhile, a less significant loss in nutrient supply is noted for type 2 injury due to the preservation of long vinculum. Though early repair is recommended, successful outcomes have been reported for as late as 3 months after surgery (Leddy and Parker 1977).

For type 3 injury, as the FDP is avulsed together with a bony fragment of the distal phalanx, retraction is not a concern and treatment can be done by fixing the bone fragment to the distal phalanx with screw(s) or Kirschner wires. Type 4 injury involves both bone avulsion and FDP rupture. Thus, both bone fixation and tendon repair are advocated. Meanwhile, for type 5 injury, the treatment plan depends on the severity of the distal phalanx fractures. Fixation of fracture can be performed in some cases. In severe comminuted fracture cases, direct tendon to bone repair may be chosen instead. The DIPJ may need to be stabilized based on the involvement of the articular surface and the stability of the joint (Tuttle et al. 2006).

Tendon to bone repair can be achieved by bringing the stump of the tendon to the bone by either using suture anchor(s) or using osseous tunnels with pullout button on the finger nail. The technique of using pullout button has enjoyed a long history of successful outcome (Bunnell 1948; Leddy 1985; Skoff et al. 1995). However, due to the irritation of the button, people are now shifting to the use of suture anchor(s). While it has proven to have a comparable load to failure strength with the pullout button, its fatigue to failure of the anchor bone interface has yet to be confirmed (Brustein et al. 2001). The adjustment of tendon tension in tendon to bone repair is important. A normal resting cascade of the fingers needs to be achieved after the repair. An excessive tension of the FDP repaired tendon may give rise to quadriga phenomenon (Schreuders 2012).

Regardless of the treatment methods, rehabilitation after the repair of the tendon is long, as protection to prevent forced extension and gripping activities is needed for around 12 weeks. Some athletes opt to treat this condition either in a delayed manner, i.e. to wait for the completion of a season or nonoperatively. This may be feasible if the patient has a full range of movement of the proximal interphalangeal joint (PIPJ) of the finger and a stable DIPJ (Goldfarb et al. 2016). The stump of the retracted FDP may be excised if discomfort is noted.

23.1.2 Mallet Finger

Mallet finger is the failure of the terminal extensor digitorum tendon, instead of the FDP tendon as of the jersey finger. It occurs when the DIPJ is forcefully flexed in an actively extended position or in axial loading. It is commonly seen in sport injuries like football, basketball or volleyball games (Wehbe and Schneider 1984). Like the jersey finger, it can be a result of either a detachment of the tendon from the bone or a bone avulsion of the dorsal base of the distal phalanx.

Mallet finger can be presented with a swelling of the DIPJ and a flexion deformity of the DIPJ of the affected finger. When tested, a failure to actively extend the DIPJ can be observed. Radiograph is often needed to assess whether there is a bony component to the injury (Fig. 23.2a) and whether there is an associated DIPJ palmar subluxation.

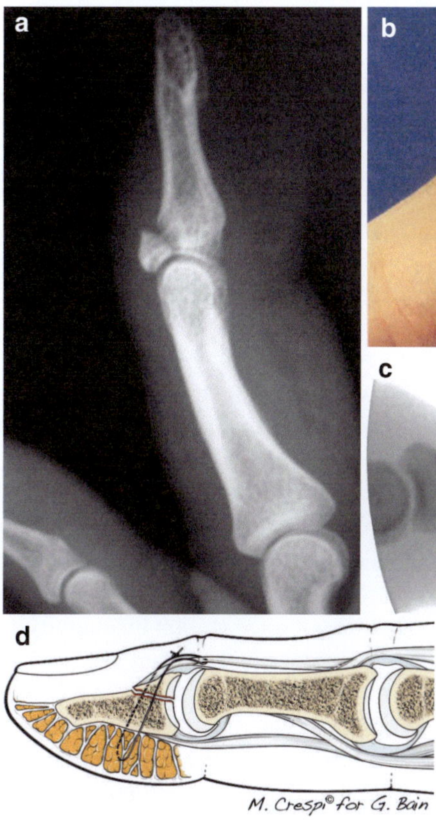

Fig. 23.2 (**a**) Mallet finger x-ray, (**b**) mallet splint and (**c**) Ishiguro technique, which involves an extension block wire to hold the fragment and a longitudinal wire across the DIP joint. Note there is still some dorsal subluxation in this image. (**d**) Internal tension band suture technique for mallet finger fracture. The suture captures the septae of the finger and secures the extensor mechanism to it. A neutralization K wire is also required (copyright Dr. Gregory Bain). (**e**) Small dorsal plate and neutralization of K wire

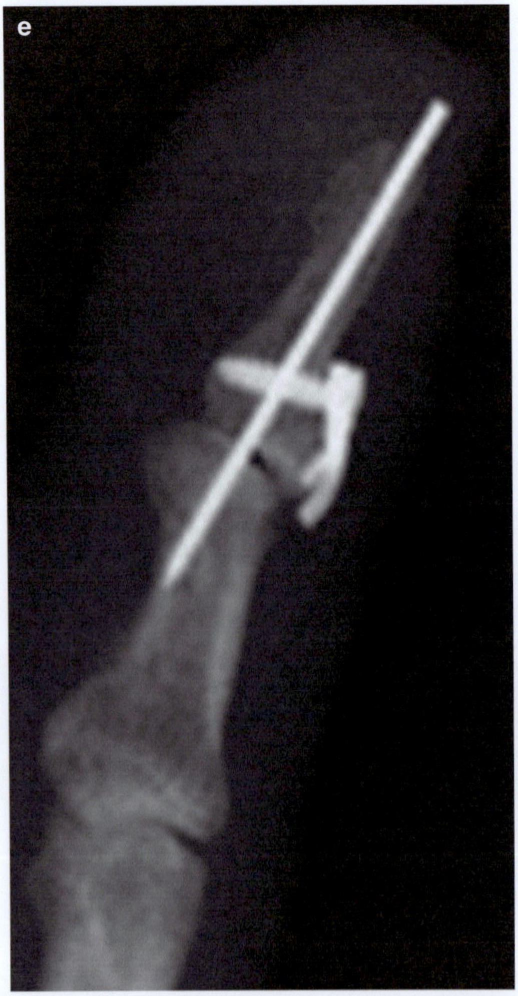

Fig. 23.2 (continued)

23.1.2.1 Management

Unlike jersey finger, most mallet fingers can be satisfactorily treated with splint only (Fig. 23.2b) (Okafor et al. 1997; Stern and Kastrup 1988). This is even applicable for patients with delayed presentation. A short mallet splint to keep the DIPJ in extension for 6–8 weeks is often advocated (Crawford 1984; Kinninmonth and Holburn 1986). Garberman et al. showed that satisfactory outcome can be achieved with splint in mallet fingers of an average of 53 days from injury (Garberman et al. 1994). In the presence of a fracture, a lateral radiograph of the affected finger, together with the splint, is needed to ensure that no joint subluxation is created post application of the splint. It is well known that they can subluxate up to 3 weeks, so repeat imaging is required (Crawford 1984).

Surgical treatment has previously been recommended for fractures which involve more than 30% of the articular surface and palmar subluxation of DIPJ (Hamas et al. 1978). Kirschner wires and screws may be used (Damron et al. 1993; Hofmeister et al. 2003; Tuttle et al. 2006). This can restore the articular surface and prevent secondary degenerative changes. Moreover, early mobilization of the joint and prevention of skin complications, created by splint, have been proposed (Nakamura and Nanjyo 1994). Nevertheless, despite the presence of a large articular fragment and even joint subluxation, studies have shown satisfactory results with splint alone (Okafor et al. 1997; Wehbe and Schneider 1984). If there is marked subluxation, we would often use the Ishiguro technique, which involves an extension block wire to hold the fragment and a longitudinal wire across the DIP joint (Ishiguro et al. 1997) (Fig. 23.2c). If it is a delayed presentation, then it may not be possible to reduce the fracture with this percutaneous technique, in which case we use an internal tension band suture technique (Bauze and Bain 1999) (Fig. 23.2d) or a small hooked plate protected by neutralization k-wire (Fig. 23.2e).

Both conservative and operative treatments for mallet finger have been associated with a high complication rates (Stern and Kastrup 1988; Wehbe and Schneider 1984). While the complications of conservative therapy are often transient like skin ulceration from the splint, the complications of surgical intervention are often more long term, e.g. joint incongruity, infection, nail deformity and implant failure. It is known that a residual extension lag of an average of 8^0 is observed with the treatment of splint (Okafor et al. 1997). While this will not lead to any functional deficit, patient may regard this as a poor cosmetic outcome. Thus, we recommend reserving surgery for a specific group of patients who desire to have early mobilization and better cosmetic outcome.

23.1.3 Extensor Tendon Subluxation

Traumatic subluxation of the extensor tendon at the metacarpophalangeal joint (MCPJ) is a relatively less common sport injury when compare to mallet finger and jersey finger. It is caused by the rupture of sagittal band, the primary stabilizer of the extensor tendon at the MCPJ level (Fig. 23.3a). The mechanisms of injury are usually direct trauma, forced flexion or resisted extension of the MCPJ (Inoue and Tamura 1996; Lin and Strauch 2014).

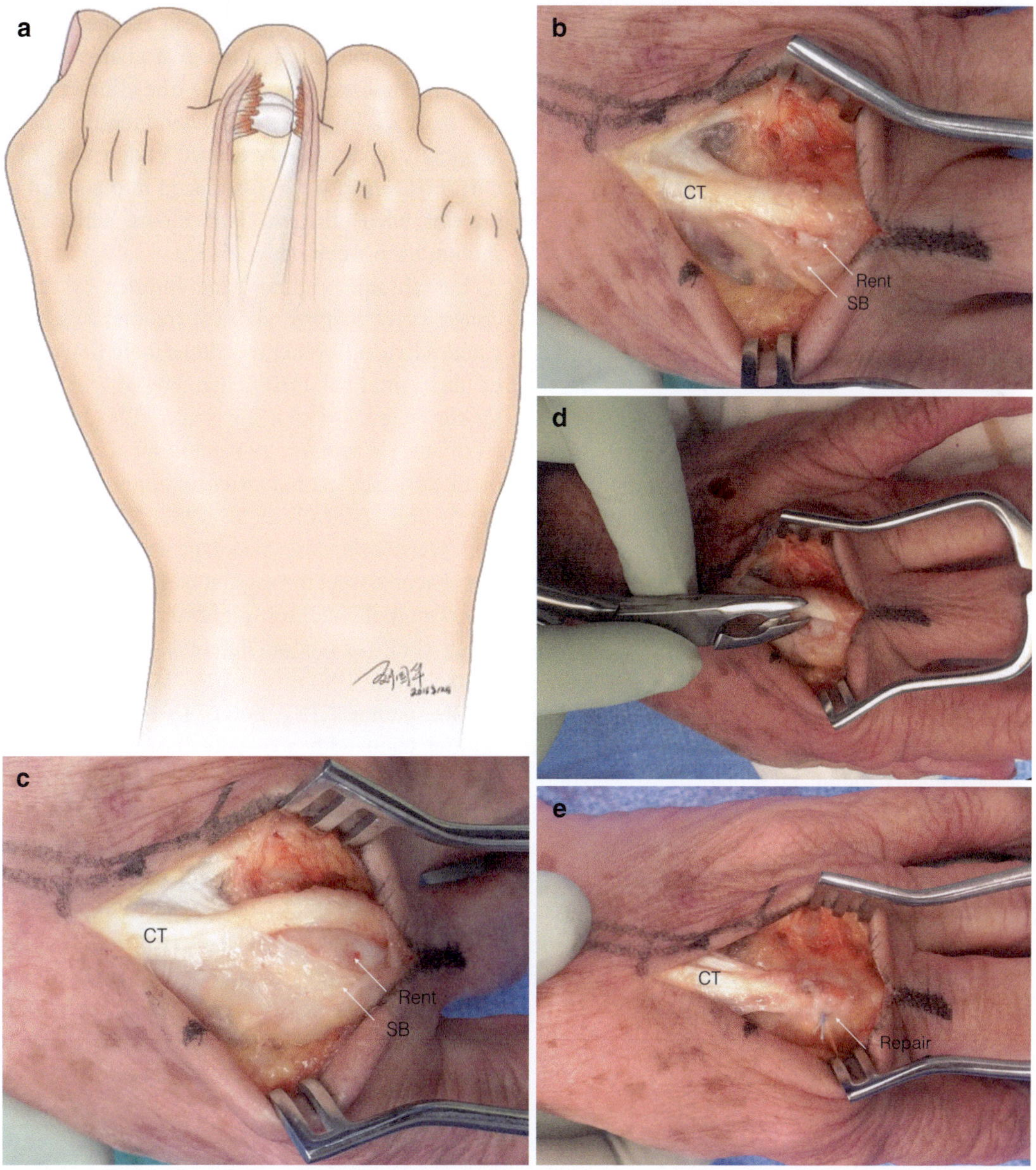

Fig. 23.3 (**a**) Radial sagittal band rupture causing extensor tendon subluxation to the ulnar side (copyright Dr. Margaret Fok). (**b**) Intraoperative view, with the rent in the sagittal band identified (*white arrow*). As the finger is straight, the central tendon is in the midline. (**c**) With finger flexion the rent opens and allows the tendon to subluxate to the ulnar side. (**d**) The granulation tissue is debrided, including any synovium. (**e**) The sagittal band is sutured to the central tendon. (**f**) With finger flexion the central tendon remains stable. (**g**) A dynamic splint is required for 6 weeks until the tendon heals. This splint keeps the MCP joint extended but allows the PIP to mobilize (Fig. 23.3b–g: copyright Dr. Gregory Bain)

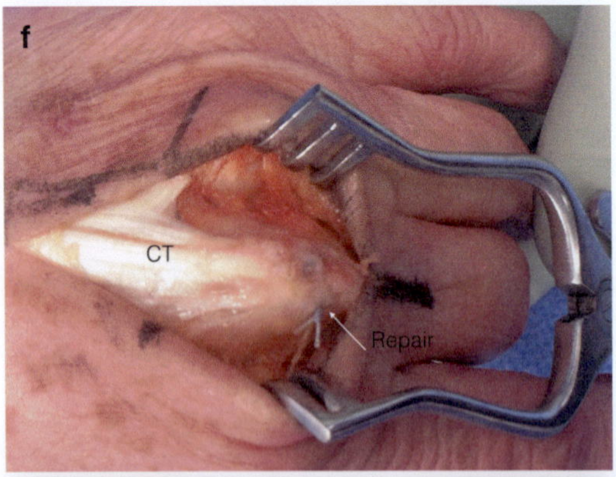

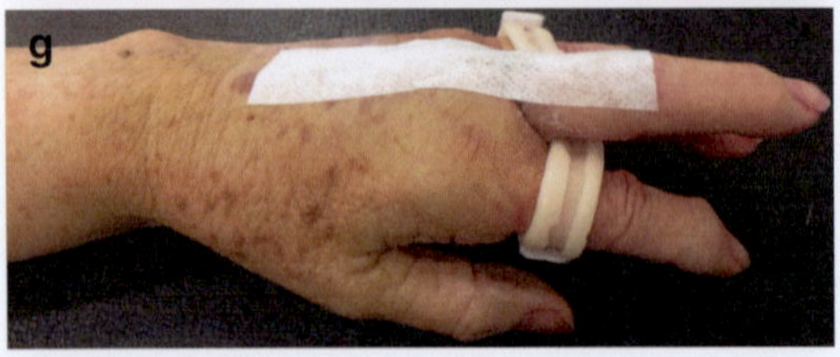

Fig. 23.3 (continued)

Patient often presents with a snapping pain in the MCPJ of the affected finger. They may either observe the subluxation of the tendon on active finger flexion or complain of a loss in active extension of the affected finger. Passive finger extending position can be maintained. As the radial sagittal band is longer and thinner than the ulnar counterpart, the rupture usually occurs on the radial side, resulting in an ulnar subluxation of the tendon (Young and Rayan 2000). The middle finger is most commonly affected (Inoue and Tamura 1996). There is also a related condition that occurs commonly in boxers and karate practitioners named boxer's knuckle (Nagaoka et al. 2006). It is a chronic condition which occurs due to repeated punching motion and involves a tear of the MCPJ and sagittal band rupture.

23.1.3.1 Management

Treatment for extensor tendon subluxation can be conservative in the acute stage, i.e. within 3 weeks from injury (Rayan and Murray 1994). After the reduction of the extensor tendon into its designated route with MCPJ in extension, splint is applied to block MCPJ from flexion while freeing PIPJ. Buddy splint may also be added. The splint is applied for 6–8 weeks. Catalano et al. (2006) reported 8 of 11 injuries had no pain and either minimal or no subluxation at an average of a 14-month follow-up, while Rayan and Murry (1994) reported 12 of 18 injuries had no pain and tendon subluxation at an average of a 13-month follow-up.

In the subacute group, it is possible to still repair the sagittal band, without the need for a full reconstruction. This does give a better insight into the pathoanatomy and the true clinical problem (Fig. 23.3b). The sagittal band requires to be surgically repaired to the central tendon (Fig. 23.3 c–f). Post-operatively it is placed into a splint to prevent MCP flexion, but allows active PIP motion for 6 weeks (Fig. 23.3g).

For chronic sagittal band injuries or failed conservative therapy, surgical treatment is indicated. Many different procedures including repair of the sagittal band (Kettelkamp et al. 1971) and tendon stabilization using grafts like juncturae tendinum (Wheeldon 1954) and local proximal- or distal-based partial extensor digitorum communis slips (Carroll et al. 1987; Watson et al. 1997) have been described. One author (MF) prefers to reconstruct the sagittal band with a distally based partial extensor digitorum to create the radial sling for tendon stabilization (Fig. 23.4a) (Carroll et al. 1987).

One author (GB) prefers to reconstruct the sagittal band with a distally based strip of the common extensor tendon to the deep intermetacarpal ligament (DIML). The advantage of this technique is that it reconstructs the sagittal band, without compromising the adjacent anatomical structures (Fig. 23.4b). The opposite half of the extensor tendon is chosen and then passed through the central tendon at the level of the proximal border of the sagittal band. We pass it through the midsection of the tendon, so that it translates the tendon back to the central position, without rolling the tendon. The free end of the tendon is then passed under the DIML with a Lahey curved clamp. It is then passed back to perforate the central tendon in the line of the distal aspect of the sagittal band. It is taken through a range of motion and ligated so that it will control the position of the central tendon throughout the motion.

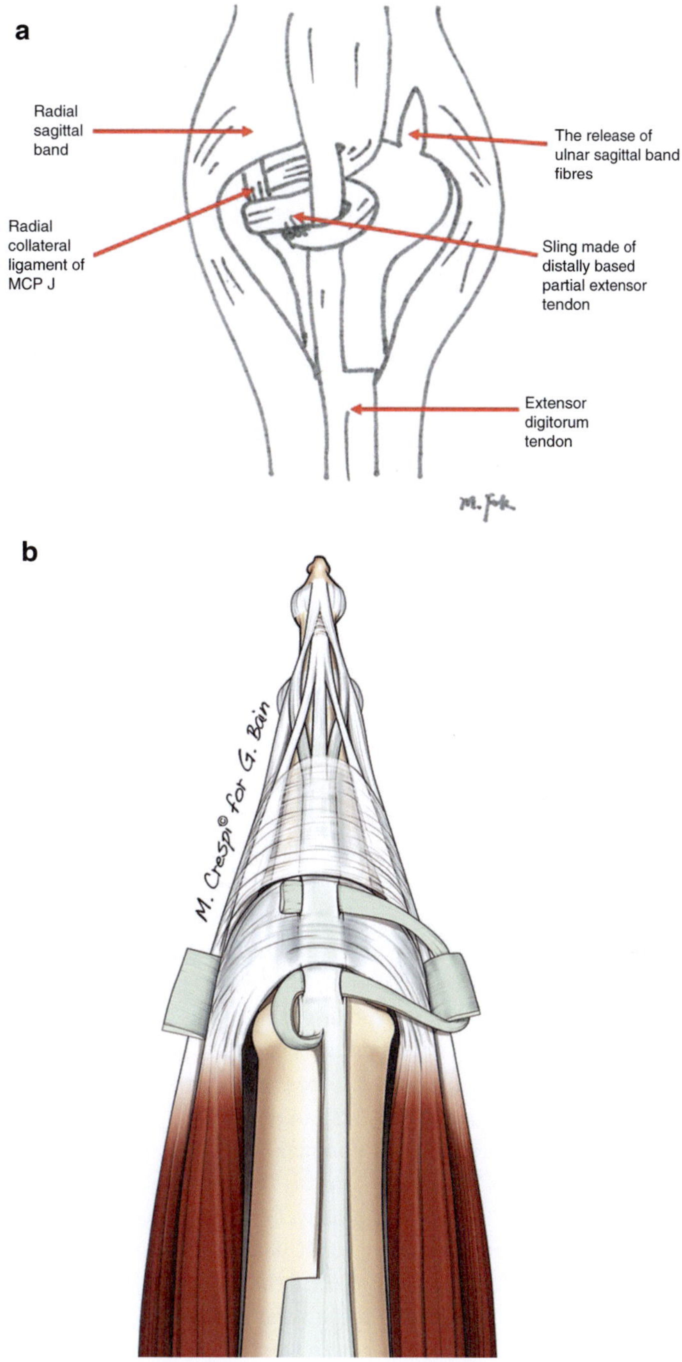

Fig. 23.4 (**a**) Reconstruction of the sagittal band with half of the central tendon, passed around the collateral ligament (copyright Dr. Margaret Fok). (**b**) Sagittal band reconstruction with a half strip of the common extensor tendon. The half strip passes through the central tendon, at the proximal edge of the sagittal band. It then passes deep to the DIML and back through the central tendon at the level of the distal margin of the sagittal band (copyright Dr. Gregory Bain)

23.2 Chronic Conditions

Apart from acute traumatic injuries, there are numerous hand and wrist tendinopathies that are precipitated by repetitive use in sport activities. The most common conditions are extensor carpi ulnaris (ECU) subluxation, de Quervain's disease and trigger finger.

23.2.1 Extensor Carpi Ulnaris (ECU) Subluxation

Extensor carpi ulnaris subluxation is a condition that is usually missed after a traumatic event. With subsequent repetitive stress on the wrist in selected sport activities, it may lead to symptomatic recurrent ECU subluxation, presented as painful snapping of the tendon during wrist rotation. The incidence of this condition reported in the literature has been low, likely owing to its missed diagnosis as wrist sprain. With the recent increase interest in the causes of ulnar wrist pain and distal radioulnar joint instability, the condition is being better recognized.

The ECU tendon is part of the sixth extensor compartment of the wrist and is bound by the fibro-osseous tunnel, with the ulnar groove as the floor and the extensor retinaculum and ECU sub-sheath as the roof (Campbell et al. 2013). It acts as a wrist extensor when the forearm is in supination and an ulnar deviator when the forearm is in pronation. It also contributes to the stability of the distal radioulnar joint (DRUJ), together with the triangular fibrocartilage complex (TFCC). Significant tension is created on the ECU retinaculum and sub-sheath during activities involving the forearm in supination, wrist flexion and ulnar deviation. In turn, it may lead to the rupture of the ECU tendon sheath and the volar subluxation of the tendon. Patients playing tennis, golf and rugby may suffer from this condition (Campbell et al. 2013).

Patient with ECU subluxation may complain of painful snapping or clicking sensation over the dorso-ulnar wrist during wrist supination and pronation. This may limit his ability to perform activities of daily living, sports and hobbies. In some instances, patients may be able to voluntarily subluxate the tendon. Physical examination reveals tenderness along the length of the ECU tendon. Pain on resisted active wrist extension and ulnar deviation can be observed. It is noted that the tendon is only subluxable under active contraction of the ECU. Thus, active supination with the affected wrist head in maximal flexion and ulnar deviation will produce visible subluxation of the tendon, while passive movement will not produce this sign.

Imaging like ultrasound and MRI may be used to supplement the clinical diagnosis. In addition, MRI can be used to rule out other causes of ulnar wrist pain like TFCC tear, while ultrasound may provide a dynamic assessment, showing the subluxation of the tendon on movement (MacLennan et al. 2008).

23.2.1.1 Management

For early diagnosis of an acute ECU tendon subluxation, conservative therapy with short arm cast or splint, for 1–3 months, can be done (Campbell et al. 2013; Montalvan et al. 2006). Montalvan et al. study showed that all 12 patients had stabilized ECU tendon even under stressed condition, after a period of up to 4 months of immobilization. However, for chronic symptomatic cases or athletes who are reluctant to undergo prolonged period of splinting, surgical stabilization is indicated. Numerous techniques have been described to reconstruct the ECU sub-sheath with satisfactory results noted (Burkhart 1982; MacLennan et al. 2008). Our preferred method is using Burkhart's technique, of which it uses part of the extensor retinaculum to reconstruct and stabilize the ECU in the dorsal aspect of the wrist (Fig. 23.5) (Burkhart 1982).

23.2.2 de Quervain's Disease

de Quervain's disease is stenosing tenosynovitis which affects the first extensor compartment of the wrist, i.e. the extensor pollicis brevis (EPB) and abductor pollicis longus (APL) (Fig. 23.6a).

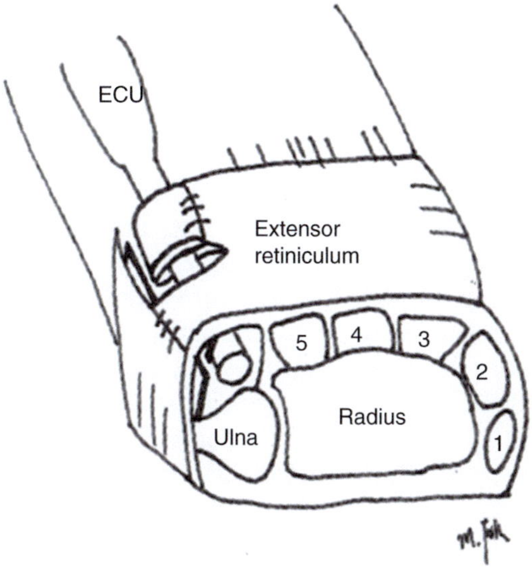

Fig. 23.5 ECU tendon stabilization procedure

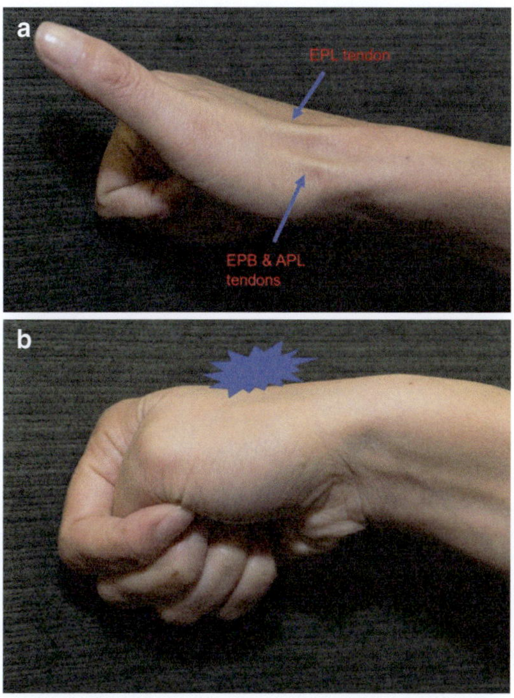

Fig. 23.6 (**a**) Affected tendons in de Quervain's disease. (**b**) Finklestein test

It is due to the repetitive use of the thumb in activities which involve radioulnar deviation such as hammering, climbing or lifting a child or pet. In sports, it is usually associated with activities that require strong thumb movement in a closed hand grip, like squash, badminton, rowing and golf (Retting 2004).

Patient typically presents with pain and swelling over the dorsal radial aspect of the wrist. These symptoms are aggravated by either resisted motion of the thumb or radial deviation and wrist extension. Physical examination of the patient reveals tenderness along the first extensor compartment. Finkelstein test causing the stretching of the tendons is usually positive (Fig. 23.6b) (Finklestein 1930).

The diagnosis of de Quervain's disease is mainly based on clinical examination and history. Radiographs of the wrist are usually unremarkable in de Quervain's disease, but it is useful in differentiating osteoarthritis of the first carpo-metacarpal joint (CMCJ) in suspicious cases. Ultrasound of the first extensor compartment may reveal distension of the tendon sheath with a surrounded fluid film.

23.2.2.1 Management

Treatment of de Quervain's disease is often started with conservative therapy including rest, non-steroidal anti-inflammatory medications and splint (Adam and Habbu 2015). The splint is a forearm-based thumb spica that is used to enforce a period of rest and prevent motions that exacerbate symptoms. Physiotherapy including cryotherapy, ultrasound and iontophoresis may be given (Hartzell et al. 2013). Corticosteroid injection is currently the most successful non-surgical treatment modality with a 62–100% success rate (Jirarattanaphochai et al. 2004; Peter-Veluthamaningal et al. 2009; Richie and Briner 2003).

Surgical release is offered for patients with de Quervain's disease, who fail conservative treatment. It involves the release of the sheath covering the first dorsal compartment, together with the sub-sheath that separates the EPB and APL tendons when present. Multiple tendon slips of APL are sometimes present (Jaskson et al. 1986). Failure to release these sub-sheaths may lead to recurrence or residual symptoms. Care also needs to be taken to identify and protect the superficial branch of the radial nerve during surgical release.

23.2.3 Trigger Finger

Trigger finger is another common condition of stenosing tenosynovitis. Due to the thickening of the A1 pulley and, to a lesser extent, the flexor tendons at the MCPJ level, the gliding of the flexor tendons is affected (Fig. 23.7a). The causes of developing trigger finger are multifactorial and include genetic basis, systemic conditions like diabetes mellitus and rheumatoid arthritis and occupational issues (Lundin et al. 2012). In sports, it may be aggravated by ball sports, especially if the ball is frequently held in one hand, e.g. handball, basketball and rugby.

Patients initially present with pain at the level of the A1 pulley, which may progress to triggering or locking. Patients may complain of a reduction in grip strength, clicking, catching or locking (Adam and Habbu 2015). In examination, a nodule may be palpated at the site of the A1 pulley.

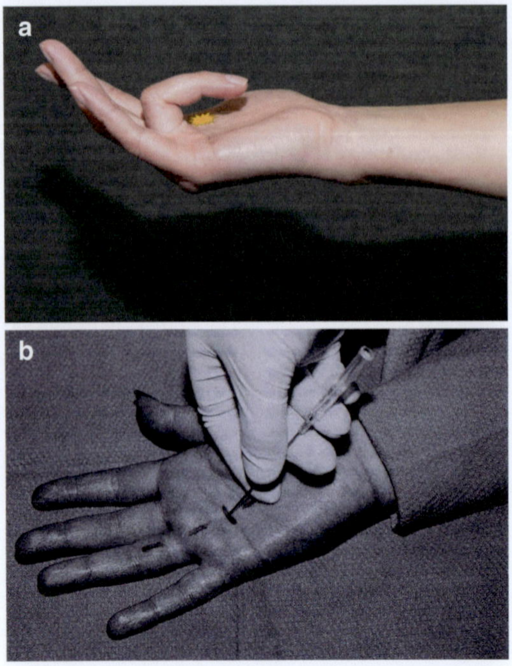

Fig. 23.7 (**a**) Trigger finger, showing catching of the finger when trying to straighten it. (**b**) Percutaneous release of a trigger finger with a 14 gauge intravenous cannular needle. Local anaesthetic is infiltrated into the area of the A1 pulley. A 14 gauge cannula is introduced just proximal to the A1 pulley land mark. The sharp bevel of the needle is then used to cut the pulley (copyright Dr. Gregory Bain)

Triggering may be felt when the finger attempts to extend from a flexed position. In chronic changes, due to the persistent locking of the finger, PIPJ contracture can develop.

23.2.3.1 Management

Like de Quervain's disease, the main stay of management in trigger finger is conservative therapy (Adam and Habbu 2015). Rest, massage and non-steroidal anti-inflammatory medication are usually advised. Physiotherapy including ultrasound, wax and magnetic pulse therapy may be given. Corticosteroid injection into the A1 pulley is a first-line treatment with a success response rate of 60–90% (Dala-Ali et al. 2012). Recurrence is high especially in the background of concomitant diabetes mellitus, multiple affected digits and other associated tendinopathies. Poor outcomes are also noted in the presence of flexion contracture.

Surgical release is advocated for failure after a course of conservative therapy or in the presence of PIPJ flexion contracture. Either percutaneous or open release of the A1 pulley can be performed under local anaesthesia (Fig. 23.7b) (Bain et al. 1995; Bain and Wallwork 1999; Turowski et al. 1997). The percutaneous release is an office-based procedure, where the 14 gauge needle is advanced just proximal to the A1 pulley and then released with the sharp edge of the needle. Excellent results can be achieved in both techniques (Gilberts et al. 2001; Saldana 2001).

23.2.4 Flexor Tendon Adhesions

Flexor tendon adhesion is not an uncommon condition after prolonged immobilization, which may be caused by both soft tissue injuries and fractures. Fingers are stiff with an inability to fully extend and flex the fingers.

23.2.4.1 Management

After a digital nerve block, the finger is approached via a Brunner incision. Nylon tapes assist in mobilizing the flexor tendons, preserving the A2 and A4 pulleys. If the pulleys are absent, then they may need to be surgically

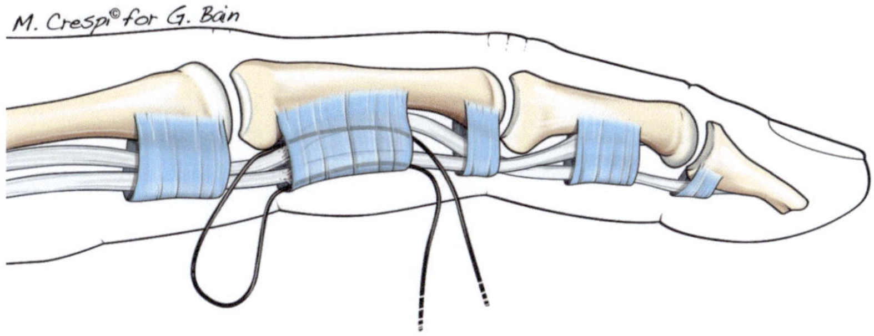

Fig. 23.8 Flexor tenolysis with a suture technique (copyright Dr. Gregory Bain). The blunt end of the suture is passed through the gutter between the flexor tendons and the flexor tendon sheath. It is then passed again on the opposite side of the finger to create a loop. Using the suture like a Gigli saw will snare the adhesions and divide them. The suture then requires to be positioned on aspects of the finger to divide the remaining adhesions

reconstructed. The tendon adhesions are released with a 2/O Prolene suture in a similar manner to a Gigli saw (Fig. 23.8) (Bain et al. 2003). The needle is introduced in the gutter between the phalanx, tendon and tendon sheath. The blunt end of the needle is inserted to avoid the sharp tip catching on the soft tissues. The needle is withdrawn and then passed down the opposite gutter.

Artery clips are placed on the suture ends, and with a sawing motion, the two ends of the suture are withdrawn. The suture catches the adhesions between the pulley and the flexor tendon. The traction is parallel to the finger, so that the adhesions are disrupted, but the tendon is not. The suture is also placed deep to both flexor tendons, so that the deep adhesions are also disrupted. The suture may need to be reinserted in other planes, to disrupt adhesions in other parts of the flexor tendon sheath.

This technique works like a "dragnet", captures the adhesions, but leaves the tendon intact. We have found this to be much better than using a beaver blade or arthroscopic knives.

23.3 The Future

Hand and wrist tendinopathies are common conditions in sports medicine. While most can be treated conservatively, a significant group of patient may opt for surgical intervention to minimize the immobilization period, so as to have an early return to sports. Minimal invasive surgical techniques including percutaneous release of soft tissue, percutaneous fixation of fracture and wrist arthroscopy have the theoretical advantage of achieving a more rapid recovery when compared with conventional open techniques. While endoscopic surgery of the shoulder and elbow is better developed, endoscopic surgery for the soft tissues around the wrist like the release of de Quervain's disease and tenosynovectomy is a relatively new form of intervention. It has potential for further expansion in the future (Bain 2016) (Fig. 23.9).

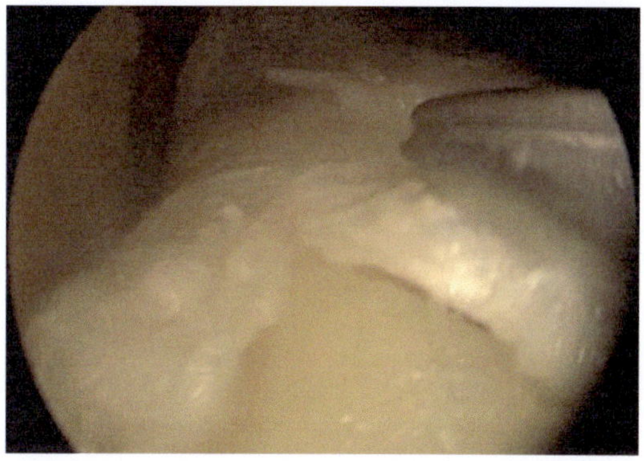

Fig. 23.9 Endoscopic release of the first extensor compartment in a cadaveric model (copyright Dr. Gregory Bain)

References

Adam JE, Habbu R (2015) Tendinopathies of the hand and wrist. JAAOS 23:741–750

Al-Qattan MM (2001) Type 5 avulsion of the insertion of the flexor digitorum profundus tendon. JS 26B: 5427–5431

Bain GI, Allen BD, Berger AC (2003) Flexor Tenolysis using a free suture. Tech Hand Up Extrem Surg 7(2):61–62

Bain G, Bhavin J (2016) The future: endoscopic surgery of the wrist and forearm. In: Savoie FH III, Field LD, Steinmann SP (eds) The elbow and wrist: AANA advanced arthroscopic surgical techniques. Healio, pp 417–424

Bain GI, Turnbull J, Charles MN, Roth JH, Richard RS (1995) Percutaneous A1 pulley release: a cadaveric study. JHS 20A:781–784

Bain GI, Wallwork NA (1999) Percutaneous A1 pulley release a clinical study. Hand Surg 4:45–50

Bauze A, Bain GI (1999) Internal suture for mallet finger fracture. J Hand Surg Br 24B(6):688–692

Brustein M, Pellegrini J, Choueka J, Heminger H, Mass D (2001) Bone suture anchors versus the pullout button for repair of distal profundus tendon injuries; a comparison of strength in human cadaveric hands. JHS 26A:489–496

Bunnell S (1948) Surgery of the hand, 5th edn. JB Limppincott, Philadelphia, pp 381–466

Burkhart SS, Wood MB, Linscheid RL (1982) Posttraumatic recurrent subluxation of the extensor carpi ulnas tendon. JHSA 7(1)1–3

Campbell D, Campbell R, O'Conner P, Hawkes R (2013) Sports-related extensor carpi ulnaris pathology: a review of functional anatomy, sports injury and management. Br J Sports Med 47:1105–1111

Carroll CT, Moore JR, Weiland AJ (1987) Post traumatic ulnar subluxation of the extensor tendons: a reconstructive technique. JHS 12A:227–231

Catalano LW III, Gupta S, Ragland R 3rd et al (2006) Closed treatment of nonrheumatoid extensor tendon dislocation at the metacarpophalangeal joint. JHS 31A:242–245

Crawford GP (1984) The molded polyethylene splint for mallet finger deformities. JHS 9A:231–237

Dala-Ali BM, Nakhdjevai A, Lloyd MA, Shreuder FB (2012) The efficacy of sterioid injection in the treatment of trigger finger. Clin Orthop Surg 4:263–268

Damron TA, Engber WD, Lange RH et al (1993) Biomechanical analysis of mallet finger fracture fixation techniques. JHS 18A:600–607

Finklestein H (1930) Stenosing tendovaginitis at the radial styloid process. JBJS 12:509–540

Garberman SF, Diao E, Peimer CA (1994) Mallet finger: results of early vs. delayed closed treatment. JHS 19A:850–852

Gilberts EC, Beekman WH, Stevens HJ, Wereldsma JC (2001) Prospective randomized trial of open versus percutaneous surgery for trigger digits. JHS 26A:497–500

Goldfarb CA, Puri SK, Carlson MG (2016) Diagnosis, treatment, and return to play for four common sports injuries of the hand and wrist. JAAOS 24:853–862

Gunter GS (1960) Traumatic avulsion of the insertion of flexor digitorum profundus. Aust NZJ Surg 30:1–9

Hamas RS, Horrell ED, Pierret GP (1978) Treatment of mallet finger due to intraarticular fracture of the distal phalanx. JHS 3A:361–363

Hartzell TL, Rubenstein R, Herman M (2013) Therapeutic modalities—an updated review for the hand surgeon. JHS 37A:597–621

Hofmeister EP, Mazurek MT, Shin AY, Bishop AT (2003) Extension block pinning for large mallet fractures. JHS 28A:453–459

Inoue G, Tamura Y (1996) Dislocation of the extensor tendons over the metecarpophlangeal joints. JHS 21A:464–469

Ishiguro T, Itoh Y, Yabe Y, Hashizume N (1997) Extension block with Kirschner wire for fracture dislocation of the distal interphalangeal joint. Tech Hand Up Extrem Surg 1(2):95–102

Jaskson WT, Viegas SF, Coon TM, Stimpson KD, Frogameni AD, Simpson JM (1986) Anatomical variations in the first extensor compartment of the wrist: a clinical and anatomical study. JBJS 68A:923–926

Jirarattanaphochai K, Saengnipanthkul S, Vipulakorn K, Jianmongkol S, Chatuparisute P, Jung S (2004) Treatemnt o de Quervain's disease with triamcinolone injection with or without nimesulide: a randomized, double-blind, placebo-controlled trial. JBJS 86A:2700–2706

Kettelkamp DB, Flatt AE, Moulds R (1971) Traumatic dislocation of the long finger extensor tendons a clnical, anatomical and biomechanical study. JBJS 53A:229–240

Kinninmonth AW, Holburn F (1986) A comparative controlled trial of a new perforated splint and a traditional splint in the treatment of mallet finger. JHS 11B:261–262

Leddy JP (1985) Avulsions of the flexor digitorm profundus. Hand Clin:77–83

Leddy JP, Parker JW (1977) Avulsions of the profundus tendon insertion in athletes. JHS 2A:66–69

Lin JD, Strauch RJ (2014) Closed soft tissue extensor mechanism injuries. JHS 39A:1005–1011

Lundin AC, Eliasson P, Aspenberg P (2012) Trigger finger and tendinosis. JHS 37:233–236

Lunn PG, Lamb DW (1984) "Rugby finger"- avulsion of profundus of ring finger. JHS 9B:69–71

MacLennan AJ, Nemechek NM, Waitayawinyu T, Trumble TE (2008) Diagnosis and anatomic reconstruction of extensor carpi ulnaris subluxation. JHS 33A:59–64

Montalvan B, Parier J, Brasseur JL, Le Viet D, Drape JL (2006) Extensor carpi ulnaris injuries in tennis players: a study of 28 cases. BJSM 40:424–429

Nagaoka M, Satoh T, Nagao S, Matsuaki H (2006) Extensor retinaculum graft for chronic boxers knuckle. JHS 31A:947–951

Nakamura K, Nanjyo B (1994) Reassessment of surgery for mallet fracture. Plastic Recon Surg 93:141–149

Okafor B, Mbubaegbu C, Munshi I, Willams DJ (1997) Mallet deformity of the finger: five-year follow-up of conservative treatment. JBJS 79B:544–547

Peter-Veluthamaningal C, van der Windt DA, Winters JC, Meyboom-de Jong B (2009) Corticosteroid injection for de Quervain's tenosynovitis. Cochrane Database Syst Rev 3:CD005616

Rayan GM, Murray D (1994) Classification and treatment of closed sagittal band injuries. JHS 19A:590–594

Retting AC (2004) Athletic injuries of the wrist and hand, part II: overuse injuries of the wrist and traumatic injuries to the hand. Am Sports Med 32:262–273

Richie CA III, Briner WW Jr (2003) Corticosteroid injection for treatment of de Quervain's tenosynovitis: a poled quantitative literature evaluation. J Am Board Fam Pract 16:102–106

Saldana MJ (2001) Rigger digits: diagnosis and treatment. JAAOS 9:246–252

Schreuder TAR (2012) The quadriga phenomenon: a review and clinical relevance. JHS 37E:513–522

Skoff HD, Hecker A, Hayes WC, Sebell-Sklar R, Straughn N (1995) Bone suture anchors in hand surgery. JHS 20B:245–248

Smith JH Jr (1981) Avulsion of a profundus tendon with simultaneous intraarticular fracture of the distal phalanx-case report. JHS 6A:600–601

Stern PJ, Kastrup JJ (1988) Complications and prognosis of treatment of mallet finger. JHS 13A:329–334

Turowski GA, Zdankiewicz PD, Thomson JG (1997) The results of surgical treatment of trigger finger. JHS 22A:145–149

Tuttle HG, Olvey SP, Stern PJ (2006) Tendon avulsion injuries of the distal phalanx. CORR 445:157–168

Watson HK, Weinzweig J, Guidera PM (1997) Sagittal band reconstruction. JHS 22A:452–456

Wehbe MA, Schneider LH (1984) Mallet fractures. JBJS 66A:658–669

Wheeldon FT (1954) Recurrent dislocation of extensor tendons in the hand. JBJS 36B:612–617

Young CM, Rayan GM (2000) The sagittal band: anatomic and biomechanical study. JHS 25A:1107–1113

Hip Tendinopathies

24

Alessandro Aprato, Andrea D'Amelio, Alessandro Bistolfi, Luigi Sabatini, and Alessandro Massè

Contents

24.1 Introduction

Groin pain is often triggered and exacerbated by sporting activities requiring rapid accelerations/decelerations or frequent changes in direction. Its aetiology is reported as multifactorial in about 27% of cases (de SA et al. 2016). Although groin pain is a frequent condition in sportive individuals, detailed epidemiological data are lacking in literature: often percentages reported about hip dysfunctions do not separate intra-articular from extra-articular pathologies. Also agreement in terminology and definitions about groin pain is still not clear and under construction among the experts (Bisciotti et al. in press; Weir et al. 2015). However hip and pelvis injuries are found in about 5–9% in high school athletes (Morelli and Weaver 2005; Morelli and Espinoza 2005), 3–11% in those competing at an Olympic level (Fricker 1997) and 10–18% in elite football players (Nicholas and Tyler 2002). In particular it has been reported that the incidence of these injuries among elite football players is 1.1 groin injuries/1000 h of athletic activity (Werner et al. 2009). Hip biomechanics is very complex during sport activities, and moreover, the mechanical relationship between the hip and spine has to be taken into consideration (Watanabe et al. 2002). With the evolution of diagnostic imaging, conservative and surgical techniques, hip dysfunctions in young active patients received a significant increase in attention. However, since tendinopathies are occasionally burdened by overlapping with intra-articular

A. Aprato (✉) • A. D'Amelio • A. Bistolfi
L. Sabatini • A. Massè
Università degli Studi di Torino, S.C.D.U. Ortopedia e Traumatologia 1, AOU Città della Salute e della Scienza di Torino, Via Zuretti 29, 10126 Torino, Italy
e-mail: ale_aprato@hotmail.com; andreadamelio.med@gmail.com; alessandro.masse@unito.it

G.L. Canata et al. (eds.), *Muscle and Tendon Injuries*, DOI 10.1007/978-3-662-54184-5_24

pathologies, accurate clinical diagnosis and appropriate management among athletes and active people remain a significant challenge (Reiman et al. 2013, 2015). Despite that each tendinopathy has different features, in general, initial treatment involves rest from the sport activities and modification in daily activities associated with non-steroidal anti-inflammatory drugs (NSAIDs). Then, depending on the severity of the injury, further management can be physical therapy (Joseph and Denegar 2015), regenerative medicine (Malanga and Nakamura 2014; Kaux et al. 2016; Zhou and Wang 2016; Fitzpatrick et al. 2016) and open or endoscopic surgical treatment (Ilizaliturri and Camacho-Galindo 2010; Chandrasekaran et al. 2015; Khan et al. 2013). Extra-articular hip endoscopy frequently follows arthroscopic evaluation and treatment of any central or peripheral hip pathology (Aprato et al. 2014). Taking into consideration muscle and tendon disorders, in this chapter pathologies have been divided according to the respective anatomical area into four groups: medial, anterior, lateral and posterior. For each pathology then it has been reported epidemiology, aetiology, clinical presentation, clinical and imaging diagnostic tests and treatment options.

24.2 Tendinopathies of the Medial Area

The hip adductor muscles, located on the anteromedial aspect of the thigh, are compounded of gracilis, pectineus, adductor magnus, adductor longus and adductor brevis. Quadratus femoris also produces adduction at the hip. Activation of the hip adductors occurs in more movements than just hip adduction. This muscle group has the secondary joint actions of hip rotation (Leighton 2006) and flexion or extension depending on initial joint position (Levangie and Norkin 2005). In addition to providing movement, the hip adductors may generate significant tension while stabilizing the hip and controlling the alignment of the lower limb (Hrysomallis 2009). A confounding issue is the definition of the injury; some studies have specific hip adductor injuries, whereas others have grouped adductor injuries along with other injuries within the "groin strain" category. Incidence of a correctly defined adductor injury, reported in some papers investigating football players and ice-hockey players, is about 7–12% over a sport season. The adductor longus is the tendon most commonly involved. Injuries usually occur at the musculotendinous junction but may also occur at the bone-tendon junction (enthesopathy) (Werner et al. 2009). The overstretching and eccentric force of the adductors attempting to decelerate the limb during rapid abduction and external rotation as occurs in ice-skating or sudden change in direction seems to be the injury mechanism (Hrysomallis 2009). Tendonitis is the most frequent disorder, while acute rupture or avulsion is less common. The risk factor is low flexibility, with a reduced ROM of the hip and adductor weakness.

Patient refers a groin pain exacerbated during the passive forced abduction and external rotation of the hip and during the active resisted adduction. Tenderness on deep palpation of the involved muscle can be observed. Specific clinical manoeuvres are the single adductor test, the squeeze test, and the bilateral adductor test (Reiman et al. 2013). The latter was found to be most diagnostic of sports-related chronic groin pain with a reported specificity of 93%, whereas the squeeze test and the single adductor test both reported a specificity of 91% (Verrall et al. 2005). Differential diagnoses are pubic osteitis, rectus-adductor syndrome and weakness of the abdominal wall in the groin region. Clinical findings can be confirmed by ultrasound (US) or magnetic resonance imaging (MRI) (Fig. 24.1). Radiographs of the pelvis can exclude intra-articular pathologies; if those images do not exclude an intra-articular disease, an ultrasound-guided intra-articular injection of anaesthetic may be used as a test.

Treatment options include the usual conservative treatment with rest and NSAIDs. Timing of the following physical rehabilitation depends on the location of the strain. If the injury is near the bone-tendon junction, physical therapy should be delayed because these areas are less vascular, and some healing is needed before starting exercises. If the tear is close to the musculotendinous junction or in the muscle belly, which are highly vascular zones, early and aggressive rehabilitation can be instituted (Elattar et al. 2016). Return to sports after acute strains is generally recommended when ath-

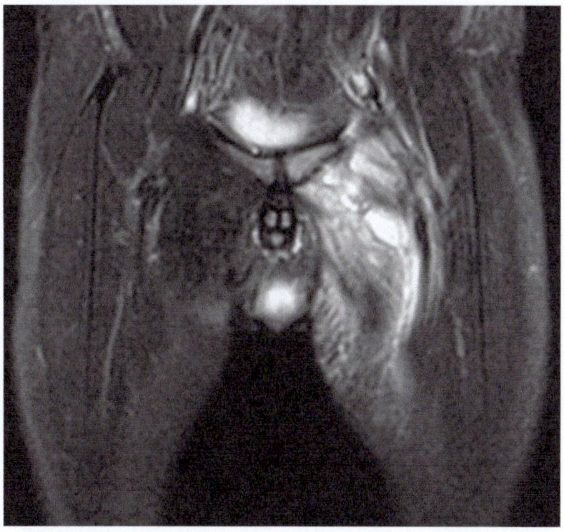

Fig. 24.1 MRI scan showing an hematoma of the left thigh adductors

letes regain 70% of strength and a painless range of motion, usually by 4–8 weeks, while for chronic strains, the recovery period and return to sports may be as long as 6 months (Holmich et al. 1999). Acute complete adductor tears in athletes generally require surgical repair with suture anchors, but it is not a so frequent procedure (de SA et al. 2016). The role of steroid injection in adductor strains remains controversial and it is not supported by an adequate good evidence. For chronic recalcitrant adductor tears with failed conservative treatment for a minimum of 6 months, surgical treatment with tenotomy may improve the pain (Gill et al. 2014). However, even if the pain relief is reported in about 73% of patients, the athletes able to return to their previous sport after surgery are only slightly more than 50% (Atkinson et al. 2010).

24.3 Tendinopathies of the Anterior Area

24.3.1 Iliopsoas

The iliopsoas musculotendinous unit is composed of three muscles: the iliacus, psoas major and psoas minor (only present in 60–65% of individuals). Significant anatomic variability has been reported in the literature, and controversy exists regarding the number of tendons and the relative contributions of the different muscle fibres to each tendon (Anderson 2016). The iliopsoas bursa, or iliopectineal bursa, is positioned between the iliopsoas unit and the bony surfaces of the pelvis and proximal femur. It is the largest bursa in the human body, typically extending from the iliopectineal eminence to the lower portion of the femoral head, with an average length of 5–6 cm and width of 3 cm (Tatu et al. 2001). Communications of the bursa with the hip joint, through a congenital defect between the iliofemoral and pubofemoral ligaments, have been reported. The iliopsoas unit functions primarily as hip flexor. It also provides femoral external rotation, with lateral bending, flexion and balance of the trunk. The iliacus is important for stabilizing the pelvis and for early rapid hip flexion while running. The psoas major is important for sitting in an erect position and stability of the spine in the frontal plane. Variable contribution of each muscle is observed during sit-ups depending on the angle of hip flexion (Fitzgerald 1969; Andersson et al. 1995). The psoas minor distally attaches both to the iliac fascia and psoas major tendon, having also another attachment to the iliopectineal eminence. This gives a partial control of the position and mechanical stability of the underlying iliopsoas as it crosses the femoral head. Pathologic conditions of the iliopsoas have been implicated as a significant source of anterior hip pain. Iliopsoas disorders have been shown to be the primary cause of chronic groin pain in 12–36% of athletes and are observed in 25–30% of athletes presenting with an acute groin injury (Serner et al. 2015; Holmich 2007; Holmich et al. 2014; Rankin et al. 2015). Described pathologic conditions include iliopsoas bursitis, tendonitis, impingement and snapping. These conditions coexist so frequently that Johnston reported an “iliopsoas syndrome” (Johnston et al. 1998), with a common diagnostic and therapeutic process. Therefore, diagnosis and treatment of the iliopsoas disorders are reported together later in this paragraph. Less frequent are acute trauma that may result in tendon injury or avulsion fracture of the lesser trochanter.

Internal Extra-Articular Snapping Hip This syndrome was originally attributed to snapping of the iliopsoas tendon over the iliopectineal eminence of the pelvis. Other mechanisms that have been then proposed include accessory iliopsoas tendon slips, iliopsoas snapping over a ridge at the lesser trochanter, snapping of the iliofemoral ligament over the femoral head and subluxation of the long head of the biceps at the ischium snapping at the anterior inferior iliac spine (Yen et al. 2015). However, most commonly, it is produced by the iliopsoas tendon snapping over the iliopectineal eminence or the femoral head. The snapping phenomenon usually occurs when the hip is brought back to extension from a flexed position (usually flexion of more than 90°). The iliopectineal eminence and the anterior edge of the pelvis work as a pulley for the iliopsoas muscle (Lyons and Peterson 1984). The iliopsoas tendon is located lateral to the iliopectineal eminence when the hip is in full flexion, with hip extension the tendon is displaced medially until it positions medial to the iliopectineal eminence when the hip is in neutral position. The psoas tendon seems to be in contact with the iliopectineal eminence at approximately 50° of hip flexion (Yoshio et al. 2002). The snapping phenomenon can occur without pain in up to 10% of the general population (Byrd 2006). In the symptomatic internal snapping hip syndrome, patients report snapping while stair climbing or standing from a chair associated with groin pain.

Iliopsoas Bursitis and Tendonitis Iliopsoas bursitis and tendonitis have been shown to be closely associated with the repetitive pathologic movement of the tendon observed in symptomatic internal snapping hip. This can cause irritation and inflammation of the underlying bursa (Fig. 24.2). Even so, some studies demonstrate no objective abnormality of the bursa in patients undergoing open surgery for symptomatic snapping (Anderson 2016).

Iliopsoas Impingement First described by Heyworth in 2007, iliopsoas impingement is a conflict between an excessively tight iliopsoas tendon impinges and the underlying acetabular labrum (Heyworth et al. 2007). The location of the anterior labral abnormality corresponded to the iliopsoas notch, significantly differs from the traditional location observed in FAI (Blankenbaker et al. 2007). Sometimes the labrum appears inflamed without frank tearing, which was referred to as the "iliopsoas impingement sign". Furthermore, adjacent tendinous inflammation and scarring with adherence of the tendon to the anterior capsule were observed in some patients. Iliopsoas impingement occurs most frequently in young active women, many who participate in regular sports. Patients typically present with anterior groin pain that worsens with athletic activities and activities of daily living, such as active hip flexion, prolonged sitting and getting out of a car (Anderson 2016). Internal snapping is less commonly observed in iliopsoas impingement but has been reported in up to 17% of cases (Blankenbaker et al. 2012).

Physical examination of the internal snapping phenomenon is carried out with the patient supine by flexing the affected hip more than 90° and extending to neutral position. This may be accentuated with abduction and external rotation in flexion and adducting and internally rotating while extending. The snapping may be audible and may be palpated by placing the hand over the affected groin while performing the examination test. Commonly, weakness of the gluteus medius

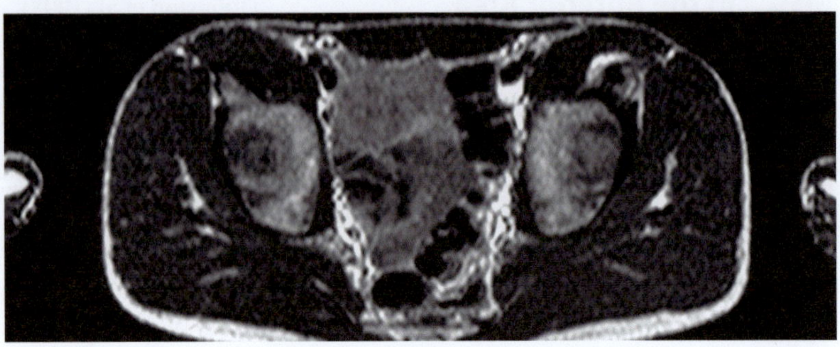

Fig. 24.2 MRI scan showing a left psoas tendonitis

with a Trendelenburg sign is found and the Thomas test, which tests for psoas contracture, is often positive, as well (Yen et al. 2015). If the snapping is produced by the iliopsoas tendon over the femoral head, plain radiographs can reveal a large anterior cam deformity at the head-neck passage of the femur. Regarding iliopsoas impingement on physical examination, patients typically have a positive impingement test (flexion, adduction and internal rotation—FADIR), scour sign and tenderness with manual compression over the iliopsoas. Approximately half of them have pain with flexion, abduction and external rotation (FABER) and resisted straight leg raise testing (RSLR) (Anderson 2016). Ultrasound exam of the iliopsoas tendon is a dynamic non-invasive study that may document the snapping phenomenon as well as pathologic changes of the iliopsoas tendon and its bursa, but the ability and experience of the examiner are fundamental. MRI scan can reveal an unspecific inflammation of the iliopsoas area, but it can be useful to detect any concomitant intra-articular hip pathology, since almost half of the patients with internal snapping hip syndrome have associated intra-articular hip pathology (Ilizaliturri et al. 2005). In case of iliopsoas impingement the most pertinent radiographic finding is a labral tear at or near the 3/9 o'clock position seen on MRI (Blankenbaker et al. 2012). Diagnostic injection test with anaesthetic can be performed, but it is important to consider the possible communication between the hip joint and the iliopectineal bursa, because the drugs can expand in both compartments, confounding the results of the test (Anderson 2016).

Treatment should be reserved for symptomatic patients and has to be initially conservative with NSAID therapy and stretching, if the tendon is too short, or lengthening, if the muscle is too active. Sometimes steroid injection in the iliopectineal bursa can give pain relief. If there is no positive response to conservative treatment surgical treatment is indicated to lengthen the iliopsoas musculotendinous unit, in order to prevent snapping and mechanical overpressure on the underlying bursa. In the past open procedures for lengthening or release of the iliopsoas tendon at different levels along its course have been proposed: results were generally good, with very high percentages (about 77%) of symptoms resolution (Khan et al. 2013). However some cases of recurrence and a significant percentage (15–45%) of post-operative subjective weakness have been reported (Yen et al. 2015). These procedures have increased morbidity and inferior results compared with recently proposed endoscopic techniques. In a recent review, there has been reported a complication rate of 21% in open procedures compared with 2.3% using arthroscopic techniques (Khan et al. 2013). Endoscopic release of the iliopsoas tendon has become more common. Three different endoscopic techniques have been described to treat this condition. First technique is a transcapsular release of the iliopsoas tendon at the level of the hip joint with an anterior hip capsulotomy during the central compartment phase of the procedure. This procedure is also used for iliopsoas impingement in association with concurrent labral abnormality debridement or repair, with generally reported favourable results (Domb et al. 2011; Cascio et al. 2013). The second technique is a release at femoral neck level trough an anterior capsulotomy in the peripheral compartment, this method is not routinely used because of the technique to find the psoas is demanding. The third option is to cut the tendon on the lesser trochanter, with this technique the iliopsoas bursa is accessed directly. Results of the endoscopic techniques are encouraging and seem to be better than those reported for open procedures, with a success rate up to 100% (Ilizaliturri et al. 2014). However, remembering the frequent intra-articular coexistent pathology in this condition, these results may be confounded by a concomitant hip arthroscopy (Yen et al. 2015; Ilizaliturri et al. 2005).

24.3.2 Rectus Femoris

Quadriceps muscle strains frequently occur in sports that require repetitive kicking and sprinting efforts, such as track and field, rugby and football. The rectus femoris is a fusiform and biarticular long muscle designed to execute movements that require significant length change or high shortening velocity. It has a high demand for eccentric muscle contraction and has a high percentage of rapid-contraction muscular fibres (approximately 65%) that can make it more prone to injury (Mendiguchia et al. 2013). Rectus femoris has two heads of origin: the direct or straight head, which arises from the anterior inferior iliac spine (AIIS), and the indirect or reflected head, which arises from the superior acetabular rim. The two heads form the conjoined tendon slightly below their origin, with the direct head contributing mostly to the superficial component of the conjoined tendon and blends anteriorly with its fascia (Hasselman et al. 1995). The rectus femoris extends the knee, flexes the hip and stabilizes the pelvis on the femur in weight bearing. Proximal rectus femoris lesions most commonly occur during hip hyperextension and knee flexion or as a result of a sharp eccentric contraction of the quadriceps. Proved risk factors include previous injury (with a recurrence rate of about 17%), short height associated with a high body weight and a low flexibility (Mendiguchia et al. 2013). According to a study evaluating 3160 hips on MRI scan, the average frequency of proximal rectus femoris origin injury was about 0.5% (Ouellette et al. 2006). Tendon avulsions are rare and account for approximately 1.5% of hip lesions that occur during sports (Dean et al. 2016). Calcification of the proximal rectus femoris tendon could follow an avulsion or a tendon rupture (partial or complete) of the rectus femoris, and a similar condition has been also described after an avulsion of the AIIS bony fragment. The healing process could lead to a protuberance, secondary to changes of ossification centres with a course following the axis of traction forces of the rectus femoris. This inferiorly prominent bony protuberance can anteriorly conflict with the femoral neck of a flexed hip. This condition has been referred to as iliac spine impingement or subspine impingement (Zini et al. 2014). Acute calcific tendinitis of the rectus femoris is extremely rare (IKobayashi et al. 2015). In acute injuries the patient feels a tearing sensation and stops playing any activity. In subacute conditions patients report gradual onset of pain during activities like running and kicking. At the clinical examination, pain is exacerbated by stretching, regional palpation, hip flexion and resisted knee extension. Sometimes a complete rupture is responsible for a local mass-like syndrome. Plain radiographs can reveal any bony involvement, as the AIIS avulsion in the childhood. In those cases a gap of more than 2 cm between the native bone and avulsed fragment is a factor of poor prognosis (Pesquer et al. 2016). Associated MRI scan, investigating the presence of a possible surrounding oedema, could reveal the acute or chronic character of the lesion. For other tendon disorders, US can be useful, even if MRI remains the gold standard allowing a more global assessment of the pathologic conditions. Regarding rectus femoris avulsion, in most of the cases tears are treated conservatively. However, indication for surgical repair may be considered in high-level athletes with significant demand for repetitive explosive hip flexion or in patients with failure of nonoperative treatment and continued pain or weakness for more than 3 months. Surgical procedure is carried on through a Smith-Petersen approach. Once identified both the proximal heads of the tendon, the lesion is pointed out and all of the devitalized and degenerated fibres should be removed from the tendon stump. The footprint of the direct arm of the rectus (on the AIIS) is then prepared by removing the soft tissues to expose subchondral bone, creating a bleeding bony bed to support healing. Then reattachment is performed with two suture anchors placed on the AIIS, with the right tension so that tissues are reduced and compressed against the bone. After surgery a knee brace locked in extension is recommended with no weight bearing and no active hip flexion for 6 weeks. Strength-training exercises and running typically begin after 8 weeks, while return to sport occurs between 4 and 6 months after surgery (Dean et al. 2016). In case of an AIIS avulsion in a skeletally immature patient, more often a nonoperative treatment is chosen, with a brief period of rest followed by protected weight bearing, progressive stretching and strengthening and gradual return to sports. Operative treatment with open reduction and internal fixation has been recommended for fractures with a displacement wider than 2 cm to prevent nonunion, exostosis formation and chronic pain and disability (Schuett et al. 2015). For tendon calcification the management starts with conservative treatment with injection of anaesthetic and corticosteroids. In case of symptoms persistence, surgery can be performed with open excision of the lesion through a Smith-Petersen approach, as described before for the tendon reattachment or with a less invasive endoscopic procedure. These two options are also used to treat the subspine impingement. Despite good results in treating pathology, open procedures are burdened by wound discomfort. For endoscopic treatment of either calcific tendonitis or subspine impingement, a standard fracture table is used with the patient in a supine position. The operative limb was placed with the hip in slight abduction and internal rotation. Two standard portals are used: the anterolateral that provides a complete view of the central compartment for the treatment of possible associated intra-articular pathologies and the midanterior portal. After concomitant intra-articular lesions are evaluated and eventually treated, the traction is removed and a shaver is used to clear all soft tissue to better delimit the plane between the acetabular rim and the calcification. After complete exposure of the calcification is achieved, using the image intensifier as a guide in addition to the direct view, the calcification is removed using a bur. After surgery, weight bearing is permitted as tolerated, but extension of the hip was forbidden for 3 weeks to avoid excessive elongation of the tendon, and prophylaxis versus heterotopic ossification is given to avoid recurrence. Outcome data reported are satisfactory with a significant improvement in terms of pain, hip flexion ROM and function, without any complication (Zini et al. 2014; Hetsroni et al. 2012).

24.4 Tendinopathies of the Lateral Area

The term greater trochanteric pain syndrome (GTPS) references a variety of diagnoses with a localized lateral hip pain and focal point tenderness over the greater trochanter. These conditions typically include external snapping hip, trochanteric bursitis and gluteus medius and minimus tendinopathies (Strauss et al. 2010), often with a coexistence of both bursitis and tendinopathy. Prevalence is about 10–25% in population between 40 and 60 years. Female are 2–5 times more frequently affected: this seemed to be related to the greater prominence of the trochanters and the associated increased tension of the iliotibial band (ITB) over them. Other predisposing factors could be an increased acetabular anteversion and a low femoral neck shaft angle. However, about 22% of the elderly individuals present some form of gluteus tear (Kagan 1999). A concurrent or past history of low back pain have been reported in 20–62% of patients with GTPS diagnosis perhaps because of the functional connection between the hip and lumbopelvic complex (Segal et al. 2007). Up to 20 bursae have been described in the trochanteric area, but only three are consistently present in the majority of individuals. These include the gluteus minimus bursa, located anterosuperiorly to the greater trochanter; the subgluteus medius bursa, which lies deep to the gluteus medius tendon; and the subgluteus maximus bursa, which lies lateral to the greater trochanter between the gluteus medius and maximus and is often described as the "trochanteric bursa". Regarding muscles anatomy, the most superficial gluteal muscle, the gluteus maximus, has a broad origin including fibres from the ilium and sacrum and inserts onto the gluteal tuberosity of the femur and the ITB. The gluteus medius lies deep within this muscle, and the gluteus minimus is deeper; they both originate from the ilium and insert onto the greater trochanter of the femur. The tensor fascia lata originates from the iliac crest and inserts onto the ITB. This fibrous band of tissue inserts distally onto the lateral condyle of the tibia. The gluteus medius and minimus, both innervated by the superior gluteal nerve, are part of the abductors of the hip. The abduction, particularly its initiation, is attributable to the anterior and middle fibres of gluteus medius. Usually, tears of the gluteus medius start from medial fibres to the lateral ones (Fig. 24.3) (Reid 2016). Soft tissue structures in the trochanteric area are similar to those in the area

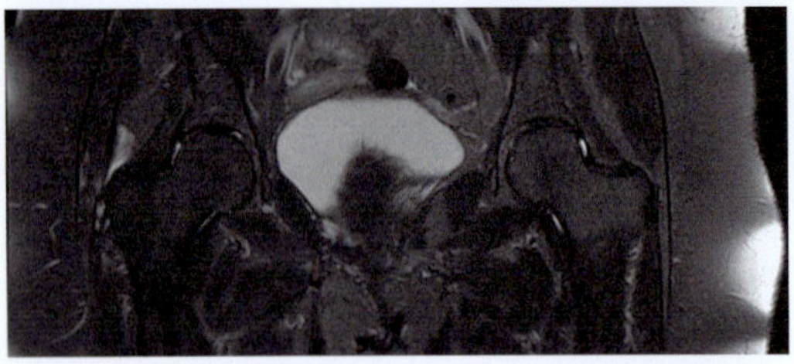

Fig. 24.3 MRI scan showing a right medius gluteus tendonitis

of the greater tuberosity of the shoulder. Gluteus medius and minimus tendons are prone degeneration or failure, and the trochanteric bursa have potential for inflammation (Ho and Howard 2012). Even if historically this syndrome has been referred to as a "bursitis", the presentation is rarely accompanied by the characteristic symptoms of inflammation including erythema, oedema and rubor. Therefore, it is now thought, also as a result of dissection, clinical and radiological studies, that bursa may be acquired as a result of friction between the greater trochanter and gluteus maximus. Bursal tissue from patients with GTPS undergoing total hip arthroplasty showed no signs of acute or chronic inflammation. This finding supports the understanding that inflammation plays a limited role in GTPS (Bird et al. 2001; Dunn et al. 2003; Silva et al. 2008). The aetiology of gluteal tendinopathy is proposed to be multifactorial with both intrinsic and extrinsic components, but the exact mechanism is unknown: repetitive activity, abnormal mechanical loads and altered cellular responses are the major suspects, but tendinopathy can occur in patients without overuse. Otherwise chronic tendinopathies seen on imaging can be asymptomatic (Kaux et al. 2011). As it regards external snapping, this phenomenon can occur as a result of a thickening of the posterior ITB, the tensor fascia lata or the gluteus maximus as they slide over the greater trochanter, during hip flexion. In more severe cases the snap may be also reproduced with hip rotations. This phenomenon is always voluntary and is the most common form of coxa saltans (Ilizaliturri and Camacho-Galindo 2010).

In GTPS pain is referred by the patient as lateral, with an insidious onset. It is persistent and often exacerbated by lying on the affected side, sitting with the legs crossed or by prolonged weight bearing in unilateral stance. Symptoms may also extend laterally down the thigh, rarely below the knee or posteriorly into the gluteal region. In case of an external snapping, patient can complain a snap while flexing or rotating the hip, often in absence of pain. At the physical examination, neurological and screening examination for the lumbosacral region is mandatory. The consistent feature of the syndrome is increased tenderness to palpation, but it has been seen that the intertester error in palpating the greater trochanter bony landmark is greater than 15 mm which is significantly larger than the dimensions of the normal bursae or footprint of the tendon insertions (Moriguchi et al. 2009). A positive FABER test and pain with resisted hip abduction can be found. The gluteal tendon pathology can be represented by pain, weakness or a lag during resisted hip abduction testing. The presence of a Trendelenburg sign is both reliable and accurate with a sensitivity of 73% and specificity of 77% in patients with MRI evidence of a torn tendon (Bird et al. 2001). Reproduction of the lateral hip pain during resisted hip internal rotation back to neutral, with hip flexed to 90°, also had a high correlation with the presence of tendon change on MRI with a sensitivity of 88% and specificity of 97% (Lequesne et al. 2008). The Ober test is described as a mechanism to evaluate for ITB (tensor fascia lata/gluteus maximus) tightness and may cause compressive pain over the trochanter but has not been studied for its accuracy as a specific predictor of GTPS (Mulligan et al. 2015). The hip lag sign, in which the ability to hold an antigravity position of hip abduction is used to detect a gluteus medius tear, is considered positive if the foot drops more than 10 cm or the patient cannot hold the internally rotated position. It seems to be 89% sensitive and 97% specific (Kaltenborn et al. 2014). For the external snapping hip, the patient could be asked to voluntarily reproduce the sign. Otherwise in a side lying position with the ITB on stretch, it can be evaluated if the snapping complaint is present as the patient actively flexes and extends the hip (Mulligan et al. 2015). Radiological investigations start as usual with a plain radiograph of the pelvis that can depict greater trochanteric enthesopathy. Ultrasound can be useful to get a dynamic imaging investigation. MRI showed good accuracy for the diagnosis of tears of the gluteus medius and gluteus minimus tendons. However, Blankenbaker found a high prevalence (50%) of peritrochanteric imaging abnormalities in patients without trochanteric pain (Blankenbaker et al. 2008). In difficult cases, injection test with local anaesthetic in the trochanteric area may be performed.

Most patients have resolution of their symptoms with conservative treatments, with surgical interventions usually appointed for refractory cases, nonrespondent to conservative treatments. Also regenerative injection therapy is also a potential treatment option for GTPS (Reid 2016). Conservative treatments start with NSAID therapy and physiotherapy with eccentric exercises. Patient treated with corticosteroid local injection showed significant early improvement up to 3 months, but often recurrence in the longer term (Mani-Babu et al. 2015). A concern for use of corticosteroid injections is the possibility for weakening the tendon structure in the long term. There is a low rate of serious adverse effects after multiple injections, while minor side effects such as skin depigmentation and post injection pain are common (Reid 2016). Shock wave therapy (SWT) has been shown to be effective in particular for GTPS, even if the mechanism of how SWT has an effect on GTPS is unclear (Mani-Babu et al. 2015). It is considered to stimulate healing, possibly by stimulating cellular activity and increasing blood flow (Kaux et al. 2011). Low-energy SWT is an effective treatment for chronic GTPS with improvement being maintained at 12 months. There is a significant improvement with repetitive low-energy SWT compared to CS injection at 4 months (Rompe et al. 2009). However, the available evidence for SWT for GTPS is still limited. Then also platelets reach plasma (PRP) or whole blood injections have been used for the treatment of tendinopathies to promote natural healing by providing/manipulating cellular mediators and growth factors. However, no studies directly relating to GTPS are present. Present in literature, but with limited evidence for efficacy and safety of use in clinical practice, are some advances in non-surgical treatments that include topical glycerol trinitrate therapy, matrix metalloproteinase-inhibitor injection, gene or stem-cell therapy, autologous tenocyte injection and sclerosant injections (Reid 2016). In case of conservative options failure surgical treatment could be taken in account for different GTPS entities. Surgery, open or by endoscopic procedure, can include bursectomy, gluteal tendon repair, ITB release or trochanteric reduction osteotomy, often with a combination of these interventions. Surgery can provide also a grading of the gluteal tears. Using open procedures, two classifications can be obtained. The first one is the Milwaukee classification, in which the trochanter is represented by a clock face and grade 1, 2, 3 and 4 tears correspond to 1 h, 2 h, 3 h and a bald trochanter (Davies et al. 2013). The other one is the Walsh classification, in which type 1 tears had a normal bursa, normal appearance of the gluteus medius tendon, deep surface detachment anteriorly only and a normal gluteus minimus; type 2 tears had a normal bursa, thickening of the tendon, greyish discoloration, loss of normal striations, detachment that may extend posteriorly and a stretched gluteus minimus; type 3 tears had a scarred bursa and may have free fluid and tendon changes as in type 2 but a small disruption exposing the underlying trochanter with a partial tear or detachment of the gluteus minimus; and type 4 tears had total disruption of the gluteus medius and minimus tendons exposing the entire trochanter front and back with ulceration of the fascia lata (Walsh et al. 2011). Using an endoscopic procedure, Domb and Carreira intraoperatively graded gluteal tears based on the percentage of the tendon involved. Grade 2 tears were repaired using a transtendinous technique and grade 4 tears with a full-thickness repair technique. Grade 3 tears were repaired with either technique depending on how near the tear was to full thickness (Walsh et al. 2011). Regarding gluteal tendon tears, surgical repair has shown good long-term improvement. A study about 72 cases reported 95% improvement, maintained at 12 months (Walsh et al. 2011). In the open procedure, patients are positioned in the lateral decubitus position, and a direct approach to the greater trochanter is performed. Then a bursectomy can be carried out or neither. The gluteus medius and minimus tendons are identified, and the ends are debrided. The trochanter is decorticated and then the tendons are sutured to bone with transosseous tunnels, or by anchors or with a combination of both these two techniques. Sutures are used in a vertical mattress configuration in the tendon or in a double-row configuration with anchor sutures securing the avulsed edge and heavy absorbable sutures to oversew the free edge to create a watertight seal. If the posterior fibres of the gluteus medius are involved, these are secured to the trochanter through a set of medial and lateral transosseous tunnels, with simple vertical stitches over the free flap to simulate a double-row repair. In addition, for retracted tears with an exposed trochanter, repair can be supplemented with a fascial allograft (Chandrasekaran et al. 2015). In the endoscopic procedure, the patient can be placed in a supine position or in a lateral position with the leg slightly abducted. A combination of direct distal-lateral and proximal portals (plus other accessory portals) are used to view the peritrochanteric space and facilitate instrumentation. A trochanteric bursectomy is performed every time to aid visualization. For partial tears, a longitudinal split is made in the gluteal tendon to create a trochanteric window for bone preparation. The gluteal tendons are mobilized by removing scar tissue and adhesions. Then anchors are placed in the greater trochanter, and horizontal mattress sutures are placed in the tendons. A double-row technique for full-thickness tears is used to provide added compression of tendon to bone. After surgery, the patient has a period of restricted weight bearing for about 6 weeks, before starting with rehabilitation protocols. Some surgeons recommend an abduction brace for the first postoperative period. Outcome results are very good for both the procedures. However, open technique has retears and wound problems in some cases (7.8% and 3.1% respectively) as disadvantages, while no complications are reported for endoscopic procedures (Chandrasekaran et al. 2015). Also bursectomy can be performed with open or endoscopic procedures. For the open surgery, a direct lateral approach is used. For the endoscopic bursectomy, the patient can be placed either in the supine or lateral position. If a supine position is preferred an anterolatral (AL) portal, slightly more superior than the standard one is created initially. Then a 30° scope is used to visualize the peritrochanteric space, which is often found to be occupied by copious amounts of thickened bursa. Then a distal AL (DAL) portal in line with the initial AL portal is created to be used as a working portal. In case of a lateral decubitus position, an anterior portal and a distal posterior portal are used to allow for visualization and adequate access to the peritrochanteric space. Bursectomy is then performed using a shaver. An ITB release either preceding or subsequent to the bursectomy has been described, with favourable results (Reich et al. 2013). Painful external snapping that is refractory to conservative treatment is rare. The goal of the surgery is to relax the tendon to eliminate the snapping. This can be obtained by a fractional lengthening or a complete release of the tendon. Various types of lengthening procedures have been described including Z-shaped release, formal Z lengthening, cross-shaped release and release of the gluteus maximus tendon insertion to the femur. All techniques can be performed both open, with a direct lateral approach, and endoscopically (Yen et al. 2015). In the endoscopic procedure the patient could be placed as usual in both supine and lateral positions. In the lateral position, working from the outside surface of the ITB, it is exposed and released with a diamond-shaped resection (Ilizaliturri et al. 2006). In another technique performed with the patient placed in a supine position, a gluteus maximus tenotomy is performed through the ITB with an inside-out technique to decrease tension on the iliotibial band (Polesello et al. 2013). All the procedures show good results at the long-term follow-up without significant complications (Reid 2016).

24.5 Tendinopathies of the Posterior Area

24.5.1 Hamstrings

With the exception of the short head of the biceps femoris, the hamstring complex originates from the ischial tuberosity and inserts distally below the knee on the proximal tibia. The tibial branch of the sciatic nerve innervates the semitendinosus, semimembranosus and the long head of biceps femoris, while the short head is innervated by the peroneal branch of the sciatic nerve. The proximal hamstring complex has a strong bony attachment on the ischial tuberosity. The footprint on the ischium includes the semitendinosus and the long head of biceps femoris, beginning in a common proximal tendon, while there is a distinct semimembranosus footprint. The semimembranosus footprint is lateral (and anterior) to the crescent-shaped footprint of the common insertion of the semitendinosus and long head of the biceps femoris (Guanche 2015). Among acute injuries states range from benign hamstring strain injuries to severe total ruptures of all the three tendons (Fig. 24.4). There is then a chronic proximal hamstring tendinopathy (PHT). Acute injuries usually derived from a traumatic event with forced hip flexion and knee in extension. Otherwise in the chronic tendinopaty, the onset is more insidious. Proximal hamstring tendinopathy is considered to be an insertional tendinopathy and compression of the tendon at its attachment during hip flexion/adduction is thought to be a key etiological factor (Cook and Purdam 2012). Shear force between the hamstring attachment and ischial tuberosity has been reported when replicating in vivo loading as well as increased displacement of proximal hamstring tendon with increased hip flexion angle. Extrinsic aetiological factors include training errors such as increasing volume or intensity too quickly, particularly the sudden introduction of sprint work, lunging, hurdles or hills. These activities require the hamstring to contract or lengthen while in hip flexion and may result in provocative tensile and compressive load at the tendon insertion (Docking et al. 2013). Symptoms may also occur due to excessive use of static stretches, for example, in yoga and Pilates involving sustained end-range hip flexion postures. Systemic factors, as loss of oestrogen at menopause, are thought to negatively influence tendon homeostasis and to reduce the threshold for tendon pain and pathology from load-related factors (Goom et al. 2016). Commonly, patients with proximal hamstring tendon tears describe a popping or tearing sensation with associated acute pain and bruising over the posterior hip. They may also complain of a pins and needles sensation in the sciatic nerve distribution, much like sciatica. This may be due to the acute compression of a hematoma in the proximity of the sciatic nerve or chronic scarring and tethering of the tendon to the nerve. Similarly, symptoms of ischial bursitis include buttock pain or hip pain and localized tenderness overlying the ischial tuberosity with occasional sciatica symptoms (Guanche 2015). The main symptom is pain in the lower gluteal region, sometimes radiating along the hamstrings to the posterior thigh. The pain mainly manifests during running at a faster pace or while sitting for a

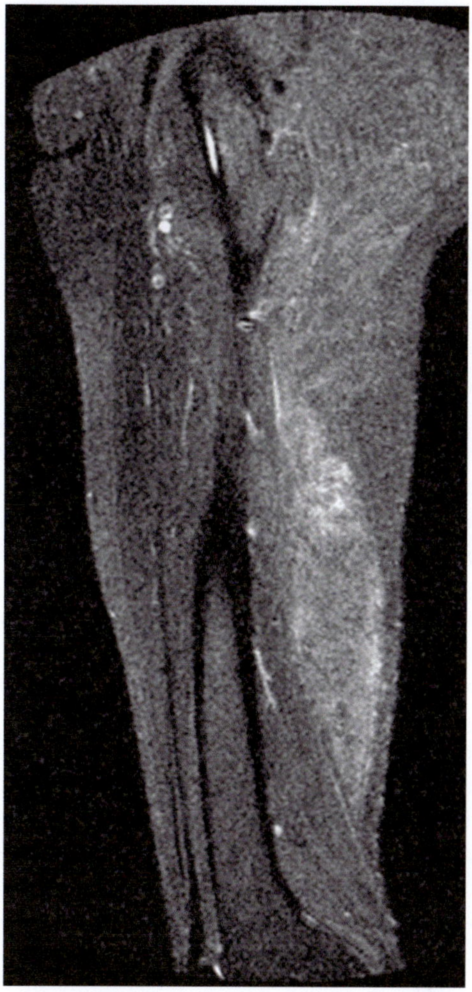

Fig. 24.4 MRI scan showing an hematoma of the right hamstrings

prolonged time. Typically, the pain appears without any sudden trauma and gradually becomes worse. However, sometimes patients also report history of repetitive hamstring injuries. In general, continued training and stretching of the hamstrings make the situation gradually worse. On clinical examination, there is often palpable tenderness and pain over the ischial tuberosity against resisted knee flexion. Furthermore, active stretching of the hamstrings recreates the pain at the site of the ischial tuberosity as well. Typically, peripheral neurological tests are normal and no strength deficiencies are noted in knee flexion or in hip extension (Lempainen et al. 2015). In case of an acute injury is suspected, standard radiographs of the pelvis and a lateral of the affected hip are performed to rule out any apophyseal avulsions, particularly to the ischial tuberosity in younger patients. Most commonly, no fractures are identified and MRI is used to assess the proximal hamstring insertion on the ischial tuberosity, where several types of injuries may be seen. A complete rupture of all three tendons is common and is easily identified on MRI. Partial hamstring origin tears, however, are more difficult to delineate. The most common situation is an avulsion of the common semitendinosus and biceps origin, with the semimembranosus remaining intact (Guanche 2015). MRI and ultrasound are the methods of choice for the visualization of the hamstring tendon complex. Ultrasound is a readily available and cost-effective imaging technique that allows dynamic evaluation for hamstring tendons. The advantage of MRI is better soft tissue contrast. It is more sensitive than US in detecting tendinopathy and peritendinous oedema of the proximal hamstring tendons. Peritendinous oedema with a distal feathery pattern is a more reliable sign of tendinopathy. Changes that mimic bone marrow oedema and thickening of tendons are also often seen. However, all these changes can also be seen in asymptomatic tendons, and therefore, a close correlation between imaging and the clinical findings is paramount (Lempainen et al. 2015). Nonoperative treatment for acute injuries is most commonly recommended in case of lowgrade partial tears. In general, nonoperative treatment in higher-level athletes has not been effective, as up to 80% complain of ongoing cramping and weakness (Lempainen et al. 2009). Initial treatment consists as usual of rest, NSAID therapy and physiotherapy rehabilitation. An ultrasound-guided corticosteroid injection may be used and has been shown to provide initial relief in up to 50% of patients at 1 month (Zissen et al. 2010). The time to full recovery is normally between 1 and 3 months. Recently a safe endoscopic procedure for the management of proximal hamstring tears has been described. The patient is placed in the prone position and two portals are then created, 2 cm medial and lateral to the palpable ischial tuberosity. The lateral portal is established first, penetrating the gluteus maximus. The medial portal is then established, taking care to palpate the medial aspect of the ischium. The lateral aspect is then exposed with the use of a switching stick as a soft tissue dissector. With the lateral aspect identified, the dissection continues anteriorly and laterally towards the sciatic nerve, with a very careful and methodical release of any soft tissue bands. The nerve is then identified and protected and the tendinous origin inspected. In acute tears, the area is obvious and the tendon is often retracted distally. In these cases, there is occasionally a large hematoma that requires evacuation. Once the area of pathology is identified, the devitalized tissue is removed and a bleeding corticocancellous bed is prepared in anticipation of the tendon repair. A third portal is then created approximately 4 cm distal to the tip of the ischium and equidistant from the medial and lateral portals. This portal is used for insertion of suture anchors, as well as suture management. Post-operatively, the patient is fitted with a hinged knee brace that is fixed at 90° of flexion for 4 weeks. After the knee is gradually extended by about 30° per week to allow full weight bearing by 6–8 weeks, while maintaining the use of crutches. Full and unrestricted activity is allowed, after a physiotherapy period, at approximately 4 months (Guanche 2015). Conservative treatment is comparable to those of other chronic tendinopathies, including reduction or pause of sports activity, soft tissue mobilization, physiotherapy and continuous home exercise programme focusing on progressive eccentric hamstring strengthening and core stabilization. Then additional physical therapies have been described as soft tissue mobilization, lumbopelvic stabilization exercises, trigger point dry needling and electrical muscle stimulation combined with US (Jayaseelan et al. 2013). As options for recalcitrant disease refractory to conventional treatment some other approaches including shockwave (SWT) and ultrasound (US) therapy, ultrasound-guided corticosteroid and Platelet rich plasma (PRP) injection have been purposed (Cacchio et al. 2011; Zissen et al. 2010; Wetzel et al. 2013). Peritendinous corticosteroid injection has been associated with a low rate of symptoms. PRP injection, despite a limited evidence and waiting for further robust clinical trials, has been reported to have therapeutic potential for several tendinopathies. In case of failure of the conservative treatment, surgical indication should be considered. Sciatic Nerve's close relation to the proximal hamstring tendons has to be taken into consideration, with adhesions or direct compression by the swollen tendons (Miller et al. 2007). Technically a partial tenotomy is performed. With the patient in a prone position the ischial tuberosity is exposed either via a transverse gluteal crease incision or via a longitudinal posterior incision by retracting superiorly the gluteus maximus muscle. The proximal attachment sites of the hamstring muscles is identified and a transverse tenotomy is done to the thickened semimembranosus tendon 3–4 cm distal to its origin. The biceps femoris and semitendinosus muscles are normally left intact. The partially tenotomised semimembranosus tendon is then sutured to the biceps femoris tendon to prevent excessive retraction. After tenotomy the sciatic nerve is explored and freed from adhesions if necessary. After surgery the patient is allowed to begin full weight bearing gradually during the first two post-operative weeks. All kind of stretching and pressure to the hamstrings are avoided first three to four weeks. Light swimming and aqua training are allowed 2–3 weeks after surgery. Bicycling with gradually increasing time and intensity is begun after 4 weeks. Running and heavier weight training are typically allowed 2 months after the operation (Lempainen et al. 2015). Results reported are good with 80 out of 90 patients being able to return to the same level of sporting activity as before the onset of the symptoms after surgery (Lempainen et al. 2009). This took an average of 5 months (range, 2–12). Similar results have also been reported after surgery in nonathletic patients with chronic PHT symptoms (Saikku et al. 2010).

24.5.2 Piriformis

The piriformis muscle is biarticular, constituting a bridge in front of the sacroiliac joint and behind the coxofemoral joint. It has a triangular shape with the base inserted on each side of the ventral surface of the sacrum at the edges of the 2nd and 3rd sacral foramens. The piriformis muscle exits the pelvic cavity by sliding under the greater sciatic notch, above the sacral spinal ligament. It then runs diagonally downwards through the gluteal region and culminates on the upper side of the greater trochanter of the femur. In the gluteal region it is located under the gluteus maximus and above the internal obturator muscle ending. It delimits the two zones of musculoligamentous passages known as the supra-piriformis and infra-piriformis foramens. The superior gluteal nerves and vessels traverse the supra-piriformis foramen. Along with the inferior gluteal and pudendal nerves, the sciatic nerve passes through the infra-piriformis canal. Less frequently, the sciatic nerve can go so far as to span the piriformis muscle. The piriformis muscle is essentially a lateral hip rotator, but it is also an extensor. It may take on a secondary role as an abductor when its point of support on the sacrum is proximal (Michel et al. 2013). The piriformis muscle syndrome (PMS) is defined as an entrapment neuropathy involving compression of the sciatic nerve by the piriformis muscle and entailing a number of symptoms with truncal sciatic pain, initially in the muscles of the buttocks (Robinson 1947). Complex proximal insertion appears likely to create zones of conflict. The distal femoral insertions of the piriformis muscle also constitute the locus of tendinous expansion towards the different structures located at the posterior superior edge of the greater trochanter. The stabilizing role of the piriformis muscle on the sacroiliac joint has been described (Snijders et al. 2006). Positional factors such as prolonged sitting and intense physical activity such as long-distance or cross-country running have been associated with piriformis syndrome. In the seated position, especially when the torso is sagittally straight, the pelvis carries out an anteversion movement provoking tension in the sacrotuberal ligament strongly associated with the piriformis muscle. During a footrace, the constraints endured by the sacroiliac joints drive the lower extremity of the sacrum upwards, and yet, it is held back by several ligaments, including the sacrotuberal (Michel et al. 2013). Patients complain pain in the buttock that may refer down the back of the leg in a sciatic distribution and is aggravated with sitting. Onset is typically insidious but may involve a traumatic impact, such as a fall. Its fluctuating development is favoured by intense effort and, more particularly, by "trigger" postures. Initial clinical assessment must preclude lombosciatica of discal origin, coxofemoral joint pain or sacroiliac joint pathology. There are some risky sport activities (distance running, cycling, horse riding) and exposed professions involving prolonged periods in a seated position (truck driver, taxi driver). During palpation of the gluteal region can be perceived an indurated and painful cord along the trajectory of the piriformis muscle. In a patient in a contralateral lateral decubitus position, the examiner places the hip of the painful lower member at 45° of flexion and in light internal rotation. The piriformis muscle is palpated 1–2 cm below the middle third of a line drawn between the posterior superior iliac spine and the upper boundary of the greater trochanter. Different manoeuvres can reproduce the pain experienced by the patient: buttock pain and sciatic torpor accompanied sometimes by distal paresthesia. Prolonging these manoeuvres, the sciatic pain may appear. In the Freiberg manoeuvre with a patient in supine position, the examiner provokes internal rotation and adduction of the affected lower limb, with the hip in 45° flexion and the knee in extension. Also a FADIR test can evoke symptoms. In the Pace and Nagle manoeuvre with his legs dangling over the edge of the examination table, the seated patient is asked to separate his knees against the manual resistance of the examiner. In the Beatty manoeuvre, the patient is placed in lateral decubitus position on the healthy side. On the painful side, the hip and the knee are in flexion, thereby allowing the medial surface of the knee to be propped on the examination table and the foot to be hooked behind the leg of the healthy limb. The patient is asked to carry out a movement of lateral rotation and hip abduction against the manual resistance of the examiner. From the same starting position, in the Fishman FADIR test, a foot is hooked behind the heel of the healthy limb. The patient actively raises the foot along the dorsal side of the leg (Michel et al. 2013). Imaging studies (standard X-ray, scanner, MRI) of the spine, the hips and the pelvis facilitate elimination of differential diagnoses. A pelvis MRI scan is necessary to detect on the affected side a possible hypertrophy of the piriformis muscle, which is a potential source of compression of the sciatic nerve (Pecina et al. 2008). In the context of a differential diagnosis, electroneuromyography (ENMG) allows for visualization of electrical signs in connection with a truncal injury of the sciatic or root nerve L5 or S1. Piriformis syndrome usually responds to conservative treatments, including physical therapy, lifestyle modification and NSAIDs. Mobilization of soft tissue restrictions and trigger points is useful. Aggressive piriformis stretching should be avoided when symptoms are irritable. Hip and lumbosacral mobilizations may also be useful if restricted motion is observed. Image-guided injections (corticosteroid, anaesthetic or botulinum toxin A) may be used for refractory cases to obtain short-term relief and determine potential surgical benefit (Filler et al. 2005; Jankovic et al. 2013). A pelvic neurogram is recommended in refractory cases to better assess for anomalous sciatic nerve anatomy causing piriformis syndrome. When the diagnosis is clear, cases that fail conservative treatment may benefit from endoscopic release of the piriformis and sciatic nerve decompression. Access to the subgluteal region begins with development and inspection of the peritrochanteric region. Then, viewing from the peritrochanteric space, posterolaterally based portals can safely be positioned. These must be posterior enough to pass behind the posterior border of the greater trochanter. The hip is placed in full internal rotation that brings the greater trochanter more anterior and eases access to the subgluteal region. Once complete visualization has been achieved by clearing out various membranous layers, the piriformis is divided at its myotendinous junction. This is lateral to the sciatic nerve and typically results in approximately 3 cm tendinous insertion stump that is excised. The sciatic nerve can be visualized coursing from the notch distally into the proximal thigh, and other sites of compression or tethering can be identified. Mobilization of the nerve always begins on its lateral border, from which no nerve branches exit that could possibly be harmed. Postoperatively, crutches are used only for a couple of weeks to normalize gait. Range of motion is emphasized, especially for mobilization of the sciatic nerve to prevent adhesions. Prolonged sitting is avoided with resumption of activities after 2 months as symptoms allow (Byrd 2015).

References

Anderson CN (2016) Iliopsoas: pathology, diagnosis, and treatment. Clin Sports Med 35(3):419–433

Andersson E, Oddsson L, Grundström H et al (1995) The role of the psoas and iliacus muscles for stability and movement of the lumbar spine, pelvis and hip. Scand J Med Sci Sports 5(1):10–16

Aprato A, Jayasekera N, Bajwa A, Villar RN (2014) Peri-articular diseases of the hip: emerging frontiers in arthroscopic and endoscopic treatments. J Orthop Traumatol 15(1):1–11

Atkinson HD, Johal P, Falworth MS et al (2010) Adductor tenotomy: its role in the management of sports-related chronic groin pain. Arch Orthop Trauma Surg 130(8):965–970

Bird PA, Oakley SP, Shnier R, Kirkham BW (2001) Prospective evaluation of magnetic resonance imaging and physical examination findings in patients with greater trochanteric pain syndrome. Arthritis Rheum 44(9):2138–2145

Bisciotti GN, Volpi P, Zini R, et al (2016) Groin Pain Syndrome Italian Consensus Conference on terminology, clinical evaluation and imaging assessment in groin pain in athlete. BMJ Open Sport & Exercise Medicine 2:e000142. doi: 10.1136/bmjsem-2016-000142

Blankenbaker DG, De Smet AA, Keene JS et al (2007 May) Classification and localization of acetabular labral tears. Skelet Radiol 36(5):391–397

Blankenbaker DG, Tuite MJ, Keene JS et al (2012 Oct) Labral injuries due to iliopsoas impingement: can they be diagnosed on MR arthrography? AJR Am J Roentgenol 199(4):894–900

Blankenbaker DG, Ullrick SR, Davis KW et al (2008) Correlation of MRI findings with clinical findings of trochanteric pain syndrome. Skelet Radiol 37(10):903–909

Byrd JW (2006) Evaluation and management of the snapping iliopsoas tendon. Instr Course Lect 55:347–355

Byrd JW (2015) Disorders of the peritrochanteric and deep gluteal space: new frontiers for arthroscopy. Sports Med Arthrosc 23(4):221–231

Cacchio A, Rompe JD, Furia JP et al (2011) Shockwave therapy for the treatment of chronic proximal hamstring tendinopathy in professional athletes. Am J Sports Med 39(1):146–153

Cascio BM, King D, Yen Y-M (2013) Psoas impingement causing labrum tear: a series from three tertiary hip arthroscopy centres. J La State Med Soc 165(2):88–93

Chandrasekaran S, Lodhia P, Gui C et al (2015) Outcomes of open versus endoscopic repair of abductor muscle tears of the hip: a systematic review. Arthroscopy 31(10):2057–2067

Cook JL, Purdam C (2012) Is compressive load a factor in the development of tendinopathy? Br J Sports Med 46(3):163–168

Davies JF, Stiehl JB, Davies JA, Geiger PB (2013) Surgical treatment of hip abductor tendon tears. J Bone Joint Surg Am 95(15):1420–1425

Dean CS, Arbeloa-Gutierrez L, Chahla J, Pascual-Garrido C (2016) Proximal rectus femoris avulsion repair. Arthrosc Tech 5(3):e545–e549

Docking S, Samiric T, Scase E et al (2013) Relationship between compressive loading and ECM changes in tendons. Muscles Ligaments Tendons J 3:7–11

Domb BG, Shindle MK, McArthur B et al (2011) Iliopsoas impingement: a newly identified cause of labral pathology in the hip. HSS J 7(2):145–150

Dunn T, Heller CA, McCarthy SW et al (2003) Anatomical study of the "trochanteric bursa". Clin Anat 16(3):233–240

Elattar O, Choi HR, Dills VD, Busconi B (2016) Groin injuries (Athletic Pubalgia) and return to play. Sports Health 8(4):313–323

Filler AG, Haynes J, Jordan SE et al (2005) Sciatica of nondisc origin and piriformis syndrome: diagnosis by magnetic resonance neurography and interventional magnetic resonance imaging with outcome study of resulting treatment. J Neurosurg Spine 2(2):99–115

Fitzgerald P (1969) The action of the iliopsoas muscle. Ir J Med Sci 8(1):31–33

Fitzpatrick J, Bulsara M, Zheng MH. The effectiveness of platelet-rich plasma in the treatment of tendinopathy: a meta-analysis of randomized controlled clinical trials. June 2016;pii:0363546516643716. [Epub ahead of print]

Fricker PA (1997) Management of groin pain in athletes. Br J Sports Med 31(2):97–101

Gill TJ, Carroll KM, Makani A et al (2014) Surgical technique for treatment of recalcitrant adductor longus tendinopathy. Arthrosc Tech 3(2):e293–e297

Goom TS, Malliaras P, Reiman MP, Purdam CR (2016) Proximal hamstring tendinopathy: clinical aspects of assessment and management. J Orthop Sports Phys Ther 46(6):483–493

Guanche CA (2015) Hamstring injuries. J Hip Preserv Surg 2(2):116–122

Hasselman CT, Best TM, Hughes C et al (1995) An explanation for various rectus femoris strain injuries using previously undescribed muscle architecture. Am J Sports Med 23(4):493–499

Hetsroni I, Larson CM, Dela Torre K et al (2012) Anterior inferior iliac spine deformity as an extra-articular source for hip impingement: a series of 10 patients treated with arthroscopic decompression. Arthroscopy 28(11):1644–1653

Heyworth BE, Shindle MK, Voos JE et al (2007 Dec) Radiologic and intraoperative findings in revision hip arthroscopy. Arthroscopy 23(12):1295–1302

Ho GW, Howard TM (2012) Greater trochanteric pain syndrome: more than bursitis and iliotibial tract friction. Curr Sports Med Rep 11(5):232–238

Holmich P (2007) Long-standing groin pain in sportspeople falls into three primary patterns, a "clinical entity" approach: a prospective study of 207 patients. Br J Sports Med 41(4):247–252

Holmich P, Thorborg K, Dehlendorff C et al (2014) Incidence and clinical presentation of groin injuries in sub-elite male soccer. Br J Sports Med 48(16):1245–1250

Holmich P, Uhrskou P, Ulnits L et al (1999) Effectiveness of active physical training as treatment for long-standing adductor-related groin pain in athletes: randomised trial. Lancet 353(9151):439–443

Hrysomallis C (2009) Hip adductors' strength, flexibility, and injury risk. J Strength Cond Res 23(5):1514–1517

IKobayashi H, Kaneko H, Homma Y et al (2015) Acute calcific tendinitis of the rectus femoris: a case series. J Orthop Case Rep 5(3):32–34

Ilizaliturri VM Jr, Buganza-Tepole M, Olivos-Meza A et al (2014) Central compartment release versus lesser trochanter release of the iliopsoas tendon for the treatment of internal snapping hip: a comparative study. Arthroscopy 30(7):790–795

Ilizaliturri VM Jr, Camacho-Galindo J (2010 Jun) Endoscopic treatment of snapping hips, iliotibial band, and iliopsoas tendon. Sports Med Arthrosc 18(2):120–127

Ilizaliturri VM Jr, Martinez-Escalante FA, Chaidez PA, Camacho-Galindo J (2006) Endoscopic iliotibial band release for external snapping hip syndrome. Arthroscopy 22(5):505–510

Ilizaliturri VM Jr, Villalobos FE, Chaidez PA et al (2005) Internal snapping hip syndrome: treatment by endoscopic release of the iliopsoas tendon. Arthroscopy 21(11):1375–1380

Jankovic D, Peng P, van Zundert A (2013) Brief review: Piriformis syndrome: etiology, diagnosis, and management. Can J Anaesth 60(10):1003–1012

Jayaseelan DJ, Moats N, Ricardo CR (2013) Rehabilitation of proximal hamstring tendinopathy utilizing eccentric training, lumbopelvic stabilization, and trigger point dry needling: 2 case reports. J Orthop Sports Phys Ther 44(3):198–205

Johnston CA, Wiley JP, Lindsay DM et al (1998) Iliopsoas bursitis and tendinitis. A review. Sports Med 25(4):271–283

Joseph MF, Denegar CR (2015) Treating tendinopathy: perspective on anti-inflammatory intervention and therapeutic exercise. Clin Sports Med 34(2):363–374

Kagan A (1999) Rotator cuff tears of the hip. Clin Orthop Relat Res 368:135–140

Kaltenborn A, Bourg CM, Gutzeit A, Kalberer F (2014) The Hip Lag Sign-prospective blinded trial of a new clinical sign to predict hip abductor damage. PLoS One 9(3):e91560.ù

Kaux JF, Forthomme B, Le Goff C et al (2011) Current opinions on tendinopathy. J Sports Sci Med 10(2):238–253

Kaux JF, Samson A, Crielaard JM (2016 Feb) Hyaluronic acid and tendon lesions. Muscles Ligaments Tendons J 5(4):264–269

Khan M, Adamich J, Simunovic N et al (2013) Surgical management of internal snapping hip syndrome: a systematic review evaluating open and arthroscopic approaches. Arthroscopy 29(5):942–948

Leighton RD (2006) A functional model to describe the action of the adductor muscles at the hip in the transverse plane. Physiother Theory Pract 22(5):251–262

Lempainen L, Johansson K, Banke IJ et al (2015) Expert opinion: diagnosis and treatment of proximal hamstring tendinopathy. Muscles Ligaments Tendons J 5(1):23–28

Lempainen L, Sarimo J, Mattila K et al (2009) Proximal hamstring tendinopathy: results of surgical management and histopathologic findings. Am J Sports Med 37(4):727–734

Lequesne M, Mathieu P, Vuillemin-Bodaghi V et al (2008) Gluteal tendinopathy in refractory greater trochanter pain syndrome: diagnostic value of two clinical tests. Arthritis Rheum 59(2):241–246

Levangie PK, Norkin CC (2005) Joint structure and function: a comprehensive analysis, 4th edn. F.A. Davis Company, Philadelphia, PA, p 375

Lyons JC, Peterson LF (1984 May) The snapping iliopsoas tendon. Mayo Clin Proc 59:327–329

Malanga G, Nakamura R (2014 Nov) The role of regenerative medicine in the treatment of sports injuries. Phys Med Rehabil Clin N Am 25(4):881–895

Mani-Babu S, Morrissey D, Waugh C et al (2015) The effectiveness and dose-response relationship of extracorporeal shock wave therapy in lower limb tendinopathy: a systematic review. Am J Sports Med 43(3):752–761

Mendiguchia J, Alentorn-Geli E, Idoate F, Myer GD (2013 Apr) Rectus femoris muscle injuries in football: a clinically relevant review of mechanisms of injury, risk factors and preventive strategies. Br J Sports Med 47(6):359–366

Michel F, Decavel P, Toussirot E et al (2013) The piriformis muscle syndrome: an exploration of anatomical context, pathophysiological hypotheses and diagnostic criteria. Ann Phys Rehabil Med 56(4):300–311

Miller SL, Gill J, Webb GR (2007) The proximal origin of the hamstrings and surrounding anatomy encountered during repair. A cadaveric study. J Bone Joint Surg Am 89(1):44–48

Morelli V, Espinoza L (2005) Groin injuries and groin pain in athletes: part 2. Prim Care 32(1):185–200

Morelli V, Weaver V (2005) Groin injuries and groin pain in athletes: part 1. Prim Care 32(1):163–183

Moriguchi CS, Carnaz L, Silva LC et al (2009) Reliability of intra- and inter-rater palpation discrepancy and estimation of its effects on joint angle measurements. Man Ther 14(3):299–305

Mulligan EP, Middleton EF, Brunette M (2015) Evaluation and management of greater trochanter pain syndrome. Phys Ther Sport 16(3):205–214

Nicholas SJ, Tyler TF (2002) Adductor muscle strains in sport. Sports Med 32(5):339–344

Ouellette H, Thomas BJ, Nelson E, Torriani M (2006) MR imaging of rectus femoris origin injuries. Skelet Radiol 35(9):665–672

Pecina HI, Boric I, Smoljanovic T et al (2008) Surgical evaluation of magnetic resonance imaging findings in piriformis muscle syndrome. Skelet Radiol 37(11):1019–1023

Pesquer L, Poussange N, Sonnery-Cottet B et al (2016) Imaging of rectus femoris proximal tendinopathies. Skelet Radiol 45(7):889–897

Polesello GC, Queiroz MC, Domb BG et al (2013) Surgical technique: endoscopic gluteus maximus tendon release for external snapping hip syndrome. Clin Orthop Relat Res 471(8):2471–2476

Rankin AT, Bleakley CM, Cullen M (2015) Hip joint pathology as a leading cause of groin pain in the sporting population: a 6-year review of 894 cases. Am J Sports Med 43(7):1698–1703

Reich MS, Shannon C, Tsai E, Salata MJ (2013) Hip arthroscopy for extra-articular hip disease. Curr Rev Musculoskelet Med 6(3):250–257

Reid D (2016) The management of greater trochanteric pain syndrome: a systematic literature review. J Orthop 13(1):15–28

Reiman MP, Goode AP, Hegedus EJ et al (2013) Diagnostic accuracy of clinical tests of the hip: a systematic review with meta-analysis. Br J Sports Med 47(12):893–902

Reiman MP, Mather RC III, Cook CE (2015) Physical examination tests for hip dysfunction and injury. Br J Sports Med 49(6):357–361

Robinson DR (1947) Piriformis syndrome in relation to sciatic pain. Am J Surg 73(3):355–358

Rompe JD, Segal NA, Cacchio A et al (2009) Home training, local corticosteroid injection, or radial shock wave therapy for greater trochanter pain syndrome. Am J Sports Med 37(10):1981–1989

de SA D, Hölmich P, Phillips M et al (2016) Athletic groin pain: a systematic review of surgical diagnoses, investigations and treatment. Br J Sports Med 50(19):1181–1186

Saikku K, Vasenius J, Saar P (2010) Entrapment of the proximal sciatic nerve by the hamstring tendons. Acta Orthop Belg 76(3):321–324

Schuett DJ, Bomar JD, Pennock AT (2015) Pelvic apophyseal avulsion fractures: a retrospective review of 228 cases. J Pediatr Orthop 35(6):617–623

Segal NA, Felson DT, Torner JC et al (2007) Greater trochanteric pain syndrome: epidemiology and associated factors. Arch Phys Med Rehabil 88(8):988–992

Serner A, Tol JL, Jomaah N et al (2015) Diagnosis of acute groin injuries: a prospective study of 110 athletes. Am J Sports Med 43(8):1857–1864

Silva F, Adams T, Feinstein J et al (2008) Trochanteric bursitis: refuting the myth of inflammation. J Clin Rheumatol 14(2):82–86

Snijders CJ, Hermans PFG, Kleinrensink GJ (2006) Functional aspects of cross-legged sitting with special attention to piriformis muscles and sacroiliac joints. Clin Biomech 21(2):116–121

Strauss EJ, Nho SJ, Kelly BT (2010) Greater trochanteric pain syndrome. Sports Med Arthrosc 18(2):113–119

Tatu L, Parratte B, Vuillier F et al (2001) Descriptive anatomy of the femoral portion of the iliopsoas muscle. Anatomical basis of anterior snapping of the hip. Surg Radiol Anat 23(6):371–374

Verrall GM, Slavotinek JP, Barnes PG et al (2005) Description of pain provocation tests used for the diagnosis of sports-related chronic groin pain: relationship of tests to defined clinical (pain and tenderness) and MRI (pubic bone marrow oedema) criteria. Scand J Med Sci Sports 15(1):36–42

Walsh MJ, Walton JR, Walsh NA (2011) Surgical repair of the gluteal tendons. A report of 72 cases. J Arthroplast 26(8):1514–1519

Watanabe W, Sato K, Itoi E et al (2002) Posterior pelvic tilt in patients with decreased lumbar lordosis decreases acetabular femoral head covering. Orthopedics 25(3):321–324

Weir A, Hölmich P, Schache AG et al (2015 Jun) Terminology and definitions on groin pain in athletes: building agreement using a short Delphi method. Br J Sports Med 49(12):825–827

Werner J, Hägglund M, Waldén M et al (2009) UEFA injury study: a prospective study of hip and groin injuries in professional football over seven consecutive seasons. Br J Sports Med 43(13):1036–1040

Wetzel RJ, Patel RM, Terry MA (2013) Platelet-rich plasma as an effective treatment for proximal hamstring injuries. Orthopedics 36(1):e64–e70

Yen YM, Lewis CL, Kim YJ (2015) Understanding and treating the snapping hip. Sports Med Arthrosc 23(4):194–199

Yoshio M, Murakami G, Sato T et al (2002) The function of the psoas major muscle: passive kinetics and morphological studies using donated cadavers. J Orthop Sci 7(2):199–207

Zhou Y, Wang JH (2016) PRP treatment efficacy for tendinopathy: a review of basic science studies. Biomed Res Int 2016:9103792

Zini R, Panascì M, Papalia R et al (2014) Rectus femoris tendon calcification: arthroscopic excision in 6 top amateur athletes. Orthop J Sports Med 2(12):2325967114561585

Zissen MH, Wallace G, Steven KJ et al (2010) High hamstring tendinopathy: MRI and ultrasound imaging and therapeutic efficacy of percutaneous corticosteroid injection. AJR Am J Roentgenol 195(4):993–998

The Groin Pain Syndrome

25

G.N. Bisciotti and P. Volpi

Contents

G.N. Bisciotti (✉)
Qatar Orthopaedic and Sport Medicine Hospital, FIFA Center of Excellence, Doha, Qatar
e-mail: bisciotti@libero.it

P. Volpi
Department of knee Orthopedic and Sports Traumatology Unit, Humanitas Research Hospital, Rozzano, Italy

FC Internazionale Medical Staff, Milan, Italy
e-mail: piero.volpi@humanitas.it

25.1 Introduction

Groin pain syndrome (GPS) is a widely known issue among professional and amateur athletes and is a very significant problematic situation that can be associated with an important time loss from sports (Engebretsen et al. 2010; Hölmich et al. 2014). Despite his incidence in athletic population being high (5–28%), the debate regarding his nomenclature diagnosis and management has not still reached a consensus (Weir et al. 2015). This poor definition of GPS means that its management has varied widely. It is important to underline that the term "groin pain," like all the other terms that are used worldwide describing these types of clinical situation like groin disruption, sport hernia, athletic pubalgia, etc., describes a symptom (i.e., "pain in the groin area") and does not represent a diagnosis. The definition concerning GPS established during the first Groin Pain Syndrome Italian Consensus Conference (GPSICC), organized by the Italian Society of Arthroscopy in Milan, on February 5, 2016 (Bisciotti et al. 2016), was:

> *Any clinical symptom reported by the patient, located at the inguinal-pubic-adductor area, affecting sports activities and/or interfering with Activities of Daily Living (ADL), and requiring medical attention.*

The term "symptomis" adopted during the GPSICC is justified by the fact that in GPS a frequent overlapping of different clinical frameworks that strongly interact with each other is

G.L. Canata et al. (eds.), *Muscle and Tendon Injuries*, DOI 10.1007/978-3-662-54184-5_25

present (Vidalin et al. 2004; Bisciotti et al. 2013a, 2015). For this reason GPS is often a diagnostic challenge. One reason of this diagnostic difficulty is the anatomical complexity of the groin area and the frequent overlapping of different diseases which makes extremely complicated a correct diagnosis (Bradshaw et al. 2008; Werner et al. 2009; Nicholson and Scott 2012; Kemp et al. 2012).

25.2 The Different Causes of GPS

During GPSICC, a document was discussed and approved in which, after a deep examination and discussion concerning the literature, a subdivision of GPS in 11 different categories was proposed, including 63 most common and probable diseases that can cause GPS (Table 25.1) as follows:

(1) Articular causes
1. Acetabular labrum tear
2. Femoroacetabular impingement(I)
3. Hip anterosuperior labral tear with avulsion of rectus femoris (HALTAR)
4. Hip osteoarthritis
5. Intra-articular loose bodies
6. Hip instability
7. Adhesive capsulitis
8. Legg-Calvé-Perthes disease and its outcomes
9. Dysplasia and its outcomes
10. Epiphysiolysis and its outcomes
11. Avascular necrosis of the femoral head
12. Sacroiliac joint disorders
13. Lumbar spine disorders
14. Synovitis

Table 25.1 The most likely causes of GPS (Hahn 1989) grouped into 11 different categories

Categories	Number of pathologies
Articular causes	14
Visceral causes	3
Bone causes	4
Musculotendineous causes	14
Pubic symphysis-related causes	3
Neurological causes	1
Developmental causes	2
Genitourinary disease-related causes (inflammatory and not)	15
Neoplastic causes	3
Infectious causes	2
Systemic causes	2
Total: 11	Total: 63

Notes:

(I): Cam-FAI, pincer-FAI, subspine impingement (or anterior inferior iliac spine (AIIS) impingement)

- Visceral causes
  1. Inguinal hernia(I)
  2. Other types of abdominal hernia
  3. Intestinal diseases

Notes:

(I): Concerning inguinal hernia, it is recommended to adopt the classification proposed by the European Hernia Society (Nicholson and Scott 2012).

- Bone causes
  1. Fractures and their outcomes
  2. Stress fractures(I)
  3. Avulsion fractures(II)
  4. Iliac crest contusion (hip pointers)(III)

Notes:

(I): Substantially concerning the pubic ramus or the femoral neck.

(II): Mainly pediatric avulsion fractures involving the anterior inferior iliac spine (AIIS), the anterior superior iliac spine (ASIS), and the ischial tuberosity (ANIT).

(III): Iliac crest contusions or hip pointers result from direct trauma at the level of the iliac crest with subsequent formation of a periosteal hematoma. Such a hematoma can compress the lateral femoro-cutaneous nerve and cause paresthesia.

- Musculotendineous causes
  1. Rectus abdominis injuries
  2. Rectus abdominis tendinopathy
  3. Adductor muscles injuries
  4. Adductor tendinopathy

5. Rectus abdominis—adductor longus common aponeurosis injuries
6. Iliopsoas injuries
7. Iliopsoas tendinopathy
8. Other indirect muscle injuries and their outcomes
9. Direct muscle injuries
10. Iliopsoas impingement(I)
11. Snapping internal hip
12. Snapping external hip
13. Bursitis(II)
14. Weakness of the inguinal canal posterior wall(III)

Notes:

(I): Iliopsoas impingement with the medial portion of the acetabular rim.

(II): Specifically concerning the ileopectineal bursa and greater trochanter seromucous bursa.

(III): Indicated by tenderness on palpation of the inguinal canal, tenderness on palpation at the level of the pubic tubercle, and superficial inguinal ring dilatation. In addition, in general manner, in case of conservative treatment failure, the clinician must consider signs and symptoms that may suggest a serious disease.

- Pubic symphysis-related causes
  1. Osteitis pubis
  2. Symphysis instability(I)
  3. Symphysis degenerative arthropathy

Notes:

(I): The radiological sign of symphyseal instability is represented by an asymmetry of pubic rami greater than 2 mm visible in the Flamingo X-ray view.

- Neurological causes(I)
  - Nerve entrapment syndrome (II)

Notes:

(I): The category "neurological causes" should be divided into two further subcategories. In the first category, there is nerve injury due to overloading or overstretching (neurological causes category A). In the second category, there is nerve injury due to an acute compression mechanism or tear of the nerve (neurological causes category B).

(II): Specifically concerning the lateral femoral cutaneous nerve, genitofemoral nerve (genital branch), ilioinguinal nerve, iliohypogastric nerve, femoral nerve, obturator nerve, and pudendal nerve.

- Developmental causes
  1. Apophysitis(I)
  2. Growth plate at pubic level(II)

Notes:

(I): Specifically concerning the pubic ramus and less frequently the anterior inferior iliac spine (AIIS) and anterior superior iliac spine (ASIS).

(II) Below 20 years of age, it is common to observe anteromedial foci of endochondral ossification centers. These findings become particularly evident in MR arthrography (Omar et al. 2008).

- Genitourinary disease-related causes (inflammatory and noninflammatory)
  1. Prostatitis
  2. Epididymitis
  3. Corditis
  4. Orchitis
  5. Varicocele
  6. Hydrocele
  7. Urethritis
  8. Other infections of the urinary tract
  9. Cystitis
  10. Ovarian cysts
  11. Endometriosis
  12. Ectopic pregnancy
  13. Round ligament entrapment
  14. Testicular/ovarian torsion
  15. Ureteral lithiasis

- Neoplastic causes
  1. Testicular carcinoma
  2. Osteoid osteoma
  3. Other carcinomas
- Infectious causes
  1. Osteomyelitis
  2. Septic arthritis

- Systemic causes
  1. Inguinal lymphadenopathy
  2. Rheumatic diseases

Obviously since, as previously mentioned, also GPS term represents an "umbrella term," and it must be necessarily accompanied by a well-defined diagnosis. In other words, a correct definition of the diagnosis should include the following sentence: "GPS caused by…" or "GPS caused by the association…."

25.3 The Most Frequent Causes of GPS in Athletes

In athletes the most frequent causes of GPS must be classified into articular causes, musculotendinous causes, and pubic symphysis-related causes.

In the first category (i.e., articular causes) , we must underline the importance of cam-FAI syndrome that can not only cause labrum tear and cartilage damage (Zhang et al. 2015) but also be the "starter" of inguinal disease, as we will discuss later (Larson et al. 2011). Furthermore, hip pathology includes also extra-articular disease like iliopsoas bursitis, trochanteric bursitis, external snapping hip syndrome, and stress fracture (Zhang et al. 2015).

In the second category (i.e., musculotendinous causes), the most frequent clinical frameworks are adductor muscle injuries and adductor tendinopathy especially at adductor longus tendon level (Harr 2016). Nevertheless, it is important to note that radiological signs of adductor longus tendinopathy are present in 71% of asymptomatic football players in comparison to a 72% of incidence in a population of symptomatic football players (Branci et al. 2015). For this reason it is paramount to distinguish a "true" adductor longus tendinopathy causing GPS from a simple functional adaptation.

In the last category (i.e., pubic symphysis-related causes), it is important to remember that the source of pain should be divided in to three zones of focal pain:

(1) First zone (suprapubic sources of pain): regarding the periosteum of the superior portion of the superior pubic rami (corresponding to abdominis rectus muscle insertion)
(2) Second zone (intrapubic sources of pain): regarding the pubic symphysis branches and its fibrocartilaginous interpubic disk. Intrapubic pain is the sign of "true" osteitis pubis.
(3) Third zone (infrapubic sources of pain): regarding the periosteum of the inferior portion of superior pubic rami (corresponding to the adductor longus muscle insertion).

25.4 The Different Types of GPS

The clinical presentation of GPS must be very different especially regarding both the etiopathogenesis (by traumatic or by overuse origin) and the temporal length of the symptoms reported by patients. Basing on these two aspects, we propose (Bisciotti et al. 2016) to subdivide the GPS into the following three categories:

(1) GPS of traumatic origin, in which the onset of pain was due to any acute trauma. This hypothesis is supported by medical history, clinical examination, and imaging.
(2) GPS due to functional overload, characterized by insidious and progressive onset, without an acute trauma, or a situation to which the onset of pain symptoms can be attributed with certainty.
(3) Long-standing GPS (LSGPS) or chronic GPS, in which the cohort of symptoms complained by the patient continues for a long period (over 12 weeks) and is recalcitrant to any conservative therapy.

25.5 The Particular Case of LSGPS

The typical patient who complains LSGP is a subject with a long history of groin pain (more than 3 months) that has already performed several clinical and imaging assessments and that, above all, has already performed unsuccessfully many types of conservative treatments. In this case it must be strongly suspected an inguinal disease (Bisciotti et al. 2015; Gilmore et al. 2014). With the term "inguinal disease," we mean a series of clinical conditions like true hernia, occult hernia, weakness of the inguinal canal posterior wall, microtear at conjoint tendon, inguinal ligament, and Cooper ligament level (Bisciotti et al. 2015; Gilmore et al. 2014) that often can cause a situation of "groin disruption" (Garvey and Hazard 2014). In the most part of the cases, this situation of groin disruption is caused by the presence of a cam-FAI syndrome (Bisciotti et al. 2015; Rambani and Hackney 2015; Griffin et al. 2016). Cam-FAI is an abnormal conformation of femoral head. In other words, cam-FAI is an osteochondral bump at femoral head-neck junction leading to a diminution of the normal femoral head-neck offset (Economopoulos et al. 2014; Satpathy et al. 2015; Fairley et al. 2016). Cam-FAI syndrome is identified by measuring the alpha angle on the Dunn view X-ray, as showed in Fig. 25.1. An alpha

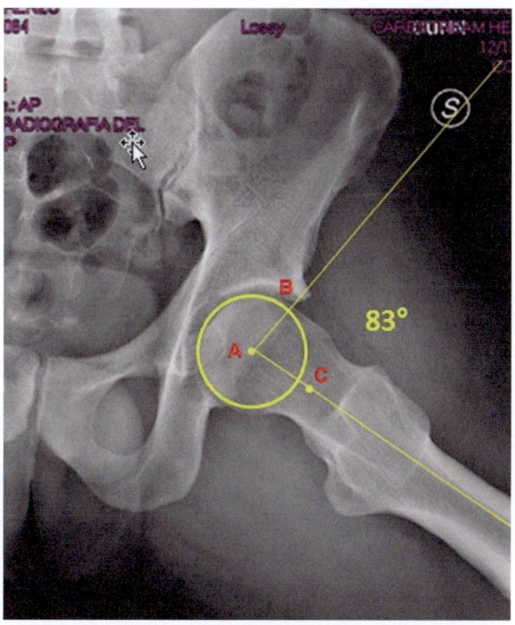

Fig. 25.1 Dunn view X-ray in which the alpha angle is calculated. The alpha angle is defined by drawing the best-fit circle (i.e., the circle that best suits the sphericity of the femoral head) and identifying the point where the femoral head profile leaves this circle; a line is drawn between the center of this circle (*A*) and the identified point (*B*). A second line is drawn between the point *A* and the center of femoral neck (*C*). The angle between these two lines is the alpha angle. An alpha angle measuring 55° or greater is considered a radiographic evidence of cam-FAI syndrome

angle measuring 55° or greater is considered radiographic evidence of cam-FAI (Beck et al. 2005). Cam-FAI syndrome can cause both hip articular cartilage and labral lesion (Griffin et al. 2016) and limitation of hip joint intra-rotation (Hammoud et al. 2012; Hammoud et al. 2014). Recently cam-FAI has been shown to be associated in GPS especially in young high-level athletes (Hammoud et al. 2012; Philippon et al. 2007; Philippon et al. 2010; Kapron et al. 2011; Weir et al. 2011; Siebenrock et al. 2011; Larson et al. 2013).

This association may be explained by the fact that in the athlete suffering from cam-FAI syndrome, the functional range of motion (ROM) required in athletic competition is often greater than the limited physiologic motion (Hammoud et al. 2012, 2014). This limitation of ROM can be compensated by an iper-mobility of the symphyseal articulation. This iper-mobility of the symphyseal articulation can stress the posterior inguinal wall and favor the onset of inguinal pathology (Bisciotti et al. 2016; Hammoud et al. 2012, 2014). The inguinal pathology shows a low rate of positive outcome with conservative treatment (Omar et al. 2008; Ahumada et al. 2005); in these cases it is necessary to consider a surgical treatment. Nowadays, the most utilized surgical treatment in inguinal pathology is Shouldice repair, open all-suture repair technique, Lichtenstein repair, transabdominal preperitoneal (TAPP) repair, total extraperitoneal (TEP) repair, transinguinal preperitoneal repair (TIPP), minimal repair, and inguinal ligament release procedure (Muschaweck and Berger 2010; Lange 2016; Lloyd 2016).

Sometimes this procedures may be completed with a single or double tenotomy at longus adductor level and/or a triple or selective neurectomy of ilioinguinal, iliohypogastric, and genital branch of femorogenital nerves (Harr 2016; Muschaweck and Berger 2010; Rossidis et al. 2015; Santilli et al. 2016). Following surgical repair, independently by the surgical technique used, most of the series report that >90% of athletes return to full sport activity within 2–4 months after surgery (Rossidis et al. 2015). In any case this high number of techniques used demonstrates that the pathophysiology of GPS is still controversial.

25.6 The Complication of Inguinal Hernia Surgical Repair

In the past the hernia surgical repair showed complication of recurrence rate of up to 67% (Vahedifar and Kamrava 2016). Nowadays, after mesh placement, the problem of recurrence is greatly reduced, and the rate of recurrence is currently between 1% and 10% for all the most used surgical techniques (Felix 2001; Pironi et al. 2008), while chronic groin pain represents a frequent problem after hernia repair with an incidence ranging from 10% to 19% (Vahedifar and Kamrava 2016; O'Dwyer et al. 2005), also if some series describe an incidence rate as high as 62.9% (Poobalan et al. 2001) with up to 10% of patients falling into moderate to severe pain (Hakeem and Shanmugam 2011). Usually secondary inguinodynia—that is the technical term for chronic groin pain after hernia repair that has continued for more than three months—is mild but in 3% of the subjects is severe and shows dramatic effect on patient's work and life daily activities (O'Dwyer et al. 2005). SI may be classified as neuropathic or non-neuropathic, with approximately 50% of patients belonging to each category (Loos et al. 2007). Then, ironically now SI is the most important complication after inguinal hernia repair replacing the old problem of recurrence of the past. SI may be caused by several situations among which the most frequent are:

(1) During hernia dissection it is possible to produce a stimulation, an entrapment, or a true injury to the nerves. This neuropathic pain may be caused by direct nerve injury due to granuloma formation, excess fibrotic reaction, direct contact of nerves with mesh, and nerve entrapment by sutures, staples, tacks, and folded or wrinkled mesh also known as meshoma (Aasvang and Kehlet 2005). Also the mesh attachment to the pubic tubercle by tack or staple may cause a periosteal reaction and be a source of SI (Miller et al. 2016). In these cases the sequelae are represented by neuralgia, paresthesia, hypoesthesia, or hyperesthesia. With an open approach, the nerves at risk are the genital branch of the genitofemoral nerve, the ilioinguinal nerve, and the iliohypogastric nerve, while with a laparoscopic (TAPP or TEP) approach, the nerves at risk are the genital nerve, the femoral branch of the genitofemoral nerve, and, more rarely, the lateral femoral cutaneous nerve, and the anterior femoral cutaneous nerve (O'Dwyer et al. 2005; Ferzli et al. 2007; Ma and Ramaswamy 2016).

(2) A remnant cord lipoma (CL) from an original surgery. It is important to remember that a cord lipoma does not represent a recurrence. CL in the most part of the cases does not show a peritoneal sac, but despite this can cause the same symptoms of a groin hernia (Lilly and Arregui 2002). It is important to note that spermatic CL is found also in the absence of a true inguinal hernia in 36–75% of the cases during male subject autopsies, while lipomas of the round ligament are present in 21–73% of the cases during herniorrhaphy. For these reasons they have often considered incidental findings during hernia repair (Heller et al. 2002; Fataar 2011). During TAPP inguinal hernia repair, it is more likely that CL or round ligament lipoma will be missed (Gersin et al. 1999). Then given the increasing popularity of laparoscopic inguinal hernia repair, the presence of a missed CL or round ligament lipoma should be considered if the patient is still experiencing pain after laparoscopic inguinal herniorrhaphy (Lilly and Arregui 2002; Nasr et al. 2005).

(3) The onset of nociceptive pain, transmitted to the brain via A-delta and C-fibers, is caused by activation of nociceptors by nociceptive molecules due to tissue injury or inflammatory reaction (Jacob et al. 2016).

In case of post-surgery neuropathic pain, the first line of treatment is represented by NSAIDs whose purpose is decreasing the inflammation process, while for moderate to severe SI, opioid analgesia may be necessary (Palumbo et al. 2007).

Antidepressants are another first-line therapy used for chronic neuropathic pain (Hansen et al. 2010). Also the use of corticosteroid drugs in the early stage of SI has proven its effectiveness showing improvement in 60–80% of the patients after a period comprising between 2 weeks and 4 months (Kozin et al. 1976; Christensen et al. 1982).

Only after failure of pharmacological treatment may surgical treatment be taken into consideration that consists in partial or complete mesh removal, foreign body removal (Öberg et al. 2016), and/or a triple (genital branch of the genitofemoral nerve, ilioinguinal nerve, and iliohypogastric nerve) or selective neurectomy. The neurectomy may be eventually preceded by nerve blocks with local anesthetics (Thomassen et al. 2013) and pulsed radiofrequency therapy (Misra et al. 2009). Neurectomy success rate is between 70 and 95% (Hahn 1989; Starling and Harms 1989; Bradshaw et al. 1997; Alfieri et al. 2011). In any case, it is important to underline that neurectomy must be avoided for the obturator nerve since its main function is motor innervations. In case of problem at obturator nerve level, the best option is represented by surgical neurolysis or nerve decompression (Bradshaw et al. 1997).

A specific clinical framework in the context of post-surgery neuropathic pain is represented by chronic testicular pain or orchialgia (OR). Very often the etiopathogenesis of OR is different from that of SI both from neuroanatomical and causative points of view. OR can arise after all types of surgical inguinal repair and his management remains a challenge. Triple neurectomy is typically ineffective for OR, and the best solution is the resection of the parabasal fibers or spermatic cord denervation (Strom and Levine 2008; Levine 2010; Dunkin 2016).

25.7 The Association Between Inguinal Hernia and Adductor Tendinopathy

The symphysis instability due to the presence of a cam-FAI syndrome often causes the association of three different pathologies: osteitis pubis, severe longus adductor tendinopathy, and weakness of the inguinal canal posterior wall or inguinal hernia (Bisciotti et al. 2016). In these particular cases, it becomes necessary for a double surgical intervention. The first consists in a mesh positioning, or otherwise in a surgical reinforcing inguinal canal posterior wall technique, coupled to adductor longus, partial, or total tenotomy (Harr 2016; Rossidis et al. 2015). The adductor longus tenotomy presents the multiple vantage points to relieve the mechanical stress at adductor and at rectus abdominis level as well as the inguinal floor weakness and therefore may be the most optimal management especially in the case of severe adductor tendinopathy coupled to inguinal pathology (Rossidis et al. 2015). Recent studies show that open and laparoscopic inguinal hernia repair, with or without mesh placement, coupled to adductor tenotomy demonstrates a return to full activity rate of 95–100% in 3–4 months (Harr 2016; Rossidis et al. 2015). It is important to remember that some electromyographic studies demonstrate that adductor longus muscle shows minimal activity during sprint (Mann et al. 1986) or cutting movements (Neptune et al. 1999). For this reason more recent studies demonstrate that the release of the longus adductor tendon does not compromise the high-level sports performance (Bisciotti et al. 2013a, 2013b; Schlegel et al. 2009).

25.8 The Problematic of Double (Hernia and Cam-FAI) Surgical Intervention

Given the relationship between cam-FAI syndrome and inguinal pathologies, a problem arises if an athlete shows both pathologies, if the surgeon must limit the surgical intervention only to the inguinal pathology, or if he must also consider a second surgery intervention concerning the cam-FAI deformity. This problematic had already been raised by other authors (Larson et al. 2011; Hammoud et al. 2012).

Larson et al. (2011) evaluated 37 subjects that were diagnosed with both symptomatic GPS and associated intra-articular hip pathology (30 cases of FAI, 1 traumatic labral tear, and 1 borderline dysplasia). The subject was evaluated at a mean of 29 months (range, 12–78 months) after surgery. The results showed that when surgery only addressed either GPS or intra-articular hip pathology, the outcomes were suboptimal. On the contrary surgical management of both disorders concurrently or in a staged manner led to improved postoperative outcomes scoring and an unrestricted return to sporting activity in 89% of the subjects.

Hammoud et al. (2012) report a series of 38 professional athletes surgically treated for symptomatic cam-FAI, with 12 of the considered subjects (32%) having previous surgical intervention for inguinal pathologies (IP). After additional surgical treatment for cam-FAI, all the patients were able to return to their sport activity. Moreover, of the 26 remaining patients, 15 had symptoms of IP that were resolved with surgical treatment. In this study, 39% (15/39) of athletes with both IP and cam-FAI symptoms had complete resolution of pain and return to their sport activity with cam-FAI surgery alone.

Therefore, it is possible that there exists a degree of impingement, and consequently an alpha angle value, beyond which it is necessary to consider the double surgery. Furthermore, it is also reasonable to suggest the hypothesis that a surgery mesh intervention in the presence of a high degree of hip impingement may have on the long follow-up a negative outcome due to the persistence of mechanical stress. However, further studies of more evidence are needed to confirm this hypothesis.

Conclusions

The GPS is sometimes a true diagnostic challenge for clinician because of the anatomical complexity of the groin area and the frequent overlapping of the different clinical frameworks causing GPS. Nevertheless, the reference to the main causes of GPS established during the first GPSICC may be an important help for the clinician in establishing a correct diagnosis. Furthermore, it is important to remember that the strong association between cam-FAI syndrome and inguinal pathologies and the increased diffusion of laparoscopic and open techniques for inguinal hernia repair will require in the future for the clinician to address new and challenging clinical frameworks.

References

Aasvang E, Kehlet H (2005) Surgical management of chronic pain after inguinal hernia repair. Br J Surg 92(7):795–801

Ahumada LA, Ashruf S, Espinosa-de-los-Monteros A, Long JN, de la Torre JI, Garth WP, Vasconez LO (2005) Athletic pubalgia: definition and surgical treatment. Ann Plast Surg 55(4):393–396

Alfieri S, Amid PK, Campanelli G, Izard G, Kehlet H, Wijsmuller AR et al (2011) International guidelines for prevention and management of post-operative chronic pain following inguinal hernia surgery. Hernia 15(3):239–249

Beck M, Kalhor M, Leunig M, Ganz R (2005) Hip morphology influences the pattern of damage to the acetabular cartilage: femoroacetabular impingement as a cause of early osteoarthritis of the hip. J Bone Joint Surg Br 87:1012–1018.3

Bisciotti GN, Auci A, Di Marzo F, Galli R, Pulici L, Carimati G, Quaglia A, Volpi P (2015) Groin pain syndrome: an association of different pathologies and a case presentation. Muscle, Tendon Ligament J 5(3):214–222

Bisciotti GN, Eirale C, Cassaghi G (2013b) Lesioni acute degli adduttori: chirurgia o riabilitazione? Il fisioterapista 6:5–10

Bisciotti GN, Eirale C, Vuckovic Z, Le Picard P, D'Hooge P, Chalabi H (2013a) La pubalgia dell'atleta: una revisione della letteratura. Med Sport 66(1):119–133

Bisciotti GN., Volpi P, Zini R, Auci A, Di Marzo F, Carimati G et al. (2016) Groin pain syndrome italian consensus conference on terminology, clinical evaluation and imaging assessment in groin pain in athlete. BMJ, in press.

Bradshaw CJ, Bundy M, Falvey E (2008) The diagnosis of longstanding groin pain: a prospective clinical cohort study. Br J Sports Med 42:851–854.43

Bradshaw C, McCrory P, Bell S, Brukner P (1997) Obturator nerve entrapment: a cause of groin pain in athletes. Am J Sports Med 25(3):402–408

Branci S, Thorborg K, Bech BH, Boesen M, Nielsen MB, Hölmich P (2015) MRI findings in soccer players with long-standing adductor-related groin pain and asymptomatic controls. Br J Sports Med 49(10):681–691

Christensen K, Jensen EM, Noer I (1982) The reflex dystrophy syndrome response to treatment with systemic corticosteroids. Acta Chir Scand 148(8):653–655

Dunkin JB (2016) Perioperative Pain Management: Multimodalities to Prevent Postoperative Chronic Pain. In:

Jacob BP, Chen DC, Ramshaw B, Towfigh S (eds) The SAGES manual of groin pain. Springer, New York
Economopoulos KJ, Milewski MD, Hanks JB, Hart JM, Diduch DR (2014) Radiographic evidence of femoroacetabular impingement in athletes with athletic pubalgia. Sports Health 6(2):171–177
Engebretsen AH, Myklebust G, Holme I, Engebretsen L, Bahr R (2010) Intrinsic risk factors for groin injuries among male soccer players: a prospective cohort study. Am J Sports Med 38(10):2051–2057
Fairley J, Wang Y, Teichtahl AJ, Seneviwickrama M, Wluka AE, Brady SR, Hussain SM, Liew S, Cicuttini FM. Management options for femoroacetabular impingement: a systematic review of symptom and structural outcomes. Osteoarthr Cartil. 2016. pii:S1063–4584(16)30048–6
Fataar S (2011) CT of inguinal canal lipomas and fat-containing inguinal hernias. J Med Imaging Radiat Oncol 55(5):485–492
Felix EL (2001) A unified approach to recurrent laparoscopic hernia repairs. Surg Endosc 15:969–971
Ferzli GS, Edwards ED, Khoury GE (2007) Chronic pain after inguinal herniorrhaphy. J Am Coll Surg 205(2):333–341
Garvey JF, Hazard H (2014) Sports hernia or groin disruption injury? Chronic athletic groin pain: a retrospective study of 100 patients with long-term follow-up. Hernia 18(6)
Gersin KS, Heniford BT, Garcia-Ruiz A, Ponsky JL (1999) Missed lipoma of the spermatic cord. A pitfall of transabdominal preperitoneal laparoscopic hernia repair. Surg Endosc 13(6):585–587
Gilmore CJ, Diduch DR, Handley MV, Hanks JB (2014) Sports Hernia-History and physical examination: making the diagnosis with confidence. In: Diduch DR, Brunt LM (eds) . Springer, New York
Griffin DR, Dickenson EJ, O'Donnell J, Agricola R, Awan T, Bennell KL et al (2016) The Warwick Agreement on femoroacetabular impingement syndrome (FAI syndrome):an international consensus statement. Br J Sports Med 50(19):1169–1176
Hahn L (1989) Clinical findings and results of operative treatment in ilioinguinal nerve entrapment syndrome. Br J Obstet Gynaecol 96(9):1080–1083
Hakeem A, Shanmugam V (2011) Inguinodynia following Lichtenstein tension-free hernia repair: a review. World J Gastroenterol 17(14):1791–1796
Hammoud S, Bedi A, Magennis E, Meyers WC, Kelly BT (2012) High incidence of athletic pubalgia symptoms in professional athletes with symptomatic femoroacetabular impingement. Arthroscopy 28(10):1388–1395
Hammoud S, Bedi A, Voos JE, Mauro CS, Kelly BT (2014) The recognition and evaluation of patterns of compensatory injury in patients with mechanical hip pain. Sports Health 6(2):108–118
Hansen MB, Andersen KG, Crawford ME (2010) Pain following the repair of an abdominal hernia. Surg Today 40(1):8–21
Harr JN (2016) Brody F. Sports hernia repair with adductor tenotomy, Hernia. [Epub ahead of print]
Heller CA, Marucci DD, Dunn T, Barr EM, Houang M, Dos Remedios C (2002) Inguinal canal "lipoma". Clin Anat 15(4):280–285
Hölmich P, Thorborg K, Dehlendorff C, Krogsgaard K, Gluud C (2014) Incidence and clinical presentation of groin injuries in subelite male soccer. Br J Sports Med 48(16):1245–1250
Jacob BP, Chen DC, Ramshaw B, Towfigh S (2016) Introduction to Primary and Secondary Groin Pain: What Is Inguinodynia? In: Jacob BP, Chen DC, Ramshaw B, Towfigh S (eds) The SAGES manual of groin pain. Springer, New York
Kapron AL, Anderson AE, Aoki SK, Phillips LG, Petron DJ, Toth R, Peters CL (2011) Radiographic prevalence of femoroacetabular impingement in collegiate football players: AAOS Exhibit Selection. J Bone Joint Surg Am 93(19):e111(1–10)
Kemp JL, Crossley KM, Schache AG, Pritchard M (2012) Hip-related pain. In: Brukner PD, Bahr R, Blair S, Cook JL, Crossley KM, McConnell J et al (eds) Clinical Sports Medicine, 4th edn. McGraw-Hill, Sydney, pp 510–544
Kozin F, McCarty DJ, Sims J, Genant H (1976) The reflex sympathetic dystrophy syndrome: I. Clinical and histological studies: evidence for bilaterality, response to corticosteroids and articular involvement. Am J Med 60(3):321–331
Lange FM (2016) Algorithmic approach to the workup and management of chronic postoperative inguinal pain. In: Jacob BP, Chen DC, Ramshaw B, Towfigh S (eds) The SAGES manual of groin pain. Springer, New York
Larson CM, Pierce BR, Giveans MR (2011) Treatment of athletes with symptomatic intra-articular hip pathology and athletic pubalgia/sports hernia: a case series. Arthroscopy 27:768–775
Larson CM, Sikka RS, Sardelli MC, Byrd JW, Kelly BT, Jain RK, Giveans MR (2013) Increasing alpha angle is predictive of athletic-related "hip" and "groin" pain in collegiate National Football League prospects. Arthroscopy 29:405–410
Levine L (2010) Chronic orchialgia: evaluation and discussion of treatment options. Ther Adv Urol 2(5–06):209–214
Lilly MC, Arregui ME (2002) Lipomas of the cord and round ligament. Ann Surg 235(4):586–590
Lloyd DM (2016) Sportman's groin and the inguinal ligament release procedure. In: Jacob BP, Chen DC, Ramshaw B, Towfigh S (eds) The SAGES manual of groin pain. Springer, New York
Loos MJ, Roumen RM, Scheltinga MR (2007) Classifying post-herniorrhaphy pain syndromes following elective inguinal hernia repair. World J Surg 31(9):1760–1765. Discussion 1766–7
Ma C, Ramaswamy A (2016) Groin pain: an overview of the broad differential diagnosis. In: Jacob BP, Chen DC, Ramshaw B, Towfigh S (eds) The SAGES manual of groin pain. Springer, New York
Mann RA, Moran GT, Dougherty SE (1986) Comparative electromyography of the lower extremity in jogging, running, and sprinting. Am J Sports Med 14(6):501–510

Miller JM, Ishimitsu DN, Saouaf R (2016) Radiologic Evaluation for Postoperative Groin Pain. In: Jacob BP, Chen DC, Ramshaw B, Towfigh S (eds) The SAGES manual of groin pain. Springer, New York
Misra S, Ward S, Coker C (2009) Pulsed radiofrequency for chronic testicular pain-a preliminary report. Pain Med 10(4):673–678
Muschaweck U, Berger L (2010) Minimal Repair technique of sportsmen's groin: an innovative open-suture repair to treat chronic inguinal pain. Hernia 14(1):27–33
Nasr AO, Tormey S, Walsh TN (2005) Lipoma of the cord and round ligament: an overlooked diagnosis? Hernia 9(3):245–247
Neptune RR, Wright IA, Van Den Bogert AJ (1999) Muscle coordination and function during cutting movements. Med Sci Sports Exerc 31(2):294–302
Nicholson J, Scott M (2012) Conjoint tendon disruption: redefining and recognizing "Golmore's groin" a review of 1200 cases. Hernia 16:143–240
O'Dwyer PJ, Alani A, McConnachie A (2005) Groin hernia repair: postherniorrhaphy pain. World J Surg 29(8):1062–1065
Öberg S, Andresen K, Rosenberg J (2016) How to Surgically Remove the Permanent Mesh Ring after the Onstep Procedure for Alleviation of Chronic Pain following Inguinal Hernia Repair. Case Rep Surg 2016:5209095
Omar IM, Zoga AC, Kavanagh EC, Koulouris G, Bergin D, Gopez AG, Morrison WB, Meyers WC (2008) Athletic pubalgia and "sports hernia": optimal MR imaging technique and findings. Radiographics 28:1415–1438
Palumbo P, Minicucci A, Nasti AG, Simonelli I, Vietri F, Angelici AM (2007) Treatment for persistent chronic neuralgia after inguinal hernioplasty. Hernia 11(6):527–531
Philippon MJ, Maxwell RB, Johnston TL, Schenker M, Briggs KK (2007) Clinical presentation of femoroacetabular impingement. Knee Surg Sports Traumatol Arthrosc 15(8):1041–1047
Philippon MJ, Weiss DR, Kuppersmith DA, Briggs KK, Hay CJ (2010) Arthroscopic labral repair and treatment of femoroacetabular impingement in professional hockey players. Am J Sports Med 38(1):99–104
Pironi D, Palazzini G, Panarese A, La Gioia G, Vendettuoli M, Romani AM, Filippini G (2008) Tecnica open versus TAPP nel trattamento dell'ernia inguinale. Nostra esperienza. G Chir 29(11/12):497–504
Poobalan AS, Bruce J, King PM, Chambers WA, Krukowski ZH, Smith WC (2001) Chronic pain and quality of life following open inguinal hernia repair. Br J Surg 88(8):1122–1126
Rambani R, Hackney R (2015) Loss of range of motion of the hip joint: a hypothesis for etiology of sports hernia. Muscles Ligaments Tendons J 5(1):29–32
Rossidis G, Perry A, Abbas H, Motamarry I, Lux T, Farmer K, Moser M, Clugston J, Caban A, Ben-David K (2015a) Laparoscopic hernia repair with adductor tenotomy for athletic pubalgia: an established procedure for an obscure entity. Surg Endosc 29:381–386
Santilli OL, Nardelli N, Santilli HA, Tripoloni DE (2016) Sports hernias: experience in a sports medicine center. Hernia 20:77–84
Satpathy J, Kannan A, Owen JR, Wayne JS, Hull JR, Jiranek WA (2015) Hip contact stress and femoral neck retroversion: a biomechanical study to evaluate implication of femoroacetabular impingement. J Hip Preserv Surg 2(3):287–294
Schlegel TF, Bushnell BD, Godfrey J, Boublik M (2009) Success of nonoperative management of adductor longus tendon ruptures in National Football League athletes. Am J Sports Med 37(7):1394–1399
Siebenrock KA, Ferner F, Noble PC, Santore RF, Werlen S, Mamisch TC (2011) The cam-type deformity of the proximal femur arises in childhood in response to vigorous sporting activity. Clin Orthop Relat Res 469(11):3229–3240
Starling JR, Harms BA (1989) Diagnosis and treatment of genitofemoral and ilioinguinal neuralgia. World J Surg 13(5):586–591
Strom KH, Levine LA (2008) Microsurgical denervation of the spermatic cord for chronic orchialgia: long-term results from a single center. J Urol 180(3):949–953
Thomassen I, van Suijlekom JA, van de Gaag A, Ponten JE, Neinhuijs SW (2013) Ultrasound-guided ilioinguinal/iliohypogastric nerve blocks for chronic pain after inguinal hernia repair. Hernia 17(3):329–332
Vahedifar P, Kamrava E (2016) Complex regional pain syndrome types I and II. In: Jacob BP, Chen DC, Ramshaw B, Towfigh S (eds) The SAGES manual of groin pain. Springer, New York
Vidalin H, Neouze G, Petit J, Brunet-Guedj E (2004) Prise en charge chirurgicale des pubalgies du sportif. J Traumatol Sport 21:166–137
Weir A, Brukner P, Delahunt E, Ekstrand J, Griffin D, Khan KM, Lovell G, Meyers WC, Muschaweck U, Orchard J, Paajanen H, Philippon M, Reboul G, Robinson P, Schache AG, Schilders E, Serner A, Silvers H, Thorborg K, Tyler T, Verrall G, de Vos RJ, Vuckovic Z, Hölmich P (2015) Doha agreement meeting on terminology and definitions in groin pain in athletes. Br J Sports Med 49:768–774
Weir A, de Vos RJ, Moen M, Hölmich P, Tol JL (2011) Prevalence of radiological signs of femoroacetabular impingement in patients presenting with long-standing adductor-related groin pain. Br J Sports Med 45(1):6–9
Werner J, Hägglund M, Waldén M, Ekstrand J (2009) UEFA injury study: a prospective study of hip and groin injuries in professional football over seven consecutive seasons. Br J Sports Med 43(13):1036–1040
Zhang C, Li L, Forster BB, Kopec JA, Ratzlaff C, Halai L, Cibere J, Esdaile JM (2015) Femoroacetabular impingement and osteoarthritis of the hip. Can Fam Phys 61(12):1055–1060

Indications for Surgical Treatment in Hamstring Tears

26

Lasse Lempainen, Janne Sarimo, Pekka Niemi, and Sakari Orava

Contents

L. Lempainen (✉) • J. Sarimo • P. Niemi • S. Orava
Sports Trauma Research Center, Hospital NEO, Joukahaisenkatu 6, 20520 Turku, Finland
e-mail: lasse.lempainen@utu.fi; sakari.orava@sairaalaneo.fi

26.1 Introduction

Most hamstring injuries are treated conservatively with good results. However, there are cases in which surgery should be considered already in the acute phase. Also there are cases in which surgery should be considered later if nonoperative treatment appears to be unsuccessful.

26.2 Terminology

Nomenclature of the injury should be muscle/tendon specific. Concerning injury classification, the term "partial tear" comprising collectively all the three hamstring muscles is nowadays not accurate enough. Instead of talking about a partial hamstring tear, we should talk about a partial biceps femoris (BF) tear, for example. Furthermore, more information would be obtained if isolated muscle/tendon ruptures were categorized also proximally as complete ones (grade III injury), for example, complete proximal semimembranosus (SM) rupture. Also the location of the tear is of importance. A proximal avulsion is often treated differently than a tear in the muscular part.

A term "central tendon" has been suggested regarding injuries in the muscular part where then tendon is surrounded by the muscle belly. The term has been applied also in other than hamstring injuries, e.g., in the rectus femoris. In the hamstrings especially, the tendon is typically not com-

G.L. Canata et al. (eds.), *Muscle and Tendon Injuries*, DOI 10.1007/978-3-662-54184-5_26

pletely surrounded by muscle tissue and therefore we suggest a term "paramuscular tendon" for these cases instead. This would refer to injuries of any tendon in a location where the tendon is not an isolated structure but has muscle fibers attaching to it.

26.3 Absolute Indications for Surgery

In an athlete a proximal one tendon avulsion with retraction of more than about 5 mm should be treated surgically regardless of the hamstring tendon (BF, SM, or ST) (Fig. 26.1a, b) (Lempainen 2015). If two or all three of the hamstring muscles are avulsed, surgery should be considered in all patients if there are no major contraindications to surgery (Figs. 26.2 and 26.3) (Lempainen 2006; Sarimo 2008; Sarimo 2009). Suture anchors are typically used to reattach the tendon to bone.

Distal tears of the hamstrings are rare (Lempainen 2007a). The BF is most commonly affected and most of the tears are incomplete. The BF or the semitendinosus (ST) may, however, rupture completely from the distal bony insertion or at the distal myotendinous junction (Fig. 26.4a, b). To our knowledge there are no reports of complete SM avulsions. An acute complete rupture (BF or ST) with a retraction should be repaired anatomically. In our opinion the behavior of an acute distal ST avulsion is not similar to that of harvesting the tendon for graft purposes (Lempainen 2007a).

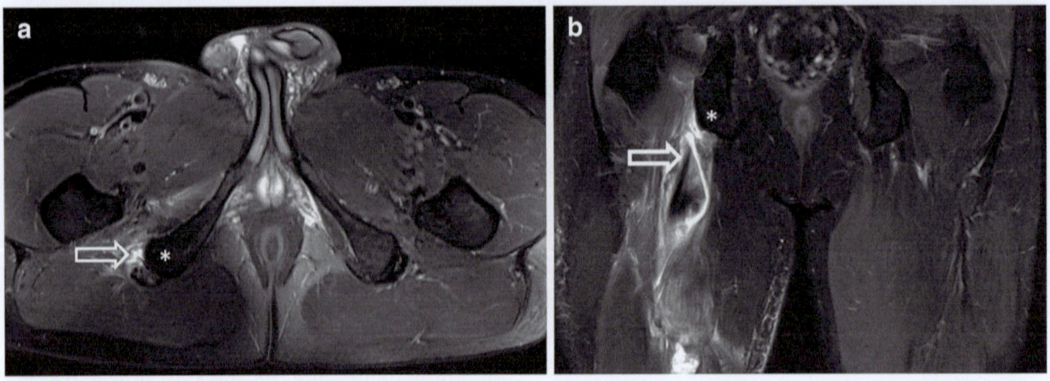

Fig. 26.1 (**a**, **b**) Isolated tear of the semimembranosus tendon at right. (**a**) On an axial MR image, the tendon is absent (*arrow*) at the level of the ischial tuberosity (*asterisk*). (**b**) A coronal image shows the retracted tendon (*arrow*) distal to the tuberosity (*asterisk*)

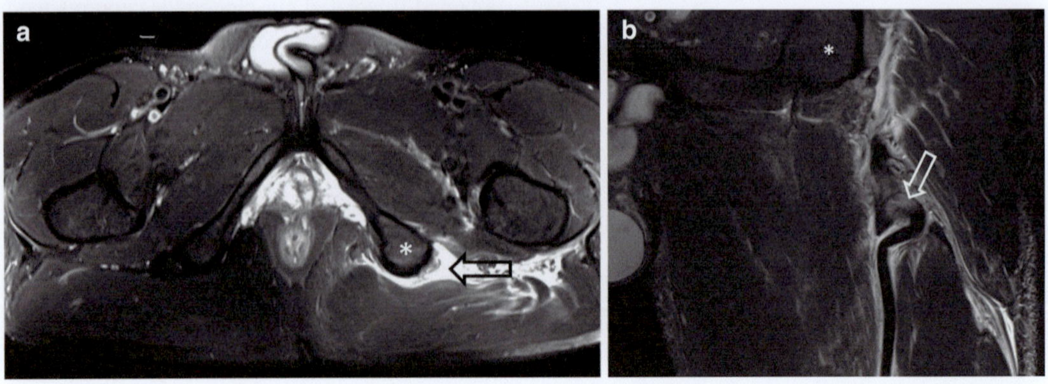

Fig. 26.2 (**a**, **b**) MR images showing a complete tear of the hamstring tendons at left. (**a**) On an axial image, the tendons are absent (*arrow*) at the level of the ischial tuberosity (*asterisk*). (**b**) As seen on an oblique sagittal image, the tendons are retracted and coiled a few centimeters distal to the tuberosity (*asterisk*)

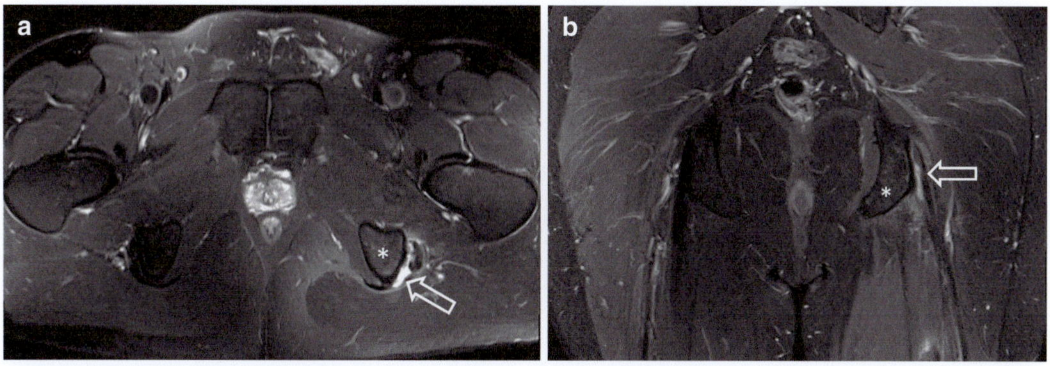

Fig. 26.3 (**a**, **b**) MR images showing a complete tear of the hamstring tendons at left. (**a**) On an axial image, only the conjoint tendon of biceps and semitendinosus is absent (*arrow*) at the level of the ischial tuberosity (*asterisk*). (**b**) A coronal image reveals that, although the semimembranosus tendon is not retracted (*arrow*), it is detached from the tuberosity (*asterisk*)

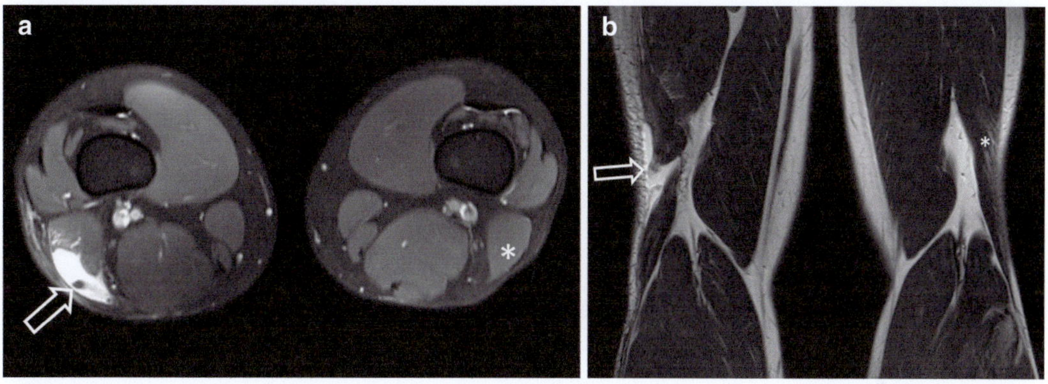

Fig. 26.4 (**a**, **b**) Distal tear of the long head of the biceps femoris tendon at right. (**a**) An axial MR image shows the torn tendon (*arrow*) surrounded by fluid. Intact biceps femoris muscle and tendon can be seen at left (*asterisk*). (**b**) A coronal image shows the retracted muscle (*arrow*). Normal muscle is seen at the contralateral side (*asterisk*)

26.4 Relative Indications for Surgery

Occasionally incomplete tears especially when recurrent form scar tissue and adhesions that cause persistent symptoms and are nonresponsive to conservative treatment (Lempainen 2006). This can occur in the proximal or distal bone-tendon interface or in the proximal or distal tendinous part or in the paramuscular area. In proximal incomplete avulsions that remain symptomatic, the MRI may show liquid between the bone and the tendon which is a sign of incomplete healing.

In surgery typically a debridement and suturing is done and sometimes in distal tears the ST is attached to the SM if continuity cannot be restored anatomically.

It has been suggested that paramuscular injuries especially in the BF may have a higher risk of poor healing with conservative treatment. Also the risk of a recurrent injury may be high. In these injuries there is often an incomplete tear of the paramuscular tendon typically in the area of 5–20 cm from the proximal origin. Often the muscle tissue is torn off from the tendon also. When a tear like this remains symptomatic after adequate conservative treatment or there are recurrences, surgery should be considered (Fig. 26.5a, b). Full continuity of the paramuscular tendon is restored with sutures, and the attachment of the muscle to

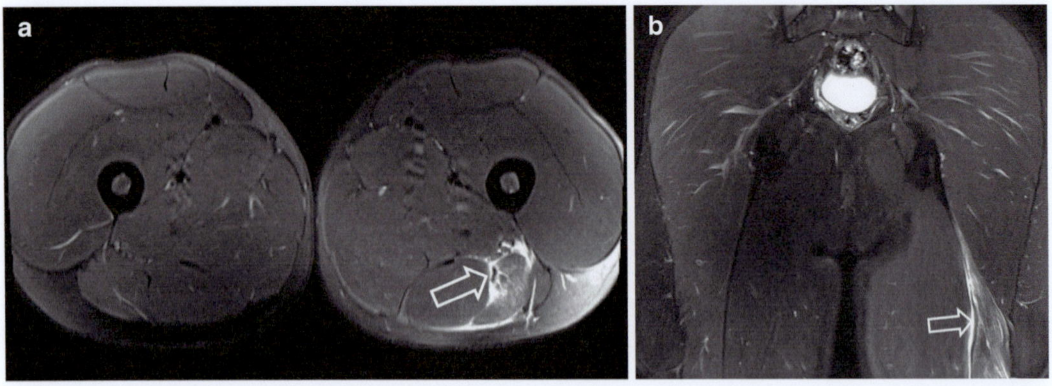

Fig. 26.5 (**a**, **b**) Longitudinal tear of the biceps femoris paramuscular tendon at left. (**a**) On an axial MR image, the torn tendon is surrounded by fluid (*arrow*). (**b**) A coronal image shows thickened and slack paramuscular tendon (*arrow*)

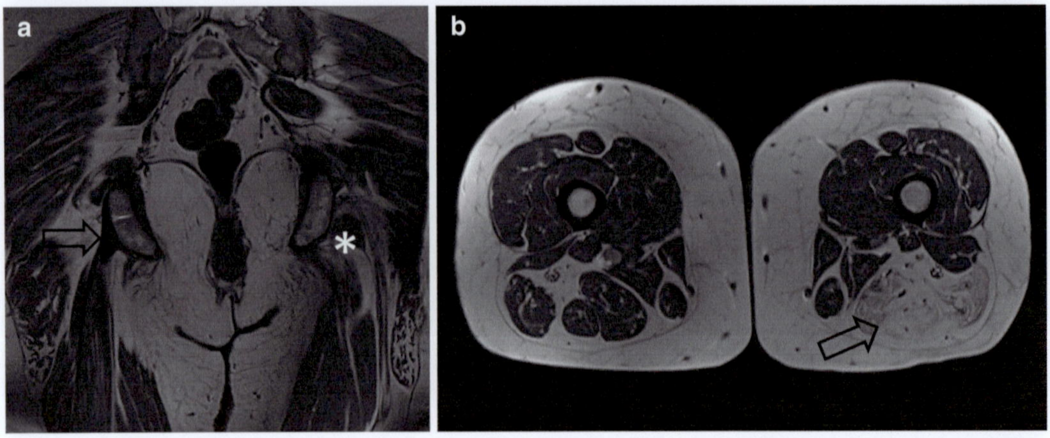

Fig. 26.6 (**a**, **b**) MR images showing a chronic tear of the hamstring tendons at left. (**a**) On a coronal image, the tendons are absent (*asterisk*) at the level of the ischial tuberosity. Normal tendons are seen at the contralateral side (*arrow*). (**b**) An axial image at midthigh level reveals a total atrophy of the hamstring muscles (*arrow*)

the tendon is reinforced. It is important to avoid overtightening of the repaired tendon. Scar tissue may be removed. Suture anchors may be used if the tear is located close to the bony origin.

26.5 Chronic Injuries

In chronic proximal hamstring ruptures and in some rerupture cases, anatomic apposition of the retracted muscles cannot always be achieved (Lempainen 2007b). In those cases we have used fascia lata autograft augmentation to connect the retracted hamstrings to ischial tuberosity. It seems that late reconstruction of complete proximal hamstring avulsion with fascia lata autograft augmentation results in enhancement of muscle strength, better function of the hamstrings, and improved leg control (Fig. 26.6a, b). Also symptoms derived from retracted hamstrings causing stretching to the sciatic nerve could be alleviated.

References

Lempainen L, Sarimo J, Heikkilä J, Mattila K, Orava S (2006) Surgical treatment of partial tears of the proximal origin of the hamstring muscles. Br J Sports Med 40:688–691

Lempainen L, Sarimo J, Mattila K, Heikkilä J, Orava S (2007a) Distal tears of the hamstring muscles: review of the literature and our results of surgical treatment. Br J Sports Med 41:80–83

Lempainen L, Sarimo J, Orava S (2007b) Recurrent and chronic complete ruptures of the proximal origin of the hamstring muscles repaired with fascia lata autograft augmentation. Arthroscopy 23:441.e1–441.e5

Lempainen L, Banke IJ, Johansson K, Brucker PU, Sarimo J, Orava S, Imhoff AB (2015) Clinical principles in the management of hamstring injuries. Knee Surg Sports Traumatol Arthrosc 23:2449–2456

Sarimo J, Lempainen L, Mattila K, Orava S (2008) Complete proximal hamstring avulsions: a series of 41 patients with operative treatment. Am J Sports Med 36:1110–1115

Sarimo J, Lempainen L, Mattila K, Orava S (2009) Diagnosis and surgical treatment of partial (one- and two-tendon) proximal hamstring avulsions. Oper Tech Sports Med 17:229–233

Patellar Tendon Rupture

27

Piero Volpi, Emanuele Prospero, Antonio Orgiani, and Alessandro Quaglia

Contents

27.1 Introduction

The rupture of patellar tendon (PT) is a pathological condition of the extensor mechanism of the knee. The PT lesions are rare, often occurring between the 2nd and 4th decade of life (Clayton and Court-Brown 2008; White et al. 2007), in active and sports patients. The aetiology of the PT lesions is multifactorial: a complete rupture of the PT could be the result of a chronic tendinopathy, or it may be caused by direct or indirect high-energy trauma of the knee. Sport practice in patients older than 40 years of age determines many cases of PT ruptures in the elderly (Chautems et al. 2001). Frequently, these patients may present concomitant systemic pathologies like metabolic or connective tissue disorders and may sustain bilateral ruptures of the PT (Wang et al. 2010; Cree et al. 2007). Rarely, PT rupture occurs in young patients.

A particular situation is the PT rupture in patients that have undergone knee surgery: PT ruptures have been reported in patients undergoing knee replacement or after PT harvesting for ligamentous reconstruction of the knee; in these cases, the aetiology of the PT rupture is multifactorial.

27.2 Biomechanics and Physiopathology

High loading forces are transmitted to the patella–PT–tibia (PPTT) complex during knee flexion, extension or hyperextension and daily life activities.

P. Volpi (✉) • E. Prospero • A. Orgiani • A. Quaglia
Knee surgery and Sport Traumatology Unit, Humanitas Research Hospital, IRCCS, Rozzano, Milan, Italy
e-mail: piero.volpi@humanitas.it

G.L. Canata et al. (eds.), *Muscle and Tendon Injuries*, DOI 10.1007/978-3-662-54184-5_27

In sports patients with strong muscles sustaining repetitive high-energy motions of the knee like jumping or running, the frequency and the entity of the stresses on the PT are two major factors involved in the pathogenesis of PT rupture.

The PT presents the capacity to resist to traction forces (Rauh and Parker 2009), and it has been proved that a high energy is necessary to determine a complete rupture of the tendon (Zernicke et al. 1977).

The extensor mechanism of the knee sustains both concentric and eccentric training. The degrees on knee flexion influence the stresses on the PT: when the knee flexion ranges from 45° to 60°, the PT is majorly exposed to sustain trauma, especially during eccentric training (Lee et al. 2013).

The clinical presentation of the lesions of the PPTT can occur in different ways: rupture of the PT associated with avulsion fracture of the patella, PT complete rupture (proximal–distal–middle part) and PT rupture associated with avulsion fracture of the anterior tuberosity of the tibia.

In cases of isolated PT rupture, the literature suggests an association of degenerative changes of the tendon structure including calcific or mucoid tendinopathy or fatty infiltration of the tendon (Kannus and Józsa 1991).

27.3 Clinical Presentation

The history, clinical presentation and imaging investigations are crucial in patients with PT rupture.

The history should be collected paying attention on work activity, sports practice and metabolic disorders. It is fundamental to find any risk factors and to understand the mechanism of trauma. Moreover, information on the postoperative functional request of the patients should be obtained.

The collection of the past medical history should focus on metabolic disorders, systemic pathologies, corticosteroids injections and episodes of tendinopathy. It is also important to ask the patients about the assumption of any medications which can be dangerous for tendon tissue such as antibiotics.

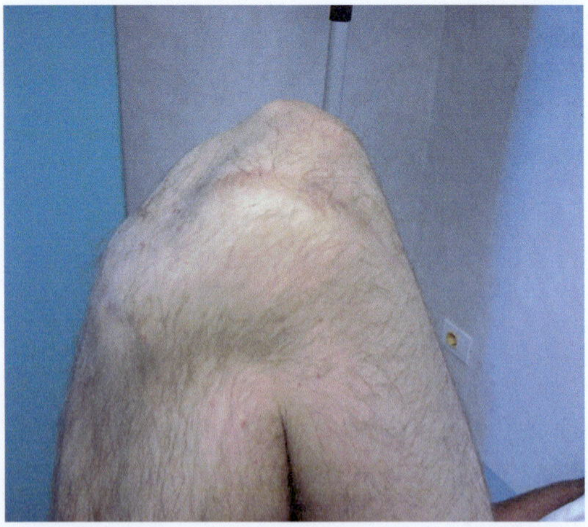

Fig. 27.1 Chronic patellar tendon rupture

Patients with PT often present swelling in the anterior aspect of the knee or may present haemarthrosis. Often the tendon gap is not appreciable due to swelling in the area of the lesion.

The most important clinical manifestation of the PT rupture is the loss of active extension of the leg and the inability to walk, also with the use of crutches. In patients with partial lesions of the PT, functional impairment could be absent.

In patients who sustained traumatic PT rupture caused by high-energy trauma, it is fundamental to evaluate the skin integrity and the presence of associated lesions of the knee like meniscal tears or ligamentous injuries (McKinney et al. 2008).

Patients with chronic patellar tendon rupture often presents with significant modifications of the patellar tendon and the height of the patella (Fig. 27.1)

27.4 Imaging Diagnosis

The following imaging investigations should be performed in patients with suspected lesion of the PT: X-ray, ultrasound and MRI.

Radiographs must be performed in both the anteroposterior and lateral views. It is important

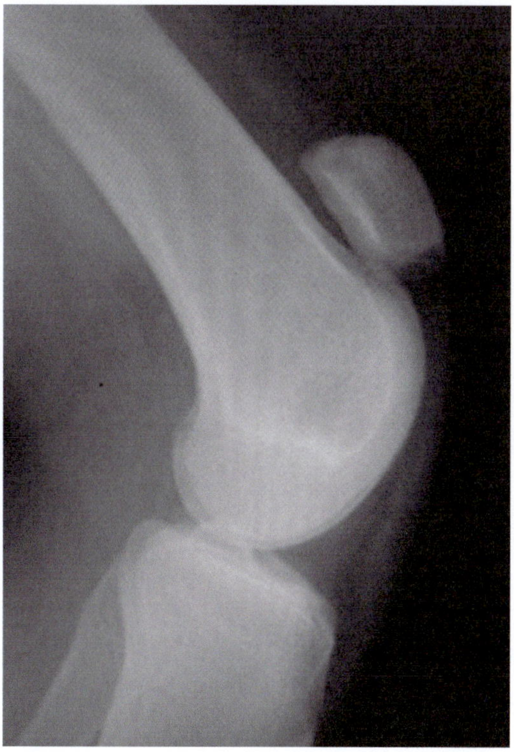

Fig. 27.2 Ascent of patella in PT rupture

to pay attention to the evaluation of the location of the patella. In case of PT rupture, the patella is dislocated proximally respect to the knee joint line (Fig. 27.2).

In case of dubious images, or especially in patients with "patella alta", it can be useful to perform the X-ray of the contralateral knee. Moreover, radiographs show any avulsion fractures of both patella and anterior tuberosity of the tibia (Fig. 27.3).

With ultrasound it is possible to appreciate the extension, shape and location of the PT rupture (Phillips and Costantino 2014). Furthermore, ultrasound allows the visualization of the haemorrhagic spreading into the surrounding soft tissues. However, there is no agreement on the use of ultrasound in case of partial and chronic tears of the PT, as well as in obese patients (Swamy et al. 2012).

The MRI is the most sensible imaging investigation for the diagnosis of PT rupture: the tendon is represented by a low-intensity homogeneous signal, and in case of rupture, the signal becomes inhomogeneous with interruptions of the tendon structure or within the osteotendinous junction (Fig. 27.4).

The MRI should be performed in case of dubious ultrasound imaging or to diagnose intra-articular and extra-articular associated lesions.

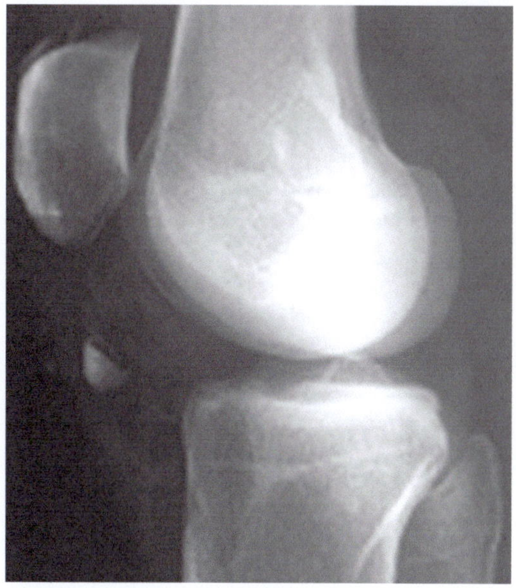

Fig. 27.3 Avulsion of the patellar inferior pole

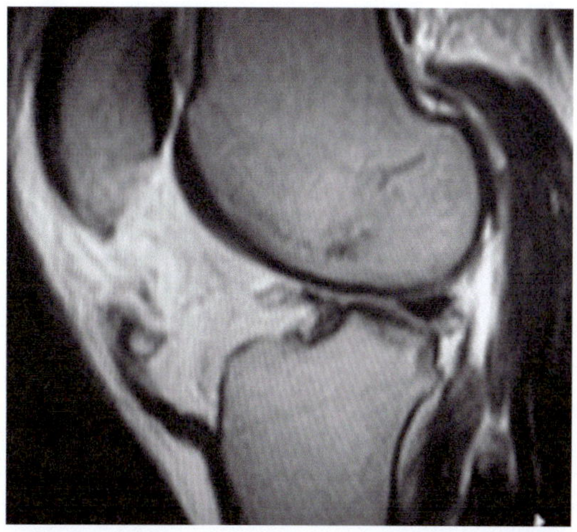

Fig. 27.4 MRI

27.5 Treatment of PT Lesions

The PT ruptures can be classified into acute and chronic.

With acute lesion we mean a lesion usually treated within 2 weeks of injury (Siwek and Rao 1981).

Chronic lesions are seen by the surgeon some weeks after the injury, especially in patients who present associated osseous and ligamentous lesions of the knee. Patients with initial diagnosis of partial tears of the PT turned into total lesion or with early failure of surgery or with septic complications are assigned to this category. Some cases of incomplete rupture of the PT, which are not associated with functional impairment, could be managed conservatively, using knee brace locked in extension for 4–6 week, followed by progressive physiotherapy based on gradual knee flexion (Rauh and Parker 2009).

Surgical management in acute PT rupture is indicated in complete lesions of the PT or in patients with partial lesions associated with functional impairment (loss of active knee extension). Surgical repair in the acute setting significantly influences tendon healing (Lee et al. 2013).

The first step in surgical treatment of acute lesions of the proximal or distal portion of the PT is to reinsert the tendon to the bone; the reinsertion can be done with transosseous sutures or through the execution of transosseous tunnels like modified Krakow technique (Fig. 27.5) or with suture anchors (Capiola and Re 2007).

The goal of surgery is to restore the osteotendinous continuity and replace the patella at the original position.

Several authors proposed the use of reinforcement with autologous or homologous grafts (Larson and Simonian 1995) or synthetic materials (Kasten et al. 2001).

In case of acute lesions of the middle part of the PT, the first step consists in an end-to-end suture of the tendon to restore the tendon continuity.

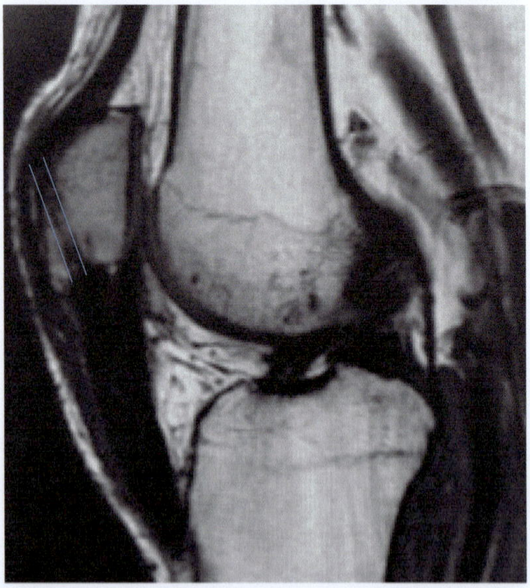

Fig. 27.5 Patellar transosseous tunnel

Even in these cases, it is essential to restore also the height of the patella, and it is possible to associate with autologous or homologous or synthetic augmentations.

The management of chronic lesions of the PT is more complex because of the presence of scar tissues surrounding the lesions and also because they are often associated with post-traumatic anatomic deformity of the knee. In this case it may be difficult to restore the normal height of the patella, because of scar retraction of the tendon, or because of tendon substance loss.

The first step consists into the removal of scar tissue or calcifications (Fig. 27.6) preserving as much healthy tissue as possible; it is very important to evaluate the relationship between the tendon residuals and the possible tendon gap.

In the majority of cases, in addition to suture of tendon residuals, it is necessary to use biological or bioabsorbable augmentations, to reinforce the tendon, thus facilitating also the vascularization of the residual tendon tissue (Fig. 27.7).

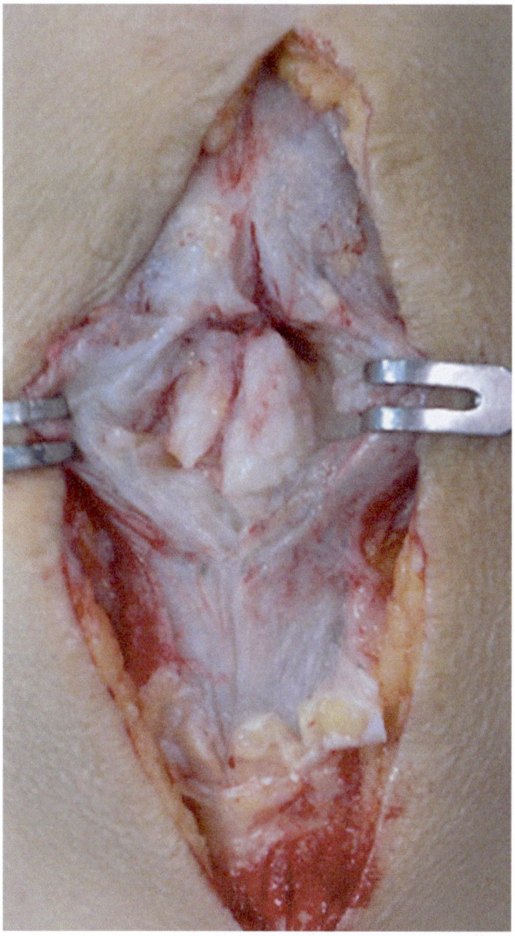

Fig. 27.6 Calcification and scar tissue in chronic PT rupture

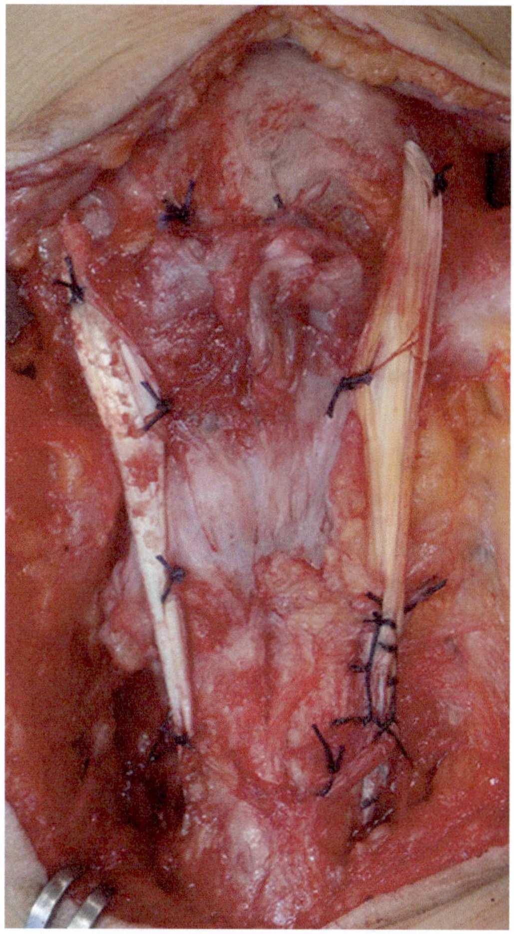

Fig. 27.7 Autologous augmentation with semitendinosus tendon

In other cases, with large loss of tendon substance, the use of allograft including complete extensor mechanism allograft or contralateral autograft is indicated (Saragaglia et al. 2013).

The patients presenting PT rupture after knee surgery (e.g. anterior cruciate ligament reconstruction with PT or knee replacement) should be treated with the techniques described previously. The suture of the PT in patients with patella prosthesis with tibial nails may be challenging due to poor osseous quality.

References

Capiola D, Re L (2007) Repair of patellar tendon rupture with suture anchors. Arthroscopy 23(8):e1–e4

Chautems R, Michel J, Barraud GE, Burdet A (2001) Bifocal avulsion of the patellar tendon in an adult: a case report. Rev Chir Orthop Reparatrice Appar Mot 87(4):388–391

Clayton RAE, Court-Brown CM (2008) The epidemiology of musculoskeletal tendinous and ligamentous injuries. Injury 39(12):1338–1344

Cree C, Pillai A, Jones B, Blyth M (2007) Bilateral patellar tendon ruptures: a missed diagnosis: case report and literature review. Knee Surg Sports Traumatol Arthrosc 15(11):1350–1354. Epub 2007 Jun 29

Kannus P, Józsa L (1991) Histopathological changes preceding spontaneous rupture of a tendon. A controlled study of 891 patients. J Bone Joint Surg Am 73(10):1507–1525

Kasten P, Schewe B, Maurer F, Gösling T, Krettek C, Weise K (2001) Rupture of the patellar tendon: a review of 68 cases and a retrospective study of 29 ruptures comparing two methods of augmentation. Arch Orthop Trauma Surg 121(10):578–582

Larson RV, Simonian PT (1995) Semitendinosus augmentation of acute patellar tendon repair with immediate mobilization. Am J Sports Med 23(1):82–86

Lee D, Stinner D, Mir H (2013) Quadriceps and patellar tendon ruptures. J Knee Surg 26:301–308

McKinney B, Cherney S, Penna J (2008) Intra-articular knee injuries in patients with knee extensor mechanism ruptures. Knee Surg Sports Traumatol Arthrosc 16(7):633–638

Phillips K, Costantino TG (2014) Diagnosis of patellar tendon rupture by emergency ultrasound. J Emerg Med 16. doi:10.1016/j.jemermed.2014.02.012pi i:S0736-4679(14)00187-5

Rauh M, Parker R (2009) Patellar and quadriceps tendinopathies and ruptures. In: DeLee JC (ed) DeLee and Drez's orthopaedic sports medicine. Saunders, Philadelphia, PA, pp 192–200

Saragaglia D, Pison A, Rubens-Duval B (2013) Acute and old ruptures of the extensor apparatus of the knee in adults (excluding knee replacement). Orthop Traumatol Surg Res 99(1 Suppl):S67–S76

Siwek CW, Rao JP (1981) Ruptures of the extensor mechanism of the knee joint. J Bone Joint Surg Am 63:932–937

Swamy GN, Nanjayan SK, Yallappa S, Bishnoi A, Pickering SA (2012) Is ultrasound diagnosis reliable in acute extensor tendon injuries of the knee? Acta Orthop Belg 78(6):764–770

Wang Z, Wang Q, Tang H, Kang Y (2010) Extensor mechanism repair and reconstruction using Achilles tendon allograft after bilateral patellar tendon rupture in a patient with rheumatoid arthritis. Knee Surg Sports Traumatol Arthrosc 18(8):1113–1115

White DW, Wenke JC, Mosely DS, Mountcastle SB, Basamania CJ (2007) Incidence of major tendon ruptures and anterior cruciate ligament tears in US Army soldiers. Am J Sports Med 35(8):1308–1314. Epub 2007 Apr 27

Zernicke RF, Garhammer J, Jobe FW (1977) Human patellar tendon rupture: a kinetic analysis. J Bone Joint Surg Am 59(2):179–183

28 Pathogenesis and Treatment of Patellar Tendinopathy

Ryohei Uchida, Norimasa Nakamura, and Shuji Horibe

Contents

R. Uchida, M.D., Ph.D.
Department of Orthopaedic Sports Medicine, Seifu Hospital, Osaka, Japan
e-mail: uchida3847@gmail.com

N. Nakamura, M.D., Ph.D., FRCS
Institute for Medical Science in Sports, Osaka Health Science University, Osaka, Japan
e-mail: viader7jp@yahoo.co.jp

S. Horibe, M.D., Ph.D. (Japan) (✉)
Faculty of Comprehensive Rehabilitation, Osaka Prefecture University, Osaka, Japan
e-mail: s-horibe@rehab.osakafu-u.ac.jp

28.1 Concept of Tendinopathy

Prior to the 1990s, pain and/or disability arising from tendons caused by overuse was referred to as tendinitis, implying that inflammation was responsible for the pathological process (Khan et al. 2002). However, this pathological condition of the tendon is widely described with the term *tendinopathy*, which is caused by a degenerative process devoid of inflammation in histological findings (Rees et al. 2014; Maffulli et al. 2010). The lesion of tendinopathy is found at the enthesis of some major tendons in both the upper and lower limbs. Achilles and patellar tendinopathy are most popular. The main symptom of tendinopathy is pain, which leads to disability not only in sports activities but also in activities of daily life.

For treatment of tendinopathy, its pathogenesis should be well understood. Although many theories are associated with the pathogenesis of tendinopathy, the genuine pathogenesis remains unclear. Current studies described the process that leads to chronic tendinopathy (Rees et al. 2014; Maffulli et al. 2010). In their theories, microtears at tendon attachment initially occur by overload, and then these microtears usual heal spontaneously, but in some cases with intrinsic or extrinsic risk factors for tendinopathy, repetitive overload to the tendon causes imbalance between synthesis and degradation of collagen. In such cases, the tendon undergoes degenerative changes, which is called chronic tendinopathy. In this chronic status, there is absence of acute inflammatory cells, but

G.L. Canata et al. (eds.), *Muscle and Tendon Injuries*, DOI 10.1007/978-3-662-54184-5_28

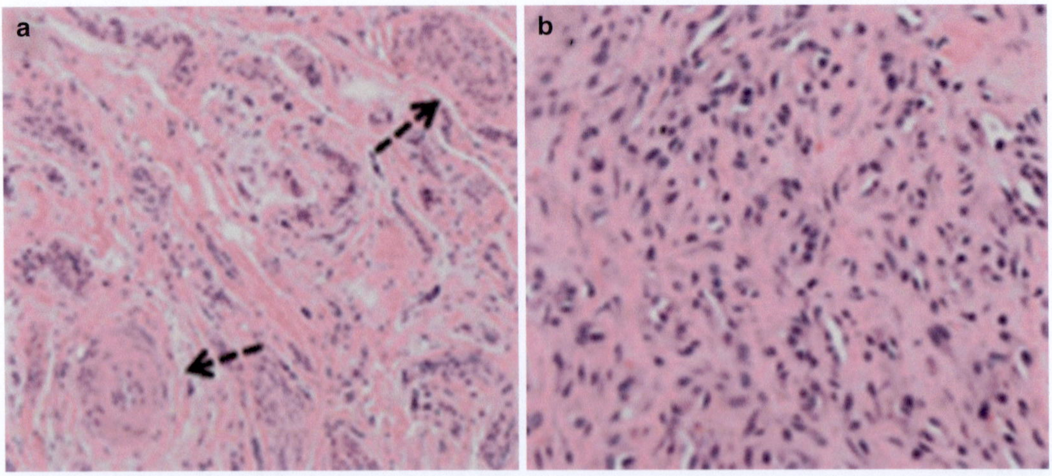

Fig. 28.1 Characteristic microscopic images of patellar tendinopathy. Neovessels (*black dotted arrows*) in the peritenon (**a**) and increased number of cells in the damaged tendon (**b**) stained with hematoxylin and eosin (H&E)

pathological neovascularization and nerve ingrowth, which are considered causes of pain, are present (Rees et al. 2014; Maffulli et al. 2010; Leal et al. 2015) (Fig. 28.1). However, Fredberg et al. (2004) reported a significant reduction in pain and tendon thickening only a week after ultrasonography-guided peritendinous corticosteroid injections in chronic Achilles and patellar tendinopathy. These corticosteroid-induced changes are difficult to explain if the process is degenerative because the time frame is too short to change degenerative tendon tissue to normal tendon tissue by corticosteroids. Therefore, the anti-inflammatory effect of corticosteroid could influence these short dramatic changes of symptom and tendon morphology. Moreover, a recent report showed that pro-inflammatory agents (VEGF or PGE2) in chronic tendinopathies were associated with pain (Fredberg and Stengaard-Pedersen 2008). In the literature reviews, the authors showed that, inflammation was also confirmed in acute tendon injury (Fredberg and Stengaard-Pedersen 2008; Sharma and Maffulli 2006). Abate et al. (2009) concluded that "it is conceivable that inflammation and degeneration are not mutually exclusive, but work together in the pathogenic cascade of tendinopathy." According to their "iceberg theory," the time course from asymptomatic to symptomatic tendinopathy is long. Therefore, whether inflammation is in early acute tendinopathy or not cannot be verified because we did not histologically investigate the tendon in patients without symptoms in the early acute phase.

28.2 Staging and Treatment

Regarding the staging classification in patellar tendinopathy, Blanzina et al. (1973) reported the first classification, which has been used over 40 years. Except for stage 4, which is complete tendon rupture, they classified three stages based on symptoms and dysfunction. In the twenty-first century, Cook and Purdam et al. (2009) classified tendinopathy into three stages, namely, reactive tendinopathy, early or late tendon disrepair, and degenerative tendinopathy. This classification was based on microstructural changes of the damaged tendon; thus, it can indicate the degree of microstructural damage that requires treatment intervention. They divided these three stages into two groups. For the tendinopathies in the first group, including reactive tendinopathy, only load management was enough for healing, whereas for the tendinopathies in the second group, including degenerative tendinopathy, treatment intervention, including eccentric exercise, should be applied. If the tendinopathies in the second group were resistant to eccentric exercise, more-invasive treatments such as extracorporeal shockwave therapy and surgery are necessary.

28.3 Pathomechanism of Patellar Tendinopathy

Patellar tendinopathy is one of the most popular tendinopathies. Generally, the region of pathological change in patellar tendinopathy is the posteromedial tendon substance at the insertion to the inferior patellar pole (Johnson et al. 1996; Lavagnino et al. 2008; Khan et al. 1996) (Fig. 28.2). This region specificity is closely related with the mechanical and structural characteristics of the patellar tendon. First, the proximal patellar tendon cross-sectional area (CSA) was smaller than the mid- or distal tendon CSA (Kongsgaard et al. 2007). Therefore, the force per unit area at the proximal patellar tendon was larger than that at the mid- or distal tendon. This is one of the reasons for the tendency of patellar tendinopathy

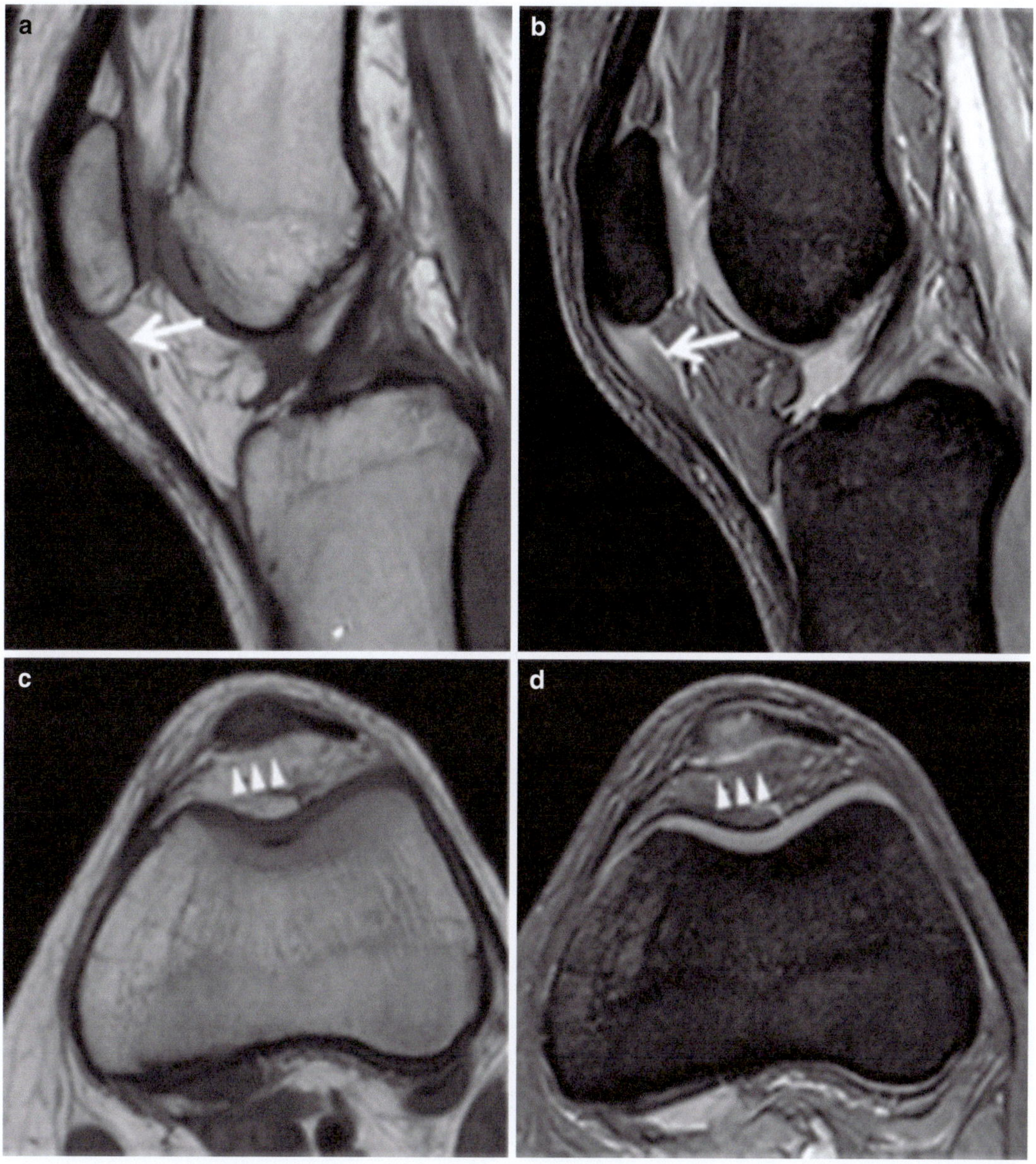

Fig. 28.2 Magnetic resonance images of the lesion of patellar tendinopathy. A lesion of proximal patellar tendinopathy at the posteromedial portion with signal change and tendon thickening (*white arrows and arrowheads*). Sagittal planes of T1- (**a**) and T2*-weighted images (**b**) and axial plane of T1- (**c**) and T2*-weighted images (**d**)

to occur at the proximal tendon attachment to the patella. Second, some reports investigated the mechanism of pathological changes in the posterior potion of the proximal patellar tendon (Basso et al. 2002; Dillon et al. 2008; Pearson and Hussain 2014; Hansen et al. 1985). In both cadaveric and experimental studies, mechanical stress was higher at the posterior region than at the anterior region of the proximal tendon owing to the lever arm (Basso et al. 2002; Dillon et al. 2008). The finite element model findings also showed maximum strain at the classical tendinopathy lesion, at the posterior region of the proximal patellar tendon attachment to patella (Lavagnino et al. 2008). Moreover, regarding the mechanical properties of the proximal tendon, posterior fascicles were markedly weaker and micro-damages are likely to occur at the posterior tendon (Hansen et al. 1985). Finally, the reason why most tendinopathy lesions are located at the medial side was explained in the study on regional structural differences at the enthesis of the proximal patellar tendon. Toumi et al. (2006) reported that bone quality, trabecular thickness, and uncalcified fibrocartilage were greatest medially and that the subchondral plate was thinner laterally. These results indicate that mechanical stress at the proximal patellar tendon enthesis is greater on the medial than on the lateral side, leading to the tendency of exposure with overload on the proximal medial tendon. Overall, the posteromedial site of the proximal patellar tendon has weak mechanical properties with large mechanical stress, which explains why the lesion of proximal patellar tendinopathy occurs at the posteromedial portion.

28.4 Treatment of Patellar Tendinopathy

Although many treatment methods are available for patellar tendinopathy, evidence-based therapies are limited. Therefore, no consensus has been reached on the appropriate use of these therapies. According to a recent systematic review (Larsson et al. 2012), only eccentric exercise has strong evidence for patellar tendinopathy.

Table 28.1 Evidence for each therapy for patellar tendinopathy (Larsson et al. 2012)

Quality of evidence	Therapy
Strong evidence	Eccentric exercise
Moderate evidence	Heavy slow resistance training
Limited evidence	Sclerosing injection Shockwave therapy Surgery

Moderate evidence was found on heavy slow resistance training as an alternative to eccentric exercise. Moreover, evidence is limited for sclerosing injection, shockwave therapy, and surgery (Table 28.1).

28.4.1 Eccentric Exercise

Many reports on eccentric exercise have been published, and these reports support the existing evidence of the effectiveness of eccentric exercise. Some reports showed that treatment with eccentric exercise had significantly better clinical results than treatment with concentric exercise (Jonsson and Alfredson 2005; Stasinopoulos and Stasinopoulos 2004; Cannell et al. 2001). In these reports, 80–100% of patients with eccentric exercise were satisfied and could return to sports within short-term follow-up. Regarding its mechanism, eccentric exercise could act both metabolically and mechanically (Maffulli and Longo 2008; Maffulli et al. 2004). However, only a few studies investigated the mechanism of eccentric exercise in detail (Boesen et al. 2006; Wasielewski and Kotsko 2007; Graham et al. 2000). Eccentric exercise affected tendons metabolically, increasing cross-linking among collagen fibers and thereby improving the elasticity and tensile strength of the patellar tendon (Graham et al. 2000). This exercise also affected tendons mechanically, stopping blood flow and reducing neoangiogenesis, similarly to sclerosing therapy during deep flexion of joints (Boesen et al. 2006; Wasielewski and Kotsko 2007).

The most widely used eccentric exercise protocols for patellar tendinopathy consisted of three sets of 15 repetitions performed twice daily with a 25° decline board (Wasielewski and Kotsko

2007). However, the most effective treatment protocol, including sets, repetitions, motion speed, and times per day, remains unknown (Pearson and Hussain 2014). How patients engage in sports activities during treatment with eccentric exercise is also unclear. Whether they should continue to participate in sports activities with limitation or discontinue sports activity completely remains to be clarified. To decide on the best eccentric exercise protocol, more randomized controlled trials are needed.

28.4.2 Heavy Slow Resistance Training

Kongsgaard et al. (2010) found that heavy slow resistance training (HSR) improved the clinical outcome of patellar tendinopathy at 12 weeks after training. They reported that these improvements were associated with normalization of fibril morphology due to new fibril production promoted by HSR. In a recent systematic review (Malliaras et al. 2013), the clinical result after HSR was equivalent to that after eccentric exercise for patellar tendinopathy. However, the definitive superiority of HSR to eccentric exercise was not proven.

28.4.3 Sclerosing Agents

Only few cases of patellar or Achilles tendinopathy treated with sclerosing agents have been reported (Lind et al. 2006; Ohberg and Alfredson 2002; Alfredson and Ohberg 2005; Hoksrud et al. 1738). Sclerosing therapy for Achilles tendinopathy reduces pain and restores function owing to its effect on new vessels and nerve destruction. Therefore, authors concluded that this treatment should be applied for advanced chronic tendinopathy with neovessel formation and neural ingrowth (Lind et al. 2006; Ohberg and Alfredson 2002). For patellar tendinopathy, however, these effects of sclerosing agents have not been confirmed, with good clinical results in >80% of patients with patellar tendinopathy at 6–12 months after injection of sclerosing agents (Alfredson and Ohberg 2005; Hoksrud et al. 1738).

28.4.4 Extracorporeal Shockwave Therapy

Extracorporeal shockwave therapy (ESWT) was initially used for treatment of patellar tendinopathy in 2001, and its use has gradually widely increased (Leal et al. 2015). According to the previous studies, symptoms improved after ESWT in 61–77% of patients (Leal et al. 2015; Taunton et al. 2003; Zwerver et al. 2010). Compared with the clinical results after surgery, those at 24 months after ESWT treatment were equivalent (Peers et al. 2003). However, the success rate of conventional conservative treatment for tendinopathy including eccentric exercise was over 80%, and thus ESWT should not be used as a first-line therapy for tendinopathy.

28.4.5 Surgical Treatment

Various open and arthroscopic procedures have been described in the operative treatment of patellar tendinopathy. Smillie (1962) published the first report on open surgical treatment with drilling multiple holes into the inferior pole of the patella. Following this report, Blazina et al. (1973) reported about open excision of the extra-articular inferior pole of the patella and reinsertion of the patellar tendon. Thereafter, open resection procedures of the damaged portion of the patellar tendon without an osseous procedure were reported (Fritschy and Wallensten 1993; Verheyden et al. 1997; Ferretti et al. 2002). One procedure was removal of the pathological tissue in a longitudinal strip (Fritschy and Wallensten 1993; Verheyden et al. 1997) and another was to excise only tissue identified as abnormal (Ferretti et al. 2002). Followed by open excision of damaged tendon, arthroscopic procedure to stimulate the healing response of patellar tendon was reported by Romeo et al. (Romeo and Larson 1999) Thereafter, various arthroscopic procedures have been developed. The most common procedure was debridement of the patellar tendon. Additional arthroscopic procedures include denervation or resection of the inferior patellar pole and synovectomy (Romeo and Larson 1999; Kelly 2009; Ogon et al. 2006).

The surgical success rate for patellar tendinopathy was 60–90% (Brockmeyer et al. 2015). According to the latest systematic review, the average success rate of open surgery was 87% and that of arthroscopic surgery was 91% (Brockmeyer et al. 2015). The average return-to-sport rate was 78.4% after open surgery and 82.3% after arthroscopic surgery. These were not statistically significantly different. However, the average time to return to sport after arthroscopic surgery was significantly shorter than that after open surgery (3.9 vs 8.3 months). Moreover, the average duration of symptoms after arthroscopic surgery was significantly shorter than that after open surgery (14.5 vs 25.8 months).

The long-term clinical results after surgery for patellar tendinopathy were evaluated in a few reports (Pascarella et al. 2011; Maffulli et al. 2014). Pascarella et al. (2011) showed significant improvements in Victorian Institute of Sports Assessment Patellar (VISA-P) score at 1 and 3 years after arthroscopic surgery, from the preoperative scores. These improvements in score were maintained within 5–10 years after surgery. A study on the long-term clinical results after open surgery reported excellent or good results, with a VISA-P score of 91% and return-to-sport rate of 86.3% (Maffulli et al. 2014). The two studies suggested that the efficacy of both open and arthroscopic surgeries for patellar tendinopathy could continue throughout a long-term follow-up period.

28.4.6 Other Treatments

In addition to the abovementioned evidence-based therapies, many other therapies are available but without consensus for their use. However, some therapies, including hyaluronic acid (HA) and corticosteroid injections, nonsteroidal anti-inflammatory drugs (NSAIDs), and load management, are considered relatively useful and reasonable for tendinopathy under limited conditions such as short-term period or acute phase.

Recently, studies on treatment using HA have been reported. These studies showed improvement of pain and knee function in short-term follow-up and no serious adverse events during the study period (Kumai et al. 2014; Muneta et al. 2012), although the number of reports is not enough to provide firm evidence. Considering its efficacy and safety, HA injection should be applied for patellar tendinopathy at least once during treatment with eccentric exercise.

Corticosteroid injections have also short-term effects on tendinopathy at relieving pain, reducing swelling, and improving function (Rees et al. 2014). However, corticosteroid injections increased the risk of tendon rupture and conferred greater risk of long-term recurrence (Khan et al. 1998). Therefore, corticosteroids should be used with caution in the management of tendinopathy in the acute phase.

A Cochrane review of interventions for treating acute and chronic Achilles tendinopathy also found weak evidence of a moderate effect of NSAIDs on acute tendon pain (McLauchlan and Handoll 2001). However, administration of NSAIDs showed no effect to promote tendon healing, and the management of patellar tendinopathy was controversial (Rees et al. 2014).

Platelet-rich plasma (PRP) has also applied for the treatment of tendinopathy. According to the recent systematic review of patellar tendinopathy treated using PRP, pain and knee function were improved in short term after PRP injection (Liddle and Rodríguez-Merchán 2015). But two randomized control studies showed that the treatment of PRP has no superiority compared to other conservative therapies (Dragoo et al. 2014; Vetrano et al. 2013).

Other than the use of these pharmaceutical agents, one approach to promoting the healing of tendon tissue in athletes with acute tendinopathy is to decrease loading by adjusting the athlete's style of playing and decreasing frequency, intensity, and exercise duration. However, how frequency, intensity, and exercise duration affect load management in tendinopathy is unknown (Khan et al. 1998).

28.5 Our Treatment Regimen

As described earlier, evidence-based therapies, including eccentric training, shockwave therapy, and surgery, should be recommended. However, in treatment using these evidence-based therapies, the disease course of tendinopathy should be considered. Cook and Purdam et al. (2009) classified tendinopathy into three stages and two groups to determine the degree of microstructural damage that require treatment intervention. However, this classification was insufficient to decide which therapy should be applied. Therefore, we suggest a new concept based on healing response of the tendon in addition to their classification for decision-making regarding the appropriate treatment method. For acute tendinopathy (reactive tendinopathy), Cook and Purdam et al. (2009) recommended load management and NSAIDs, but we consider that, as the tendon are inflamed, NSAIDs and corticosteroid injection are effective. However, in consideration of the risk of tendon rupture, attention should be given to the use of corticosteroid injection.

In chronic tendinopathy with degenerative damage to the tendon, healing ability is low and partially fails. The damaged tendons could be divided into two phases based on response to mechanical stimulus. If tendons respond to mechanical load and resume healing ability, they are considered to be in the reversible phase. On the other hand, if the damaged tendon do not respond to mechanical loading and have poor healing potential, they are assumed to be in the irreversible phase. In reversible phase, mechanical loading by eccentric exercise stimulates mechanoreceptors in the damaged tendon and then promotes collagen synthesis, which leads to healing of the degenerated tendon to normal. However, when tendinopathy progresses to the irreversible phase, the tendon completely loses its healing ability by mechanical loading by exercise alone. For tendinopathy in this phase, ESWT or surgical intervention should be indicated (Fig. 28.3). This classification is considered useful for decision-making regarding treatment methods for chronic tendinopathy. However, histological and clinical evidence are insufficient to

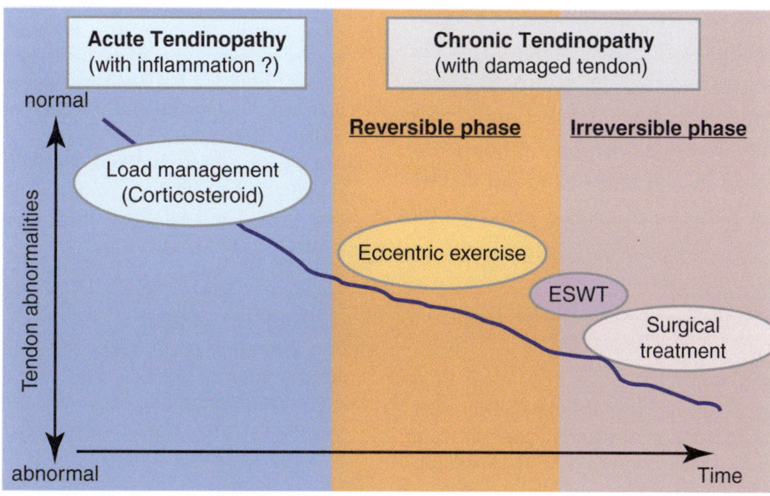

Fig. 28.3 The new concept based on healing response of the tendon for decision-making regarding the appropriate treatment method. Tendinopathy is classified into two stages, namely, acute (*blue square*) and chronic (*orange and pink squares*). For the acute stage, only load management, including reduction in frequency or intensity of tendon load (and/or corticosteroid injection), can improve tendon to normal, whereas physical or surgical treatment is needed for the chronic stage. Moreover, we propose to classify chronic tendinopathy into reversible and irreversible phases. In the reversible phase, damaged tendon can improve to normal tendon with eccentric exercise. However, in the irreversible phase, damaged tendon cannot be improved with mechanical loading alone. In this phase, ESWT or surgical intervention is needed. This figure shows that tendon abnormalities progress gradually. The vertical axis represents the degree of tendon abnormalities; and the horizontal axis, the elapsed time

distinguish reversible and irreversible phases. Further research studies are required in the future.

28.6 Summary

Patellar tendinopathy is one of the most common injuries caused by overuse. Generally, histological findings in tendinopathy indicate a degenerative process and loss of healing response. The symptoms of tendinopathy are pain and/or disability due to pain. Although many treatment methods are available for patellar tendinopathy, no consensus has been reached as to the proper use of these therapies because of the limited evidence from their application. Only eccentric exercise has strong evidence of effectiveness for patellar tendinopathy. Moderate evidence was found for heavy slow resistance training. Moreover, the evidence for sclerosing injections, shockwave therapy, and surgery is limited. The success rate of conventional conservative treatment of tendinopathy, including eccentric exercise, was >80%. For the remaining patients, invasive therapies such as arthroscopic and open surgeries are needed. The success rate of surgery for patellar tendinopathy was reported to be 60–90%. The mean period of return to sports after arthroscopic surgery was significantly shorter than that after open surgery, although the success and return-to-play rates were not significantly different between open and arthroscopic surgeries.

References

Abate M, Gravare Silbernagel K, Siljeholm C, Di Iorio A, De Amicis D, Salini V et al (2009) Pathogenesis of tendinopathies: inflammation or degeneration? Arthritis Res Ther 11(3):235

Alfredson H, Ohberg L (2005 Mar) Neovascularisation in chronic painful patellar tendinosis—promising results after sclerosing neovessels outside the tendon challenge the need for surgery. Knee Surg Sports Traumatol Arthrosc 13(2):74–80

Basso O, Amis AA, Race A et al (2002) Patellar tendon fiber strains: their differential responses to quadriceps tension. Clin Orthop Relat Res 400:246–253

Blazina ME, Kerlan RK, Jobe FW, Carter VS, Carlson GJ (1973) Jumper's knee. Orthop Clin N Am 4(3):665–678

Boesen MI, Koenig MJ, Torp-Pedersen S, Bliddal H, Langberg H (2006) Tendinopathy and Doppler activity: the vascular response of the Achilles tendon to exercise. Scand J Med Sci Sports 16:463–469

Brockmeyer M, Diehl N, Schmitt C, Kohn DM, Lorbach O (2015) Results of surgical treatment of chronic patellar tendinosis (jumper's knee): a systematic review of the literature. Arthroscopy 31(12):2424-9.e3

Cannell LJ, Taunton JE, Clement DB et al (2001) A randomised clinical trial of the efficacy of drop squats or leg extension/leg curl exercises to treat clinically diagnosed jumper's knee in athletes: pilot study. Br J Sports Med 35:60–64

Cook JL, Purdam CR (2009) Is tendon pathology a continuum? A pathology model to explain the clinical presentation of load-induced tendinopathy. Br J Sports Med 43(6):409–416

Dillon EM, Erasmus PJ, Müller JH et al (2008) Differential forces within the proximal patellar tendon as an explanation for the characteristic lesion of patellar tendinopathy: an in vivo descriptive experimental study. Am J Sports Med 36(11):2119–2127

Dragoo JL, Wasterlain AS, Braun HJ, Nead KT (2014) Platelet-rich plasma as a treatment for patellar tendinopathy: a double-blind, randomized controlled trial. Am J Sports Med 42(3):610–618

Ferretti A, Conteduca F, Camerucci E, Morelli F (2002) Patellar tendinosis: a follow-up study of surgical treatment. J Bone Joint Surg Am 84:2179–2185

Fredberg U, Bolvig L, Pfeiffer-Jensen M, Clemmensen D, Jakobsen BW, Stengaard-Pedersen K (2004) Ultrasonography as a tool for diagnosis, guidance of local steroid injection and together with pressure algometry monitoring of the treatment of athletes with chronic Jumper's knee and Achilles tendinitis: a randomised, double-blind, placebo-controlled study. Scand J Rheumatol 33:94–101

Fredberg U, Stengaard-Pedersen K (2008) Chronic tendinopathy tissue pathology, pain mechanisms, and etiology with a special focus on inflammation. Scand J Med Sci Sports 18(1):3–15

Fritschy D, Wallensten R (1993) Surgical treatment of patellar tendinitis. Knee Surg Sports Traumatol Arthrosc 1:131–133

Graham HK, Holmes DF, Watson RB, Kadler KE (2000) Identification of collagen fibril fusion during vertebrate tendon morphogenesis. The process relies on unipolar fibrils and is regulated by collagen-proteoglycan interaction. J Mol Biol 295:891–902

Hansen P, Haraldsson BT, Aagaard P, Kovanen V, Avery NC, Qvortrup K, Larsen JO, Krogsgaard M, Kjaer M, Peter MS (1985/2010) Lower strength of the human posterior patellar tendon seems unrelated to mature collagen cross-linking and fibril morphology. J Appl Physiol 108(1):47–52

Hoksrud A, Ohberg L, Alfredson H, Bahr R (2006) Ultrasound-guided sclerosis of neovessels in painful chronic patellar tendinopathy: a randomized controlled trial. Am J Sports Med 34(11):1738–1746. Epub 2006 Jul 10. Erratum in: Am J Sports Med. 2011 Jul;39(7)

Johnson DP, Wakeley CJ, Watt I (1996) Magnetic resonance imaging of patellar tendonitis. J Bone Joint Surg Br 78(3):452–457

Jonsson P, Alfredson H (2005) Superior results with eccentric compared to concentric quadriceps training in patients with jumper's knee: a prospective randomized study. Br J Sports Med 39:847–850

Kelly JD IV. (2009) Arthroscopic excision of distal pole of patella for refractory patellar tendinitis. Orthopedics 32:504

Khan KM, Bonar F, Desmond PM, Cook JL, Young DA, Visentini PJ, Fehrmann MW, Kiss ZS, O'Brien PA et al (1996) Patellar tendinosis (jumper's knee): findings at histopathologic examination, US, and MR imaging. Victorian Institute of Sport Tendon Study Group. Radiology 200(3):821–827

Khan KM, Cook JL, Maffulli N et al (2002) Time to abandon the "tendinitis" myth. BMJ 16:626–627

Khan KM, Maffulli N, Coleman BD, Cook JL, Taunton JE (1998) Patellar tendinopathy: some aspects of basic science and clinical management. Br J Sports Med 32(4):346–355

Kongsgaard M, Qvortrup K, Larsen J et al (2010) Fibril morphology and tendon mechanical properties in patellar tendinopathy: effects of heavy slow resistance training. Am J Sports Med 38(4):749–756

Kongsgaard M, Reitelseder S, Pedersen TG et al (2007) Region specific patellar tendon hypertrophy in humans following resistance training. Acta Physiol 191(2):111–121

Kumai T, Muneta T, Tsuchiya A, Shiraishi M, Ishizaki Y, Sugimoto K, Samoto N, Isomoto S, Tanaka Y, Takakura Y (2014) The short-term effect after a single injection of high-molecular-weight hyaluronic acid in patients with enthesopathies (lateral epicondylitis, patellar tendinopathy, insertional Achilles tendinopathy, and plantar fasciitis): a preliminary study. J Orthop Sci 19(4):603–611

Larsson ME, Käll I, Nilsson-Helander K (2012) Treatment of patellar tendinopathy—a systematic review of randomized controlled trials. Knee Surg Sports Traumatol Arthrosc 20(8):1632–1646

Lavagnino M, Arnoczky SP, Elvin N, Dodds J (2008 Nov) Patellar tendon strain is increased at the site of the jumper's knee lesion during knee flexion and tendon loading: results and cadaveric testing of a computational model. Am J Sports Med 36(11):2110–2118

Leal C, Ramon S, Furia J, Fernandez A, Romero L, Hernandez-Sierra L (2015) Current concepts of shockwave therapy in chronic patellar tendinopathy. Int J Surg 24(Pt B):160–164

Liddle AD, Rodríguez-Merchán EC (2015) Platelet-rich plasma in the treatment of patellar tendinopathy: a systematic review. Am J Sports Med 43(10):2583–2590

Lind B, Ohberg L, Alson H (2006) Sclerosing polidocanol injections in mid-portion Achilles tendinosis: remaining good clinical results and decreased tendon thickness at 2-year follow-up. Knee Surg Sports Traumatol Arthrosc 14:1327–1332

Maffulli N, Longo UG (2008) How do eccentric exercises work in tendinopathy? Rheumatology 47:1444–1445

Maffulli N, Longo UG, Denaro V (2010) Novel approaches for the management of tendinopathy. J Bone Joint Surg Am 92(15):2604–2613

Maffulli N, Oliva F, Maffulli G, King JB, Del Buono A (2014) Surgery for unilateral and bilateral patellar tendinopathy: a seven year comparative study. Int Orthop 38(8):1717–1722

Maffulli N, Sharma P, Luscombe KL (2004) Achilles tendinopathy: aetiology and management. J R Soc Med 97:472–476

Malliaras P, Barton CJ, Reeves ND et al (2013) Achilles and patellar tendinopathy loading programmes: a systematic review comparing clinical outcomes and identifying potential mechanisms for effectiveness. Sports Med 43(4):267–286

McLauchlan GJ, Handoll HH (2001) Interventions for treating acute and chronic Achilles tendinitis. Cochrane Database Syst Rev (2):CD000232

Muneta T, Koga H, Ju YJ, Mochizuki T, Sekiya I (2012) Hyaluronan injection therapy for athletic patients with patellar tendinopathy. J Orthop Sci 17:425–431

Ogon P, Maier D, Jaeger A, Suedkamp NP (2006) Arthroscopic patellar release for the treatment of chronic patellar tendinopathy. Arthroscopy 22:462.e1–462.e5

Ohberg L, Alfredson H (2002) Ultrasound guided sclerosis of neovessels in painful chronic Achilles tendinosis: pilot study of a new treatment. Br J Sports Med 36:173–175

Pascarella A, Alam M, Pascarella F, Latte C, Di Salvatore MG, Maffulli N (2011) Arthroscopic management of chronic patellar tendinopathy. Am J Sports Med 39(9):1975–1983

Pearson SJ, Hussain SR (2014) Region-specific tendon properties and patellar tendinopathy: a wider understanding. Sports Med 44(8):1101–1112

Peers KH, Lysens RJ, Brys P, Bellemans J (2003) Cross-sectional outcome analysis of athletes with chronic patellar tendinopathy treated surgically and by extracorporeal shock wave therapy. Clin J Sport Med 13:79–83

Rees JD, Stride M, Scott A (2014 Nov) Tendons—time to revisit inflammation. Br J Sports Med 48(21):1553–1557. doi:10.1136/bjsports-2012-091957. Epub 2013 Mar 9. Review

Romeo AA, Larson RV (1999) Arthroscopic treatment of infrapatellar tendonitis. Arthroscopy 15:341–345

Sharma P, Maffulli N (2006) Biology of tendon injury: healing, modeling and remodeling. J Musculoskelet Neuronal Interact 6(2):181–190

Smillie IS (1962) Injuries of the knee joint, 3rd edn. Livingstone, Edinburgh, pp 264–267

Stasinopoulos D, Stasinopoulos I (2004) Comparison of effects of exercise programme, pulsed ultrasound and transverse friction in the treatment of chronic patellar tendinopathy. Clin Rehabil 18:347–352

Taunton KM, Taunton JE, Khan KM (2003) Treatment of patellar tendinopathy with extracorporeal shock wave therapy. B C Med J 45:500–507

Toumi H, Higashiyama I, Suzuki D, Kumai T, Bydder G, McGonagle D, Emery P, Fairclough J, Benjamin M (2006) Regional variations in human patellar trabecular architecture and the structure of the proximal patellar tendon enthesis. J Anat 208(1):47–57

Verheyden F, Geens G, Nelen G (1997) Jumper's knee: Results of surgical treatment. Acta Orthop Belg 63:102–105

Vetrano M, Castorina A, Vulpiani MC, Baldini R, Pavan A (2013) Ferretti A Platelet-rich plasma versus focused shock waves in the treatment of jumper's knee in athletes. Am J Sports Med 41(4):795–803

Wasielewski NJ, Kotsko KM (2007) Does eccentric exercise reduce pain and improve strength in physically active adults with symptomatic lower extremity tendinosis? A systematic review. J Athl Train 42:409–421

Zwerver J, Dekker F, Pepping GJ (2010) Patient guided piezo-electric extracorporeal shockwave therapy as treatment for chronic severe patellar tendinopathy: a pilot study. J Back Musculoskelet Rehabil 23:111–115

Surgical Treatment of Patellar Tendinopathy

29

Gian Luigi Canata, Valentina Casale,
Josè Huylebroek, and Alberto Vascellari

Contents

29.1 Introduction

Patellar tendinopathy is a common musculoskeletal disorder among recreational and professional athletes (Blazina et al. 1973). It has an important impact on the athletes' careers, because of its high prevalence, the resulting impairment of knee function, and its chronic clinical course (Zwerver et al. 2011) (Figs. 29.1 and 29.2).

Despite the occurrence rate of patellar tendinopathy in different sports is mostly unknown, it

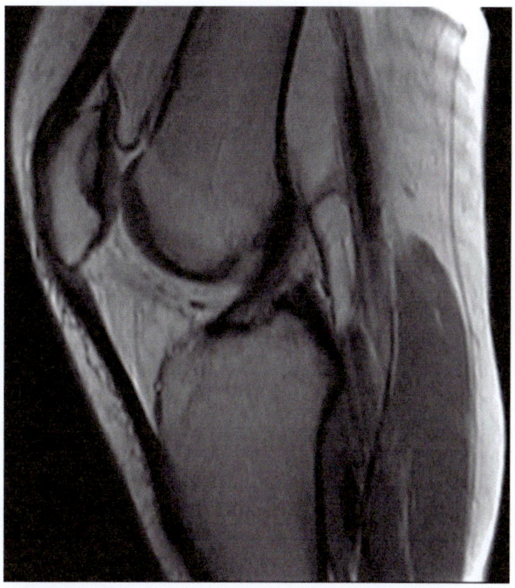

Fig. 29.1 Sagittal T1 MRI showing tendon thickening and an abnormal signal at the proximal insertion of the patellar tendon

G.L. Canata, M.D. (✉) • V. Casale, M.D.
Centre of Sports Traumatology, Koelliker Hospital, Turin, Italy
e-mail: canata@ortosport.it

J. Huylebroek, M.D.
Sportsmed—Orthopaedic Centre, Parc Leopold Hospital, Brussels, Belgium
e-mail: jose@sportsmedchirec.be

A. Vascellari, M.D.
Orthopaedic Unit Oderzo Hospital, Oderzo, Italy

G.L. Canata et al. (eds.), *Muscle and Tendon Injuries*, DOI 10.1007/978-3-662-54184-5_29

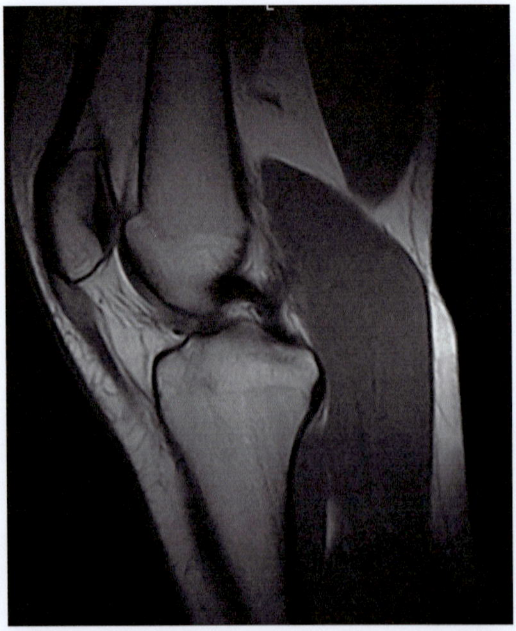

Fig. 29.2 Sagittal T1 MRI showing a marked tendon thickening and an increased signal intensity within the tendon

has been reported a prevalence in sports with high demands on speed and power for the leg extensors, such as volleyball and basketball, soccer, and athletics (Zwerver et al. 2011; Lian et al. 2005).

The management of patellar tendinopathy is controversial (Blazina et al. 1973; Nichols 1992). The conservative treatment includes several options, such as rest, anti-inflammatory drugs, physical therapy, orthoses, stretching, eccentric exercises, extracorporeal shockwave therapy, dextrose prolotherapy (Ryan et al. 2011; Topol et al. 2011), platelet-rich plasma (Filardo et al. 2010) and autologous blood injection (James et al. 2007), and ultrasound-guided sclerotherapy (Zwerver 2008; Testa et al. 1999).

If conservative treatment fails after at least 6 months of therapies, surgical treatment is recommended (Cucurulo et al. 2009) in particular for athletes whose careers are put at risk, or in the presence of a complete tendon disruption (Brockmeyer et al. 2015).

Multiple surgical techniques can be adopted, depending on the site of the tendinopathy, i.e., along the main tendon body or the insertional area, and the characteristics of the lesions such as calcifications, cysts, or tears that may be present (Cucurulo et al. 2009).

However, a general agreement on the ideal surgical management option is still lacking (Marcheggiani Muccioli et al. 2013). In their systematic review, Coleman et al. highlighted too many methodological deficiencies which negatively impact on the validity of the reported outcomes (Coleman et al. 2000).

Both open and arthroscopic procedures are effective to restore function by minimizing tissue damaging, mitigate compression and pain, and promote vascularization (Maffulli et al. 2014).

Postoperative results are satisfying: it has been reported that the mean success rate after surgical treatment of chronic patellar tendinopathy ranges between 60% and 90% (Johnson 1998). Marcheggiani Muccioli et al. (2013) have provided an overview about the different surgical options for the treatment of patellar tendinopathy. This review shows better outcomes after the arthroscopic approach, with an average success rate of 92.4% against the 87.2% rate in the open surgery group. Better results after arthroscopy have been reported also by Brockmeyer et al. in a systematic review (Brockmeyer et al. 2015), with a success rate of 91% against the 81% after the open surgery.

Similarly, the average time and rate for returning to sport show some differences between the two approaches. The mean rate of return to sport after an arthroscopic treatment is 82.3%, within a mean of 3.9 months, while the rate decreases to 78.4% within 8.3 months after an open surgery (Brockmeyer et al. 2015). Stuhlman et al. have reported satisfactory results in 81% after an open approach, and 91% after an arthroscopic surgery (Stuhlman et al. 2016), thus confirming the slightly greater effectiveness of arthroscopy.

Gill et al. (2013) have described a surgical approach which combined open and arthroscopic techniques. Starting from arthroscopy, they managed intra-articular pathologic findings if present; then they switched to the open approach, with a midline incision into the patellar tendon and excising the thickened areas of tendinosis.

Surgery was completed by performing fenestrations to encourage a healing response. The reported data were satisfying, especially in terms of time to return to sports activities.

This chapter aims to give an overview about the different surgical options for the treatment of patellar tendinopathy, describing both open and arthroscopic available techniques.

29.2 Open Surgical Techniques

Open surgical options for the treatment of patellar tendinopathy essentially include the affected tissue removal after sectioning the peritenon, as well as the removal or drilling of the patellar pole (Zhang et al. 2016). The operation may essentially involve a midline or medial parapatellar longitudinal skin incision, a paratenon incision and stripping, multiple longitudinal tenotomies and the excision of the damaged tendon tissue (Testa et al. 1999) (Figs. 29.3 and 29.4).

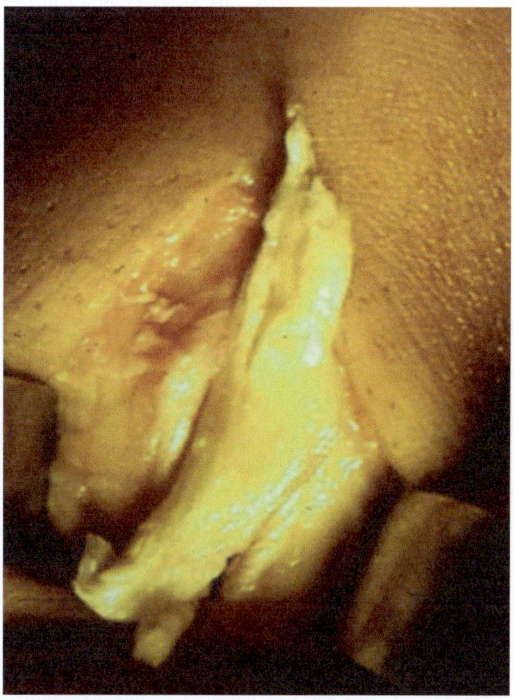

Fig. 29.3 Open surgery: resection of fibrotic tendon tissue

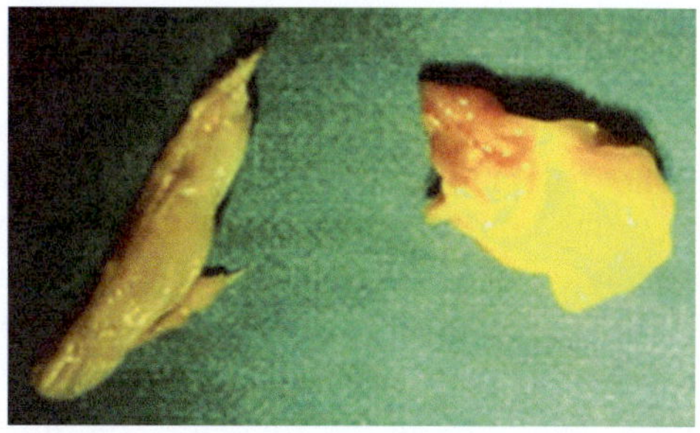

Fig. 29.4 Open surgery: pathologic patellar tendon resected and removed fibrotic synovial tissue

Whichever method is chosen, the aim of surgical management is to promote wound repair through a modulation of the tendon cell-matrix environment (Leadbetter et al. 1992).

Open surgery was firstly mentioned in 1946 by Smillie (1946), who described a technique still performed which consists in drilling multiple holes in the inferior patellar pole.

In 1973, Blazina et al. suggested excision of the extra-articular patella by opening the tendon along its axis and removing the abnormal tendinous tissue (1973).

Several derivative techniques have been developed later. The purpose essentially aimed to avoid an osseous procedure by removing the damaged part of the patella (Fritschy and Wallensten 1993; Verheyden et al. 1997), although bone-involving techniques are still performed. In fact, the technique described by Smillie is still in use (Popp et al. 1997; Raatikainen et al. 1994), while other authors prefer to create tendinoperiostal scars (Karlsson et al. 1991), or combine both the techniques (Ferretti et al. 2002).

Nevertheless, it has been demonstrated that bone excision should be avoided in the treatment of patellar tendinopathy: Kaeding et al. (2007) found a 71% success rate after approaching the inferior pole of the patella, compared to the 92% if there is no bony involvement. They also reported better outcomes if no paratenon closure was performed, as well as in case of no postoperative immobilization.

A further surgical choice consists in ultrasound-guided percutaneous longitudinal tenotomies (Testa et al. 1999; Lorbach et al. 2008): under ultrasound control, a surgical scalpel blade penetrates the whole thickness of the tendon during passive extensions and flexions of the knee leading to longitudinal and parallel tenotomies, with an average length of 2 cm. This process is repeated laterally and medially to the tendon width (Testa et al. 1999). The use of sonographic guidance in the treatment of musculoskeletal disorders has gained consensus in the literature: the ultrasound-guided percutaneous needle tenotomies reduce pain in patients with chronic patellar tendinopathy without complications (Housner et al. 2009).

An increasing number of authors choose the arthroscopic approach, not for its clinical superiority to others (Marcheggiani Muccioli et al. 2013; Rodriguez-Merchan 2013), rather because it is less invasive and provides a faster postoperative return to sport (Brockmeyer et al. 2015). Open surgery is still preferred when a calcification along the tendon is present (Fig. 29.5), or when a tendon tear has occurred (Cenni and Silva 2015).

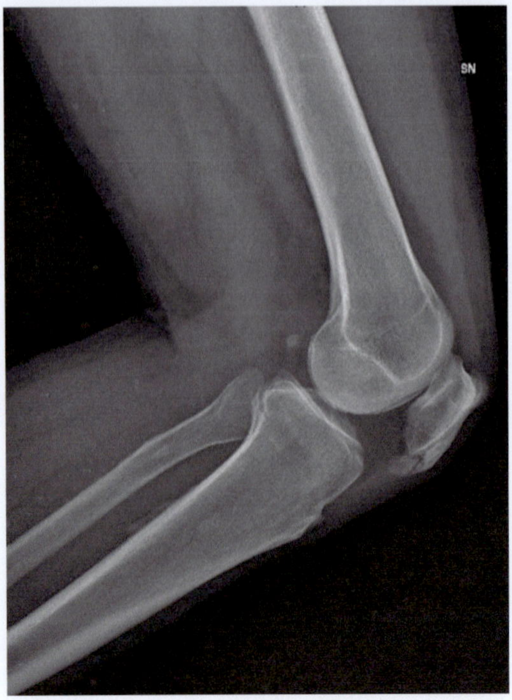

Fig. 29.5 Preoperative lateral X-ray showing osteophytes at the proximal insertion of the patellar tendon

29.3 Arthroscopic Techniques for Patellar Tendinopathy

Arthroscopic procedures for the treatment of patellar tendinopathy allows a better management of the painful areas of the proximal-posterior tendon fibers and of the infrapatellar fat pad (Pascarella et al. 2011).

New arthroscopic techniques have been developed (Coleman et al. 2000; Lorbach et al. 2008; Ogon et al. 2006; Willberg et al. 2007), even if synovectomy and/or apicectomy are the most widely used. The main purpose is to remove the damaged retrotendinous tissue through the debridement and the treatment of the patella only if necessary (Cucurulo et al. 2009). The surgeon may opt for a partial resection of Hoffa's fat and of the lower pole of the patella (Cenni and Silva 2015). The final purpose is the excision of the neovascularization and the innervation of the degenerative area (Cucurulo et al. 2009).

Willberg et al. (2007) have proposed an arthroscopic shaving technique, which involves the area of interest on the dorsal surface of the tendon, combined with Ultrasound + Doppler examinations during surgery. The ultrasound and the color Doppler guidance effectively reduce the risk of "shaving too much," thus minimizing trauma to the Hoffa's fat pad and to the tendon.

The presence of abnormal neovascularity typically arises from the fat pad, thus its debridement and partial resection is recommended, as discussed by several authors (Brockmeyer et al. 2015; Pascarella et al. 2011; Alaseirlis et al. 2012). On the other hand, a total excision of the fat pad could excessively reduce the vascularity of the patella, causing anterior impingement and anterior knee pain, as noted by Pinsornsak et al. in total knee arthroplasty (Pinsornsak et al. 2014).

A further surgical issue is whether to perform the resection of the lower patellar pole or not. An impingement or a compression of the inferior pole of the patella onto the posterior aspect of the tendon during the flexion of the knee has been reported as one of the causes of patellar tendinopathy (Lorbach et al. 2008). It is common to find an elongation of the lower patellar pole on the X-rays (Blazina et al. 1973). In this case, an abrasion of the lower patella should be performed to release the deep fiber of the tendon from the inferior pole and to excise the bony protrusion (Lorbach et al. 2008) (Fig. 29.6). The result is an arthroscopic tenolysis, highly effective in terms of postoperative recovery and time to return to sport (Cenni and Silva 2015; Pascarella et al. 2011; Alaseirlis et al. 2012).

With regard to the specific arthroscopic technique, the conventional anteromedial and anterolateral portals and an optional central transtendinous accessory portal are performed (Cenni and Silva 2015). (Figs. 29.7, 29.8, 29.9, 29.10, 29.11 and 29.12)

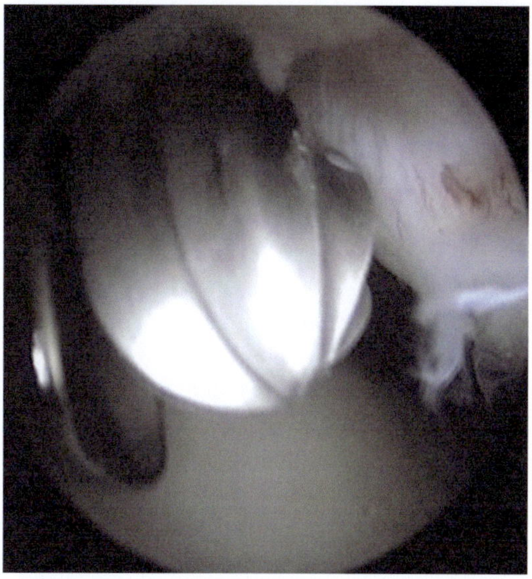

Fig. 29.6 Arthroscopic resection of distal patellar bone with a burr

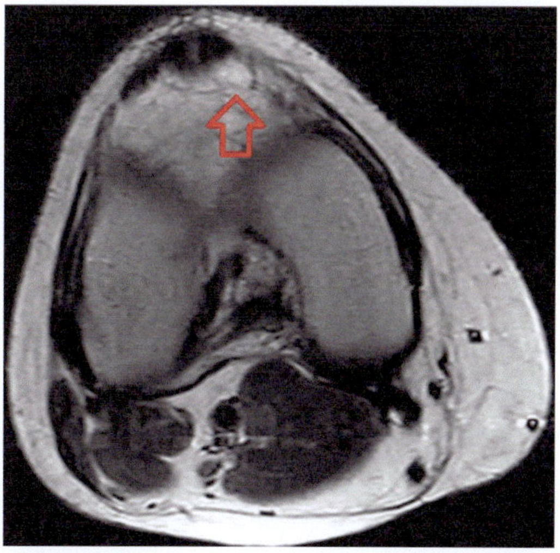

Fig. 29.7 MRI showing right knee synovial hypertrophic nodular tissue behind the tendon

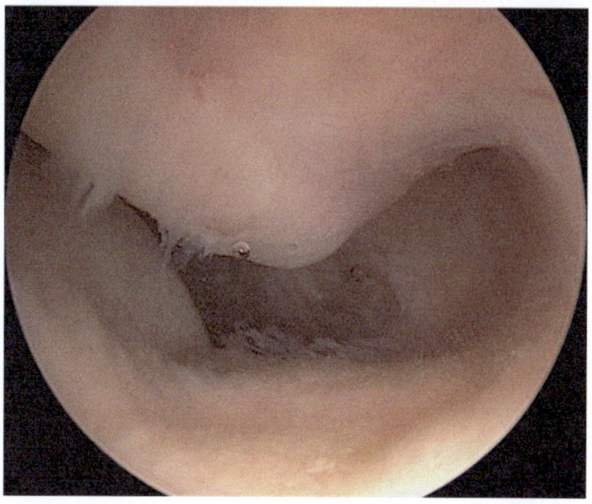

Fig. 29.8 Arthroscopic view: hypertrophic synovial tissue, right knee

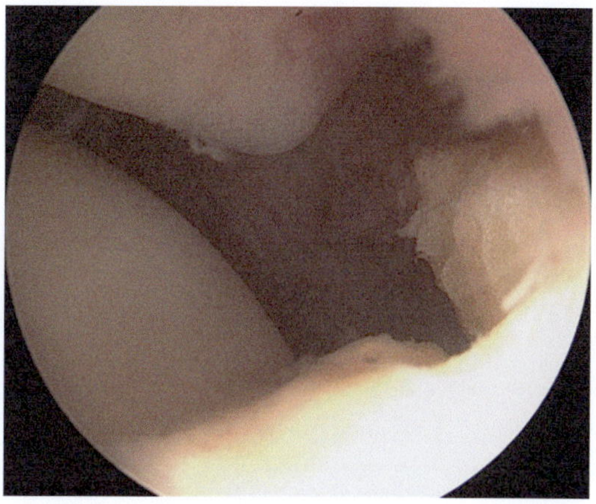

Fig. 29.9 Nodular hypertrophic tissue behind the tendon

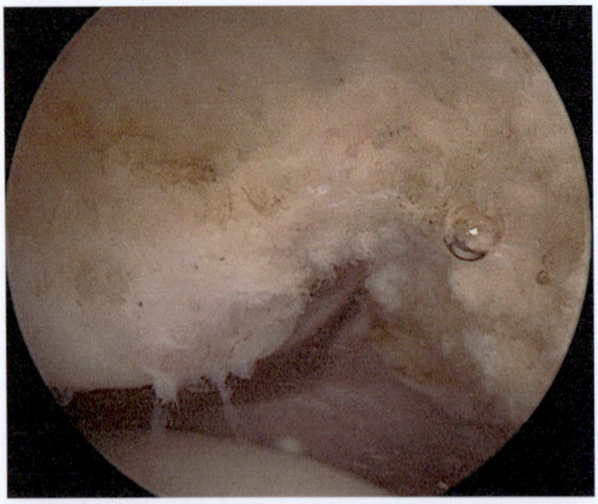

Fig. 29.10 Arthroscopic view of the inferior patellar pole after debridement, right knee

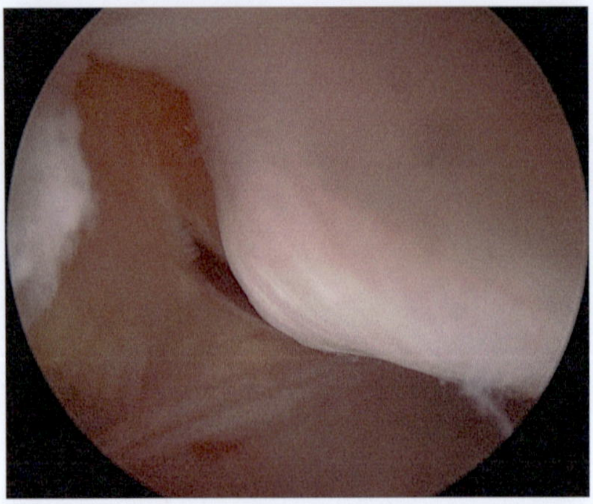

Fig. 29.11 Arthroscopic view: hypertrophic synovial tissue of the same patient, left knee

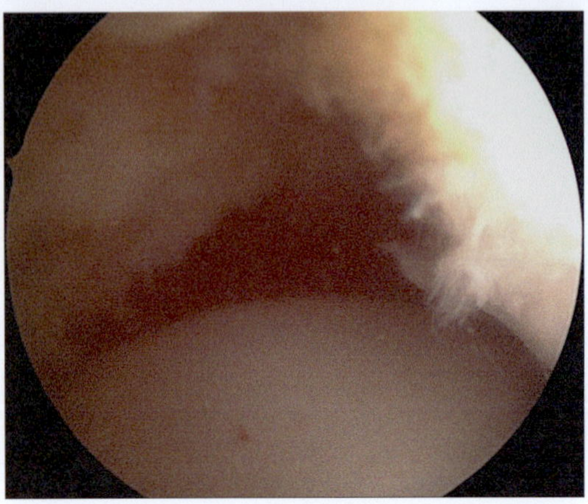

Fig. 29.12 Arthroscopic view after synovectomy with radio frequencies. No patellar bone resection, left knee

29.4 Postoperative Management and Rehabilitation Program

Surgical management and postoperative rehabilitation are paramount for a complete biological and functional recovery. Several authors consider rehabilitation as an integral part of treatment (Verheyden et al. 1997; Lorbach et al. 2008; Ogon et al. 2006; Kelly et al. 1984).

There is a great variety of postoperative protocols: as Khan and Smart (2016) have reported in a systematic review, some authors suggest a prolonged casting after surgery (Karlsson et al. 1991; Pierets et al. 1999; Peers et al. 2003), whereas others recommend early motion without any restriction (Fritschy and Wallensten 1993; Popp et al. 1997; Willberg et al. 2007; Shelbourne et al. 2006; Orava et al. 1986; Maffulli et al. 1999; Bahr et al. 2006; Maier et al. 2013; Willberg et al. 2011; Santander et al. 2012), or letting a full range of motion except for a complete knee extension, which was avoided during the first 3–4 weeks after surgery (Coleman et al. 2000; Lorbach et al. 2008; Sarimo et al. 2007).

In their retrospective study, Cucurulo et al. reported that postoperative immobilization in extension was prescribed in the 80% of cases, for 23 days on average; the rehabilitation protocol started 15 days after surgery (Cucurulo et al. 2009). However, they advocated a quick rehabilitation protocol without immobilization period, in order to achieve better functional postoperative results.

Maier et al. (2013) conducted postoperative rehabilitation in a symptom-oriented fashion. Range of motion and weight bearing were allowed immediately from day 1 as tolerated. Open kinetic chain exercises were started as soon as patients were free of symptoms. During the first two postoperative weeks, patients performed open kinetic chain exercises to preserve and strengthen the quadriceps muscles. However, physiotherapy must not have caused any symptoms of patellar tendinopathy. From week 3, patients started closed kinetic chain exercises and resumed sports-specific training but still avoided higher loads of knee extension (e.g., jumping, running, bench press). From week 5, patients started with light running and participated in training sessions. From week 7, athletes resumed sports and returned to competition if training sessions could be completed without symptoms at previous levels. Patients could return to training after 4 weeks and to competition after 6 weeks if they remained free of symptoms.

Pascarella et al. (Pascarella et al. 2011) started rehabilitation on the first day after the procedure, with continuous passive motion from 0° to 30° for a minimum of 4 h a day and isometric quadriceps exercises. The range of motion was then gradually increased as tolerated. In the second week, massage of the thigh was added, and range of motion was increased until full passive motion was achieved. A partial weight bearing was encouraged in the very first phase, with a progressive increase to full weight bearing within 7 days. At 2 weeks, hydrotherapy and light closed kinetic chain exercises with progressive loads were introduced. Running was allowed at 5–6 weeks, and patients usually returned to pivoting sports by 12 weeks. Load increases were dependent on being symptom free on the increased load. Return to sports was based on multiple factors, including being asymptomatic after at least eight sessions of full training at preinjury level over a 4-week period.

Shelbourne et al. have described an example of aggressive postoperative protocol (2006): on the basis of the ACL reconstruction rehabilitation, they suggest immediate active and passive full extension exercises with the tendon still anesthetized and the use of a low-resistance leg press machine, to be continued even after the patient has been discharged. The full weight bearing is allowed immediately after surgery. During the first week, the protocol leads to a full recovery of the range of motion, gradually reinforcing muscles. When patient's isokinetic quadriceps strength is at least 85%, return to play is allowed; this usually occurs 2 months after surgery.

The isokinetic strength improvement has been reported as an effective method for monitoring the postoperative recovery (Marcheggiani Muccioli et al. 2013).

Alaseirlis et al. (2012) proposed a further type of postoperative rehabilitation protocol which requires a postoperative knee immobilization in full extension for three weeks after. Then, the functional cast is unlocked for a passive range of motion recovery. Active motion and a full weight bearing should be progressively restored within the first four weeks after surgery. During this period, at the second week the patient may start isometric exercises, while the isotonic and kinetic chain exercises should be delayed until the fourth postoperative week. The gradual return to sports activities may be finally advised after eighth weeks.

In their review, Cucurulo et al. have reported that patients could start running an average of 5.5 months after open surgery and 4 months after arthroscopy; the training protocol began a mean of 7 months after open surgery and 5 months after arthroscopy (Cucurulo et al. 2009).

Conclusions

Surgery is recommended in the presence of patellar tendinopathy only when the conservative treatment has failed. Both open and arthroscopic procedures are widely used, even if arthroscopy is preferred due to its shorter recovery times. The surgical rationale consists in the debridement of the damaged tissue, and performing apicectomy could be an option in case of bony protrusion. The mean time to return to sports activities is 3–6 months.

The healing process requires time to avoid postoperative complications, thus the rehabilitation program should not be too aggressive.

References

Alaseirlis DA, Konstantinidis GA, Malliaropoulos N et al (2012) Arthroscopic treatment of chronic patellar tendinopathy in high-level athletes. Muscles Ligaments Tendons J 2(4):267–272

Bahr R, Fossan B, Løken S et al (2006) Surgical treatment compared with eccentric training for patellar tendinopathy (jumper's knee): a randomised controlled trial. J Bone Joint Surg Am 88(8):1689–1698

Blazina ME, Kerlan RK, Jobe FW et al (1973) Jumper's knee. Orthop Clin North Am 4(3):665–678

Brockmeyer M, Diehl N, Schmitt C et al (2015) Results of surgical treatment of chronic patellar tendinosis (Jumper's Knee): a systematic review of the literature. Arthroscopy 31(12):2424–2429

Cenni MH, Silva TD, do Nascimento BF et al (2015) Patellar tendinopathy: late-stage results from surgical treatment. Rev Bras Ortop 50(5):550–555

Coleman BD, Khan KM, Maffulli N et al (2000) Studies of surgical outcome after patellar tendinopathy: clinical significance of methodological deficiencies and guidelines for future studies. Victorian Institute of Sport Tendon Study Group. Scand J Med Sci Sports 10(1):2–11

Cucurulo T, Louis ML, Thaunat M et al (2009) Surgical treatment of patellar tendinopathy in athletes. A retrospective multicentric study. Orthop Traumatol Surg Res 95(8 suppl 1):S78–S84

Ferretti A, Conteduca F, Camerucci E et al (2002) Patellar tendinosis: a follow-up study of surgical treatment. J Bone Joint Surg Am 84-A(12):2179–2185

Filardo G, Kon E, Della Villa S et al (2010) Use of platelet-rich plasma for the treatment of refractory jumper's knee. Int Orthop 34:909–915

Fritschy D, Wallensten R (1993) Surgical treatment of patellar tendinitis. Knee Surg Sports Traumatol Arthrosc 1(2):131–133

Gill TJ 4th, Carroll KM, Hariri S (2013) Open patellar tendon debridement for treatment of recalcitrant patellar tendinopathy: indications, technique, and clinical outcomes after a 2-year minimum follow-up. Sports Health 5(3):276–280

Housner JA, Jacobson JA, Misko R (2009) Sonographically guided percutaneous needle tenotomy for the treatment of chronic tendinosis. J Ultrasound Med 28(9):1187–1192

James SL, Ali K, Pocock C et al (2007) Ultrasound guided dry needling and autologous blood injection for patellar tendinosis. Br J Sports Med 41:518–521

Johnson DP (1998) Arthroscopic surgery for patellar tendonitis. Arthroscopy 14(suppl. 1):S44

Kaeding CC, Pedroza AD, Powers BC (2007) Surgical treatment of chronic patellar tendinosis: a systematic review. Clin Orthop Relat Res 455:102–106

Karlsson J, Lundin O, Lossing IW et al (1991) Partial rupture of the patellar ligament. Results after operative treatment. Am J Sports Med 19(4):403–408

Kelly DW, Carter VS, Jobe FW et al (1984) Patellar and quadriceps tendon ruptures–jumper's knee. Am J Sports Med 12(5):375–380

Khan WS, Smart A (2016) Outcome of surgery for chronic patellar tendinopathy: a systematic review. Acta Orthop Belg 82(3):610–626

Leadbetter WB, Mooar PA, Lane GJ et al (1992) The surgical treatment of tendinitis. Clinical rationale and biological basis. Clin Sports Med 11(4):679–712

Lian OB, Engebretsen L, Bahr R (2005) Prevalence of jumper's knee among elite athletes from different sports: a cross-sectional study. Am J Sports Med 33(4):561–567

Lorbach O, Diamantopoulos A, Paessler HH (2008) Arthroscopic resection of the lower patellar pole in patients with chronic patellar tendinosis. Arthroscopy 24(2):167–173

Maffulli N, Binfield PM, Leach WJ et al (1999) Surgical management of tendinopathy of the main body of the patellar tendon in athletes. Clin J Sport Med 9(2):58–62

Maffulli N, Oliva F, Maffulli G et al (2014) Surgery for unilateral and bilateral patellar tendinopathy: a seven year comparative study. Int Orthop 38:1717–1722

Maier D, Bornebusch L, Salzmann GM et al (2013) Mid- and long-term efficacy of the arthroscopic patellar release for treatment of patellar tendinopathy unresponsive to nonoperative management. Arthroscopy 29(8):1338–1345

Marcheggiani Muccioli GM, Zaffagnini S, Tsapralis K et al (2013) Open versus arthroscopic surgical treatment of chronic proximal patellar tendinopathy. A systematic review. Knee Surg Sports Traumatol Arthrosc 21(2):351–357

Nichols CE (1992) Patellar tendon injuries. Clin Sports Med 11(4):807–813

Ogon P, Maier D, Jaeger A et al (2006) Arthroscopic patellar release for the treatment of chronic patellar tendinopathy. Arthroscopy 22(4):462.e1–462.e5

Orava S, Osterback L, Hurme M (1986) Surgical treatment of patellar tendon pain in athletes. Br J Sports Med 20(4):167–169

Pascarella A, Alam M, Pascarella F et al (2011) Arthroscopic management of chronic patellar tendinopathy. Am J Sports Med 39(9):1875–1983

Peers KH, Lysens RJ, Brys P et al (2003) Cross-sectional outcome analysis of athletes with chronic patellar tendinopathy treated surgically and by extracorporeal shock wave therapy. Clin J Sport Med 13(2):79–83

Pierets K, Verdonk R, De Muynck M et al (1999) Jumper's knee: postoperative assessment. A retrospective clinical study. Knee Surg Sports Traumatol Arthrosc 7(4):239–242

Pinsornsak P, Naratrikun K, Chumchuen S (2014) The effect of infrapatellar fat pad excision on complications after minimally invasive TKA: a randomized controlled trial. Clin Orthop Relat Res 472(2):695–701

Popp JE, Yu JS, Kaeding CC (1997) Recalcitrant patellar tendinitis. Magnetic resonance imaging, histologic evaluation, and surgical treatment. Am J Sports Med 25(2):218–222

Raatikainen T, Karpakka J, Puranen J et al (1994) Operative treatment of partial rupture of the patellar ligament. A study of 138 cases. Int J Sports Med 15(1):46–49

Rodriguez-Merchan EC (2013) The treatment of patellar tendinopathy. J Orthopaed Traumatol 14(2):77–81

Ryan M, Wong A, Rabago D et al (2011) Ultrasound-guided injections of hyperosmolar dextrose for overuse patellar tendinopathy: a pilot study. Br J Sports Med 45(12):972–977

Santander J, Zarba E, Iraporda H et al (2012) Can arthroscopically tendinopathy reduce pain and restore function? Clin Orthop Relat Res 470:993–997
Sarimo J, Sarin J, Orava S et al (2007) Distal patellar tendinosis: an unusual form of jumper's knee. Knee Surg Sports Traumatol Arthrosc 15(1):54–57
Shelbourne KD, Henne TD, Gray T (2006) Recalcitrant patellar tendinosis in elite athletes: surgical treatment in conjunction with aggressive postoperative rehabilitation. Am J Sports Med 34(7):1141–1146
Smillie IS (1946) Injuries of the knee joint, 3rd edn. E. & S, Livingstone, Edinburgh, Scotland
Stuhlman CR, Stowers K, Stowers L et al (2016) Current concepts and the role of surgery in the treatment of Jumper's knee. Orthopedics 1:1–8
Testa V, Capasso G, Maffulli N et al (1999) Ultrasound-guided percutaneous longitudinal tenotomy for the management of patellar tendinopathy. Med Sci Sports Exerc 31(11):1509–1515
Topol GA, Podesta LA, Reeves KD et al (2011) Hyperosmolar dextrose injection for recalcitrant Osgood-Schlatter disease. Pediatrics 128(5): e1121–e1128
Verheyden F, Geens G, Nelen G (1997) Jumper's knee: results of surgical treatment. Acta Orthop Belg 63(2):102–105
Willberg L, Sunding K, Forssblad M et al (2011) Sclerosing polidocanol injections or arthroscopic shaving to treat patellar tendinopathy/jumper's knee? A randomised controlled study. Br J Sports Med 45(5):411–415
Willberg L, Sunding K, Ohberg L et al (2007) Treatment of Jumper's knee: promising short-term results in a pilot study using a new arthroscopic approach based on imaging findings. Knee Surg Sports Traumatol Arthrosc 15(5):676–681
Zhang B, Qu TB, Pan J et al (2016) Open patellar tendon tenotomy and debridement combined with suture-bridging double-row technique for severe patellar tendinopathy. Othop Surg 8(1):51–59
Zwerver J (2008) Patellar tendinopaty (jumper's knee): a common and difficult-to-treat sports inhjury. Ned Tijdschr Geneeskd 152(33):1831–1837
Zwerver J, Hartgens F, Verhagen E et al (2011) No effect of extracorporeal shockwave therapy on patellar tendinopathy in jumping athletes during the competitive season: a randomized clinical trial. Am J Sports Med 39(6):1191–1199

Periarticular Tendinopathies of the Knee

30

Federico Raggi, Tommaso Roberti di Sarsina, Federico Stefanelli, Alberto Grassi, Cecilia Signorelli, and Stefano Zaffagnini

Contents

There are several knee diseases; the most cases during clinical practice concern meniscal and ligament lesions, but we must remember various disorders related to periarticular tendon inflammation, which can mime different conditions.

A correct anamnesis and an accurate physical examination are fundamental to diagnose this kind of pathologies which, if untreated, can often become chronic.

30.1 Tendonitis of the Quadriceps Tendon

30.1.1 Anatomy

The quadriceps tendon originates from the union of the four distal insertions of the femoral quadriceps muscle: the rectus femoris, the vastus lateralis, the vastus medialis, and the vastus intermedius.

The most superficial fibers of the tendon, resulting from the rectus femoris, pass ahead the patella and continue with the patellar ligament which insertion is in the tibial tuberosity; the intermediate fibers of the tendon, originated by vastus lateralis and medialis, insert in the edge of the patella; the deep fibers, which originate from

F. Raggi • T. Roberti di Sarsina • F. Stefanelli
A. Grassi • C. Signorelli • S. Zaffagnini (✉)
Clinica Ortopedica e Traumatologica II, Laboratorio di Biomeccanica ed Innovazione Tecnologica, Istituto Ortopedici Rizzoli, via di Barbiano, 1/10, 40136 Bologna, Italy

Dipartimento di Scienze Anatomiche Umane e Fisiopatologia dell'Apparato Locomotore, Università di Bologna, Alma Mater Studiorum, Bologna, Italy
e-mail: federico.raggi@studio.unibo.it; tommaso.robertidisarsina@gmail.com; federico.stefanelli@studio.unibo.it; alberto.grassi@ior.it; cecilia.signorelli@gmail.com; stefano.zaffagnini@unibo.it

G.L. Canata et al. (eds.), *Muscle and Tendon Injuries*, DOI 10.1007/978-3-662-54184-5_30

the vastus intermedius, insert in the base of the patella.

The tendon function connects the femoral quadriceps muscle, the most voluminous muscle mass of the body, to the patella, to allow the extension of the leg on the thigh, and with the rectus femoris, to flex the thigh on the pelvis.

30.1.2 Pathogenesis: Clinical Presentation

Tendinopathy of the quadriceps tendon concerns especially patients who practice activities that include running, jumping, or however situations where the extensor apparatus is strongly stressed through intense and explosive contractions.

The frequency of this disease is lower than the patellar tendinitis; probably the reason is the better vascularization of the quadriceps tendon and the lower mechanical stress which it is subjected during the activities.

The main symptom is pain, localized just above the upper pole of the patella.

Typically the onset of symptoms is insidious and often associated with a recent increase in physical activity; in some cases the pain can be mild, in others it can be so intense to force the athlete to stop the activities.

Objectively, a tumefaction at the upper pole of the patella and pain at palpation in that spot can be observed; the extension of the leg on the thigh against resistance is painful.

It's important to evaluate possible bad alignments of the lower limbs, defects of rotation, the tone of the quadriceps, and the motility of the knee.

The clinical diagnosis is sufficient if there isn't a strength deficit in the extension of the leg, otherwise it is possible to use X-rays or MRI.

Radiographies are often negative, especially in young athletes, while in older patients, there might be calcifications in the context of the tendon or an osteophyte at the upper pole of the patella. The MRI images show signs of tendon degeneration especially at the distal insertion of the quadriceps tendon (Fig. 30.1).

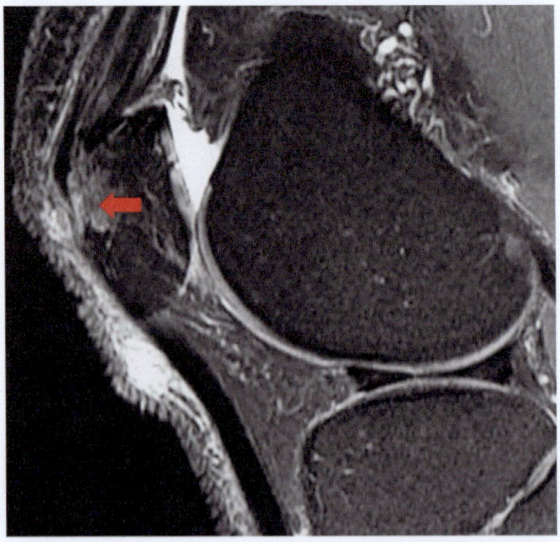

Fig. 30.1 Tendinopathy of the distal insertion of quadriceps tendon

30.1.3 Treatment

Treatment is conservative with an initial period of abstention from sports activities, the use of NSAIDs, and physical therapy (cryotherapy, laser therapy, Tecar). Later, muscle strengthening and improvement of elasticity of the tendon are important: particularly recommended in this phase is eccentric exercise of the quadriceps (Fyfe and Stanish 1992).

In most cases symptoms resolve in 2–3 weeks, only rarely it is necessary to perform surgery. Surgical treatment is indicated when conservative treatment has not given results within 3–6 months; the operation consists of the stimulation of tendon bleeding through longitudinal tenotomies.

30.1.4 Tendon Rupture

The rupture of the quadriceps tendon typically concerns subjects older than 40 years, and it's associated with multiple risk factors including pathological conditions and chronic drug therapies.

Diseases that predispose to rupture of the quadriceps tendon are kidney failure, diabetes mellitus, hyperparathyroidism, rheumatoid arthritis, SLE, gout, and obesity (Shah 2002; Preston and Adicoff 1962; Ribbans and Angus 1989; Cooney et al. 1991).

Drugs involved include statins, local corticosteroid injections, fluoroquinolones, anabolic androgens, and prolonged treatment with systemic corticosteroids.

In these groups, the tendon rupture is usually caused by a minor injury, a fall, an effort descending stairs, or even spontaneous, because there are histological changes of the tendon structure that compromise the mechanical strength (Shah 2002). In most cases the tendon breaks transversally in proximity of the osteo-tendon junction, where it is observed an abnormal distribution of collagen fibers and an increase of the type 3 collagen production by tenocytes (Preston and Adicoff 1962).

In sportsman, complete or partial tears of the quadriceps tendon are rare and not always associated with a history of tendinopathy or previous injuries of the quadriceps. The main damage mechanism consists in an eccentric overload with the knee flexed as in weightlifting or in a direct trauma as in contact sports.

Objectively, characteristic sign of tendon rupture is the inability to extend the leg, although in partial injury, this function can be maintained; in this case it is observable lower strength in the extension against resistance compared to the contralateral knee.

The patient usually is able to walk with stiff limbs and there is a compensatory attitude of hip flexion. In acute phases there is swelling of the knee associated with hemarthrosis; through palpation it is possible to identify a groove at the upper pole of the patella that corresponds to the separation of the tendon at its insertion (Ribbans and Angus 1989).

In cases of complete tendon injury, radiographies show an abnormal patella baja, while in partial lesions, they are negative.

The MRI, in case of complete rupture, confirms the diagnosis by showing in the sagittal projections the discontinuity of the tendon associated with edema of the surrounding tissues, while in the partial ruptures, it is the gold standard for the identification and localization of the lesion.

The treatment of complete ruptures of the tendon is surgical, and the best results are obtained when surgery is performed early, when the tendon is not retracted yet.

The upper pole of the patella and the tendon are freshened to increase bleeding, the tendon is set up by two Krackow sutures using nonabsorbable strand and fixed to the patella through metal anchors or trans-bone holes.

If the tendon is retracted and cannot reach the patella, it can be lengthened by the Codivilla's technique (Cooney et al. 1991). The technique involves an inverted-V incision about 1.5 cm proximal to the lesion; the two sides of the inverted V are sutured to each other, and the triangular tendon flap is distally overturned and sutured to the patella as reinforcement.

The post operation, in healthy patients who have received early reconstruction, involves the use of a brace for 6/8 weeks, initially blocked in extension, and then increasing the bending of 5°/10° every week. For patients with predisposing diseases or patients undergoing surgery late, rehabilitation must be more cautious and functional recovery expect longer times.

In selected cases of partial rupture in which the lesion affect less than 50% of the tendon, it might be undertaken a conservative treatment by immobilizing the knee with a brace locked in extension for 6/8 weeks.

30.2 Iliotibial Band (ITB) Syndrome

30.2.1 The Iliotibial Band Anatomy

The iliotibial band, or iliotibial tract, originates as common tendon of two muscles, the gluteus maximus and tensor fasciae latae, and then goes down along the thigh thickening the lateral portion of the fascia lata. Near the knees it runs superficially on lateral femoral epicondyle and inserts on the lateral side of the tibia at the tubercle of Gerdy.

Proximally iliotibial tract serves as insertion to the gluteus maximus and tensor fasciae latae, allowing their function of abductors of the thigh.

Distally, from 0° to 20° of knee flexion, it isn't forward the lateral femoral epicondyle and participates at the extension of the knee; over 30° of flexion, it climbs over the lateral femoral epicondyle and it is positioned posteriorly to it. Under the microscope the iliotibial band is separated to the epicondyle by a highly vascularized adipose tissue, without the evidence of a real bursa (Kannus and Jozsa 1991).

30.2.2 Pathogenesis and Clinical Presentation

The ITB syndrome is a common disorder among athletes, due to inflammation of the most distal tract of the iliotibial band.

The inflammatory process originates from the rubbing of ITB on the lateral femoral epicondyle during repeated flexions and extensions of the knee; the maximum impingement between these structures is between 20° and 30° of flexion, which correspond to the phase of the step when the foot is in contact with the ground (foot strike) (Maffulli et al. 2012).

This pathology concerns especially runners and cyclists, but it is common in all sports with repetitive movements of flexion-extension of the knee.

Many risk factors predispose to the development of the disease and are related to the training mode or to anatomical characteristics.

Rapid changes in the training program, increase of the distance, and running on a slope can trigger symptoms. In particular in the downhill race, the bending angle of the knee decreases during the contact of the foot to the ground, increasing the time spent in the period of maximum impingement (Boublik et al. 2013).

Anatomical factors that cause an increased tension of the ITB, predisposing to the development of the disease, are the varus knee, the excessive internal rotation of the tibia, and the foot pronation during running (Rougraff et al. 1996).

The main symptom is pain, often described as burning, to the lateral side of the knee that sometimes is well localized by the patient at the lateral femoral epicondyle but in other cases is described as widespread lateral pain.

The pain initially occurs at the end of the training or after a race and then stops to rest. If practice is continued, the pain becomes more intense, and it occurs earlier during training and may persist with the rest.

Objectively the patient has pain with palpation of the lateral femoral epicondyle (2–3 cm proximally to the lateral joint line), which is generally showed at 30° of knee flexion. In some cases, with palpation it's possible to appreciate a jerk sensation during flexion-extension that corresponds to the passage of the ITB above femoral epicondyle. The pain is also caused by asking at the patient to do a lounge with the affected limb.

The Noble's tests (Muhle et al. 1999) and the Ober's test (Terry et al. 1986) are useful in the diagnosis of the ITB syndrome.

The Noble's test consists in extending the patient's leg, starting from 90° of flexion while exercising a pressure on the femoral epicondyle. The test is positive if the patient has pain at about 30° of flexion.

Ober's test is performed with patient in lateral decubitus on the healthy side. The examiner, behind, with one hand stabilizes the pelvis, while the other flexes the knee up to 90° and abducts and extends the hip. Held this position for a while, the examiner leaves the limb. If the hip stays abducted and doesn't reach the neutral position, the test is positive for suffering of the ITB.

The differential diagnoses of this disease include lateral meniscus tears, stress fractures, tendonitis of the popliteal tendon, degenerative disorders of the lateral compartment of the knee, and sciatalgy.

The diagnosis is mainly clinical, MRI may be indicated in cases of refractoriness to conservative treatment, and it is useful in the differential diagnosis.

Resonance can show an alteration of the signal at the distal insertion of the ITB (*white arrow*) and liquid between the deepest part of the band and the external femoral epicondyle (*black arrow*) (Fig. 30.2) (Orchard et al. 1996).

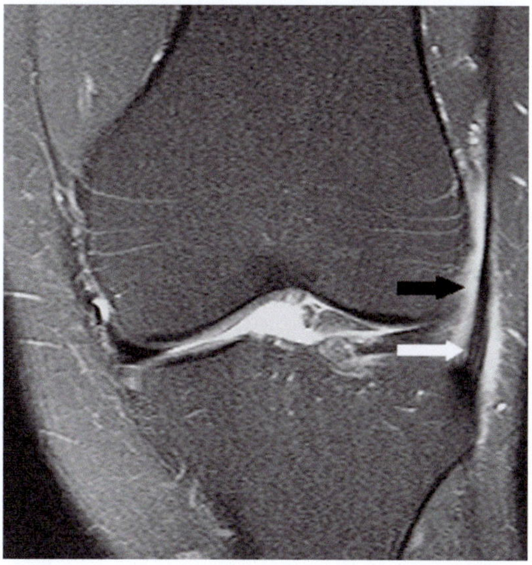

Fig. 30.2 Edema and tension at the distal insertion of ITB

30.2.3 Treatment

Most patients get well with a conservative treatment consisting in a first phase, which turn off the inflammation of the involved structures, followed by a second one focused on stretching and muscle strengthening. During the first phase, training should be suspended or replaced by activities that do not involve repetitive movements of flexion-extension of the knee (swimming); the use of NSAIDs and application of local ice are recommended. If pain does not regress after several days of treatment, a cortisone injection is indicated.

Once pain is decreased, it's important to regularly perform specific stretching exercises to stretch ITB, tensor fascia latae, and gluteus.

Moreover, when patients return to practice sport, they must continue stretching exercises and avoid running on dangerous ground and correct eventual pronation of the foot when they run with orthopedic insole.

Surgery is necessary few times, only if good results are not obtained after 6 months of conservative treatment.

The intervention consists in an inspection and a possible regularization of the bone surface of the lateral femoral epicondyle and s in a V incision of the posterior fibers of band, in order to reduce the friction with the surface of the epicondyle (Martens et al. 1989).

30.3 Tendinopathy of the Popliteal

30.3.1 Anatomy

Popliteus is a posterior muscle of the leg, the only one which does not reach the foot. It is composed of a muscle-tendon unit placed in the popliteal fossa deep to the plantar and gastrocnemius muscles. His tendon segment originates from the lateral femoral condyle forward the external collateral ligament; his fibers move down and medially and insert, with the muscular portion, on the oblique line and on the posterior face of the tibia.

The popliteus muscle is connected to the fibula through the popliteal-fibular ligament that originates in the proximal fibula and ends near the muscle-tendon junction of the popliteus. This ligament is important to control the posterior translation of the tibia, the rotations, and the stability in varus. For this reason, injuries of popliteus tendon can affect the lateral posterior stability of the knee.

The popliteus muscle intrarotates the tibia and participates at leg flexion (Noble 1980).

30.3.2 Popliteus Tendinitis

Tendinitis of the popliteus isn't a frequent pathology; it is an inflammatory process that affects the tendon in its insertion on the lateral femoral condyle.

It affects especially runners, and its development is facilitated by running on sloped funds; the tendon is more stressed when the athlete slows down while he's running downhill.

The popliteal tendinitis occurs with posterolateral knee pain, and symptoms are triggered by physical activity and, at least in the acute form, stop with rest. An excessive pronation of the foot constitutes a predisposing factor to the development of the disease.

Physical examination reveals pain with palpation of the tendon that is easier palpable with knee in position 4. The differential diagnosis should be made with lesions of the lateral meniscus or meniscal cysts, ITB syndrome, lateral collateral ligament injuries, and degenerative disorders of the lateral compartment of the knee. The MRI shows an alteration of the signal and edema in the popliteal hiatus (Figs. 30.3 and 30.4) and helps to exclude intra-articular pathologies or tendon rupture.

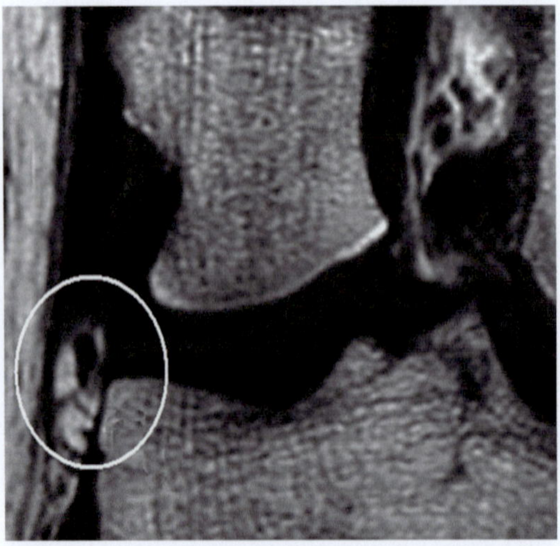

Fig. 30.3 Edema and mild effusion in the popliteal hiatus

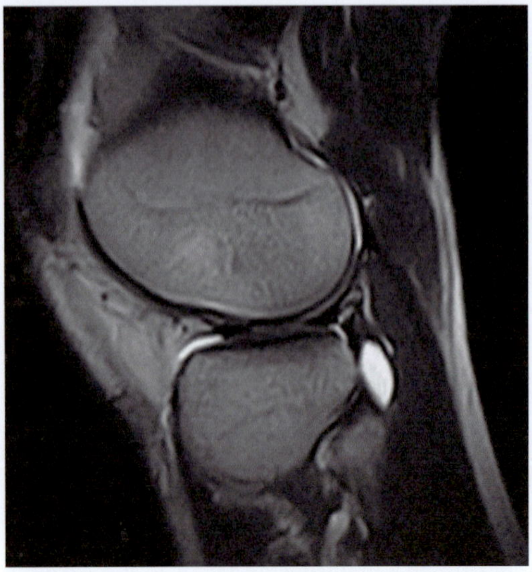

Fig. 30.4 Effusion in the muscle belly of the popliteus

People affected by the popliteal tendonitis are advised to suspend physical activity and taking NSAIDs at least for 2 weeks. If the symptoms persist, a therapeutic intervention-based infiltration with cortisone is considered. The athletes' activities should be corrected avoiding paths on inclined bottoms.

30.3.3 Popliteus Subluxation

Subluxation of the popliteus tendon has been described in young athlete (Ober n.d.).

The origin of the disease can be the result of a trauma in varus or hyperextension, or spontaneous.

The subluxation of the tendon is appreciable by palpation at 20° and 30° of flexion as a jerk between the lateral femoral epicondyle and the external joint line during the passive extension of the leg associated with a varus stress.

The MRI shows in these subjects no specific alterations of the tendon, and arthroscopy is not useful. The differential diagnosis should be made with the presence of a mobile body in the lateral compartment, hypermotility, or a lesion of the lateral meniscus.

The treatment involves abstaining from physical activities and the use of NSAIDs.

In refractory cases to conservative treatment, it can be performed by a tenodesis, anchoring the popliteal ligament to the proximal half of the lateral collateral.

30.3.4 Popliteus Tendon Rupture

The isolated popliteus tendon rupture is an extremely rare event. Usually the tendon rupture is associated with a posterolateral acute or chronic instability due to complex PLC lesions. (Ekman et al. 1994).

The rupture can be caused by a trauma of the leg in external rotation with the knee flexed or by a direct trauma, such as a kick received on the lateral side of the knee. The clinic is characterized by pain in the lateral compartment and hemarthrosis, in the absence of clinical signs of joint instability. The pain is elicited by asking the patient to intrarotate tibia against resistance or passively externally rotate the tibia at 90° of flexion.

MRI is useful to confirm the diagnosis: the tendon appears detached from its femoral insertion, with an irregular profile, and a there is degradation of the signal due to edema surrounding.

In most cases there is an osteochondral fragment due to the detachment of the tendon from its femoral insertion which can also be visible with X-rays.

The surgery involves the repositioning of the fragment and tendon repair followed by a 4-week period of immobilization with a rigid support.

30.4 Semimembranosus Tendinitis

30.4.1 Anatomy

The semimembranosus muscle originates from the ischial tuberosity with a flattened tendon which continues in an equally flattened muscle. The muscle fibers descend long the posterolateral portion of the thigh and continue with a tendon, which splits in three parts at level of the knee. The first is directed to the medial condyle of the tibia, posteriorly to the medial collateral ligament; the second goes up on the posterior side of the knee joint capsule, arrives to the lateral femoral condyle, and represents the oblique popliteal ligament; the third is part of the fascia of the popliteal muscle.

By its action the semimembranosus muscle extends the thigh on the pelvis, intrarotates the leg, and flexes it on the thigh.

30.4.2 Pathogenesis: Clinical Presentation

The semimembranosus tendinitis includes an isolated primary form, in athletes, and a secondary form due to compensatory overload in patients with osteoarthrosis, meniscal degeneration, or pathologies of the patellofemoral joint (Martens et al. 1989).

The inflammatory process that causes the disease often concerns the lower part of the tendon, which inserts in the medial condyle of the tibia. During repeated flexion-extension movements, this portion of the tendon impinges on the medial femoral condyle, the internal tibial plateau, and the tendon of the semitendinosus muscle. This causes irritation of the fibers and consequent degeneration (Veltri et al. 1996).

Valgus knee and an excessive pronation of the foot during running predispose to the development of the disease.

The patient suffering semimembranosus tendinitis has pain in the posterior-medial compartment of the knee that gets worse during physical activity. Physical examination shows pain with palpation of the posterior-medial knee portion, just below the joint line. The differential diagnosis should be made with lesions or degeneration of the internal meniscus, lesions of the medial collateral ligament, and tendonitis of the goose foot. The last one is different because pain is localized anteriorly and distally.

Particularly accurate in diagnosis is the scintigraphy which reveals an abnormal hyperaccumulation posteriorly to the medial tibial condyle, in correspondence of the tendon insertion (Martens et al. 1989).

MRI is useful to exclude lesions or degenerative alterations of the internal meniscus.

30.4.3 Treatment

The secondary semimembranosus tendinitis is treated after solving the primary joint disease. The treatment of the primary tendinitis consists in a period of abstention from physical activity, cryotherapy, stretching exercises, and NSAIDs. Surgery is recommended if the conservative treatment has not given the results after at least 3 months.

The surgery consists in the isolation of the tendon, the opening of the sheath, and the execution of some longitudinal tenotomies. The insertion site is cut to promote bleeding, and finally the tendon is repositioned and sutured to the posterior side of the medial collateral ligament; in this way the contact of the tendon with the internal tibial plateau during flexion-extension of the knee is reduced.

30.5 Tendinitis of the Goose Foot

30.5.1 Anatomy

The goose foot or pes anserinus is the insertion of the sartorius, gracilis, and semitendinosus muscles. It is located on the anterior-medial side of the proximal tibia, about 5 cm distally from the medial joint line. Its name originates from its structure, which resembles the membrane of goose's legs. Between these tendons and the medial collateral ligament there is an interposed bursa.

The three muscles that end in the goose foot are mainly flexors but also participate to the internal rotation of the tibia and control of valgus deviations of the knee.

30.5.2 Pathogenesis: Clinical Presentation

Goose foot tendinitis mainly affects long-distance runners, because it's an overload condition due to repeated rubbing of the tendons on the internal tibial condyle and the medial collateral ligament. It is not clear if the inflammatory process affects the tendon or the underlying bursa; however, the clinical presentation and the subsequent treatment of the two conditions coincides (Cooper 1999).

In the rest of the population, the disease mainly affects overweight women between 50 and 80 years, diabetics, and patients with knee arthrosis (Guha et al. 2003; Raj et al. 1988).

The knee valgus and flatfeet are risk factors for the development of the disease because they increase the tension of the tendons in their area of common insertion.

The clinic is characterized by pain at the medial knee compartment that is typically exacerbated by ascending and descending the stairs or by rising from a chair.

Objectively, there is pain with palpation in the anatomic insertion of the goose foot sometimes associated with edema.

The diagnosis is essentially clinical; X-rays have little diagnostic significance, except in cases where there are radiographic signs of osteoarthrosis of the medial compartment or an osteophyte. MRI is useful in cases of acute bursitis of the goose foot associated with important presence of liquid in correspondence of the bursa but does not reveal characteristic changes in the majority of symptomatic individuals who have already received a clinical diagnosis.

MRI is especially important for the differential diagnosis with lesions of the medial meniscus (sometimes clinically indistinguishable), osteoarthrosis of the medial compartment, semimembranosus tendinitis, or Baker's cyst.

30.5.3 Treatment

The treatment includes resting from sport, cryotherapy, stretching of the posterior muscles of the thigh, and the use of NSAIDs. Laser therapy and ultrasounds are indicated in order to reduce the inflammatory process.

Any predisposing conditions such as valgus knee and flatfeet should be corrected, in diabetic patients it is necessary to achieve a better control of glycemic levels, and a weight reduction should be suggested in overweight subjects.

If there isn't an improvement of the symptoms after 15–20 days of rest and use of NSAIDs, a therapeutic intervention-based infiltration with cortisone can be practiced.

In some rare cases unresponsive to the conservative treatment it may be necessary to perform a surgical drainage of the anserine bursa.

References

Boublik M, Schlegel TF, Koonce RC, Genuario JW, Kinkartz JD (2013) Quadriceps tendon injuries in national football league players. Am J Sports Med 41(8):1841–1846

Cooney LM, Aversa JM, Newmann JH (1991) Insidious bilateral infrapatellar tendon rupture in a patient with systemic lupus erythematosus. Arch Orthop Trauma Surg 110:22–26

Cooper DE (1999) Snapping popliteus tendon syndrome. A cause of mechanical knee popping in athletes. Am J Sports Med 27(5):671–674

Ekman EF, Pope T, Martin DF, Curl WW (1994) Magnetic resonance imaging of iliotibial band syndrome. Am J Sports Med 22(6):851–854

Fyfe I, Stanish WD (1992) The use of eccentric training and stretching in the treatment an prevention of tendon injuries. Clin Sports Med 11(3):601–624

Guha AR, Gorgees KA, Walker DI (2003) Popliteus tendon rupture: a case report and review of the literature. Br J Sports Med 37(4):358–360. Review

Kannus P, Jozsa L (1991) Histopathological changes preceding spontaneous rupture of a tendon. A controlled study of 891 patients. J Bone Joint Surg Am 73:1507–1525

Maffulli N, Del Buono A, Spiezia F, Longo UG, Denaro V (2012) Light microscopic histology of quadriceps tendon ruptures. Int Orthop 36(11):2367–2371

Martens M, Libbrecht P, Burssens A (1989) Surgical treatment of the iliotibial band friction syndrome. Am J Sport Med 17:651–654

Muhle C, Ahn JM, Yeh L, Bergman GA, Boutin RD, Schweitzer M, Jacobson JA, Haghighi P, Trudell DJ, Resnick D (1999) Iliotibial band friction syndrome: MR imaging findings in 16 patients and MR arthrographic study of six cadaveric knees. Radiology 212(1): 103–110

Noble CA (1980) Iliotibial band friction syndrome in runners. Am J Sports Med 8(4):232–234

Ober FR The role of the iliotibial band and fascia lata as a factor in the causation of low back disabilities and sciatica. J Bone Joint Surg 18:105–110

Orchard JW, Fricker PA, Abud AT, Mason BR (1996) Biomechanics of iliotibial band friction syndrome in runners. Am J Sports Med 24(3):375–379

Preston FS, Adicoff A (1962) Hyperparathyroidism with avulsion of three major tendons. Report of a case. N Engl J Med 266:968–971

Raj JM, Clancy WG, Lemon RA (1988) Semimembranous tendinitis: an overlooked cause of medial knee pain. Am J Sport Med 16:347–351

Ribbans WJ, Angus PD (1989) Simultaneous bilateral rupture of the quadriceps tendon. Br J Clin Pract 43: 122–125

Rougraff BT, Reeck CC, Essenmacher J (1996) Complete quadriceps tendon ruptures. Orthopedics 19:509–514

Shah MK (2002) Simultaneous bilateral rupture of quadriceps tendons: analysis of risk factors and associations. South Med J 95:860–866

Terry GC, Hughston JC, Norwood LA (1986) The anatomy of the iliopatellar band and iliotibial tract. Am J Sports Med 14(1):39–45

Veltri DM, Deng XH, Torzilli PA, Maynard MJ, Warren RF (1996) The role of the popliteofibular ligament in stability of the human knee. A biomechanical study. Am J Sports Med 24(1):19–27

Pitfalls and Risks of Tendon Harvest About the Knee

31

Naaman V. Mehta and Robert G. Marx

Contents

N.V. Mehta
Sports Medicine and Shoulder Service, Hospital for Special Surgery, New York, NY, USA
e-mail: mehtana@hss.edu; nmehta5893@gmail.com

R.G. Marx (✉)
Sports Medicine and Shoulder Service, Hospital for Special Surgery, New York, NY, USA

Department of Orthopedic Surgery, Weill Cornell Medicine, New York, NY, USA
e-mail: marxr@hss.edu

31.1 Introduction: The Basics of Tendon Harvest

Anterior cruciate ligament (ACL) injuries are becoming increasingly common (Griffin et al. 2006). In the early 2000s, it was estimated 100,000 to 175,000 reconstructions were performed in the United States each year (Gottlob et al. 1999; Lyman et al. 2009). ACL reconstruction involving the use of graft tissue harvested, or taken directly from the patient, is known as an autograft, while graft taken from a cadaver is known as an allograft (Mcguire and Hendricks 2007).

Autografts are most frequently made by harvesting the patient's own patellar tendon or hamstring (HT). Patellar tendon, also known as "bone–patellar tendon–bone" (BTB) grafts, is derived from the middle third of the patellar ligament. Though surgeons may have their own preferences about the best type of graft, studies have demonstrated that both BTB and HT have high rates of success (Mcguire and Hendricks 2007).

31.2 Complications Specific to BTB Autografts

Patellar tendon grafts have a lower rate of re-tear but can be associated with a more difficult recovery for some patients (Freedman et al. 2003). Complications associated with BTB autograft include tibial fractures, patellar fractures, patellar

G.L. Canata et al. (eds.), *Muscle and Tendon Injuries*, DOI 10.1007/978-3-662-54184-5_31

tendon ruptures, or patellar tendinitis. In this section, we discuss the potential complications of harvesting the patellar tendon.

31.2.1 Tibial Plateau Fracture

Fracture of the tibia after ACL reconstruction is a rare occurrence that is induced by torsional trauma to the knee (Delcogliano et al. 2001) (Fig. 31.1). In surgery, BTB autografts are placed anatomically by drilling tunnels into the tibia and the femur. The tibial tunnel results in a cortical defect that acts as a stress riser (Delcogliano et al. 2001). As such, the effects of the tibial graft harvest, combined with the tibial tunnel drilling, increase the susceptibility of the area to postoperative tibial fracture (Delcogliano et al. 2001). Tibial fracture is more common in older patients, for instance, those with osteoporosis, who already have low bone mineral density, increasing the likelihood of fractures from minor injury (Voos et al. 2008; El-Hage et al. 1998; Thaunat et al. 2006). Most tibial fractures post-ACL reconstructions are treated with the use of locked plate technology. The majority of these injuries do not require revision ACL reconstruction.

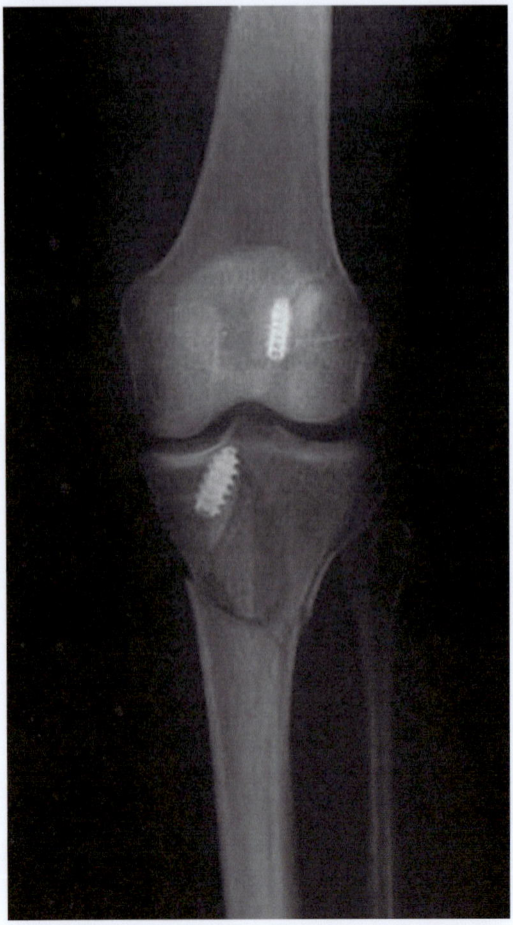

Fig. 31.1 AP radiograph of a metaphyseal fracture of the proximal tibia after ACL reconstruction (Voos et al. HSSJ, 2008) (Voos et al. 2008)

31.2.2 Patellar Fracture

Studies infrequently report on patellar fractures as a potential complication of BTB autograft: the incidence of such fractures has been reported to be between 0.23 and 2.3% (Wilson et al. 2006). Possible reasons for these fractures include a large patellar bone plug harvest (greater than 11–12 mm) or a stress riser caused by an aggressive saw cut (Christen and Jakob 1992; Stein et al. 2002).

Intraoperative patellar fractures occur due to aggressive bony resection, while postoperative patellar fractures usually occur from direct trauma to the patella in the setting of a stress riser. Intraoperative fractures tend to be longitudinal fissure fractures, with the most common being a nondisplaced vertical fissure fracture. Postoperative patella fractures are typically transverse-shaped injuries that result from an aggressive contraction of the quadriceps or direct trauma (Wilson et al. 2006).

Displaced fractures require surgical intervention, but nondisplaced fractures can typically be treated nonoperatively with rigid knee immobilization (Wilson et al. 2006).

31.2.3 Patellar Tendon Ruptures

Though uncommon, reports of patellar tendon rupture following ACL reconstruction do exist—with most describing injuries in the early postoperative period and others describing injury up to

3 years after surgery (Shelbourne et al. 2006). Most studies report only one or two cases—for instance, Lee et al. reported one rupture among 1725 BTPB reconstructions (Lee et al. 2008).

A study by Benner et al. described a subset of patients presenting with postoperative patellar tendon rupture (Benner et al. 2012). These patients all experienced an acute onset of pain and weakness after an injury to their graft knee. Injury was typically due to a "slip and fall" mechanism of injury. Patients also observed swelling around their injured knees. As well, patellar tendon ruptures result in patella alta and an inability to extend the knee. Physical examination typically reveals a palpable tendon defect (Fig. 31.2) (Benner et al. 2012).

31.2.4 Patellar Tendinitis

Shelbourne et al. reported patellar tendinitis in 21% of patients who received a BTB graft (Mastrokalos 2005; Shelbourne et al. 1994). They defined patellar tendinitis as soreness in the patellar tendon region.

31.2.5 Secondary Complications

One of the primary secondary complications following BTB graft harvest is increased anterior knee pain. Specifically, kneeling is more difficult up to 7 years postoperatively for BTB graft patients (Riaz et al. 2015).

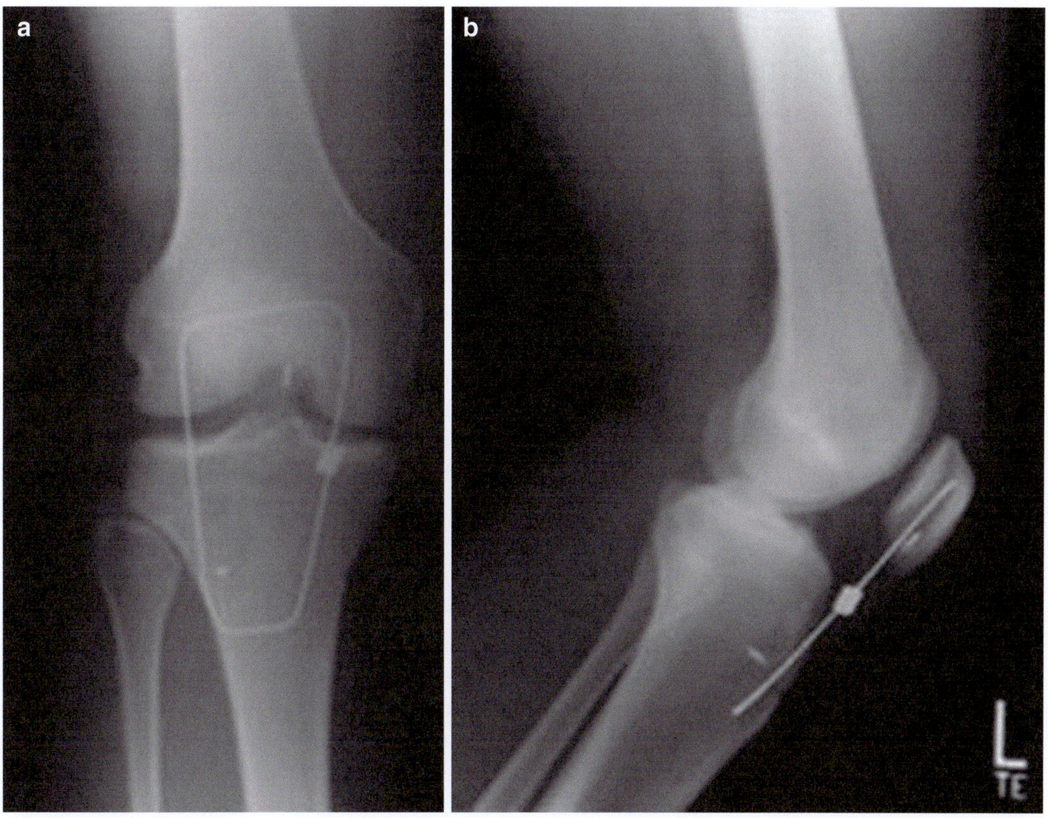

Fig. 31.2 Posteroanterior (**a**) and lateral radiographs (**b**) after repair of a proximal–medial/distal–lateral Z-type patellar tendon rupture after bone–patellar tendon–bone autograft harvest for anterior cruciate ligament reconstruction (Benner et al. AJSM, 2012) (Benner et al. 2012)

31.3 Complications Specific to Hamstring Autografts

Most of the complications specific to harvesting the semitendinosus and gracilis tendons are technical problems that are avoidable with good surgical technique (Williams et al. 2005).

31.3.1 Incomplete Tendon Harvest

The most common problem harvesting the semitendinosus and gracilis tendons occurs due to tendon amputation leading to inadequate graft issue. The tendons lie deep to the sartorius fascia and superficial to the medial collateral ligament. There are bands of tissue that must be released, including usually a very thick band running from the semitendinosus to the gastrocnemius, which can cause the tendon stripper to deviate and prematurely amputate the tendon tissue (Williams et al. 2005). With good surgical technique, it is extremely rare for the surgeon to be unable to harvest adequate graft issue for ACL reconstruction.

31.3.2 MCL Injury

The medial collateral ligament is located just deep to the insertion of the gracilis and semitendinosus tendons. Care must be taken to avoid this tissue when dividing the sartorius fascia and when releasing the gracilis semitendinosus tendons from their insertion (Wittstein et al. 2006).

31.3.3 Secondary Complications

Secondary complications of hamstring harvest typically resolve about 3 months post-op and do not require surgical intervention (Wittstein et al. 2006). Such complications include persistent weakness of the hamstrings and surrounding muscle (which compensates for the lack of hamstring tissue), as well as donor site pain. However, donor site pain appears to be temporary (Yasuda et al. 1995).

Hamstring autografts have several pros compared to BTB autografts. These include preserved quadriceps, decreased anterior knee pain, and reduced risk of patellar tendon rupture or patellar fracture. However, BTB autografts have a lower rate of re-rupture (Freedman et al. 2003).

31.4 Surgical Tips to Minimize the Risk of Pitfalls

- Bone–tendon–bone harvest requires adequate exposure, and the proximal incision is usually around the inferior pole of the patella, but varies depending on the skin mobility.
- Split the peratenon and meticulously dissect free of the tendon for later repair to promote healing.
- Always remove the tibial bone plug first in order to apply traction distally and use a retractor (such as a Richardson) to push the patella inferiorly to visualize the patella well for bone plug removal.
- When sawing the bone plugs, a vertical cut is made on the tibia angled only 10° inward so that extra bone is taken and it can be used to bone graft the patella defect at the end of the operation. On the patellar side, the vertical cuts are made at a 45° angle and the horizontal cut does not extend medial or lateral to the vertical cuts to avoid creating a stress riser.
- When cutting the tendon, use a double cutting knife and make sure to follow the fibers and not to cross them to avoid dividing the tendon, which would be disastrous.
- For hamstring harvest, when using a closed loop tendon stripper, be sure that the gracilis and semitendinosus are completely freed from surrounding tissue. The semitendinosus in particular has a large fibrous band to the medial head of gastrocnemius and that must be divided to avoid premature amputation of the tendon.

31.5 Nonoperatively Managing Effects of Major Complications

- Nondisplaced patella fractures can typically be treated nonoperatively if there is less than 2 mm displacement. The knee is immobilized in extension until clinical and radiographic signs of healing are observed, usually at 4–6 weeks (Stein et al. 2002; Wilson et al. 2006).
- Once the fracture heals, ACL rehabilitation can be continued (Stein et al. 2002).

References

Benner RW, Shelbourne KD, Urch SE, Lazarus D (2012) Tear patterns, surgical repair, and clinical outcomes of patellar tendon ruptures after anterior cruciate ligament reconstruction with a bone-patellar tendon-bone autograft. Am J Sports Med 40(8):1834–1841

Christen B, Jakob RP (1992) Fractures associated with patella ligament grafts in cruciate ligament surgery. J Bone Jt Surgery Br 74(4):617–619

Delcogliano A, Chiossi S, Caporaso A, Franzese S, Menghi A (2001) Tibial plateau fracture after arthroscopic anterior cruciate ligament reconstruction. Arthroscopy 17(4):E16

El-Hage ZM, Mohammed A, Griffiths D, Richardson JB (1998) Tibial plateau fracture following allograft anterior cruciate ligament (ACL) reconstruction. Injury 29(1):73–74

Freedman KB, D'Amato MJ, Nedeff DD, Kaz A, Bach BR (2003) Arthroscopic anterior cruciate ligament reconstruction: a metaanalysis comparing patellar tendon and hamstring tendon autografts. Am J Sports Med 31(1):2–11

Gottlob CA, Baker CL, Pellissier JM, Colvin L (1999) Cost effectiveness of anterior cruciate ligament reconstruction in young adults. Clin Orthop Relat Res 367:272–282

Griffin LY, Albohm MJ, Arendt EA et al (2006) Understanding and preventing noncontact anterior cruciate ligament injuries: a review of the Hunt Valley II meeting, January 2005. Am J Sports Med 34(9):1512–1532

Lee GH, McCulloch P, Cole BJ, Bush-Joseph CA, Bach BR (2008) The incidence of acute patellar tendon harvest complications for anterior cruciate ligament reconstruction. Arthroscopy 24(2):162–166

Lyman S, Koulouvaris P, Sherman S, Do H, Mandl LA, Marx RG (2009) Epidemiology of anterior cruciate ligament reconstruction: trends, readmissions, and subsequent knee surgery. J Bone Joint Surg Am 91(10):2321–2328

Mastrokalos DS (2005) Donor site morbidity and return to the preinjury activity level after anterior cruciate ligament reconstruction using ipsilateral and contralateral patellar tendon autograft: a retrospective, nonrandomized study. Am J Sports Med 33(1):85–93

Mcguire DA, Hendricks SD (2007) Anterior cruciate ligament reconstruction graft harvesting: pitfalls and tips. Sports Med Arthrosc 15(4):184–190

Riaz O, Nisar S, Phillips H, Siddiqui A (2015) Quantifying the problem of kneeling after a two incision bone tendon bone arthroscopic anterior cruciate ligament reconstruction. Muscles Ligaments Tendons J 5(3): 181–186

Shelbourne KD, Lawrance SE, Kerr B (2006) Patellar tendon rupture after anterior cruciate ligament surgery. Oper Tech Sports Med 14(1):8–14

Shelbourne KD, Rubinstein RAJ, VanMeter CD, McCarroll JR, Rettig AC (1994) Correlation of remaining patellar tendon width with quadriceps strength after autogenous bone-patellar tendon-bone anterior cruciate ligament reconstruction. Am J Sports Med 22(6):774–778

Stein DA, Hunt SA, Rosen JE, Sherman OH (2002) The incidence and outcome of patella fractures after anterior cruciate ligament reconstruction. Arthroscopy 18(6):578–583

Thaunat M, Nourissat G, Gaudin P, Beaufils P (2006) Tibial plateau fracture after anterior cruciate ligament reconstruction: role of the interference screw resorption in the stress riser effect. Knee 13(3): 241–243

Voos JE, Drakos MC, Lorich DG, Fealy S (2008) Proximal tibia fracture after anterior cruciate ligament reconstruction using bone-patellar tendon-bone autograft: a case report. HSS J 4(1):20–24

Williams RJ 3rd, Hyman J, Petrigliano F, Rozental T, Wickiewicz TL (2005) Anterior cruciate ligament reconstruction with a four-strand hamstring tendon autograft. JBJS 86-A(February 2004):225–232

Wilson JB, Wittstein JR, Moorman CT (2006) Patella fractures with bone-patella tendon-bone autografts for anterior cruciate ligament reconstruction. Oper Tech Sports Med 14(1):2–7

Wittstein JR, Wilson JB, Moorman CT (2006) Complications related to hamstring tendon harvest. Oper Tech Sports Med 14(1):15–19

Yasuda K, Tsujino J, Ohkoshi Y, Tanabe Y, Kaneda K (1995) Graft site morbidity with autogenous semitendinosus and gracilis tendons. Am J Sports Med 23(6):706–714

Triceps Surae Injuries

32

Fernando Radice, Ausberto Velasquez,
and Alejandro Orizola

Contents

F. Radice, M.D. (✉) • A. Velasquez, M.D.
A. Orizola, M.D.
Sports Medicine Center Clinica Las Condes/
Universidad de Chile, Santiago, Chile
e-mail: fradice@clc.cl

32.1 Introduction

The "calf muscle," or *triceps surae*, consists of three separate muscles (the gastrocnemius, soleus, and plantaris) whose aponeuroses unite to form the Achilles tendon. Clinical history and physical examination, along with imaging studies, allow localization of the injured muscle. Differentiating strains in the gastrocnemius from those in the soleus is particularly important for an accurate prognosis, appropriate treatment, and successful prevention of recurrent injury. Ninety-two percent of all muscle injuries affect the four major muscle groups of the lower limbs; strains to the triceps surae (13%) are preceded in frequency by injuries to the hamstrings (37%), adductors (23%), and quadriceps muscle group (19%). Many muscle injuries are misdiagnosed and have an insidious evolution, and athletes often have a high risk of re-injury (Ekstrand et al. 2011). Calf strains are generally regarded as common injuries, particularly in athletes, although specific data on injury rates are sparse (Coughlin et al. 2006; DeLee et al. 2003; Brukner and Khan 2002; Garrett 1996; Armfield et al. 2006). In one study of soccer players, calf strains represented 3.6% of injuries over a 5-year period (Luck et al. 2008).

G.L. Canata et al. (eds.), *Muscle and Tendon Injuries*, DOI 10.1007/978-3-662-54184-5_32

32.2 Definition of the Injury

32.2.1 Anatomy of the Calf

The posterior of the lower leg has a shallow posterior compartment that contains the plantar flexors of the ankle (gastrocnemius, soleus, and plantaris) and a deep posterior compartment that contains the tibialis posterior, flexor digitorum longus, flexor halluces longus, and popliteal muscles; an interosseous layer between the tibia and fibula isolates the deep posterior from the anterior compartments (Luck et al. 2008). The triceps surae comprises the gastrocnemius muscle (medial and lateral heads), the soleus, and the plantaris muscle (Kerkhoffs and Servien 2014).

32.2.1.1 Gastrocnemius

The gastrocnemius is the lowest muscle and crosses three joints: the knee, the ankle and the subtalar joint. A Fusiform muscle, is the lower border of the popliteal fossa and gives volume and shape to the calf (Kerkhoffs and Servien 2014; O'Brien 2005; Warwick and Williams 1973).

The medial head of the gastrocnemius emerges over the medial femoral condyle: from the popliteal surface of the femur behind the medial supracondylar line and the adductor tubercle. It is bigger, longer, and develops more distally than the lateral head (Warwick and Williams 1973). The lateral head is shorter and originates from a tendon in a fossa situated posterior to the lateral epicondyle and proximal to the insertion of the popliteal muscle tendon in the lateral supracondylar ridge. Both heads also emerge from the popliteal tendon, part of the posterior capsule of the knee joint, and are connected to the condyles of the femur by solid flat ligaments, which stretch out for a short separation on the back or the shallow surface of the muscles as an aponeurosis (O'Brien 2005). The most common variation of the gastrocnemius muscle is a third head, which arises from the posterior inferior part of the femur and joins the medial or, more often, the lateral head of the gastrocnemius, and may result in popliteal artery entrapment syndrome (Koplas et al. 2009). These anatomical variations have been reported in between 2.9% and 5.5% of the population (Garrett 1996), although a frequency of 1.9% was observed in a recent magnetic resonance imaging (MRI) series of 1039 knees (Koplas et al. 2009). The gastrocnemius muscle heads have a higher proportion of type II (fast-twitch) muscle fibers than the soleus, which may predispose the gastrocnemius to injury; in addition, this muscle spans multiple joints and has eccentric contraction, which occurs during lengthening (Counsel and Breidahl 2010; Koulouris et al. 2007). Because of these features, the gastrocnemius is used fundamentally in rapid movements such as running and jumping. Also, it acts as an agonist for the posterior cruciate ligament and as a venous pump for the lower limb (Koulouris et al. 2007).

32.2.1.2 Soleus

The soleus is a broad and flat muscle that lies deep to the gastrocnemius and plantaris and superficial to the muscles of the deep posterior compartment.

The soleus has both a fibular and tibial origin. The fibular origin is on the posterior aspect of the head and upper fourth of the diaphysis. The tibial origin is at the inferior border of the soleal line, a bony ridge running obliquely lateral-proximal to medial-distal that is situated on the upper third of the posterior aspect of the tibia, and the posteromedial border of the tibia (middle third). The popliteal vessels and the tibial nerve pass under the fibrous arch of the soleus. Each soleus muscle only crosses the ankle joint (Kerkhoffs and Servien 2014; O'Brien 2005; Warwick and Williams 1973). Distally, the soleus and gastrocnemius muscles together insert on the calcaneus via the Achilles tendon (Kerkhoffs and Servien 2014). The tendinous part of the soleus is the biggest of the fibers that add to the Achilles tendon and is the prime plantar flexor (Kvist 1991, 1994). Rotation of the Achilles tendon begins and becomes more marked in the distal 5–6 cm, where the soleus contributes fibers to the tendon. The gastrocnemius fibers rotate to lateral and the soleus fibers are positioned medial to the insertion (O'Brien 2005). Several authors have observed the pennation of the soleus, with a bipennate arrangement found in 86% of the population (right side, 83%; left side, 89% by Joshi et al. (2010), and such an arrangement found in up to 94% by Singhal et al. (2012).

The bipennate nature and orientation of the soleus muscle fibers cannot be visualized in a single orthogonal plane on MRI. Two proximal aponeuroses have been identified, medial (tibial origin) and lateral (fibular origin), penetrating deep into the medial and lateral aspects of the soleus muscle belly, while simultaneously curving toward the midline of the muscle belly and distal central tendon. The two aponeuroses are a continuation of the perimysium covering the soleus and act as rigid fibrous "struts" from which the proximal soleus muscle fibers gain origin. The aponeuroses can be considered as genuine intramuscular tendons, from an anatomical, functional, and pathological perspective (Joshi et al. 2010).

Dissimilar to the gastrocnemius, the soleus is made fundamentally of slow-twitch (type I) fibers and hence is predominantly used in postural control and low-speed actions, such as walking (Koulouris et al. 2007). Variations in standard muscle anatomy structures do occur and might be symptomatic; for example, an accessory soleus muscle is present in 0.7% to 5.6% of patients, originating from the anterior surface of the soleus muscle itself, the fibula, or the soleus line of the tibia (Luck et al. 2008) with a variable insertion into the Achilles tendon or the calcaneus, which may occur superiorly or medially and via a muscular fascicle or tendon (Luck et al. 2008; Jozsa and Kannus 1997). Other anatomical variants of the soleus muscle have been described as a soleus more distal than expected along the Achilles tendon. Anatomical variants are found in fewer than 2% of patients who require Achilles tendon surgery (Jozsa and Kannus 1997).

32.2.1.3 Plantaris

The plantaris muscle is variable in size, originates from the supracondylar ridge of the lateral femoral condyle, and is absent in 6–8% of individuals (Hollinshead 1969). It is situated between the more superficial gastrocnemius and the more profound soleus muscle. The function of this muscle is the plantar flexion of the ankle (Van Sterkenburg et al. 2011). The muscle belly is usually 5–10 cm in length, and the plantaris inserts into the medial border and anterior to the Achilles tendon. In 6% to 8% of subjects, the plantaris inserts into the flexor retinaculum (Hollinshead 1969). The plantaris can be injured at the level of the musculotendinous junction, either in isolation or simultaneously with a partial rupture of the medial head of the gastrocnemius or soleus.

The plantaris is also used as a augmentation tendon graft in surgical repair of achilles tendon rupture (Kerkhoffs and Servien 2014; O'Brien 2005; Hollinshead 1969).

32.2.2 Injury Mechanism and Epidemiology

A tear in a muscle created by the muscle being stretched past its capacity is called a strain. This injury frequently happens during powerful eccentric contractions of the muscle, and for the most part happens in the region adjacent to the musculotendinous junction. Biomechanical studies demonstrate that muscle failure occurs at strengths much greater than maximal isometric force, and stretching is important in causing harm (Garrett 1990, 1996). In contrast with a passively stretched muscle, a muscle activated by nerve contraction and stretched to failure shows little increment in force at failure, no adjustment in strain to failure, and a substantial increment in energy absorbed prior to failure. Biomechanical studies show the capacity of muscles to work as energy absorbers in preventing damage to themselves and to bones and joints. Treatment protocols indicate stress relaxation and reduction of stiffness in the muscle, taking advantage of the natural viscoelastic properties of muscle, rather than an automatic muscle protection reaction. These viscoelastic properties may be helpful in investigating how muscle damage may be prevented (Garrett 1990).

Calf strains often occur during acceleration or during an unexpected change in direction while a person is running (Bryan Dixon 2009). These strains are commonly associated with playing tennis, and are generally regarded as common injuries, particularly in athletes, although specific data on injury rates are sparse. In football players, calf strains represented 3.6% of injuries over a 5-year period (Bryan Dixon 2009). Calf muscle injuries are also commonly seen in other sports.

32.2.2.1 Gastrocnemius

The gastrocnemius is the calf muscle that is most often injured, followed by the plantaris and soleus muscles. The gastrocnemius muscle is particularly powerless against injury since it traverses three joints. Damage usually happens during unpredictable eccentric contraction when the ankle is in dorsiflexion with the knee in extension. Injury happens for the most part in racquet sports, running, basketball, football, and skiing (Kerkhoffs and Servien 2014).

In a series of 20 MRIs of the distal myotendinous junction, the medial head of the gastrocnemius muscle was more commonly involved (19/22) than the lateral head (3/22), as the medial head has been shown to be more active (Segal and Song 2005).

32.2.2.2 Distal Gastrocnemius Injury ("Tennis Leg")

Rupture of the distal musculotendinous junction of the medial head of the gastrocnemius muscle is known as "tennis leg," and it is a common clinical condition that typically occurs when the muscle is overstretched by dorsiflexion of the ankle with the knee in full extension (Counsel and Breidahl 2010; Gilbert et al. 1996; Weishaupt et al. 2001; Bencardino et al. 2000).

Tennis leg is a relatively common clinical condition, and its pathogenesis has been debated since Powell first described it in 1883 (Powell 1883). For some time, the condition was attributed to a rupture of the plantaris tendon. However, this pathogenesis is now considered to be a myth without scientific support, and recently most investigators have implicated a rupture of the medial head of the gastrocnemius muscle at the musculotendinous junction in the pathogenesis of this entity (Bencardino et al. 2000).

MRI and ultrasonography (US) are now used as the primary imaging techniques for the evaluation of patients with tennis leg (Delgado et al. 2002).With regard to US findings in 141 patients referred with clinical findings of tennis leg, the most commonly injured muscle in the calf complex was the medial head of the gastrocnemius; partial rupture of the medial head at, or no more than 2 cm from, the myotendinous junction, without rupture of the plantaris tendon, was identified in 94 patients (66.7%). Of these 94 patients, 59 (62.8%) had associated fluid collection between the medial head of the gastrocnemius muscle and the soleus muscle. In 30 patients (21.3%) liquid accumulation between the aponeurosis of the gastrocnemius and soleus muscles was evident with US, while without US there was evidence of rupture of the triceps surae musculotendinous unit. Rupture of the plantaris tendon in the middle third of the leg was seen in 2 patients (1.4%), one patient had a partial rupture of the soleus muscle (0.7%) (Delgado et al. 2002).

In another series, all of the 65 patients who had acute posttraumatic calf pain subsequent to a sports activity (51 cases) or trivial injury (14 cases), and with the clinical diagnosis of tennis leg, had tears of the medial head of the gastrocnemius, 24 of which were partial tears of <2 cm, while 27 were larger partial tears, and 14 were complete tears. Most patients reported a history of sudden intense medial calf pain, followed by local edema and impaired function (Bianchi et al. 1998).

In an MRI study of 23 injuries to the distal gastrocnemius muscle [26], the myotendinous junction was involved in 96% of cases. The medial head was more frequently involved than the lateral head (86% and 14%, respectively), and low-grade or partial tears were more common than complete tears (Boutin et al. 2002). Twenty-two patients (age, 30–45 years) with clinically suspected tears of the medial head of the gastrocnemius showed US findings of disruption of the normal regular linear hyperechoic and hypoechoic appearance of the tendon at the site of origin of the medial head of the gastrocnemius. Partial rupture of the medial head of the gastrocnemius was recognized in seven patients (31.8%); five of these patients had an associated fluid collection between the medial head of the gastrocnemius and the soleus muscle (71.4%) (Kwak et al. 2006).

The first and more generally accepted proposed mechanism of injury to the distal gastrocnemius is ankle dorsiflexion with extension of the knee, a circumstance that focuses most extreme stretching on the gastrocnemius, especially when there is a sudden change from plantar flexion to dorsiflexion, such as during descending from a jump. Another proposed mechanism is active plantar flexion of the foot with concurrent knee extension, which requires active contraction of the muscle at the same time as passive stretching (Counsel and Breidahl 2010; Weishaupt et al. 2001).

32.2.2.3 Proximal Gastrocnemius Injuries

Proximal gastrocnemius tears can happen; however, this is an unusual clinical entity. The clinical significance of proximal tears is also unclear, aside from the localization of pain to the knee instead of the midcalf, which can alter the differential diagnosis. The imaging appearance at the level of the knee is infrequently reported and is associated with injuries of the neighboring semimembranosus and biceps tendons and, additionally, popliteal and plantaris tears (Bencardino et al. 2000). If no variation from the norm exits on MRI, one ought to consider referred pain related to lower lumbar disc pathology (i.e., L5 level) (Yamazaki et al. 1995).

32.2.2.4 Injuries of the Lateral Head of the Gastrocnemius

Tears of the lateral head of the gastrocnemius are much less common than tears of the medial head. Of 39 reported strains of the triceps surae, injury to the gastrocnemius was the most common (19 out of 39, 48.7%), involving the medial head in 18 cases and the lateral head in 1 case (Koulouris et al. 2007).

32.2.2.5 Soleus and Plantaris Injuries

Injuries of the plantaris and soleus muscles are far less common than those of the gastrocnemius muscle. This striking difference in pathophysiology is due to the fact that the gastrocnemius and plantaris muscles cross the knee joint, and the soleus muscle does not. Soleus injuries occur during sports such as running and volleyball, or they may occur simply during actions such as stepping off a curb, without evident trauma (Campbell 2009). Injuries of the small plantaris muscle occur after ankle dorsiflexion while the knee is extended, similar to gastrocnemius tears (Lopez et al. 2009). In contrast, soleus tears occur when the ankle is passively dorsiflexed while the knee is flexed, because this muscle does not cross both joints (Cavalier et al. 1998). In a series of 141 patients referred for US examination after calf strain, plantaris muscle rupture (1.4%) and isolated soleus tear (0.7%) were the least frequent findings, while 67% of the patients had gastrocnemius tears, 21% had hematoma and fluid accumulation but no clear muscle tear, and 9% had deep venous thrombosis (Delgado et al. 2002).

However, MRI studies have shown the limitations of US in identifying soleus injuries. In one MRI study, the authors showed an incidence of solitary soleus lesions of 46% (18 soleus injuries in 39 patients) and there were 16 soleus injuries in the 20 patients with dual injuries (80%) (Koulouris et al. 2007).

The occurrence of strains along the proximal medial side of the soleus may be, in part, related to the expanded length of the intramuscular tendon, and such expanded length is also a generally accepted reason for the high rate of medial-sided gastrocnemius tears. The larger musculotendinous junction of the gastrocnemius compared with the soleus enables the muscle unit to generate greater force and places it at increased risk of strain injury. The presence of two proximal tendons and the central tendon that arises from the anterior aponeurosis represent the inferior muscular attachment; that is to say, the insertion of the soleus muscle fibers (whether emerging from the medial or lateral proximal tendons) (Balius et al. 2013).

32.3 Clinical Signs and Symptoms

The classical clinical history of a triceps surae strain is that of a sharp tearing or popping sensation, usually occurring when the calf muscles are stretched simultaneously over the ankle and knee joints. Clinically, there is a marked decrease in plantar flexion strength, and there are complaints of acute pain in the proximal calf, as well as cramping and muscle weakness; swelling or ecchymosis may be visible. Rarely, the swelling may be so extensive that it causes an acute compartment syndrome (Koulouris et al. 2007; Delgado et al. 2002; Campbell 2009). The condition must be differentiated, accurately, with US, from a ruptured Baker cyst, deep venous thrombosis, and, occasionally, Achilles tendon rupture (Bianchi et al. 1998).

Calf injuries occur more commonly in men than in women. These injuries usually affect athletes and people in the fourth to sixth decades of life. Medial calf injuries are most commonly seen acutely, but up to 20% of affected patients have reported calf tightness being present several days before the injury (Koulouris et al. 2007; Campbell 2009; Maffulli et al. 2011).

Clinically, it may be difficult to distinguish among gastrocnemius, plantaris, and soleus injuries. On top of that, a more distal calf injury may present as a proximal Achilles tendon rupture or strain due to the anatomical proximity. This is emphasized by the frequently described sensation of tearing and popping of the tendon or muscle or a feeling as if the calf has been kicked (Campbell 2009; Maffulli et al. 2011).

32.3.1 Physical Examination

Physical examination can help to distinguish between strains of the soleus and gastrocnemius; this allows us to isolate the site and severity of the injury. A combination of palpation, strength testing, and stretching is required to localize strains to the gastrocnemius or soleus. Palpation of the calf should occur along the entire length. It is necessary to identify tenderness, swelling, thickening, defects, and masses if present. Gastrocnemius strains typically present with tenderness in the medial belly or the musculotendinous junction. In soleus strains the pain is often lateral (Brukner and Khan 2002).

On inspection, a (horizontal) ecchymosis can be found at the location of the injury (Campbell 2009; Maffulli et al. 2011; Brukner and Khan 2002). A plantaris or soleus injury typically presents with acute swelling and ecchymosis of the calf (Campbell 2009).

A palpable defect in the muscle helps in the localization and suggests an injury of greater severity. The origins of the gastrocnemius and soleus are anatomically distinct, arising from above and below the knee, respectively (Kerkhoffs and Servien 2014). A rupture may be palpable if there is retraction of the muscle. As previously mentioned, it may be difficult to clinically distinguish a muscle tear from a proximal tear of the Achilles tendon (Kerkhoffs and Servien 2014; Campbell 2009).

According to the degree of knee flexion, the examiner can isolate the activation of the muscles. With the knee in maximal flexion, the soleus becomes the primary generator of force in plantar flexion. The gastrocnemius muscle is the primary generator of force when the knee is in full extension. This technique can also be used in testing pain and flexibility during passive movements (Koulouris et al. 2007; Fleiss 1996). The relationship between the position of the knee (full flexion or full extension) and the function of the muscles involved (soleus or gastrocnemius) allows for more accurate strength testing of the individual calf muscles and enables the clinician to better delineate which muscle has been injured. In injuries of the plantaris and soleus muscles, the pain is exacerbated on weight bearing and with passive dorsiflexion of the ankle and palpation over the site of injury, with the site usually located laterally (Brukner and Khan 2002; Fleiss 1996). It has been suggested that soleus and/or plantaris injuries can be differentiated from gastrocnemius injuries based on their less extensive pain and swelling. Additional testing that can be used during the evaluation of calf strain includes the Thompson test and functional movements such as hopping, running, and jumping (Bryan Dixon 2009).

32.3.2 Clinical and Imaging Classification

Three types of acute skeletal muscle trauma have been described: strains, tears, and contusions and hematomas. On the other hand, chronic lesions after muscle trauma include fibrous scars, muscle hernias, and heterotopic calcification (Lee and Healy 2004).

Muscular injuries are classified according to their injury mechanism as extrinsic (direct) or intrinsic (indirect). Extrinsic injuries are classified according to their severity, as light or benign (grade I), moderate (grade II), or serious (grade III). Intrinsic injuries, due to stretching, are produced by the application of a tensional force higher than the tissue resistance in an eccentric contraction. The classification of intrinsic injuries is more complex (Kerkhoffs and Servien 2014).

Clinically, injuries of the calf muscle complex are graded as 1–3 (Table 32.1), and this classification can be utilized to gauge the recovery period and to choose a suitable rehabilitation program (Lee and Healy 2004).

Table 32.1 Clinical classification of calf muscle injury

Grade 1 (mild)	Sharp pain in the posterior aspect of the leg at the time of injury or with activity May be able to continue activity Mild pain, spasm, and swelling Minimal loss of strength and range of motion (ROM) Tightness and aching for up 2–5 days
Grade 2 (moderate)	Sharp pain in the posterior aspect of the leg Unable to continue activity Swelling. Mild to moderate bruising Loss of strength and ROM Tightness and aching for about 2 weeks
Grade 3 (severe)	Severe immediate pain and disability Considerable swelling and bruising Loss of function Palpable defect

These lesions are commonly located at the musculotendinous junction in the superficial muscle layers, but the location may vary depending on the mechanism of injury. Musculotendinous strains are clinically classified as grade 1 (without loss of muscle function), grade 2 (mild loss of muscle function), or grade 3 (complete loss of muscle function) (Valle 2011). Based on the patient's disability, physical findings, and relevant pathological findings, a grade 1 muscle strain is an injury with a minor tear of up to 10% of the muscle fibers. A grade 2 injury involves tearing of up to 50% of the muscle fibers, and a grade 3 injury represents tearing of over 50% of the muscle fibers, including complete ruptures (Delgado et al. 2002; Bryan Dixon 2009).

A relatively new classification system, which differentiates between four types of acute muscle disorders and injuries, has recently been developed; this comprises the classification of indirect muscle disorders/injuries as functional muscle disorders (type 1, overexertion-related, and type 2, neuromuscular muscle disorders), and structural muscle injuries (type 3, partial tears, and type 4, (sub) total tears/tendinous avulsions) with macroscopic evidence of fiber tear; that is, structural damage (Mueller-Wohlfahrt et al. 2013) (Table 32.2).

Table 32.2 Classification of acute muscle disorders and injuries

Indirect muscle disorder/ injury	Functional muscle disorder	**Type 1**: Overexertion-related muscle disorder	**Type 1A**: Fatigue-induced muscle disorder **Type 1B**: Delayed onset muscle soreness (DOMS)
		Type 2: Neuromuscular muscle disorder	**Type 2A**: Spine-related neuromuscular muscle disorder **Type 2B**: Muscle-related neuromuscular muscle disorder
	Structural muscle injury	**Type 3**: Partial muscle tear	**Type 3A**: Minor partial muscle tear **Type 3B**: Moderate partial muscle tear
		Type 4: Total tear	Subtotal or complete muscle tear. Tendinous avulsion
Direct muscle injury		Contusion/laceration	

32.4 Imaging

In athletes, indirect injuries are the most relevant structural muscle injuries with macroscopic evidence of muscle damage; that is, stretch-induced injuries caused by a sudden forced lengthening over the viscoelastic limits of muscles occurring during a powerful contraction (Mueller-Wohlfahrt et al. 2013). Imaging plays a role in providing an accurate prognosis as well as aiding in proper management decisions. Magnetic resonance imaging (MRI) or US can be of value in both the initial assessment and follow-up of the injury (Mueller-Wohlfahrt et al. 2013; Hayashi et al. 2012).

Although US is cheap and generally accessible, it depends on the experience of the radiologist and has lower sensitivity for distinguishing ongoing muscle healing than MRI, leading to a more inaccurate prediction of convalescence time and risk of recurrent injury (Kerkhoffs and Servien 2014; Hayashi et al. 2012).

32.4.1 Modalities for Imaging of Musculotendinous Injuries

32.4.1.1 MRI

According to the sports medicine literature, MRI is a sensitive modality for confirming strain in the muscles of the calf muscle complex and for accurately identifying the location of injury within the muscle-tendon-bone unit (Koulouris et al. 2007; Menz and Lucas 1991). However, MRI would only be recommended particularly in high-performance sports in cases where a rapid and accurate diagnosis is required and in which a thorough US study does not identify any injury (Balius et al. 2014).

Previously not appreciated is the high number of dual injuries (although the most commonly injured muscle of the calf muscle complex is the medial head of the gastrocnemius in the proximal musculotendinous junction), as well as strains involving the soleus muscle, which may potentially be of prognostic significance. Soleus muscle injuries have been rarely described in the echotomography literature; it is likely that these injuries have been underdiagnosed, and thus MRI should be considered the modality of choice in elite athletes and preferred over US (Kerkhoffs and Servien 2014; Koulouris et al. 2007; Hayashi et al. 2012).

MRI is commonly used to locate the lesion and assess its severity. The extent of musculotendinous injuries and the associated architectural distortion is assessed using axial, sagittal, and coronal images arranged along the long and short axes of the included musculotendinous unit. The axial plane is helpful to evaluate muscle contours and to delineate the musculotendinous junction and its exact anatomical relation to focal lesions (Hayashi et al. 2012; Palmer et al. 1999), while the coronal and sagittal planes are utilized to survey the longitudinal extent of the injury (Valle 2011).

Musculotendinous units are commonly altered in all forms of acute traumatic injuries. Normal skeletal muscles, compared with other soft tissues, show intermediate to low signal intensity on both T1-weighted (T1-w) (short TR/TE) and T2-weighted or short tau inversion recovery (STIR) (long TR/long TE) images (Deutsch and Mink 1989).

Fluid-sensitive sequences, i.e., fat-suppressed T2-weighted (FS T2-w) or fat-suppressed proton density-weighted (FS PD-w) images, and turbo spin echo (TSE) and STIR sequences, are suitable for detecting edematous changes (hyperintense feather-shaped) in the musculotendinous unit, and for delineating and locating intramuscular or perifascial fluid collections or hematomas as hyperintensity (Hayashi et al. 2012). T1-w TSE sequences are used to visualize atrophy and fatty infiltration and to differentiate between edema (hypointensity) and hematoma (hyperintensity) (Deutsch and Mink 1989). But in chronic muscle injuries, T1-w images may not show any signal abnormalities in small tears (Hayashi et al. 2012).

32.4.1.2 MRI Features in Musculotendinous Strains and Tears

Findings in musculotendinous strains and tears include rupture or discontinuity of gastrocnemius muscle fibers, fluid signals consistent with hemorrhage and hematoma at the musculotendinous junction, and retraction of the torn muscle fibers. MRI also allows differentiation between gastrocnemius and Achilles tendon injury, which can help to improve the treatment (Campbell 2009).

In musculotendinous strains without a tear, some fiber disruptions are seen, but muscle functions are maintained. On MRI, interstitial edema and hemorrhage are present at the musculotendinous junction and extend into the adjacent muscle fascicles, producing a feathery appearance (i.e., hyperintensity) on fluid-sensitive sequences. In the presence of partial tears (without retraction), in addition to interstitial edema and hemorrhage, hematoma at the musculotendinous junction and perifascial fluid collection appear as hyperintensity on fluid-sensitive sequences. Hematoma in this region is associated with a complete musculotendinous rupture. Clinically, muscle function is completely lost, with a palpable gap and retraction of muscle fibers. MRI and US may be useful for the preoperative assessment of the extent of retraction (Hayashi et al. 2012).

In an MRI series of 23 injuries to the distal gastrocnemius that occurred in 20 patients, myotendinous strains were the most common injuries (43%); partial tears (30%) and complete tears (22%) of the myotendinous junction or proximal Achilles tendon were less frequent. Injuries to the medial head of the gastrocnemius in the myotendinous junction were more frequent than those to the lateral head (86% vs. 14%) (Weishaupt et al. 2001).

MRI is also helpful in diagnosing tears of the plantaris or soleus muscles. Soleus injuries can occur throughout the extent of the muscle; those occurring at the perimeter of the muscle and not at the tendons are classified as myofascial (epimysial) strains, those at the myofascial junction of the soleus with the gastrocnemius are classified as posterior myofascial strains, and those at the junction between the soleus and the deep posterior compartment of the leg are classified as anterior myofascial strains (Campbell 2009; Balius et al. 2013)., Soleus injuries can also occur in the musculotendinous junction, involving the distal intramuscular tendon, or the proximal medial and lateral aponeuroses. As shown in a retrospective study of 55 cases of soleus muscle strains, 31 strains were considered musculotendinous, of which 14 were located at the medial aponeurosis and 10 were located at the central tendon; 24 of the soleus muscle strains were myofascial, of which half were anterior myofascial (Balius et al. 2013).

Imaging features of plantaris injury include hemorrhage and edema in the muscle, seen on T1 and T2 imaging (27); the fluid is located between the gastrocnemius and soleus muscles. Plantaris injury may occur at the myotendinous junction with or without a partial tear of the medial head of the gastrocnemius muscle; plantaris injury may also occur as an isolated injury or in conjunction with injury to the anterior cruciate ligament (ACL) (10 of 15 patients) (Helms et al. 1995).

32.4.1.3 Echotomography

Ultrasonography has proven to be an easy to perform and a fast and safe imaging modality for evaluating the size of the tears in patients with clinically suspected tennis leg (Bianchi et al. 1998). Ultrasonography allows dynamic imaging while the injured leg is maneuvered to elicit symptoms and aid in clarifying the diagnosis. Power Doppler is useful for identifying hyperemia associated with acute injuries (Blankenbaker and Tuite 2010).

Moreover, a large hematoma may be drained under US guidance after liquefaction of the hematoma has occurred. The sensitivity of US for acute fluid collection has been shown to be equal to that of MRI in some studies (Koulouris and Connell 2005), especially in larger tears where fluid collection occurs between the injured medial head of the gastrocnemius muscle and the soleus muscle (Bianchi et al. 1998).

The disadvantages of US are seen in follow-up imaging, because is very difficult to reproduce exactly the same imaging position and plane as those at baseline, and US cannot always differentiate between old and new lesions and those on follow-up visits (Hayashi et al. 2012).

32.4.1.4 Ultrasonographic Features of Musculotendinous Strains and Tears

The US technique discriminates partial tears from complete tears of the muscle, with case reports demonstrating the rate of occurrence of incomplete injuries as 33% to 75% (Campbell 2009). At the gastrocnemius muscle myotendinous junction, US usually shows discontinuity of fibers, and follow-up US shows union of this defect with hypoechoic tissue at 4 weeks (Bianchi et al. 1998). The lesions in a gastrocnemius muscle injury produce loss of the alternating linear hyperechoic and hypoechogenic structures of muscle fibers and normal muscle septum (Delgado et al. 2002).

Fluid collections are often a useful guide to the site of injury (Bianchi et al. 1998). Edema peripheral to a gastrocnemius muscle injury appears as a poorly defined region of increased echogenicity, and this can be an important echotomographic sign of a muscle injury, especially in small tears (Lee and Healy 2004). In the presence of partial tears, these pathological features are depicted as hypoechogenicity. Disruption of muscle fibers will be depicted as notable echo-inhomogeneity (Hayashi et al. 2012).

In patients with small tears, examined within a couple of hours of the injury, the absence of a definite hypoechoic or anechoic blood collection was reported to make detection of the tear difficult. Cautious assessment of the distal segment of the medial head of the gastrocnemius, however, revealed that muscle fibers and septa did not achieve an aponeurosis. Most of these injuries affected the most anteromedial portion of the gastrocnemius medial head and could be missed if this region is not evaluated carefully (Bianchi et al. 1998).

US also offers a quick and inexpensive imaging methodology to diagnose plantaris or soleus injuries.

32.4.1.5 US in Soleus Muscle Injuries

Five sites of strain distribution have been identified within the soleus: three musculotendinous junction sites (proximal medial strains, accounting for 25.5% of all injuries, were the most common type of soleus muscle injuries, with proximal lateral strains accounting for 12.7%, and distal central tendon strains accounting for 18.2%) and two myofascial sites (anterior strains 21.8% and posterior strains 21.8%) (Balius et al. 2013).

US, compared with MRI, is not sensitive enough for detecting and assessing soleus injuries (Delgado et al. 2002; Balius et al. 2014), although the sensitivity is enhanced by thorough anatomically based US; also, the timing of the US examination (within 28.8 days of the injury in positive cases $P = 0.003$) may be important. Some authors observed that injuries at the myofascial junctions (10 out of 24; 41.7%) were more readily identified than those situated at the musculotendinous junctions (5 out of 26; 19.2%). This may be due to the presence of a fluid collection that appears to facilitate US visualization of myofascial injuries. Each type of soleus injury appears to have a characteristic US pattern based on a defect of connective expansions, the existence of small myofascial filiform collections, and the rarefaction of the fibrillar area (Balius et al. 2014).

32.4.1.6 US in Plantaris Muscle Injuries

Plantaris rupture is a strong diagnostic possibility when a mass-like structure of the same echogenicity as muscle is seen in the plane between the gastrocnemius and soleus muscles, along with fluid collection (Rohilla et al. 2013). Plantaris tears are typically located at the midcalf level at the muscle-tendon junction (Campbell 2009; Leekam et al. 1999). Less commonly, tears of the plantaris tendon without muscle involvement may show little fluid on US. US can also reveal a small soleus aponeurosis avulsion, but the fluid collection or hematoma is always located between the soleus and gastrocnemius muscles, usually the medial head. Such injuries may also be found on echotomography, obtained to rule out deep vein thrombosis, clarifying a potentially confusing clinical picture (Rohilla et al. 2013; Leekam et al. 1999). Comparison with the contralateral extremity can assist in detecting subtle differences. Fluid collection alone without an obvious tear of the muscle fibers has also been described (Leekam et al. 1999).

32.5 Treatment

The time required for recovery is often difficult to predict, and re-injury is common. The length of recovery time may be influenced by different variables, such as the part of the muscle involved. Complete recovery of strength and flexibility should be achieved prior to return to pre-injury activity. Premature return may result in a prolonged recovery or incomplete return to the pre-injury baseline.

Acute treatment is aimed at limiting hemorrhage and pain, as well as preventing complications. Over the first few days, muscle rest, achieved by limiting stretch and contraction, cryotherapy, compressive wrap or tape, and elevation of the leg are generally recommended.

The use of nonsteroidal anti-inflammatory drugs (NSAIDs) should be restricted because of increased bleeding caused by their antiplatelet effects. Cyclooxygenase (COX)-2 inhibitors have a negative effect on muscle injury recovery. Acetaminophen or opiate pain medication could also be used.

The suggested treatment regime in athletes is:

Days 0–3, Cryotherapy, electrotherapy, and draining massage

Days 3–7, Prediathermy, isometric exercises, walking/biking; postcryotherapy, active stretching

Progressive work in a swimming pool is very well tolerated. It stimulates the activity of the injured muscle and controls the load.

Days 7–14, Electrotherapy, concentric exercises, elliptical trainer/treadmill; prediathermy, Closed Kinetic Chain Exercises (CKCE): exercises performed where the foot doesn't move during the exercise. The foot remains in constant contact with a surface, usually the ground or a footplate of a machine. These exercises are typically weight-bearing exercises, where an exerciser uses their own body weight and/or external weight.

Examples: Back Squats, Front Squats, Leg Press, and Lunges

A progressive series of 22 Swiss ball exercises are planned to easily strengthen the hamstrings, thighs, buttocks and back muscles to enhance the core stability control and improve the balance.

Ten days after the injury, the developing scar has the same tensile strength as the adjacent muscle and further progression of rehabilitative exercises can begin. Isometric, isotonic, and then dynamic training exercises can be added in a consecutive manner as each type of exercise is completed without pain.

Days 14–21, Eccentric exercises, exercises to improve strength, flexibility, and balance

Exercise in the field of play

Return to training and competition if return to play (RTP) criteria are met.

32.6 Return to Play in Sports

32.6.1 Gastrocnemius

For safe return to sport following muscle strains, there are no consensus guidelines or settled-upon criteria that completely eliminate the risk of recurrence and maximize performance (Orchard et al. 2005). Some studies have shown RTP data for different types of muscle injuries. In a study by Hallén and Ekstrand (2014), 81 elite professional teams of football players in Europe were followed between 2001 and 2013, and individual player exposure and time-loss for injuries were recorded. A total of 17,371 injuries occurred, including 5603 (32%) muscle injuries. Lay-off days were correlated with the MRI grading of thigh muscle injuries ($P < 0.001$). Calf muscle injuries were responsible for a median absence of 13 days ($P < 0.001$). MRI was valuable for prognosticating RTP, with radiological grading associated with lay-off times after injury.

32.6.2 Soleus

According to a recent study, by Pedret et al. (2015), the site with the worst prognosis was the myotendinous central junction, with a mean recovery time of 44.3 ± 23.0 days, and a longer RTP than injuries in other locations. The site with the best prognosis was the myotendinous lateral junction, with a mean recovery time of 19.2 ± 13.5 days ($P < 0.05$). There was a statistically significant correlation between recovery time and age ($P < 0.001$) and between recovery time and the extent of retraction ($P < 0.05$). The most important prognostic factors were the anterior-posterior extent of the retraction or gap and the involvement of the surrounding tissue, while measurement of the extent of edema was relatively insignificant. Multivariate equations were specifically applied to different sport disciplines. For example, for the 44-included patients, a worse prognosis regarding age, transverse muscle area, and weight was found for soccer; the factors that explained RTP were the transverse muscle area and the gap; age and weight were less important because of a certain amount of homogeneity regarding these variables in soccer players (Pedret et al. 2015).

Conclusion

Muscle injuries are classified according to the degree of involvement of the muscle.

Injuries to the soleus muscle are underestimated because of their subacute clinical characteristics.

For the diagnosis of these injuries, MRI is our preferred modality.

Soleus muscle injuries show different prevalences in different sport disciplines and are more frequent in soccer.

It is important to establish the prognosis for every type of muscle injury to make correct decisions about return to sport. You need to know the exact injury location and the specific type of injury. The soleus muscle is characterized by a complex anatomy and unique mechanical properties. Injuries in the central tendon of the soleus muscle have a longer return to sports than injuries in other locations and have a worse prognosis.

In our experience in working with professional soccer players (Universidad de Chile and the National Chilean Team), the factors that define return to sports are the transverse area of the muscle and the gap, and the extent of edema.

References

Armfield DR, Kim DH, Towers JD, Bradley JP, Robertson DD (2006) Sports-related muscle injury in the lower extremity. Clin Sports Med 25:803–842. doi:10.1016/j.csm.2006.06.011

Balius R, Alomar X, Rodas G, Miguel-Pérez M, Pedret C, Dobado MC, Blasi J, Koulouris G (2013) The soleus muscle: MRI, anatomic and histologic findings in cadavers with clinical correlation of strain injury distribution. Skeletal Radiol 42(4):521–530. doi:10.1007/s00256-012-1513-3

Balius R, Rodas G, Pedret C, Capdevila L, Alomar X, Bong DA (2014) Soleus muscle injury: sensitivity of ultrasound patterns. Skelet Radiol 43(6):805–812. doi:10.1007/s00256-014-1856-z

Bencardino JT, Rosenberg ZS, Brown RR, Hassankhani A, Lustrin ES, Beltran J (2000) Traumatic musculotendinous injuries of the knee: diagnosis with MR imaging. Radiographics 20:S103–S120

Bianchi S, Martinoli C, Abdelwahab IF, Derchi LE, Damiani S (1998) Sonographic evaluation of tears of the gastrocnemius medial head ("tennis leg"). J Ultrasound Med 17(3):157–162

Blankenbaker DG, Tuite MJ (2010) Temporal changes of muscle injury. Semin Musculoskelet Radiol 14:176–193

Boutin RD, Fritz RC, Steinbach LS (2002) Imaging of sports-related muscle injuries. Radiol Clin North Am 40(2):333–62, vii. Review

Brukner P, Khan K (2002) Clinical sports medicine, Revised 2nd edn. McGraw-Hill, Australia

Bryan Dixon J (2009) Gastrocnemius vs. soleus strain: how to differentiate and deal with calf muscle injuries. Curr Rev Muscoskelet Med 2(2):74–77. doi:10.1007/s12178-009-9045-8

Campbell JT (2009) Posterior calf injury. Foot Ankle Clin 14(4):761–771

Cavalier R, Gabos PG, Bowen JR (1998) Isolated rupture of the soleus muscle: a case report. Am J Orthop 27:755–757

Coughlin MJ, Mann RA, Saltzman CL (2006) Surgery of the foot and ankle, 8th edn. Mosby, Philadelphia

Counsel P, Breidahl W (2010) Muscle injuries of the lower leg. Semin Musculoskelet Radiol 14(2):162–175. doi:10.1055/s-0030-1253158. Review

DeLee JC, Drez D, Miller MD (eds) (2003) DeLee & Drez's orthopaedic sports medicine; principles and practice, 2nd edn. Saunders, Philadelphia

Delgado GJ, Chung CB, Lektrakul N et al (2002) Tennis leg: clinical US study of 141 patients and anatomic investigation of four cadavers with MR imaging and US. Radiology 224(1):112–119

Deutsch AL, Mink JH (1989) Magnetic resonance imaging of musculoskeletal injuries. Radiol Clin North Am 27:983–1002

Ekstrand J, Hägglund M, Waldén M (2011) Epidemiology of muscle injuries in professional football (soccer). Am J Sports Med 39(6):1226–1232. doi:10.1177/0363546510395879

Fleiss DJ (1996) Tennis calf or tennis leg. Orthopedics 19(5):377

Garrett WE Jr (1990) Muscle strain injuries: clinical and basic aspects. Med Sci Sports Exerc 22(4):436–443

Garrett WE Jr (1996) Muscle strain injuries. Am J Sports Med 24(6 suppl):S2–S8

Gilbert TJ Jr, Bullis BR, Griffiths HJ (1996) Tennis calf or tennis leg. Orthopedics 19:179

Hallén A, Ekstrand J (2014) Return to play following muscle injuries in professional footballers. J Sports Sci 32(13):1229–1236. doi:10.1080/02640414.2014.905695

Hayashi D, Hamilton B, Guermazi A, de Villiers R, Crema MD, Roemer FW (2012) Traumatic injuries of thigh and calf muscles in athletes: role and clinical relevance of MR imaging and ultrasound. Insights Imaging 3(6):591–601

Helms CA, Fritz RC, Garvin GJ (1995) Plantaris muscle injury: evaluation with MR imaging. Radiology 195(1):201–203

Hollinshead WH (1969) Anatomy for surgeons, vol. 3. The back and limbs, 2nd edn. Harper and Row Publishers

Joshi SS, Joshi SD, Kishve PS (2010) Feathered fibres of human soleus. Int J Morphol 28(1):239–242

Jozsa G, Kannus P (1997) Human tendons anatomy and physiology. Human Kinetics

Kerkhoffs G, Servien E (eds) (2014) Acute muscle injuries. Springer. doi:10.1007/978-3-319-03722-6

Koplas MC, Grooff P, Piraino D, Recht M (2009) Third head of the gastrocnemius: an MR imaging study based on 1039 consecutive knee examinations. Skeletal Radiol 38(4):349–354. doi:10.1007/s00256-008-0606-5

Koulouris G, Connell D (2005) Hamstring muscle complex: an imaging review. Radiographics 25:571–586

Koulouris G, Ting AYI, Jhamb A, Connell D, Kavanagh EC (2007) Magnetic resonance imaging findings of injuries to the calf muscle complex. Skeletal Radiol 36:921–927

Kvist M (1991) *Achilles tendon overuse injuries*. Doctoral dissertation. Turku University of Turku

Kvist M (1994) Achilles tendon injuries in athletes. Sports Med 18:173–201

Kwak H-S, Han Y-M, Lee S-Y, Kim K-N, Chung GH (2006) Diagnosis and follow-up US evaluation of ruptures of the medial head of the gastrocnemius ("tennis leg"). Korean J Radiol 7(3):193–198. doi:10.3348/kjr.2006.7.3.193

Lee JC, Healy J (2004) Sonography of lower limb muscle injury. AJR Am J Roentgenol 182(2):341–351. Review

Leekam RN, Agur AM, McKee NH (1999) Using sonography to diagnose injury of plantaris muscles and tendons. AJR Am J Roentgenol 172:185–189

Lopez GJ, Hoffman RS, Davenport M (2009) Plantaris rupture: a mimic of deep venous thrombosis. J Emerg Med 40(2):e27–e30

Luck MD, Gordon AG, Blebea JS, Dalinka MK (2008) High association between accessory soleus muscle and Achilles tendonopathy. Skeletal Radiol 37(12):1129–1133

Maffulli N, Longo UG, Gougoulias N, Caine D, Denaro V (2011) Sport injuries: a review of outcomes. Br Med Bull 97:47–80

Menz MJ, Lucas GL (1991) Magnetic resonance imaging of a rupture of the medial head of the gastrocnemius muscle. A case report. J Bone Joint Surg Am 730(8):1260–1262

Mueller-Wohlfahrt H-W, Haensel L, Mithoefer K, Ekstrand J, English B, McNally S, Ueblacker P (2013) Terminology and classification of muscle injuries in sport: the Munich consensus statement. Br J Sports Med 47(6):342–350. doi:10.1136/bjsports-2012-091448

O'Brien M (2005) The anatomy of the Achilles tendon. Foot Ankle Clin 10(2):225–238. Review

Orchard J, Best TM, Verrall GM (2005) Return to play following muscle strains. Clin J Sport Med 15(6):436–441. Review

Palmer WE, Kuong SJ, Elmadbouh HM (1999) MR imaging of myotendinous strain. AJR Am J Roentgenol 173:703–709. doi:10.2214/ajr.173.3.10470908

Pedret C, Rodas G, Balius R, Capdevila L, Bossy M, Vernooij RWM, Alomar X (2015) Return to play after soleus muscle injuries. Orthop J Sports Med 3(7):2325967115595802. doi:10.1177/2325967115595802

Powell RW (1883) Lawn tennis leg. Lancet 2:44

Rohilla S, Jain N, Yadav R (2013) Plantaris rupture: why is it important? BMJ Case Rep bcr2012007840. doi:10.1136/bcr-2012-007840

Segal RL, Song AW (2005) Nonuniform activity of human calf muscles during an exercise task. Arch Phys Med Rehabil 86:2013–2017

Singhal MD, Kher NB, Gandotra A, Panwar AS (2012) Bipennate arrangement of soleus muscle in human and its relevance to the force of contraction. J Anat Soc India 61(2):246–249. doi:10.1016/S0003-2778(12)80039-6

Valle X (2011) Clinical practice guide for muscular injuries: epidemiology, diagnosis, treatment and prevention. Br J Sports Med 45(2):e2. doi:10.1136/bjsm.2010.081570.20

Van Sterkenburg M, Kerkhoffs GM, Kleipool RP, Niek van Dijk C (2011) The plantaris tendon and a potential role in mid-portion Achilles tendinopathy: an observational anatomical study. J Anat 218(3):336–341

Warwick R, Williams PC (eds) (1973) Gray's anatomy, 35th edn. Longmans, Edinburgh

Weishaupt D, Schweitzer ME, Morrison WB (2001) Injuries to the distal gastrocnemius muscle: MR findings. J Comput Assist Tomogr 25(5):677–682

Yamazaki T, Maruoka S, Takahashi S et al (1995) MR findings of avulsive cortical irregularity of the distal femur. Skeletal Radiol 24:43–46

Achilles Tendinopathy

33

Kenneth J. Hunt

Contents

K.J. Hunt, M.D.
Chief, Foot and Ankle Section, Department of Orthopaedic Surgery, University of Colorado School of Medicine, 12631 E. 17th Ave, Room 4508, Aurora, CO 80045, USA
e-mail: kenneth.j.hunt@ucdenver.edu

33.1 Introduction

The Achilles tendon is the strongest and thickest tendon in the body that endures considerable loads during athletic activities. It has been estimated that loads of up to 11 kN per cm^2 or 12 times the body weight are absorbed by the Achilles tendon during jumping and running (Fukashiro et al. 1995; Slane and Thelen 2014). In addition, the trade-off in design between the Achilles tendon's strength and stiffness and its ability to store and release energy results in a relatively low safety factor (Ker 1999). This low safety factor can lead to rupture of the Achilles tendon under certain conditions. However, Achilles tendinopathy is far more common as a result of repetitive loading, often under suboptimal physiologic or environmental conditions, and is in fact one of the most common musculoskeletal conditions in athletes.

33.2 Terminology

Clinical complaints of pain, swelling, and impaired function of the Achilles tendon are common in sports. A number of terms are applied to the chronically painful Achilles tendon, including tendinitis, tendinosis, and paratenonitis. However, histopathological studies have demonstrated that most Achilles tendon disorders are the result of an inadequate healing response, often leading to degenerative changes in the ten-

G.L. Canata et al. (eds.), *Muscle and Tendon Injuries*, DOI 10.1007/978-3-662-54184-5_33

don, rather than from inflammation. This process tends to occur in three continuous stages: reactive tendinopathy, tendon disrepair, and degenerative tendinopathy (Abate et al. 2009; Cook and Purdam 2009). An inflammatory response is not found in any of the three stages. For this reason, Maffulli et al. have suggested the use of the term "tendinopathy" as a more encompassing term to describe these intratendinous disorders (Maffulli et al. 1998).

There are two broad anatomic categories of Achilles tendinopathy: insertional (at the calcaneus-Achilles tendon junction) and non-insertional (2–6 cm proximal to the insertion of the Achilles tendon into the calcaneus) (Almekinders 1998). Kvist found that 20–25% of Achilles tendinopathy patients had insertional disorder, 66% had non-insertional, and 23% had a combination of retrocalcaneal bursitis or insertional tendinopathy (Kvist 1991).

The non-insertional variety typically involves the substance of the Achilles tendon, with or without inflammation of the paratenon and with or without adhesions. Insertional disease can commonly include a prominent enlargement of the calcaneal tuberosity above the Achilles insertion (i.e., Haglund's lesion), an inflamed retrocalcaneal bursa, and intratendinous calcifications at or near the Achilles insertion. Successful treatment is often predicated on identification of the etiologic condition(s) and addressing them with an effective, and sometime comprehensive, treatment strategy.

33.3 Functional Anatomy

The Achilles tendon originates from the merging of the soleus muscle with the two bellies of the gastrocnemius (often referred to as the *triceps surae*), and it inserts distally onto the posterior tuberosity of the calcaneus. The normal tendon is generally a rounded structure that is avascular, white, and elastic. The Achilles is primarily composed of collagen fibers (mostly type I collagen), which make up 90% of the tendon protein. Collagen forms microfibrils, fibrils, and fibers. A group of fibers constitutes a fascicle. The fascicles unite to form bundles and are surrounded by the endotenon, which carries blood vessels, lymphatics, and nerves.

The Achilles tendon receives blood supply from three sources: the muscle-tendon junction, the bone-tendon junction, and centrally from the endotenon along the length of the tendon. The blood supply to the middle portion of the tendon (referred to as a watershed area) is by way of the surrounding paratenon. The most abundant blood supply zone in the tendon is at the tendon insertion, whereas, in people older than 30 years, the most intensely vascularized zone is at the tendon origin. The area of the tendon between approximately 2 and 6 cm above the insertion into the calcaneus is the least vascularized zone at all ages, resulting in limited reparative ability at times of stress or repeated injury.

33.4 Etiology

Achilles tendinopathy is generally chronic and related to overuse. There is a good general understanding of the intrinsic and extrinsic factors that are associated with Achilles tendinopathy. Intrinsic factors include biomechanical factors involving the lower extremity, such as cavus hindfoot deformity, forefoot varus, equinus, limb length inequality, and subtalar joint stiffness (Irwin 2010). Systemic conditions are also known to contribute risk including advancing age (Tuite et al. 1997), diabetes, corticosteroid use, inflammatory arthropathies, hypertension, obesity, gout (Holmes and Lin 2006; Paavola et al. 2002), and the use of statin drugs, aromatase inhibitors, and quinolone antibiotics (Knobloch 2016). Extrinsic factors are related to excessive training errors and repeated mechanical overload, including significant increases in interval training, excessive hill training, abrupt changes in training schedule, training on hard or sloping surfaces, rapid increases in mileage, footwear or running surfaces with poor shock absorption (especially when changing from normal), and wedging from uneven wear (Irwin 2010; Kirchgesner et al. 2014). The cycle of tendinopathy is usually repetitive microtrauma to an area of the tendon at risk (due at least in part to the above factors) followed by an inability of the body to effectively heal these regions. The reduced blood supply in the central portion of the tendon is a likely contributor to Achilles tendinopathy in this area.

33.5 Epidemiology

Achilles tendinopathy is among the most frequently lower extremity overuse injuries (Sobhani et al. 2013) and is most likely to be experienced by individuals who participate in repetitive impact physical activities, such as running and jumping. The lifetime prevalence of Achilles tendinopathy in runners is up to 52% (Maffulli et al. 2003) and it can be career ending in up to 5% of professional athletes (Lysholm and Wiklander 1987). In their epidemiologic analysis of nearly 1400 nonathletic individuals, Waldecker et al. (2012) identified Achilles tendinopathy in 5.6% of the subjects (4% insertional, 3.6% non-insertional, and 1.9% a combination of both) (Waldecker et al. 2012). Chronic Achilles tendinopathy is more common in older people than in young people. In the study by Kvist (1991), only 25% of the subjects with Achilles tendinopathy patients were young athletes. In addition, insertional Achilles tendinopathy tends to occur more commonly in active persons, whereas non-insertional tendinopathy tends to occur in older, less active, and overweight people (Li and Hua 2016).

33.6 Clinical and Diagnostic Features

Patients most often present with insidious onset of pain, swelling, and stiffness. They will frequently localize symptoms to the involved region of the Achilles tendon and associated structures. In cases of insertional tendinopathy, pain is typically at the posterior midline of the calcaneal tuberosity, but there can also be pain just medial or just lateral to the Achilles insertion, particularly when there are focal enthesophytes and/or retrocalcaneal bursitis. Non-insertional tendinopathy typically involves the section of the tendon 2–6 cm above the insertion and rarely involves the calcaneus. Patients often complain that exercise, stair climbing, and running on hard surfaces can exacerbate symptoms. In the earlier stages, patients often report that symptoms occur only after a strenuous activity, but as the disease progresses and becomes more chronic, any activity may cause symptoms, including walking on flat ground, and pain can even occur at rest.

Physical examination is a critical component of diagnosis. Exam can reveal tenderness and swelling at the involved portion of the Achilles. The tendon is often thickened and the pain can be made worse with resisted plantar flexion. Calf strength is usually normal, but can be limited by pain. If the location of tenderness is isolated to the medial and/or lateral aspects of the Achilles insertion without tendon thickening, then retrocalcaneal bursitis is a likely diagnosis. It is important to utilize the physical examination to rule out other potential injuries, such as Achilles rupture, calcaneal stress fracture, and FHL pathology.

Imaging. Radiographs are not always necessary for non-insertional tendinopathy, but weight-bearing radiographs of the foot are should be obtained with insertional tendinopathy. The anteroposterior view can identify a pes planovalgus or cavovarus foot alignment (Fig. 33.1). The width of the Achilles shadow and maintenance of Kager's fat pad triangle should be evaluated on the lateral view. The presence of enthesophytes

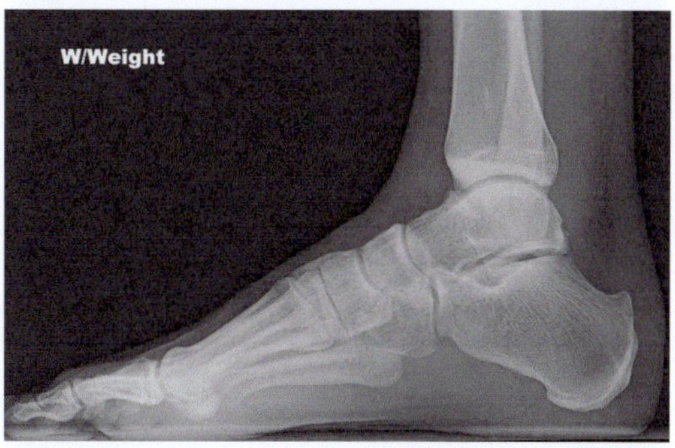

Fig. 33.1 Lateral radiograph demonstrating cavus foot and prominent Haglund's lesion on posterior calcaneal tuberosity

and intratendinous calcification is best seen on this view (Fig. 33.2) and can also be appreciated on an axial view of the calcaneus (Fig. 33.3). Haglund's lesion can also be identified on a lateral radiograph.

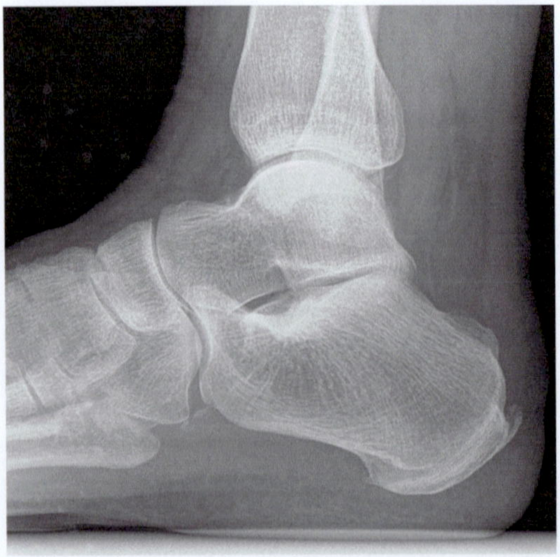

Fig. 33.2 Radiograph demonstrating calcaneal enthesophyte with intrasubstance calcifications

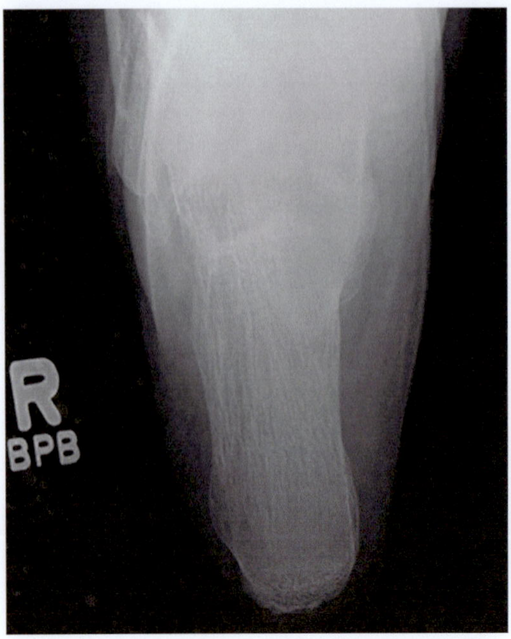

Fig. 33.3 Axial radiograph of the heel demonstrating calcaneal enthesophytes

Magnetic resonance imaging (MRI) can provide useful information regarding the Achilles tendon in both acute and chronic settings. MRI can show thickening of the Achilles tendon substance as well as intrasubstance degenerative changes (Figs. 33.4 and 33.5). MRI can also show pathology at the Achilles insertion including tendon thickening, retrocalcaneal bursitis, and the impact of Haglund's deformity (Fig. 33.6). One study evaluated 118 painful Achilles tendons and found that 15% had intrasubstance abnormalities within 2 cm of the insertion, 19% had an enlarged retrocalcaneal bursa, and 8% had increased signal in the calcaneus (Karjalainen et al. 2000). Nicholson et al. used MRI scans to classify the degree of tendon degeneration in 157 patients with insertional Achilles tendinopathy and were able to predict the success of nonoperative treatment based on these findings (Nicholson et al. 2007). They determined that tendons with confluent areas of intrasubstance signal abnormalities are unlikely to respond to nonoperative treatment.

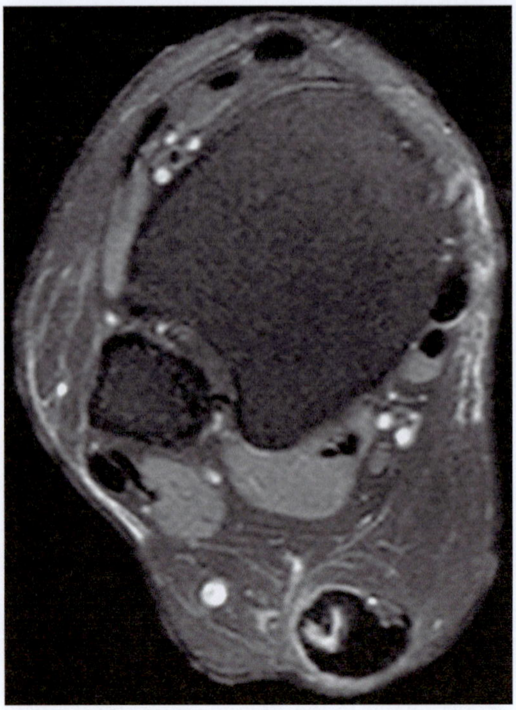

Fig. 33.4 T2-weighted axial MRI scan image demonstrating increased signal in tendon substance representing degenerative tendinosis

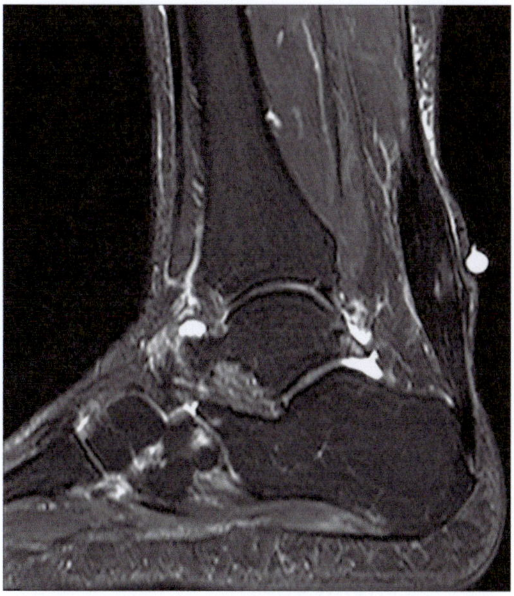

Fig. 33.5 T2-weighted sagittal MRI scan image demonstrating thickening of the midsubstance Achilles tendon with increased signal consistent with tendinosis

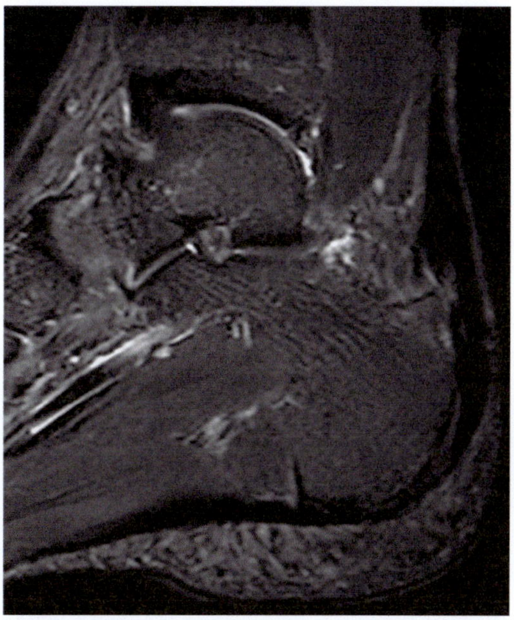

Fig. 33.6 T2-weighted sagittal MRI scan image demonstrating Haglund's lesion with surrounding edema and thickening of the Achilles tendon above the insertion

The role of **diagnostic ultrasound** has increased in recent years as a less-expensive alternative to MRI scan, allowing dynamic examination of the tendon. Astrom et al. compared ultrasound images with MRI images and surgical pathologic findings in 27 patients with chronic Achilles tendinopathy. They concluded both ultrasound and MRI provide similar useful information and both may be utilized as a prognostic instrument (Astrom et al. 1996). Bakkegaard et al. (2015) prospectively evaluated 92 patients with Achilles tendon complaints and found that ultrasound findings of tendon thickness, hypoechogenicity, and increased flow at any time point were significantly correlated to pain with activity, palpatory pain, and morning pain (Bakkegaard et al. 2015).

33.7 Conservative Treatment

Conservative treatment is commonly the first strategy in management for Achilles tendinopathy. In general, 3–6 months of conservative care is instituted before alternative options are implemented and at least 6 months before surgical option is considered. The outcome of surgical treatment after failed conservative management can be unpredictable and generally involves extensive postoperative rehabilitation before return to full activities. (Alfredson 2011; Bohu et al. 2009). Due to the invasiveness and potential pitfalls of surgical interventions, great effort has been undertaken to identify effective conservative treatment modalities in order to avoid surgery, yet achieve optimal clinical outcomes. To date, there is no single modality that has been consistently effective at eradicating symptomatic Achilles tendinopathies, but there are a number of tools that have been shown to be effective in certain patients.

Maffulli's group (Rowe et al. 2012) recently published a systematic review of conservative treatments for non-insertional Achilles tendinopathy, combining graded evidence with qualitative analysis of clinical reasoning. A brief summary of their findings is found below. They also identified important areas requiring future research, including the effectiveness of orthoses, effectiveness of manual therapy, etiological factors, optimal application of loading related to stage of presentation, and optimizing protocols for different types of patients (e.g., the older patient with the metabolic syndrome versus the athletically active).

33.7.1 Eccentric Exercises

Eccentric loading exercises have the strongest supporting evidence of all the conservative treatment modalities in the literature. A high degree of success has been shown in both sedentary and athletic patients with eccentric exercises. However, clinical outcomes vary widely and superior clinical outcomes have been reported for non-insertional tendinopathy, compared with insertional tendinopathy. Most studies use an eccentric training protocol similar to that described by Alfredson et al. (1998). In Rowe et al.'s investigation, physiotherapists commonly used eccentric training and reported using complex clinical reasoning to adapt research protocols for individual patients. As an example, eccentric loading protocols were varied for patients where pain prevented adherence to published protocols by utilizing mixed concentric/eccentric or isometric loading initially (Rowe et al. 2012).

33.7.2 Extracorporeal Shockwave Therapy (ESWT)

ESWT is one the few conservative modalities with a strong support in clinical evidence (Rowe et al. 2012). Low-energy ESWT has the most available evidence and is much less expensive than high energy. One investigation of low-energy ESWT found that VISA-A and pain scores improved at 4 months when ESWT was combined with eccentric exercise training compared with eccentric exercises alone (Rompe et al. 2009). However, at 12 months' follow-up, there was no difference in outcome between the groups. The authors suggested that ESWT might be a useful addition to eccentric exercise for athletic patients desiring a more rapid return to sport.

33.7.3 Continued Tendon Loading or Physical Activity

One excellent quality is that RCT showed no detrimental effect of continued tendon-loading activity (i.e., sporting activity), as long as pain was monitored and a threshold of 5/10 on a VAS was not exceeded (Silbernagel et al. 2007). There are no significant differences in symptomatic outcome between continued tendon loading and active rest groups at a 5 year follow-up (Silbernagel et al. 2011). However, physiotherapists frequently recommend a reduction in the level and frequency of tendon-loading activities (i.e., relative rest), citing anecdotal evidence that this improves treatment outcomes (Rowe et al. 2012).

33.8 Surgical Procedures

33.8.1 Non-insertional Achilles Tendinopathy

As discussed above, at least 6 months of conservative treatments should be tried before surgical intervention. The goal of surgery is to remove degenerative tissue and stimulate tendon healing. In cases of insufficient tendon substance, augmentation with autologous or allogeneic grafts can be implemented as well. Conventional surgical treatment consists of open removal of degenerative tissues, repair of healthy remaining tissues, and release of adhesions with or without resection of the paratenon. If greater than 50% of the tendon is unhealthy and requires debridement, augmentation or reconstruction is recommended to ensure sufficient substance to optimize function and minimize risk of rupture. Other surgical treatments include percutaneous longitudinal tenotomies, gastrocnemius lengthening, endoscopic tendon stripping and tenolysis, open tenosynovectomies, open debridement and tubularization, and tendon augmentation with flexor hallucis longus (FHL) (Fig. 33.7). Further study of most of these treatments is necessary before clear recommendations can be made in terms of their utility.

Complications are not uncommon following surgical treatment procedure. In a large series of 432 consecutive patients, Paavola et al. reported an overall complication rate of 11% of cases. These included wound necrosis in 3%, superficial

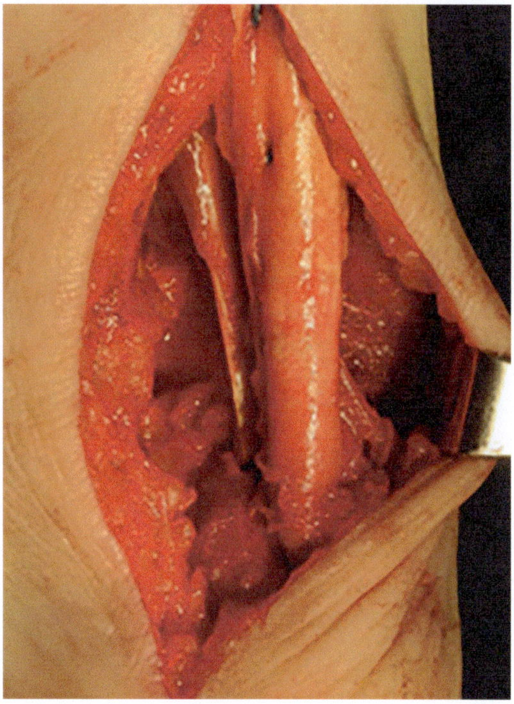

Fig. 33.7 Clinical photograph of transferred FHL tendon adjacent to the Achilles tendon

infection in 2.5%, and sural nerve injury in 1%, with other complications including hematoma, seroma, and deep vein thrombosis (Paavola et al. 2000).

Clinical **outcomes** following surgical treatment for non-insertion Achilles tendinopathy are good in general. Khan et al. performed a systematic review of 62 high-quality studies, finding that the overall success rate for surgery is 83.5%. They also noted that the quality of study methodology (as measured by the Coleman methodology score) improved over time, correlating with a decrease in success rates (Khan et al. 2015). This most likely represents an improvement in the study quality, rather than worsening of outcomes.

33.8.2 Insertional Achilles Tendinopathy

Patients who do not respond to conservative treatment for non-insertional Achilles tendinopathy may also need operative management. There is currently no consensus regarding the duration before surgery, although as in non-insertional disease, most clinicians consider 4–6 months as the minimum time necessary to evaluate the effect of conservative treatment (Kearney and Costa 2010). The surgical strategy for insertional Achilles tendinopathy is removal of all degenerative tissues contributing to pain and dysfunction. Typically this includes one or more of the following structures:

1. Excision of degenerative tendon at or above the insertion on the calcaneus, including intratendinous calcifications
2. Excision of the inflamed retrocalcaneal bursa
3. Resection of the prominent posterior calcaneal prominence (i.e., Haglund's deformity)

If there is excessive tendon degeneration and intratendinous calcification, an open surgical approach is generally required in order to sufficiently remove unhealthy tissue and repair the remaining healthy tissue (Fig. 33.8). It is rare that the majority of the Achilles tendon must be detached, although the central section is the most common site of disease. Reattachment of the insertion using drill holes and/or suture anchors as required will aid in healing and reduce scar tissue. When a significant amount of degenerative tissue is identified and removed, augmentation with a tendon transfer/graft is often warranted (Wiegerinck et al. 2013).

When symptoms are primarily related to prominent Haglund's deformity and inflamed retrocalcaneal bursa, endoscopic calcaneoplasty and resection of the retrocalcaneal bursa can be performed (Phisitkul 2012). This typically entails two endoscopic portals and the use of small joint arthroscope and shaver device to debride the retrocalcaneal bursa and remove prominent Haglund's lesion (Fig. 33.9). Intraoperative fluoroscopy is utilized to ensure sufficient removal of the bone (Fig. 33.10). Biomechanical and clinical data suggest that up to 50% of the Achilles tendon attachment can be safely debrided without compromising the strength of the insertion nor increasing risk of rupture. If greater than 50% of

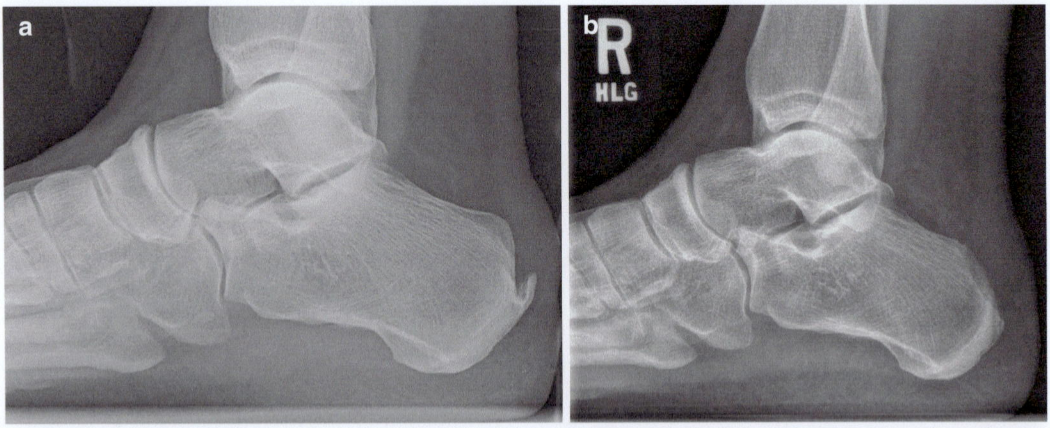

Fig. 33.8 Lateral radiographs demonstrating (**a**) prominent Haglund's lesion and insertional calcaneal enthesophyte in patient with insertional Achilles tendinopathy, (**b**) postoperative film demonstrating removal of enthesophytes and Haglund's lesion

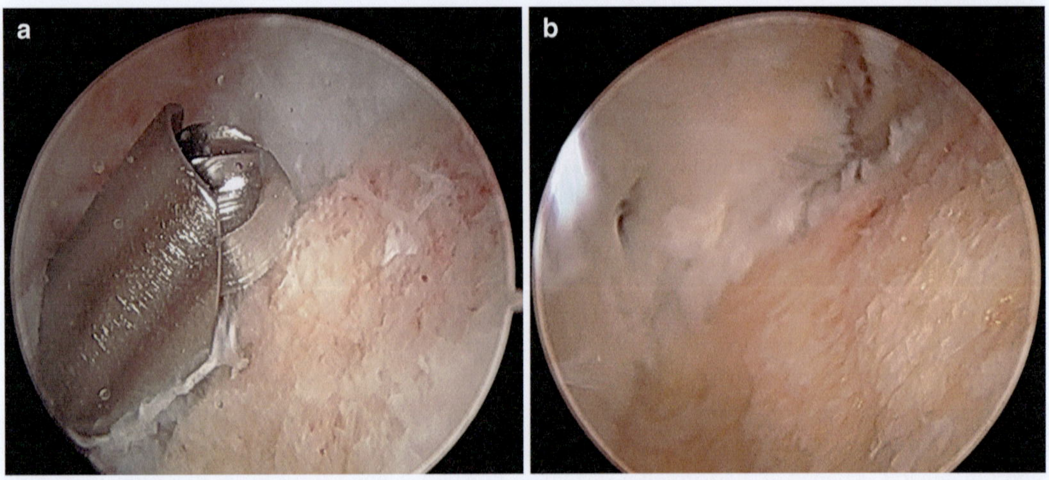

Fig. 33.9 Photographs from endoscopic removal of Haglund's lesion illustrating (**a**) a small joint burr removing prominent bone and (**b**) a healthy Achilles insertion after removal of Haglund's lesion

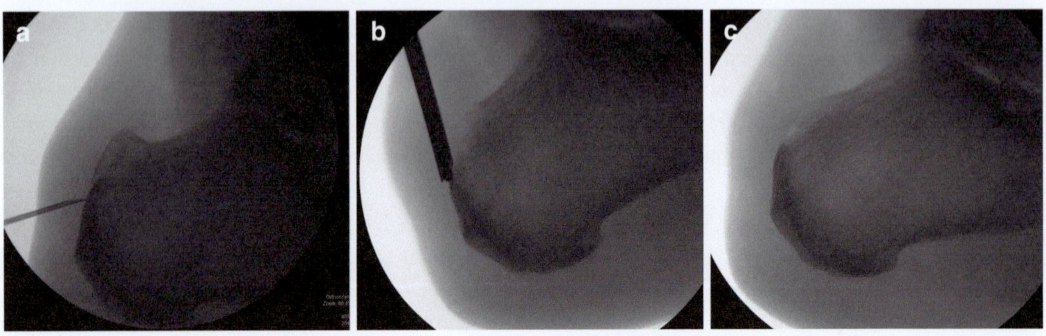

Fig. 33.10 Fluoroscopic images demonstrating (**a**) prominent Haglund's lesion, (**b**) a small joint burr utilized endoscopically to remove Haglund's lesion, and (**c**) after removal of Haglund's lesion and confirmation of a healthy Achilles insertion

the Achilles tendon must be separated from the calcaneal insertion, suture anchors are recommended to reattach the residual tendon. With extensive insertional Achilles tendon disease when as much as 75% of the tendon is excised, augmentation with the local tissue, such as the flexor hallucis longus tendon, or allograft, has been suggested (DeOrio and Easley 2008) (Fig. 33.7).

Traina et al. (2016) reported a systematic review on surgical treatments for insertional Achilles tendinopathy, having 465 surgically treated insertional Achilles tendons with a mean follow-up of 29.8 months on 16 studies. They included both studies of primary surgical debridements and those that included augmentation for excessive tendon loss. They reported that results were good or excellent in 89.6% of cases and fair or poor in 10.4%. Average complication rate was 18.3% (Traina et al. 2016; Hunt et al. 2015) published a randomized control trial comparing FHL transfer to debridement alone in patients over 50 years of age. They found no differences in pain, functional outcome (as measured by the AOFAS ankle/hindfoot scale), and patient satisfaction when comparing patients treated with Achilles debridement alone versus FHL augmentation for chronic Achilles tendinopathy. However, ankle plantar flexion strength was improved with FHL transfer, with no loss of hallux plantar flexion strength.

Conclusion

Achilles tendinopathy is a very common clinical syndrome characterized by the combination of pain, swelling, and impaired function. It can impact active and nonactive people alike, but has particularly high prevalence in running and jumping athletes. The etiology of Achilles tendinopathy is multifactorial and typically includes one or more intrinsic and extrinsic factors. Histological studies have determined this to be a degenerative process rather than an inflammatory one. The sources of pain in Achilles tendinopathy are very complicated, necessitating a careful history and physical examination to determine the appropriate course of treatment. There are a number of conservative treatments for these disorders which should be attempted before surgical intervention is considered. For patients who fail conservative treatments, surgical intervention is recommended and is associated with good success rates in most patients. However, there is no gold standard of the treatments because of the inconsistent clinical results between various studies. Additional high-quality clinical outcome studies are needed in this area, particularly to assess some of the promising new technologies making their way into the treatment armamentarium.

References

Abate M, Silbernagel KG, Siljeholm C, Di Iorio A, De Amicis D, Salini V, Werner S, Paganelli R (2009) Pathogenesis of tendinopathies: inflammation or degeneration? Arthritis Res Ther 11:235

Alfredson H (2011) Where to now with Achilles tendon treatment? Br J Sports Med 45:386

Alfredson H, Pietila T, Jonsson P, Lorentzon R (1998) Heavy-load eccentric calf muscle training for the treatment of chronic Achilles tendinosis. Am J Sports Med 26:360–366

Almekinders LC (1998) Tendinitis and other chronic tendinopathies. J Am Acad Orthop Surg 6:157–164

Astrom M, Gentz CF, Nilsson P, Rausing A, Sjoberg S, Westlin N (1996) Imaging in chronic Achilles tendinopathy: a comparison of ultrasonography, magnetic resonance imaging and surgical findings in 27 histologically verified cases. Skeletal Radiol 25:615–620

Bakkegaard M, Johannsen FE, Hojgaard B, Langberg H (2015) Ultrasonography as a prognostic and objective parameter in Achilles tendinopathy: a prospective observational study. Eur J Radiol 84:458–462

Bohu Y, Lefevre N, Bauer T, Laffenetre O, Herman S, Thaunat M, Cucurulo T, Franceschi JP, Cermolacce C, Rolland E (2009) Surgical treatment of Achilles tendinopathies in athletes. Multicenter retrospective series of open surgery and endoscopic techniques. Orthop Traumatol Surg Res 95:S72–S77

Cook JL, Purdam CR (2009) Is tendon pathology a continuum? A pathology model to explain the clinical presentation of load-induced tendinopathy. Br J Sports Med 43:409–416

DeOrio MJ, Easley ME (2008) Surgical strategies: insertional Achilles tendinopathy. Foot Ankle Int 29:542–550

Fukashiro S, Komi PV, Jarvinen M, Miyashita M (1995) In vivo Achilles tendon loading during jumping in humans. Eur J Appl Physiol Occup Physiol 71:453–458

Hunt KJ, Jones CP, Anderson RB, Cohen BE, Davis WH (2015) Surgical treatment of insertional Achilles tendinopathy with or without flexor hallucis longus tendon transfer: A prospective, randomized, clinical study. Foot Ankle Int. 36(9):998–1005

Holmes GB, Lin J (2006) Etiologic factors associated with symptomatic Achilles tendinopathy. Foot Ankle Int 27:952–959

Irwin TA (2010) Current concepts review: insertional Achilles tendinopathy. Foot Ankle Int 31: 933–939

Karjalainen PT, Soila K, Aronen HJ, Pihlajamaki HK, Tynninen O, Paavonen T, Tirman PF (2000) MR imaging of overuse injuries of the Achilles tendon. AJR Am J Roentgenol 175:251–260

Kearney R, Costa ML (2010) Insertional Achilles tendinopathy management: a systematic review. Foot Ankle Int 31:689–694

Ker RF (1999) The design of soft collagenous load-bearing tissues. J Exp Biol 202:3315–3324

Khan WS, Malvankar S, Bhamra JS, Pengas I (2015) Analysing the outcome of surgery for chronic Achilles tendinopathy over the last 50 years. World J Orthop 6:491–497

Kirchgesner T, Larbi A, Omoumi P, Malghem J, Zamali N, Manelfe J, Lecouvet F, Vande Berg B, Djebbar S, Dallaudiere B (2014) Drug-induced tendinopathy: from physiology to clinical applications. Joint Bone Spine 81:485–492

Knobloch K (2016) Drug-induced tendon disorders. Adv Exp Med Biol 920:229–238

Kvist M (1991) Achilles tendon injuries in athletes. Ann Chir Gynaecol 80:188–201

Li HY, Hua YH (2016) Achilles tendinopathy: current concepts about the basic science and clinical treatments. Biomed Res Int 2016:6492597

Lysholm J, Wiklander J (1987) Injuries in runners. Am J Sports Med 15:168–171

Maffulli N, Khan KM, Puddu G (1998) Overuse tendon conditions: time to change a confusing terminology. Arthroscopy 14:840–843

Maffulli N, Wong J, Almekinders LC (2003) Types and epidemiology of tendinopathy. Clin Sports Med 22:675–692

Nicholson CW, Berlet GC, Lee TH (2007) Prediction of the success of nonoperative treatment of insertional Achilles tendinosis based on MRI. Foot Ankle Int 28:472–477

Paavola M, Kannus P, Jarvinen TA, Khan K, Jozsa L, Jarvinen M (2002) Achilles tendinopathy. J Bone Joint Surg Am 84-A:2062–2076

Paavola M, Orava S, Leppilahti J, Kannus P, Jarvinen M (2000) Chronic Achilles tendon overuse injury: complications after surgical treatment. An analysis of 432 consecutive patients. Am J Sports Med 28:77–82

Phisitkul P (2012) Endoscopic surgery of the Achilles tendon. Curr Rev Musculoskelet Med 5:156–163

Rompe JD, Furia J, Maffulli N (2009) Eccentric loading versus eccentric loading plus shock-wave treatment for midportion Achilles tendinopathy: a randomized controlled trial. Am J Sports Med 37:463–470

Rowe V, Hemmings S, Barton C, Malliaras P, Maffulli N, Morrissey D (2012) Conservative management of midportion Achilles tendinopathy: a mixed methods study, integrating systematic review and clinical reasoning. Sports Med 42:941–967

Silbernagel KG, Brorsson A, Lundberg M (2011) The majority of patients with Achilles tendinopathy recover fully when treated with exercise alone: a 5-year follow-up. Am J Sports Med 39:607–613

Silbernagel KG, Thomee R, Eriksson BI, Karlsson J (2007) Continued sports activity, using a pain-monitoring model, during rehabilitation in patients with Achilles tendinopathy: a randomized controlled study. Am J Sports Med 35:897–906

Slane LC, Thelen DG (2014) Non-uniform displacements within the Achilles tendon observed during passive and eccentric loading. J Biomech 47:2831–2835

Sobhani S, Dekker R, Postema K, Dijkstra PU (2013) Epidemiology of ankle and foot overuse injuries in sports: a systematic review. Scand J Med Sci Sports 23:669–686

Traina F, Ruffilli A, Mazzotti A, Meliconi R, Berti L, Faldini C (2016) Surgical treatment of insertional Achilles tendinopathy: a systematic review. J Biol Regul Homeost Agents 30:131–138

Tuite DJ, Renstrom PA, O'Brien M (1997) The aging tendon. Scand J Med Sci Sports 7:72–77

Waldecker U, Hofmann G, Drewitz S (2012) Epidemiologic investigation of 1394 feet: coincidence of hindfoot malalignment and Achilles tendon disorders. Foot Ankle Surg 18:119–123

Wiegerinck JI, Kerkhoffs GM, van Sterkenburg MN, Sierevelt IN, van Dijk CN (2013) Treatment for insertional Achilles tendinopathy: a systematic review. Knee Surg Sports Traumatol Arthrosc 21:1345–1355

Tibialis Posterior and Anterior Tendons

34

Hélder Pereira, Manuel Resende Sousa, Daniel Mendes, Joaquim M. Oliveira, Rui L. Reis, João Espregueira-Mendes, J. Batista, and Pedro Luís Ripoll

Contents

H. Pereira (✉)
Orthopedic Department Centro Hospitalar Póvoa de Varzim, Vila do Conde, Portugal

Ripoll y De Prado Sport Clinic—FIFA Medical Centre of Excellence, Murcia-Madrid, Spain

3B's Research Group–Biomaterials, Biodegradables and Biomimetics, University of Minho, Headquarters of the European Institute of Excellence on Tissue Engineering and Regenerative Medicine, AvePark, S. Cláudio de Barco, 4806-909 Taipas, Guimarães, Portugal

ICVS/3B's–PT Government Associate Laboratory, Braga/Guimarães, Portugal
e-mail: helderduartepereira@gmail.com

M.R. Sousa
Foot and Ankle Unit, Hospital Beatriz Ângelo, Lisbon, Portugal

Foot and Ankle Unit, Hospital da Luz, Lisbon, Portugal

Sporting Clube de Portugal, Lisbon, Portugal

D. Mendes
Foot and Ankle Unit, Hospital Beatriz Ângelo, Lisbon, Portugal

Foot and Ankle Unit, Hospital da Luz Setúbal, Setubal, Portugal

J.M. Oliveira • R.L. Reis
3B's Research Group–Biomaterials, Biodegradables and Biomimetics, University of Minho, Headquarters of the European Institute of Excellence on Tissue Engineering and Regenerative Medicine, AvePark, S. Cláudio de Barco, 4806-909 Taipas, Guimarães, Portugal

ICVS/3B's–PT Government Associate Laboratory, Braga/Guimarães, Portugal

J. Espregueira-Mendes
3B's Research Group–Biomaterials, Biodegradables and Biomimetics, University of Minho, Headquarters of the European Institute of Excellence on Tissue Engineering and Regenerative Medicine, AvePark, S. Cláudio de Barco, 4806-909 Taipas, Guimarães, Portugal

ICVS/3B's–PT Government Associate Laboratory, Braga/Guimarães, Portugal

Clínica do Dragão, Espregueira-Mendes Sports Centre—FIFA Medical Centre of Excellence, Porto, Portugal
e-mail: jem@espregueira.com

G.L. Canata et al. (eds.), *Muscle and Tendon Injuries*, DOI 10.1007/978-3-662-54184-5_34

J. Batista
Clinical Department Club Atletico Boca Juniores and CAJB—Centro Artroscopico,
Buenos Aires, Argentina

P.L. Ripoll
Ripoll y De Prado Sport Clinic—FIFA Medical Centre of Excellence, Murcia-Madrid, Spain

34.1 Introduction

Sports activities are increasing worldwide as a promoter of global health (Palacios-Cena et al. 2012). Enhanced proprioception and fine-tuned neuromuscular control around the foot and ankle are particularly required for gait in uneven ground and most types of sports (Cote et al. 2005). This includes fine balance between dorsiflexion-plantarflexion and pronation-supination. General population is presenting increased and earlier attention to foot and ankle tendon-related disorders probably led by their higher functional demand. This fact might play a role in earlier diagnosis of some condition in its primary stages thus also influencing the clinical outcome. This is of paramount relevance in the herein described conditions.

The ankle joint complex comprises the tibiotalar (talocrural), talocalcaneal (subtalar), and transverse tarsal (talocalcaneonavicular) joints (Brockett and Chapman 2016).

Plantar- and dorsiflexion occur predominantly at the tibiotalar joint (Brockett and Chapman 2016). Pronation-supination mostly depends on subtalar joint but tibiotalar and talocalcaneonavicular participate at different levels. Foot pronation is a complex movement which combines abduction of the forefoot, eversion of the hindfoot, and dorsiflexion (Gluck et al. 2010). Supination also happens in the three planes while combining internal ankle rotation, hindfoot adduction, forefoot inversion, and medial arch elevation. Pronation provides some degree of flexibility opposing to supination which increases foot stability (Cote et al. 2005).

The *tibialis anterior* (together with the *extensor hallucis longus*) produces dorsiflexion and some degree of inversion of the foot (Brockett and Chapman 2016). The *extensor digitorum longus* only produces dorsiflexion of the foot. The *tibialis posterior* (together with the *flexor digitorum longus* and the *flexor hallucis longus*) produces plantarflexion and inversion of the foot (Otis and Gage 2001; Brockett and Chapman 2016). Conversely, peroneal muscles (PMs), including *peroneus longus*, *brevis*, and *tertius*, are the active evertors of the foot (Selmani et al. 2006). Plantarflexion of the foot is furthermore provided by the *triceps surae* and *plantaris muscles*. These muscles play a key role controlling ankle motion (Brockett and Chapman 2016).

In order to understand and properly deal with physiopathology, it is mandatory to comprehend the fundamental biomechanics of the foot and ankle. The navicular bone is considered a "key bone" providing distal support to the talus. It is the highest structure of the longitudinal medial arch in the standing position. In the static position, the balance of these structures relies on the surrounding bones and the spring ligament (calcaneonavicular). In motion, the action of the posterior tibial muscle (PTM) preserves the superior position of the navicular thus assisting in the support of the medial arch. Therefore, a weakened PTM (e.g., neurologic conditions) or an insufficient posterior tibial tendon (PTT) is incapable to sustain the navicular in place, and a collapse of the medial arch might happen (acquired flatfoot condition) (Lhoste-Trouilloud 2012). From gait analysis, one observes a dorsiflexion moment at heel strike as the dorsiflexors (e.g., *tibialis anterior*) eccentrically contract to control the rotation of the foot and avoids the foot from slapping the ground (Brockett and Chapman 2016). These basic examples are representatives of the paramount relevance of biomechanical phenomena in this field.

Some principles of clinical assessment are common to both groups of pathology. Clinical examination while standing and gait analysis are critical in any foot and ankle conditions. Moreover, global assessment, including alignment, of inferior limbs is required.

Radiological study must always include standing foot and ankle x-rays. Further views might be considered according to the clinical findings and local experience. Ultrasound and MRI might be useful (Fig. 34.1); however, limitations exist and

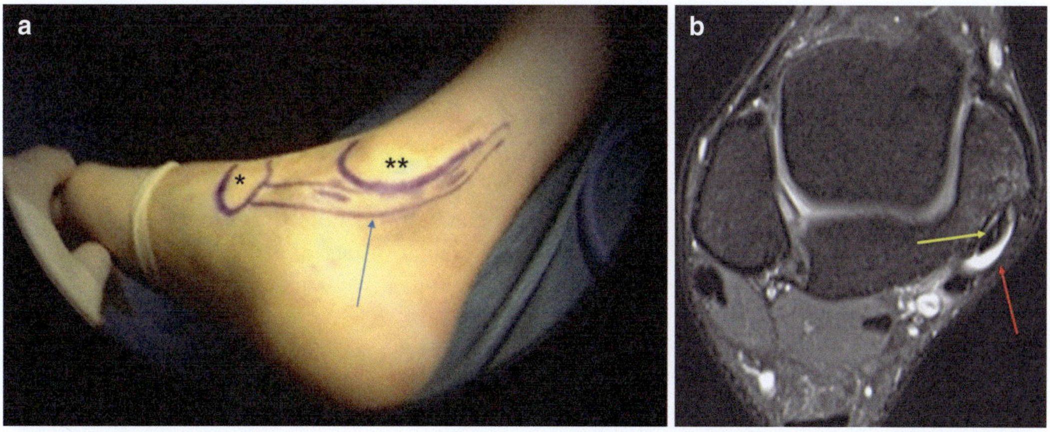

Fig. 34.1 (**a**) Surface anatomy with *blue arrow* representing hypovascular zone along with posterior tibial tendon course, (*asterisk*) navicular bone, and (*double asterisk*) medial malleolus. (**b**) MRI axial view with intratendon signal changes in the hypovascular zone (*yellow arrow*) and fluid within its sheath (*red arrow*)

must be acknowledged. Ultrasound is known to be operator dependent while providing dynamic evaluation (Nallamshetty et al. 2005). MRI is considered diagnostically specific but not highly sensitive for some tendon-related disorders (Park et al. 2012; van Sterkenburg et al. 2010b). Local anesthetic injection might be helpful to confirm the origin of pain (Cooper et al. 2007). CT scans are particularly useful in the study of bony structures which might be suspected (e.g., navicular deformities, bone ossicles/spurs). Endoscopic/tendoscopic evaluation provides direct inspection and is gaining popularity in either diagnostic or therapeutic approaches (van Sterkenburg et al. 2010b; Park et al. 2012).

Shoewear inspection is also required either because of its possible contribution to pathology (e.g., shoes-related compression might cause inflammatory reaction) or because it might reflect some conditions (e.g., uneven wear of shoe soles might reflect malalignment) (Kulig et al. 2009).

Listening to the patient's complaints is critical. The targets are to identify its cause, worsening, and relief factors and understand its functional implication. Moreover, clinicians must understand patient's expectations and provide "realistic" information of therapeutic options.

Herein, the most common conditions affecting anterior tibial tendon (ATT) and PTT will be discussed. Despite being rare, simultaneous affections of both tendons resulting in severe flatfoot and dropfoot gait have been described requiring surgical treatment (Frigg et al. 2006).

The concepts of tendinopathy are described elsewhere and thus are out of the scope of this work.

34.2 Posterior Tibial Tendon Pathology

34.2.1 Clinical Anatomy

Tibialis posterior muscle arises from the posterior aspect of the tibia and fibula and from the interosseous membrane. PTT passes immediately behind the medial malleolus, through a fibrous tunnel which is covered by the flexor retinaculum. After contouring the malleolus, the tendon begins to fan out. It has a wide insertion including the navicular, the *sustentaculum tali*, first cuneiform bones, and the bases of the second, third, and fourth metatarsals. The PTT is an important dynamic stabilizer of the medial arch and the most powerful inverter of the foot (Gluck et al. 2010). The spring ligament complex is the static soft tissue support of the talonavicular joint and also plays a key role in its biomechanics (Boss and Hintermann 2002). The PTT does not have a mesotenon.

A retromalleolar hypovascular region (Fig. 34.1) has been observed and can be implicated in degenerative changes of the tendon (Frey et al. 1990; Manske et al. 2015). The posterior tibial tendon is usually supplied by two vessels entering the tendon approximately 4.5 cm proximal and 2.0 cm distal to the medial malleolus (Manske et al. 2015).

34.2.2 Etiology and Pathogenesis

Inflammatory, degenerative, functional, and traumatic processes might lead to PTT dysfunction at different levels (Yao et al. 2015). Inflammatory diseases (e.g., lupus or rheumatoid arthritis) are more common in younger patients (Myerson 1997; Otis and Gage 2001). Chronic overuse and consequent tendon deterioration have been noticed to occur more often and more frequently in late to middle age, women, and obese (Myerson 1997; Otis and Gage 2001). However, degeneration due to overtraining with repetitive microtrauma has also been described among young athletes, particularly in running and sports requiring repeated and rapid changes in direction (Ribbans and Garde 2013; Supple et al. 1992). Inflammatory changes, tendon tears, and tenosynovitis have been connected to activity levels around 1500 to 2000 cycles per hour (Bare and Haddad 2001).

Other risk factors include hyperpronation or anomalous anatomy, ligamentous laxity, diabetes mellitus, hypertension, and corticosteroid therapy (Yao et al. 2015). Moreover, Probasco et al. recently stated that an increased valgus orientation of the subtalar joint is more frequent among patients with adult acquired flatfoot when compared to controls (Probasco et al. 2015). Acute trauma is rarely the cause of tendon dysfunction or rupture (Trnka 2004).

The precise mechanisms leading to PTT degeneration remain unclear. The combination of the hypovascular zone and abnormal mechanical forces experienced behind the medial malleolus where the tendon acutely changes direction in several activities might play a role (Trnka 2004).

The summary of sequential events might be summarized: loss of posterior tibialis function results in collapse of the medial longitudinal arch and increased stress in the medial structures of the foot. Gradually, there is weakening of the medial ligaments: the spring ligament (connects the anterior margin of the *sustentaculum tali* to the plantar surface of the navicular) gradually ails with repetitive loading, leading to a flatfoot deformity. The deltoid ligament also might become insufficient, permitting the talus to tilt into valgus. In the hindfoot valgus, the Achilles tendon becomes an evertor due to its position lateral to the axis of the subtalar joint and also might become shortened/contracted, resulting in an equinus deformity.

34.2.3 Clinical Presentation and Imaging

A patient suffering from PTT tendinopathy might refer isolated posteromedial ankle pain. The natural history is usually slow, with insidious onset of complaints which can cause delay in searching for assistance. However, on clinical examination one can find local tenderness, medial pain (sometimes irradiating to the calf), positive PTT provocation test, or inability to walk on tiptoes. Over time, patients may notice progressive collapse of the medial longitudinal arch (acquired flatfoot) and increased hindfoot valgus. The shoe soles may show signs of increased wear on the medial side, and they may report difficulty standing on their toes due to pain and weakness.

Pain usually worsens with walking and progressively affects sports and activities of daily living (Trnka 2004). On later stages of the disease, patients often report that pain shifts laterally as the fibula begins to impinge against the calcaneus while the medial pain often disappears (Yao et al. 2015). At these stages sports activities are severely compromised if possible at all.

Examination (Fig. 34.2) should begin with inspection through all sides while standing (including podoscope for plantar view). The examiner should search for increased valgus angulation of the hindfoot and abduction of the

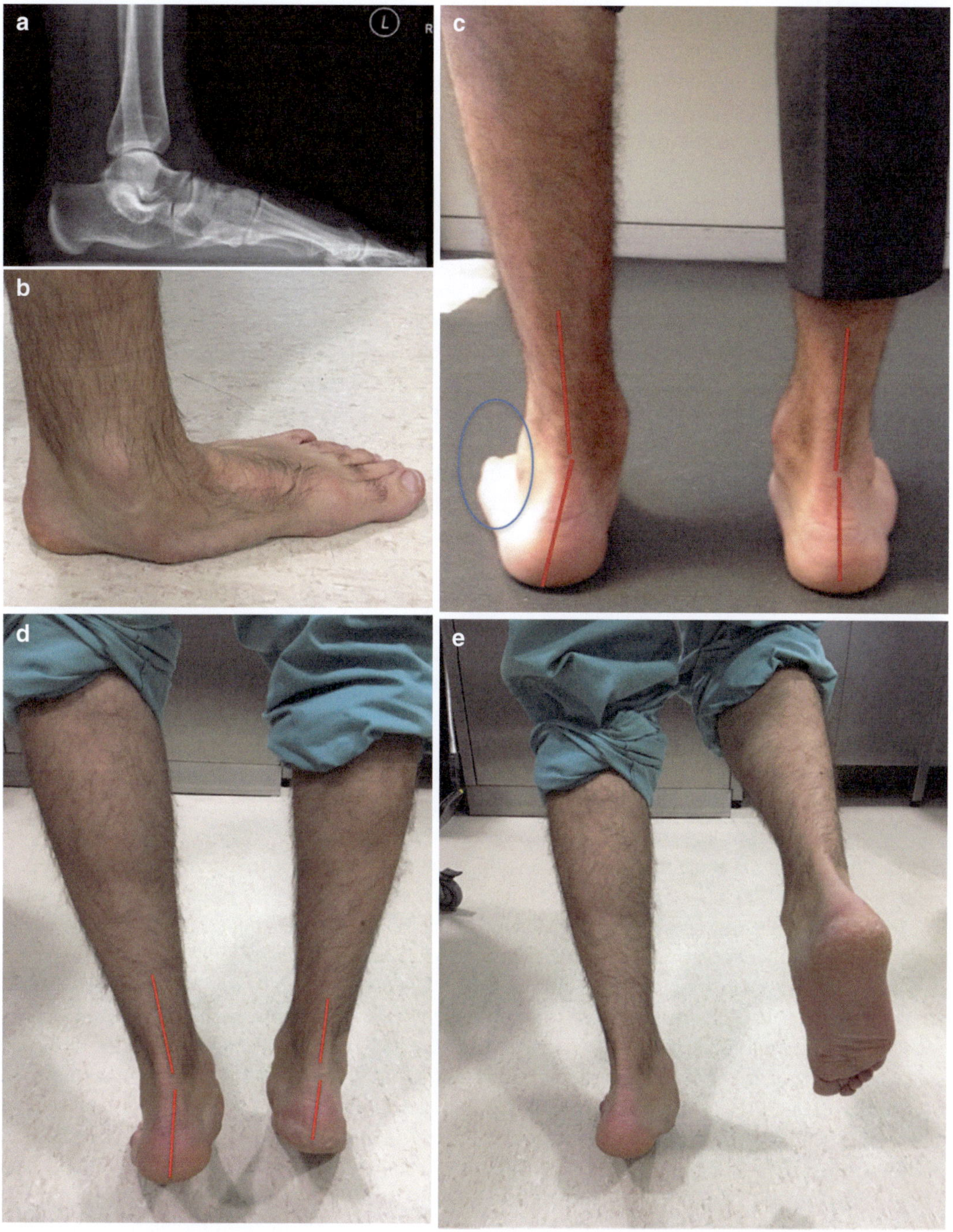

Fig. 34.2 (**a**) X-ray lateral view with characteristic changes of adult flatfoot; (**b**) lateral view of the foot with visible collapse of medial arch; (**c**) posterior view with hindfoot valgus and "to many toes sign" on the *left* foot opposing to neutral alignment of the *right* foot (*red lines* represent hindfoot alignment); (**d**) the valgus alignment is not corrected when raising the heels; (**e**) positive single "heel raise test" on the *left* foot. The patient is incapable to raise and experiences pain, and the valgus does not correct during the attempt

forefoot. Both these features are reflected in a positive "too many toes" sign, in which more toes are visible on the lateral side of the affected foot when viewed from behind given the increased hindfoot valgus and forefoot abduction (Johnson 1983).

Next, the "heel-rise test" (Fig. 34.2) is performed to assess severity of the condition (Johnson 1983). The patient is asked to attempt to rise onto the ball of the affected foot while keeping the contralateral foot lifted off the ground. The normal foot is also tested for comparison. A positive test is considered if the affected hindfoot will either remain in valgus abduction during the heel raise (once the PTT fails to invert it) or the patient will refer important pain limiting this movement. It might be required to repeat the test a few times for proper assessment. Hintermann and Gächter have described another useful test: the first metatarsal rise sign (Hintermann and Gachter 1996). The patient is asked to stand in full weight bearing on both feet. The examiner will then externally rotate the shin of the affected foot with one hand. In the presence of marked PTT insufficiency, the head of the first metatarsal will be lifted off the floor (fixed supination of the first ray).

Subsequent clinical examination can be managed with the patient seated. The PTT should be palpated throughout its course to assess for a palpable gap, crepitation, tenderness, or swelling. The lateral side of the foot should also be palpated once subfibular tenderness may be an indication of calcaneofibular impingement. Palpation and strength assessment should be repeated with resisted inversion and compared to the opposite side. The foot is held in slight plantarflexion and eversion to isolate the posterior tibialis from the synergistic action of tibialis anterior (Myerson and Corrigan 1996). The patient is then asked to invert and further plantarflex the foot against resistance, while the examiner palpates for the posterior tibialis tendon to determine its integrity and the painful site. The mobility of the ankle and the subtalar joint should be carefully assessed given the implication in the method of treatment. Range of motion at the subtalar joint will progressively decrease with the progression of the condition, and eventually the hindfoot will assume a fixed valgus deformity. The forefoot and midfoot will try to compensate for this by progressively adopting a supinated position, which is best appreciated with the heel in a neutral position. This is another critical part of the examination because a fixed supination deformity of the forefoot is an important consideration in the subsequent selection of treatment (Yao et al. 2015).

It is also mandatory to assess the Achilles tendon for contracture. This is often associated with chronic hindfoot valgus once the Achilles tendon adopts an abnormal position lateral to the axis of the subtalar joint, leading to tendon shortening over time (Yao et al. 2015).

Radiographies assess global foot and ankle morphology and alignment and are helpful in later stages of these disorders. In early stages, they are often normal.

Standing anteroposterior and lateral view (Fig. 34.2) radiographs of both feet and ankles as well as mortise views of the ankle joint should be ordered. The collapse of the longitudinal arch on a lateral weight-bearing radiograph might be noticed in any of the following measurements, especially if asymmetric: calcaneal inclination angle (angle between the calcaneal inclination axis and the supporting surface, considered low if less than 20°), talometatarsal angle (angle between the axis of the talus and the axis of the first metatarsal, normally between 0° and 10°), or the distance of the medial cuneiform from the floor (normally between 15 and 25 mm) (Slovenkai 1997).

Uncovering of the talar head might be recognizable on an anteroposterior view. With increased forefoot abduction deformity, the navicular slides laterally, leading to subluxation of the talonavicular joint which is abnormal if more than 15% of the talar head is uncovered (Slovenkai 1997). Plain radiographs might also show talar tilt; calcaneofibular impingement; arthritic changes of the tibiotalar, subtalar, and talonavicular joints; and signs of enthesopathy in the form of bony irregularities and hypertrophic changes at the navicular insertion site of the posterior tibialis tendon (Kong and Van Der Vliet 2008).

MRI (Fig. 34.3) and ultrasound, despite known limitations in low-grade PTT disease, are

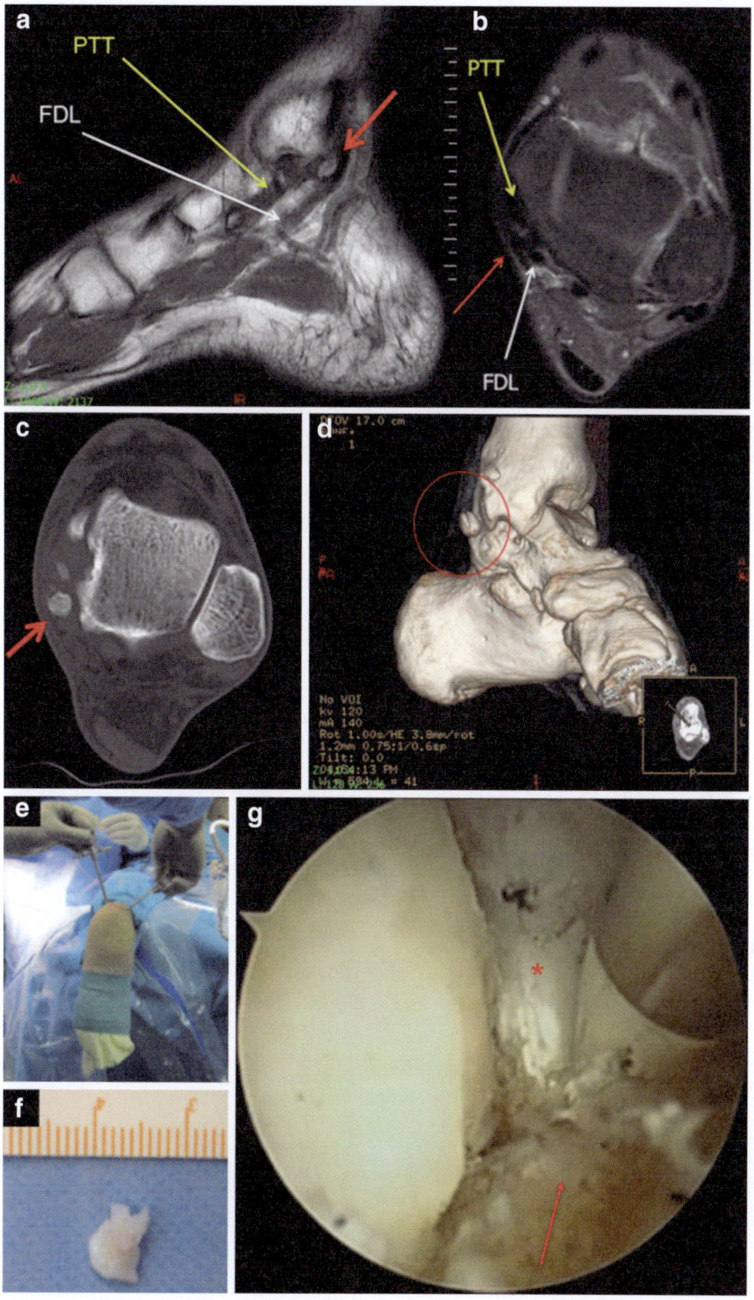

Fig. 34.3 (**a** and **b**) represent MRI views (sagittal and axial, respectively) of posterior tibial tendon (PTT) and flexor digitorum longus (FDL). (**c** and **d**) show CT axial and 3D images. *Red arrows* and *red circle* indicate bone ossicle causing tendon's irritation. (**e**) shows posterior ankle arthroscopic approach. (**f**) The removed ossicle. (**g**) Arthroscopic view where PTT (*red* *) and the ossicle (*red arrow*) are visible, with distal tibia on the *left* and surgical instrument on the *right*

useful in identifying different pathologies, such as tenosynovitis (longitudinal) ruptures, degenerative changes, or adhesions (Cooper et al. 2007; Lhoste-Trouilloud 2012). Moreover, MRI can be useful in identifying spring and deltoid ligament injuries (Kong and Van Der Vliet 2008; Nallamshetty et al. 2005).

CT scan is useful in identifying bone ossicles (Fig. 34.3) and deformities, namely, secondary to fractures which might cause persistent damage to the tendon (Kong and Van Der Vliet 2008).

When dealing with diagnosis of PTT disorders, one must also consider and rule out subtalar arthritis, Müller-Weiss disease, Lisfranc joint pathology, consequences of fractures or bone ossicles, PTT subluxation, coalition, Charcot arthropathy, spring ligament injury, and deltoid ligament injury.

34.2.4 Principles for Treatment

Johnson and Strom proposed a classification system correlating the severity of PTT dysfunction and subsequent adaptations of the foot to treatment recommendations (Johnson and Strom 1989). This classification was further refined by Myerson (Myerson 1997) and Bluman (Bluman et al. 2007) (Table 34.1 summarizes one of the most popular classification systems). Further classifications have been proposed, and all try to correlate major clinical findings and treatment options (Haddad et al. 2011). Treatments of PTT disorders include conservative and surgical options depending on the severity of the condition.

In the early stages of the disease, conservative treatment is recommended. This comprises modification of activity, cryotherapy, physiotherapy, medication, insoles, corrective shoes (medial heel and sole wedge), and orthosis (Kulig et al. 2009).

In common patients, when a trial of 3–6 months of conservative treatment has failed with progression of symptoms (Ribbans and Garde 2013; Bare and Haddad 2001), tendoscopy represents an option with increased popularity (Khazen and Khazen 2012; van Dijk et al. 1997). Tendoscopy (Fig. 34.4) is considered in grade I

Table 34.1 PTT disease classification of Johnson and Strom (1989) modified by Myerson and Bluman (Bluman et al. 2007)

	Clinical findings	Physical examination	Radiographs
Stage I	• Tenosynovitis • No deformity	• Single-heel raise+ • Too many toes sign(−)	• Normal
Stage IIA	• Flatfoot deformity • Flexible hindfoot • Normal forefoot	• Single-leg heel raise(−) • Too many toes sign+ • Mild sinus tarsi pain	• Medial arch collapse deformity
Stage IIB	• Flatfoot deformity • Flexible hindfoot • Forefoot abduction ("too many toes," >40% talonavicular uncoverage)		
Stage IIC	• Flatfoot deformity • Flexible hindfoot • Forefoot abduction • Medial ray instability (not corrected with ankle plantarflexion)		
Stage III	• Flatfoot deformity • Rigid forefoot abduction • Rigid hindfoot valgus	• Single-leg heel raise(−) • Too many toes sign+ • Severe sinus tarsi pain	• Medial arch collapse deformity • Subtalar arthritis
Stage IV	• Flatfoot deformity • Rigid forefoot abduction • Rigid hindfoot valgus • Deltoid ligament injury	• Single-leg heel raise(−) • Too many toes sign+ • Severe sinus tarsi pain • Ankle pain	• Medial arch collapse deformity • Subtalar arthritis • Talar tilt

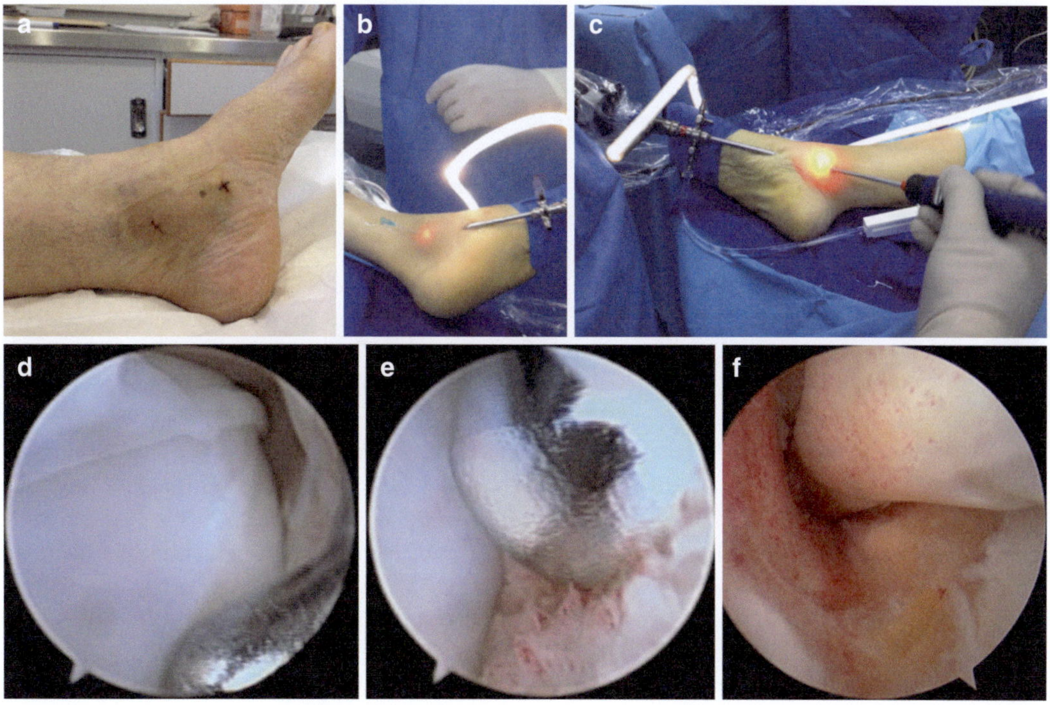

Fig. 34.4 Posterior tibial tendon tendoscopy (PTT) with portal placement (**a**), arthroscope introduced by the distal portal and proximal portable created using transillumination and a needle (**b**). With arthroscope and shaver (**c**) the debridement of partial longitudinal ruptures (**d**) or synovectomy is possible (**e**). Inflammatory changes in the synovia and the tendon are often found in rheumatoid patients (**f**)

(Khazen and Khazen 2012; Chow et al. 2005; van Dijk et al. 1997) and selected cases of early grade II cases (Lui 2007). However, one must consider that particularly in patients with inflammatory diseases, the process of tendon degradation secondary to synovitis might be more aggressive, and surgical treatment is considered earlier (6-week trial of conservative treatment) (Myerson et al. 1989).

More complex approaches include the combined treatment of spring and deltoid ligaments as recently described by Lui et al. (Lui 2015, 2016a). Posterior arthroscopic approach (Fig. 34.3) has also been described and might also be used for the removal of bone ossicles in post-traumatic cases (Hua et al. 2015). However, these approaches should be further validated by clinical evidence before widespread recommendation.

Currently, indications for posterior tibial tendon tendoscopy (van Dijk et al. 1997; Pereira et al. 2014) include:

- Tenosynovectomy
- Tendon sheath release
- Tendon debridement and cleaning of partial rupture
- Resection of pathological vincula
- Removal of exostosis/irregularity of posterior tibial sliding tunnel
- Endoscopic removal of implants (screws/anchors) from medial malleolus
- Adhesiolysis
- Diagnostic procedure

PTT tendoscopy enables diagnostic confirmation of symptomatic partial tendon tear (false positives and false negatives have been described on MRI and ultrasound) (van Sterkenburg et al. 2010b). Partial tendon tears can be definitively treated endoscopically. However, if that is not the case, it will help to diminish open surgical approach thus contributing in the worst-case scenario to lower the incision, diminish postoperative pain, and contribute to earlier rehabilitation. The tendoscopic procedure can be converted to a "guided" mini-open approach, which is still less invasive than the standard open procedure (Pereira et al. 2014).

34.3 Technique for Posterior Tibial Tendoscopy (van Dijk et al. 1997)

Patient is positioned supine. For superficial landmarks the patient should be questioned before being anesthetized to actively invert the foot. In this way, the painful site can be identified as well as the course of the PTT facilitating the placement of the portals. The distal portal is performed first, 2.5 cm distal to the posterior edge of the medial malleolus. A 2.7 or 4.0 mm arthroscope is introduced, and the complete tendon sheath should be inspected. The proximal portal is made under direct vision. Tissue debridement by means of shaver or tendon repair by using recently developed suture tools can be used. At the end of the procedure, the portals are sutured, and a bandage is applied. Active range of motion of the ankle (plantarflexion-dorsiflexion) is encouraged since the first day. Partial weight bearing is advised for 2–3 days and gradually resumption of daily activities as tolerated. Sutures are removed from 10 to 14 days.

34.4 Operative Treatment Guidelines

The goals for treatment depend on the severity of the disease and include: control of symptoms, restore function, stop progression of the deformity, and obtain adequate alignment.

- Stage I—Endoscopic or open (McCormack et al. 2003) tendon debridement or synovectomy (Fig. 34.4) is a valid option in symptom controls after failed conservative treatment. Tendon repair with or without augmentation by flexor tendon transfer (most commonly using the flexor digitorum longus) might be considered (Vora et al. 2006). Some authors combine medial sliding calcaneal osteotomy (Fig. 34.5) when in the presence of a flatfoot (Vora et al. 2006).
- Stage II—Upon PTT insufficiency and subsequent deformity, flexor tendon transfer (Fig. 34.6) combined with a calcaneal osteotomy (most commonly of the medial slide type) is used. In the presence of a fixed elevation of the first ray, the medial cuneiform open-wedge osteotomy (Cotton osteotomy) is considered (Aiyer et al. 2016). If the first ray is unstable, a first metatarsal-tarsal fusion is considered. Fusion of the navicular cuneiform joint is rarely required and difficult to achieve (Mosier-LaClair et al. 2001). Treatment of Stage IIB

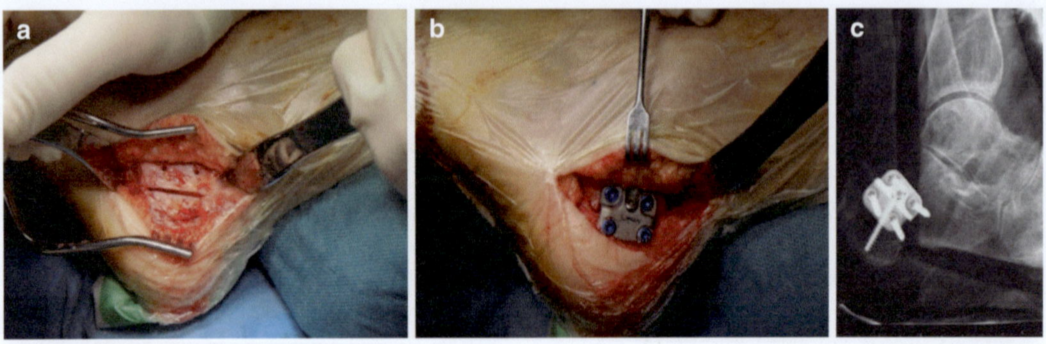

Fig. 34.5 Surgical approach (**a** and **b**) and x-ray (**c**) of medial sliding calcaneal osteotomy

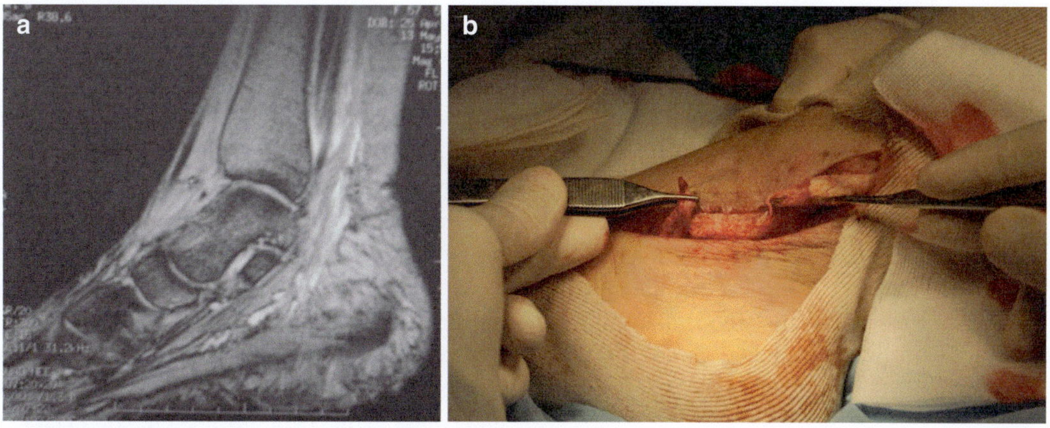

Fig. 34.6 Posterior tibial tendon rupture on MRI (**a**) and direct surgical repair (**b**) which was further augmented by *flexor digitorum longus* transfer

deformity is particularly controversial, with some clinicians performing a lateral column lengthening for this stage while others choose other options (Lee 2005). The amount of abduction requiring a lateral column lengthening has not been established (Chi et al. 1999). Besides the previously described, spring ligament repair/reconstruction can also be used when required (Palmanovich et al. 2015). The formerly described correction can be combined with arthroereisis in selected cases (Soomekh and Baravarian 2006). Subtalar fusion with correction of alignment represents another valid option in more severe cases (Yao et al. 2015).

- Stage III—The most frequent treatment at this stage involves a triple arthrodesis (Catanzariti et al. 2014) (triple joint complex—subtalar, talonavicular, and calcaneocuboid). Overcorrection of deformity should be avoided. The talonavicular joint should be fused in neutral position without excessive abduction, but also without supination (varus of the midfoot and forefoot). The metatarsal heads should be even to the floor with the heel in neutral position. If the excessive heel valgus remains after triple arthrodesis, a medial heel slide is added to provide good alignment and avoid excessive stress on the deltoid and progression to Stage IV.
- Stage IV—There is limited clinical evidence on the outcome of Stage IV patients (Deland et al. 2004). Correction of alignment in the foot is critical. Flexible deformities in the foot, if present, should be corrected as described for Stage II. Correction of fixed deformity should be addressed as described for Stage III. Consideration for reconstruction of the deltoid ligament with tendon graft can be done and may give correction to the alignment at the ankle (Catanzariti et al. 2014). When symptomatic ankle arthritis develops, ankle fusion is required to relieve pain (Toullec 2015). Total ankle replacement is also an option (Ketz et al. 2012). However, inadequate function of the deltoid ligament after total ankle replacement can result in failure of the arthroplasty (Toullec 2015; Yao et al. 2015).

As previously described, in all stages, assessment of the Achilles tendon is critical. If shortened, an Achilles lengthening or gastrocnemius recession should be considered. Furthermore, we emphasize that instability or hypermobility of the first ray must also be considered. If that is the case, a first metatarsal-tarsal fusion or Cotton osteotomy should be considered (Yao et al. 2015).

34.5 Anterior Tibial Tendon Pathology

34.5.1 Anterior Tibial Tendon (ATT) Clinical Anatomy

The tibialis anterior muscle (Fig. 34.7) originates from the lateral tibial condyle and interosseous membrane. The musculotendinous junction occurs at the transition of the middle and distal thirds of the tibia. The ATT has its main insertions at the medial cuneiform and the inferomedial base of the first metatarsal; however, different types of distal insertions have been described in the literature (Varghese and Bianchi 2014). The ATT courses within a synovial sheath during most of its course, deep to the extensor retinaculum of the ankle and foot. It is the strongest dorsiflexor of the foot (accounts for more than 80% of the strength required for this movement) while also contributing to inversion (Ouzounian and Anderson 1995). It also controls deceleration of the foot after heel strike. It is innervated by the deep peroneal nerve. Peterson et al. described a zone of hypovascularity (Petersen et al. 2000); however, Geppert et al. had opposed to this theory stating that ATT has no sustainable hypovascular zones (Geppert et al. 1993). It receives vascular supply from the anterior tibial artery proximally and the medial tarsal arteries distally. The ATT's bursa is found close to its insertion, between the tibialis anterior tendon and the medial cuneiform bone.

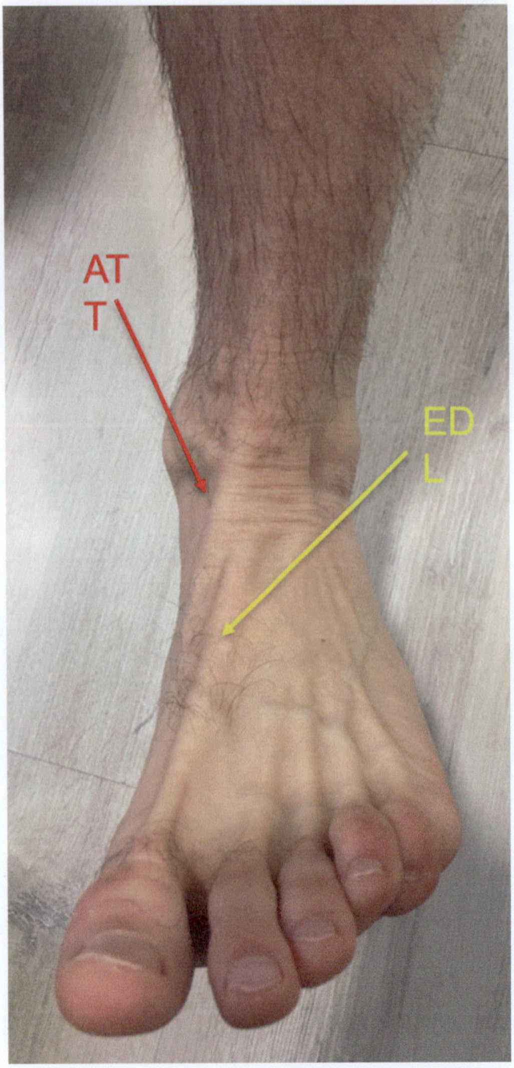

Fig. 34.7 Surface anatomy where anterior tibial tendon (ATT) and extensor digitorum longus (EDL) are identified

34.5.2 Etiology and Clinical Presentations

Lesions of the tibialis anterior muscle and tendon are not frequently found in international literature (Varghese and Bianchi 2014). However, most likely being unreported, tibialis anterior tendinopathy or rupture might not be that rare. Pathology can be spontaneous, trauma related, associated with arthropathy or more generalized conditions (Varghese and Bianchi 2014). Either local or systemic diseases can be considered as risk factors: corticosteroid injection, diabetes mellitus, hyperparathyroidism, or aging. In most cases, a careful history and a thorough physical examination are sufficient for achieving the diagnosis. Clinical assessment alone, however, may not be sufficient for distinguishing conditions like tendinopathy, tears (Fig. 34.8), bursitis, calcifications, and cysts (Fig. 34.8), among others (Ouzounian and Anderson 1995). Insertional tendinopathy has been described, more often in ballet dancers or jumpers. Tendinopathy might derive from repetitive compression from footwear

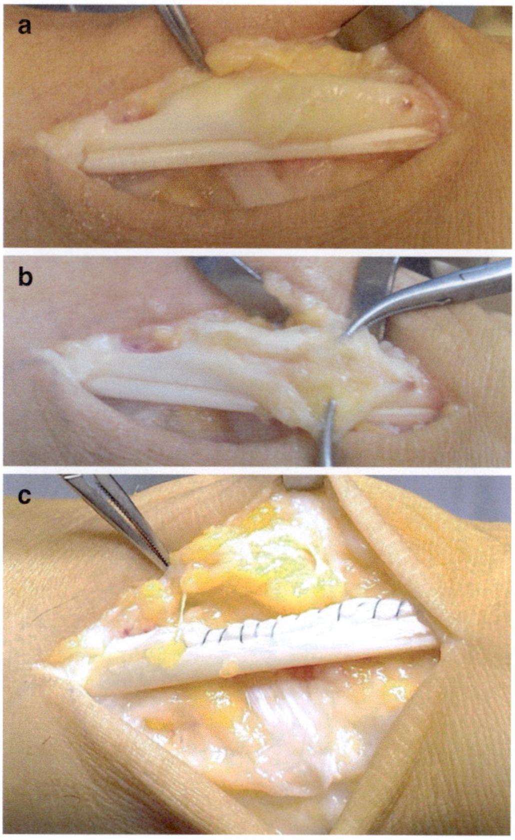

Fig. 34.8 Cystic degeneration with rupture of the anterior tibial tendon (**a** and **b**). After debridement, tubulization and direct repair have been performed (**c**)

or overuse leading to inflammatory changes. Patients describe pain on the medial cuneiform particularly when loading the foot immediately after heel strike or during swing phase of gait (Ritter and Moore 2008). Bursitis can occur as a result of excessive local friction, infection, or direct trauma.

The tibialis anterior tendon may rupture spontaneously or by open or closed trauma. TAT rupture may present as an acute lesion or as a chronic, painless foot drop which is usually late diagnosed (Varghese and Bianchi 2014). Younger patients without degenerative tendon changes rarely suffer spontaneous rupture. Their most frequent injury mechanism is laceration following penetrating trauma or tibial fracture (Sammarco et al. 2009). Spontaneous ruptures typically occur in older patients with tendon degeneration. Minor trauma by plantarflexion-eversion might be the precipitating event.

Clinical examination includes inspection for swelling or palpable mass. Closed tibialis anterior ruptures might present with a bulbous mass at the anterior medial aspect of the ankle joint due to the proximal retraction of the ruptured tendon (Dooley et al. 1980). A gap might be felt indicating rupture. Analysis of gait pattern in chronic ruptures might range from slight changes, with limitation only on uneven ground, up to slap-foot gait or foot drop. Incapacity to walk on heels suggests ATT dysfunction. During the swing phase of gait patients might hyperflex the hip and knee to compensate loss of ankle dorsiflexion. Diminished ankle dorsiflexion strength is another sign. When asked to dorsiflex the ankle, patients will exhibit toe hyperextension. In chronic cases, Achilles contracture might also occur. A minimum of 10° dorsiflexion must be preserved in order to permit ATT repair. For this reason, in some cases, repair is combined with Achilles lengthening (Ouzounian and Anderson 1995).

Radiography can be useful in conditions like *myositis ossificans* or to assess arthropathy. Magnetic resonance imaging, due to its excellent tissue contrast, allows simultaneous assessment of the muscle, joint, and bone. It remains a second-line study due to its high cost (Varghese and Bianchi 2014). Ultrasound, which enables dynamic evaluation, despite the fact that it is operator dependent, can also be useful for final diagnosis (Varghese and Bianchi 2014).

Differential diagnosis includes peroneal nerve palsy, lumbar radiculopathy, or peripheral neurologic conditions affecting ATT function.

34.5.3 Principles for Treatment

Concerning ATT tendinopathy, the principles of treatment are common to other tendons. Conservative treatment is the first line of treatment. The former includes rest, ice, immobilization, analgesics, appropriate physiotherapy protocol, change in footwear, injection therapy, etc. Upon failure of conservative treatment, endoscopy is being presented as a promising possibility, including bursectomy, synovitis, or debridement (Lui 2016b). However, in this less reported group of pathology, increased experience and evidence are required before more definitive conclusions.

Although the treatment for ATT ruptures is somewhat controversial, most literature recommends conservative management for most longstanding chronic ruptures, as well as ruptures occurring in the elderly or sedentary patients (Funk et al. 2016). Treatment of this clinical entity must be tailored to the individual.

Conservative therapy may consist of shoe modifications, bracing, and a non-weight-bearing short leg cast with the foot in a dorsiflexed and inverted position for 4 to 6 weeks. An ankle foot orthosis may be indicated in these patients after therapy due to some loss in muscle strength and ankle joint dorsiflexion (Markarian et al. 1998).

Surgical management is indicated for younger, more active patients, who present an acute ATT rupture, or preferably within 3 to 4 months after injury (Trout et al. 2000; Christman-Skieller et al. 2015). The age of the patient, functional status and demands, stage of rupture, and chronicity should be considered when developing a treatment plan (Trout et al. 2000; Christman-Skieller et al. 2015).

Some authors recommend direct primary repair for acute tibialis anterior ruptures (Dooley et al. 1980; Markarian et al. 1998). Primary tendon repair may be accomplished with nonabsorbable suture (Fig. 34.8) using Bunnell, Krakow, or modified Kessler suture techniques (Harvey and Rockett 2000). Fixation using EndoButton® has also been described (Funk et al. 2016). In case it is not possible to perform a direct suture of the tendon or reinsert the tendon (Mao and Xu 2015) into its native insertion, a tendon reconstruction technique can be used. The extensor retinaculum should always be reconstructed to prevent the bowstringing phenomenon and cicatricial adhesions to the subcutaneous tissue (Sammarco et al. 2009). After surgery, a period of 6 weeks of immobilization with plaster cast is recommended before the patient begins active mobilization and physical therapy rehabilitation.

Several surgical techniques have been described to treat anterior tibial tendon ruptures. Available options include direct primary repair (less viable in chronic cases), augmentation by tendon grafts, tendon transfers, and tendon reconstruction. Considering the latter, Trout et al. utilized the central one third of the anterior tibial tendon to bridge the ruptured gap (Trout et al. 2000). The flap was rotated posteriorly and distally and tenodesed into the medial cuneiform using a 4–0 mm cancellous screw with washer. Another option is interposing an allograft (Huh et al. 2015) or autologous graft, such as the *plantaris* tendon, *extensor digitorum longus* tendon, *peroneus tertius* tendon, Achilles tendon, or semitendinosus tendon (Christman-Skieller et al. 2015). *Extensor hallucis longus* transfer to medial cuneiform is probably the most popular tendon transfer/augmentation technique (Sammarco et al. 2009; Christman-Skieller et al. 2015).

Studies have shown that patients treated surgically were more likely to develop a normal gait, with more dorsiflexion strength and motion compared to patients treated conservatively (Markarian et al. 1998; Christman-Skieller et al. 2015). Surgical intervention appears to achieve a better functional outcome when compared to conservative treatment. Mild to moderate flatfoot deformity, decrease in ankle joint range of motion, lack in coordination or a slapping type gait, and Achilles tendon contraction were more frequent among patients treated conservatively (Trout et al. 2000).

However, we must emphasize the paucity of the available literature and methodological limitation of the small sample series reported.

34.6 Injection Therapy in Tendinopathies

Injection treatments for controlling painful tendon-related disorders (Fig. 34.9) have been increasing its popularity, particularly among populations with higher functional demand.

Through time, several agents have been studied such as corticosteroids (Johnson et al. 2011),

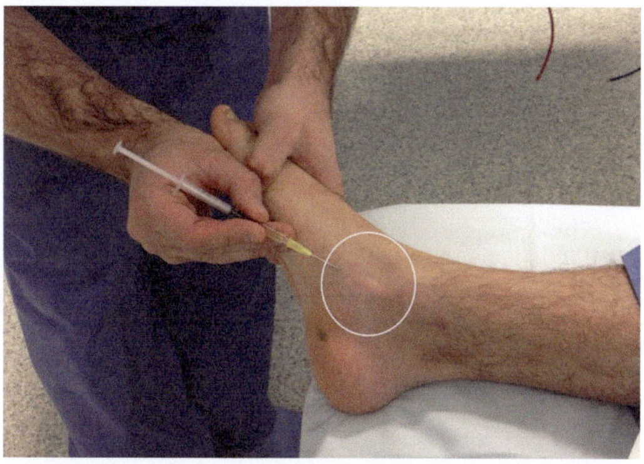

Fig. 34.9 Injection therapy around in the posterior tibial tendon (PTT) sheath. The PTT is visible (*white circle*) by asking the patient to actively invert the foot against resistance from the examiner. Ultrasound can be a useful tool to perform these treatments under visual control

polidocanol, platelet-rich plasma (PRP), high-volume injections, hyperosmolar dextrose, brisement, aprotinin, and low-dose heparin (van Sterkenburg and van Dijk 2011).

One must understand that each agent and technique presents its specific implications, and until now there is no such thing as a securely effective and harmless percutaneous "panacea" capable to cure all sources of pain.

There is controversial data in literature related to percutaneous treatment/prolotherapy. Often, the cause-effect rationale supporting its application, particularly in tendons, is not completely understood, so despite being open-minded, we must evaluate them with necessary caution.

Many limitations persist concerning clinical and biological aspects of tendon healing. The main goal in tendon repair is to achieve a faster rehabilitation with tissue healing with similar or better characteristics than those of normal tendons. Tissue engineering and regenerative medicine research envisions new perspectives for the future (Hogan et al. 2011).

Corticosteroids are powerful anti-inflammatory medications which were previously injected around tendons. Its use in tendinopathies is currently discouraged given the risk of subsequent tendon degeneration and/or rupture (Speed 2001).

Polidocanol has been proposed as a method to abolish neovascularity within and around inflamed tendons (Ohberg and Alfredson 2002). However, the role of this neovascularization phenomenon is not completely comprehended. Moreover, there have been inconsistent results obtained from the method (van Sterkenburg et al. 2010a).

Currently, the most popular injectable therapy is probably PRP in one of its different preparations (with inherent different effects) (Papalia et al. 2012). It proposes a wide range of favorable effects in several tissues including tendon pathologies, muscle injuries, or even cartilage and joint arthritis. However, besides its proven safety profile, there has been some controversy around clinical outcome (Tinsley et al. 2012). Results have been obtained from pathologies, considering different tissues and different preparations of PRP (e.g., with/without leukocyte and platelet concentration) which limits the possibility for further assumptions regarding clinical use (Martinez-Zapata et al. 2012). It should be acknowledged that this is a most promising technique. Growth factors have provided consistent laboratorial results; however, it has not been easy to replicate such results in the clinics (Boswell et al. 2013). Improved research methodology and more clinical trials assessing outcome of PRP technology are still required (Engebretsen and Schamasch 2012).

"It is necessary to develop appropriate guidelines and increase evidence-level prior to its widespread application as treatment option for joint" (Sheth et al. 2012).

Conclusions

Tendinopathies around the foot and ankle are frequently associated with overuse and/or traumatic events. Anterior and posterior tibial tendon pathologies require a complete understanding of foot and ankle anatomy and biomechanics. Tendoscopy has been significantly developed in recent years. Posterior tibial tendon insufficiency requires diagnosis on an early phase of the disease in order to diminish further consequences and limitations. In later stages the prognosis is significantly worst and therapeutic options more aggressive and of more uncertain outcome.

On the other hand, ruptures of the anterior tibial tendon are unusual injuries but probably occur with greater frequency than reported. The fact that there is regularly a delay of several months in the diagnosis of ATT rupture indicates the need for an increased awareness of this entity. Ruptures of the ATT might have significant implications on gait and ambulation. The proper treatment option must be tailored to individual aspects. However, there seems to be improved outcome in the surgically treated group.

Injection therapy is under development aiming to control degeneration and achieve or enhance healing, particularly in the early stages of tendon's disease.

References

Aiyer A, Dall GF, Shub J, Myerson MS (2016) Radiographic correction following reconstruction of adult acquired flat foot deformity using the cotton medial cuneiform osteotomy. Foot Ankle Int 37(5):508–513. doi:10.1177/1071100715620894

Bare AA, Haddad SL (2001) Tenosynovitis of the posterior tibial tendon. Foot Ankle Clin 6(1):37–66

Bluman EM, Title CI, Myerson MS (2007) Posterior tibial tendon rupture: a refined classification system. Foot Ankle Clin 12(2):233–249, v. doi:10.1016/j.fcl.2007.03.003

Boss AP, Hintermann B (2002) Anatomical study of the medial ankle ligament complex. Foot Ankle Int 23(6):547–553

Boswell SG, Schnabel LV, Mohammed HO, Sundman EA, Minas T, Fortier LA (2013) Increasing platelet concentrations in leukocyte-reduced platelet-rich plasma decrease collagen gene synthesis in tendons. Am J Sports Med. doi:10.1177/0363546513507566

Brockett CL, Chapman GJ (2016) Biomechanics of the ankle. Orthop Trauma 30(3):232–238. doi:10.1016/j.mporth.2016.04.015

Catanzariti AR, Dix BT, Richardson PE, Mendicino RW (2014) Triple arthrodesis for adult acquired flatfoot. Clin Podiatr Med Surg 31(3):415–433. doi:10.1016/j.cpm.2014.03.004

Chi TD, Toolan BC, Sangeorzan BJ, Hansen ST Jr (1999) The lateral column lengthening and medial column stabilization procedures. Clin Orthop Relat Res 365:81–90

Chow HT, Chan KB, Lui TH (2005) Tendoscopic debridement for stage I posterior tibial tendon dysfunction. Knee Surg Sports Traumatol Arthrosc 13(8):695–698. doi:10.1007/s00167-005-0635-8

Christman-Skieller C, Merz MK, Tansey JP (2015) A systematic review of tibialis anterior tendon rupture treatments and outcomes. Am J Orthop (Belle Mead NJ) 44(4):E94–E99

Cooper AJ, Mizel MS, Patel PD, Steinmetz ND, Clifford PD (2007) Comparison of MRI and local anesthetic tendon sheath injection in the diagnosis of posterior tibial tendon tenosynovitis. Foot Ankle Int 28(11):1124–1127. doi:10.3113/FAI.2007.1124

Cote KP, Brunet ME, Gansneder BM, Shultz SJ (2005) Effects of pronated and supinated foot postures on static and dynamic postural stability. J Athl Train 40(1):41–46

Deland JT, de Asla RJ, Segal A (2004) Reconstruction of the chronically failed deltoid ligament: a new technique. Foot Ankle Int 25(11):795–799

Dooley BJ, Kudelka P, Menelaus MB (1980) Subcutaneous rupture of the tendon of tibialis anterior. J Bone Joint Surg Br 62-B(4):471–472

Engebretsen L, Schamasch S (2012) The use of platelet-rich plasma in sports medicine—the International Olympic Committee opinion. Oper Tech Orthop 22(1):43–48

Frey C, Shereff M, Greenidge N (1990) Vascularity of the posterior tibial tendon. J Bone Joint Surg Am 72(6):884–888

Frigg AM, Valderrabano V, Kundert HP, Hintermann B (2006) Combined anterior tibial tendon rupture and posterior tibial tendon dysfunction in advanced flatfoot. J Foot Ankle Surg 45(6):431–435. doi:10.1053/j.jfas.2006.09.007

Funk SS, Gallagher B, Thomson AB (2016) Repair of chronic tibialis anterior tendon ruptures. Orthopedics 39(2):e386–e390. doi:10.3928/01477447-20160307-05

Geppert MJ, Sobel M, Bohne WH (1993) Lateral ankle instability as a cause of superior peroneal retinacular laxity: an anatomic and biomechanical study of cadaveric feet. Foot Ankle 14(6):330–334

Gluck GS, Heckman DS, Parekh SG (2010) Tendon disorders of the foot and ankle, part 3: the posterior tibial tendon. Am J Sports Med 38(10):2133–2144. doi:10.1177/0363546509359492

Haddad SL, Myerson MS, Younger A, Anderson RB, Davis WH, Manoli A 2nd (2011) Symposium: adult acquired flatfoot deformity. Foot Ankle Int 32(1):95–111. doi:10.3113/FAI.2011.0095

Harvey L, Rockett MS (2000) Mechanical comparison of two extensor tendon repairs of ankle tendons. J Foot Ankle Surg 39(4):232–238

Hintermann B, Gachter A (1996) The first metatarsal rise sign: a simple, sensitive sign of tibialis posterior tendon dysfunction. Foot Ankle Int 17(4):236–241

Hogan MV, Bagayoko N, James R, Starnes T, Katz A, Chhabra AB (2011) Tissue engineering solutions for tendon repair. J Am Acad Orthop Surg 19(3):134–142

Hua Y, Chen S, Li Y, Wu Z (2015) Arthroscopic treatment for posterior tibial tendon lesions with a posterior approach. Knee Surg Sports Traumatol Arthrosc 23(3):879–883. doi:10.1007/s00167-013-2629-2

Huh J, Boyette DM, Parekh SG, Nunley JA 2nd (2015) Allograft reconstruction of chronic tibialis anterior tendon ruptures. Foot Ankle Int 36(10):1180–1189. doi:10.1177/1071100715589006

Johnson JE, Klein SE, Putnam RM (2011) Corticosteroid injections in the treatment of foot & ankle disorders: an AOFAS survey. Foot Ankle Int 32(4):394–399. doi:10.3113/FAI.2011.0394

Johnson KA (1983) Tibialis posterior tendon rupture. Clin Orthop Relat Res 177:140–147

Johnson KA, Strom DE (1989) Tibialis posterior tendon dysfunction. Clin Orthop Relat Res 239:196–206

Ketz J, Myerson M, Sanders R (2012) The salvage of complex hindfoot problems with use of a custom talar total ankle prosthesis. J Bone Joint Surg Am 94(13):1194–1200. doi:10.2106/JBJS.K.00421

Khazen G, Khazen C (2012) Tendoscopy in stage I posterior tibial tendon dysfunction. Foot Ankle Clin 17(3):399–406. doi:10.1016/j.fcl.2012.06.002

Kong A, Van Der Vliet A (2008) Imaging of tibialis posterior dysfunction. Br J Radiol 81(970):826–836. doi:10.1259/bjr/78613086

Kulig K, Reischl SF, Pomrantz AB, Burnfield JM, Mais-Requejo S, Thordarson DB, Smith RW (2009) Nonsurgical management of posterior tibial tendon dysfunction with orthoses and resistive exercise: a randomized controlled trial. Phys Ther 89(1):26–37. doi:10.2522/ptj.20070242

Lee MS (2005) Posterior calcaneal displacement osteotomy for the adult acquired flatfoot. Clin Podiatr Med Surg 22(2):277–289, vii. doi:10.1016/j.cpm.2004.11.002

Lhoste-Trouilloud A (2012) The tibialis posterior tendon. J Ultrasound 15(1):2–6. doi:10.1016/j.jus.2012.02.001

Lui TH (2007) Endoscopic assisted posterior tibial tendon reconstruction for stage 2 posterior tibial tendon insufficiency. Knee Surg Sports Traumatol Arthrosc 15(10):1228–1234.doi:10.1007/s00167-006-0282-8

Lui TH (2015) Posterior tibial tendoscopy: endoscopic synovectomy and assessment of the spring (calcaneonavicular) ligament. Arthrosc Tech 4(6):e819–e823. doi:10.1016/j.eats.2015.08.006

Lui TH (2016a) Endoscopic repair of the superficial deltoid ligament and spring ligament. Arthrosc Tech 5(3):e621–e625. doi:10.1016/j.eats.2016.02.004

Lui TH (2016b) Endoscopic resection of the tibialis anterior tendon bursa. Arthrosc Tech 5(5):e1029–e1032. doi:10.1016/j.eats.2016.05.008

Manske MC, McKeon KE, Johnson JE, McCormick JJ, Klein SE (2015) Arterial anatomy of the tibialis posterior tendon. Foot Ankle Int 36(4):436–443. doi:10.1177/1071100714559271

Mao H, Xu G (2015) Soft tissue repair for tibialis anterior tendon ruptures using plate and screw fixation technique in combination with anterolateral thigh flaps transplantation. J Orthop Surg Res 10:143. doi:10.1186/s13018-015-0278-5

Markarian GG, Kelikian AS, Brage M, Trainor T, Dias L (1998) Anterior tibialis tendon ruptures: an outcome analysis of operative versus nonoperative treatment. Foot Ankle Int 19(12):792–802

Martinez-Zapata MJ, Marti-Carvajal AJ, Sola I, Exposito JA, Bolibar I, Rodriguez L, Garcia J (2012) Autologous platelet-rich plasma for treating chronic wounds. Cochrane Database Syst Rev 10:CD006899. doi:10.1002/14651858.CD006899.pub2

McCormack AP, Varner KE, Marymont JV (2003) Surgical treatment for posterior tibial tendonitis in young competitive athletes. Foot Ankle Int 24(7):535–538

Mosier-LaClair S, Pomeroy G, Manoli A 2nd (2001) Operative treatment of the difficult stage 2 adult acquired flatfoot deformity. Foot Ankle Clin 6(1):95–119

Myerson M, Solomon G, Shereff M (1989) Posterior tibial tendon dysfunction: its association with seronegative inflammatory disease. Foot Ankle 9(5):219–225

Myerson MS (1997) Adult acquired flatfoot deformity: treatment of dysfunction of the posterior tibial tendon. Instr Course Lect 46:393–405

Myerson MS, Corrigan J (1996) Treatment of posterior tibial tendon dysfunction with flexor digitorum longus tendon transfer and calcaneal osteotomy. Orthopedics 19(5):383–388

Nallamshetty L, Nazarian LN, Schweitzer ME, Morrison WB, Parellada JA, Articolo GA, Rawool NM, Abidi NA (2005) Evaluation of posterior tibial pathology: comparison of sonography and MR imaging. Skelet Radiol 34(7):375–380. doi:10.1007/s00256-005-0903-1

Ohberg L, Alfredson H (2002) Ultrasound guided sclerosis of neovessels in painful chronic Achilles tendinosis: pilot study of a new treatment. Br J Sports Med 36(3):173–175. discussion 176–177

Otis JC, Gage T (2001) Function of the posterior tibial tendon muscle. Foot Ankle Clin 6(1):1–14, v

Ouzounian TJ, Anderson R (1995) Anterior tibial tendon rupture. Foot Ankle Int 16(7):406–410

Palacios-Cena D, Fernandez-de-Las-Penas C, Hernandez-Barrera V, Jimenez-Garcia R, Alonso-Blanco C, Carrasco-Garrido P (2012) Sports participation increased in Spain: a population-based time trend study of 21 381 adults in the years 2000, 2005 and 2010. Br J Sports Med 46(16):1137–1139. doi:10.1136/bjsports-2012-091076

Palmanovich E, Shabat S, Brin YS, Feldman V, Kish B, Nyska M (2015) Anatomic reconstruction technique for a plantar calcaneonavicular (spring) ligament tear. J Foot Ankle Surg 54(6):1124–1126. doi:10.1053/j.jfas.2015.06.013

Papalia R, Vasta S, Zampogna B, Tecam A, Maffulli N (2012) Platelet-rich plasma injections and surgery: short-term outcomes and long-term prognosis. Oper Tech Orthop 22(2):71–77

Park HJ, Lee SY, Park NH, Rho MH, Chung EC, Kwag HJ (2012) Accuracy of MR findings in characterizing peroneal tendons disorders in comparison with surgery. Acta Radiol 53(7):795–801. doi:10.1258/ar.2012.120184

Pereira H, Ripoll PL, Oliveira JM, Reis LR, Espregueira-Mendes J, van Dijk CN (2014) Peroneal and posterior tibial tendon pathology. In: d'Hooghe PPRN, Kerkhoffs GMMJ (eds) The ankle in football. Springer-Verlag Paris

Petersen W, Stein V, Bobka T (2000) Structure of the human tibialis anterior tendon. J Anat 197(Pt 4):617–625
Probasco W, Haleem AM, Yu J, Sangeorzan BJ, Deland JT, Ellis SJ (2015) Assessment of coronal plane subtalar joint alignment in peritalar subluxation via weight-bearing multiplanar imaging. Foot Ankle Int 36(3):302–309. doi:10.1177/1071100714557861
Ribbans WJ, Garde A (2013) Tibialis posterior tendon and deltoid and spring ligament injuries in the elite athlete. Foot Ankle Clin 18(2):255–291. doi:10.1016/j.fcl.2013.02.006
Ritter S, Moore M (2008) The relationship between lateral ankle sprain and ankle tendinitis in ballet dancers. J Dance Med Sci 12(1):23–31
Sammarco VJ, Sammarco GJ, Henning C, Chaim S (2009) Surgical repair of acute and chronic tibialis anterior tendon ruptures. J Bone Joint Surg Am 91(2):325–332. doi:10.2106/JBJS.G.01386
Selmani E, Gjata V, Gjika E (2006) Current concepts review: peroneal tendon disorders. Foot Ankle Int 27(3):221–228
Sheth U, Simunovic N, Klein G, Fu F, Einhorn TA, Schemitsch E, Ayeni OR, Bhandari M (2012) Efficacy of autologous platelet-rich plasma use for orthopaedic indications: a meta-analysis. J Bone Joint Surg Am 94(4):298–307. doi:10.2106/JBJS.K.00154
Slovenkai MP (1997) Clinical and radiographic evaluation. Foot Ankle Clin 2:241–260
Soomekh DJ, Baravarian B (2006) Pediatric and adult flatfoot reconstruction: subtalar arthroereisis versus realignment osteotomy surgical options. Clin Podiatr Med Surg 23(4):695–708, v. doi:10.1016/j.cpm.2006.08.003
Speed CA (2001) Fortnightly review: corticosteroid injections in tendon lesions. BMJ 323(7309):382–386
Supple KM, Hanft JR, Murphy BJ, Janecki CJ, Kogler GF (1992) Posterior tibial tendon dysfunction. Semin Arthritis Rheum 22(2):106–113
Tinsley BA, Ferreira JV, Dukas AG, Mazzocca AD (2012) Platelet-rich plasma nonoperative injection therapy—a review of indications and evidence. Oper Tech Sports Med 20(2):192–200
Toullec E (2015) Adult flatfoot. Orthop Traumatol Surg Res 101(1 Suppl):S11–S17. doi:10.1016/j.otsr.2014.07.030
Trnka HJ (2004) Dysfunction of the tendon of tibialis posterior. J Bone Joint Surg Br 86(7):939–946
Trout BM, Hosey G, Wertheimer SJ (2000) Rupture of the tibialis anterior tendon. J Foot Ankle Surg 39(1):54–58
van Dijk CN, Kort N, Scholten PE (1997) Tendoscopy of the posterior tibial tendon. Arthroscopy 13(6):692–698
van Sterkenburg MN, de Jonge MC, Sierevelt IN, van Dijk CN (2010a) Less promising results with sclerosing ethoxysclerol injections for midportion achilles tendinopathy: a retrospective study. Am J Sports Med 38(11):2226–2232. doi:10.1177/0363546510373467
van Sterkenburg MN, Haverkamp D, van Dijk CN, Kerkhoffs GM (2010b) A posterior tibial tendon skipping rope. Knee Surg Sports Traumatol Arthrosc 18(12):1664–1666. doi:10.1007/s00167-010-1194-1
van Sterkenburg MN, van Dijk CN (2011) Injection treatment for chronic midportion Achilles tendinopathy: do we need that many alternatives? Knee Surgery Sports Traumatol Arthrosc 19(4):513–515. doi:10.1007/s00167-011-1415-2
Varghese A, Bianchi S (2014) Ultrasound of tibialis anterior muscle and tendon: anatomy, technique of examination, normal and pathologic appearance. J Ultrasound 17(2):113–123. doi:10.1007/s40477-013-0060-7
Vora AM, Tien TR, Parks BG, Schon LC (2006) Correction of moderate and severe acquired flexible flatfoot with medializing calcaneal osteotomy and flexor digitorum longus transfer. J Bone Joint Surg Am 88(8):1726–1734. doi:10.2106/JBJS.E.00045
Yao K, Yang TX, Yew WP (2015) Posterior tibialis tendon dysfunction: overview of evaluation and management. Orthopedics 38(6):385–391. doi:10.3928/01477447-20150603-06

Peroneal Tendons

35

P.A.D. van Dijk and C.N. van Dijk

Contents

P.A.D. van Dijk
Department of Orthopedic Surgery—Academic Medical Center,
Meibergdreef 9, 1105 AZ, Amsterdam,
The Netherlands

Academic Center for Evidence Based Sports Medicine (ACES),
Meibergdreef 9, 1105 AZ, Amsterdam,
The Netherlands

Amsterdam Collaboration for Health and Safety in Sports (ACHSS),
Meibergdreef 9, 1105 AZ, Amsterdam,
The Netherlands

C.N. van Dijk (✉)
Department of Orthopedic Surgery—Academic Medical Center,
Meibergdreef 9, 1105 AZ, Amsterdam,
The Netherlands

Academic Center for Evidence Based Sports Medicine (ACES),
Meibergdreef 9, 1105 AZ, Amsterdam,
The Netherlands

Amsterdam Collaboration for Health and Safety in Sports (ACHSS),
Meibergdreef 9, 1105 AZ, Amsterdam,
The Netherlands
FIFA Medical Center of Excellence, Madrid, Spain
e-mail: c.niekvandijk@anklecare.org

35.1 Introduction

Peroneal tendon injuries account for a significant number of posterolateral ankle complaints following acute ankle inversion trauma and are often a result of chronic lateral ankle instability or predisposing anatomical abnormalities (DiGiovanni et al. 2000; Krause and Brodsky 1998). In turn, peroneal tendon injuries can be associated with significant disability and thus warrant close attention to diagnosis and treatment (Krause and Brodsky 1998; Redfern and Myerson 2004). Injuries to the peroneal tendons, however, are often misdiagnosed as a lateral ankle sprain, resulting in inadequate initial treatment. While acute peroneal tendon injuries can often be treated with conservative management, late diagnosis often leads to chronic damage that needs surgical treatment. Adequate knowledge of

G.L. Canata et al. (eds.), *Muscle and Tendon Injuries*, DOI 10.1007/978-3-662-54184-5_35

the peroneal anatomy and clinical presentation of the associated pathologies are essential for early diagnosis and treatment of peroneal tendon disorders. This chapter provides an overview on the anatomy, diagnosis and management of peroneal tendon injuries.

35.2 Anatomy and Function

The peroneal brevis (PB) and longus muscles (PL) form the lateral compartment of the lower leg, or 'the peroneal compartment', and act as the primary abductors and evertors of the foot. Furthermore, they play an important role in the stability of the lateral ankle. The PL originates at the lateral condyle of the tibia, the lateral aspect of proximal fibular head, the intramuscular septa and the adjacent fascia. The PB originates more distally on the fibular shaft and interosseous membrane. Approximately 3–4 cm proximal to the distal fibular tip, the PL becomes completely tendinous, whereas the muscle fibres of the PB tend to extend more distally (Edwards 1928). In some cases, the PB musculotendinous junction occurs more distally around the fibular tip, an anatomical variation known as a low-lying muscle belly (Freccero and Berkowitz 2006; Saupe et al. 2007).

Around the tip of the fibula, the tendons share a common tendon sheath. At this level, the PB is anteromedially located from the PL and is flattened against the fibula. The tendons descend posterior to the distal fibular tip, passing through the superior retromalleolar tunnel formed by the retromalleolar groove of the fibula and buttressed by a fibrocartilaginous ridge (Mota and Rosenberg 1998). The tendons are secured to the posterior side of the distal fibula by the superior peroneal retinaculum (SPR), which plays a critical role in maintaining stability of the tendons (Kumai and Benjamin 2003). The SPR originates laterally along the posterior aspect of the distal fibula and extends to its tip where it becomes contiguous with the periosteum. Medially, the retinaculum is merged with the deep transverse fascia of the posterior compartment of the lower leg (Athavale et al. 2011).

After leaving the superior peroneal tunnel distally to the fibular tip, the tendons are separated by the calcaneal peroneal tubercle, and the common tendon sheath splits into two separated sheaths. Each tendon enters an individual fibrous tunnel and is secured by the inferior peroneal retinaculum. The insertion of the PB is found at the base of the fifth metatarsal. The PL tendon runs more distally; after turning plantarly at the cuboid groove, it inserts at the plantar side of the medial cuneiform and the first metatarsal base.

The tendons are innervated by the superficial peroneal nerve which innervates both tendons, and blood is supplied by the peroneal artery and branches of the anterior tibial artery. Branches run through a common vincula formed by the distal fibres of the PB muscle belly and penetrate both tendons over their entire length along the posterolateral side (Scholten and van Dijk 2006; van Dijk et al. 2016). For many years it has been assumed that the peroneal tendons have critical avascular zones around the distal fibular tip and the cuboid bone, playing a role in the development of pathologies of the tendons (Petersen et al. 2000). Recent work by our group, however, found no evidence to support these avascular zones (van Dijk et al. 2016).

35.3 Peroneal Tendon Pathologies

Given their important role in the stabilization of the lateral ankle, the peroneal tendons remain under significant tension. During inversion of the ankle, the tendons are exposed to high mechanical loads (DiGiovanni et al. 2000; Molloy and Tisdel 2003; Sammarco and DiRaimondo 1989). Recurrent ankle sprains exacerbate these loads, leading to potential damage of the tendons. Chronic ankle instability has been described in 77% of the patients who are surgically treated for a peroneal tendon injury (Bassett and Speer 1993). Chronic ankle inversion or instability may cause chronic squeezing of the PB tendon between the PL tendon and the fibula, predisposing the PB to potential pathologies such as hypertrophic tendinopathy, recurrent stenosis and eventually tendon tears (DiGiovanni et al. 2000). Also, in patients with malalignment of the hindfoot, i.e., cavovarus feet, the tendons encounter significant overload (Younger and Hansen 2005). Other predisposing factors of peroneal tendon injuries include rheumatoid arthritis, psoriatic arthritis, diabetic neuropathy, calcaneal fractures, fluoroquinolone use and local steroid injections (Borton et al. 1998; Brandes and Smith 2000; Rosenberg et al. 1987; Truong et al. 1995; Vainio 1991; Wright and Sangeorzan 1996).

Tendinopathies related to the peroneal tendons are generally classified into three categories: (1) tendinitis, tenosynovitis, tendinosis and stenosis; (2) (partial) tears and ruptures; and (3) subluxation and dislocation (Cardone et al. 1993; DiGiovanni et al. 2000; Strauss et al. 2007). Other diagnoses for posterolateral ankle pain include posterior ankle impingement, chronic laxity of the lateral ankle ligaments, avulsion or calcification of the posterior talofibular ligament (PFTL), bony spurs, rheumatoid arthritis and disorders of the posterior compartment of the subtalar joint (van Dijk 2006).

35.3.1 Tendinitis, Tenosynovitis, Tendinosis and Stenosis

Tendinitis and tenosynovitis involve inflammation of the tendon and tendon sheath, respectively, and may lead to noninflammatory degeneration of the collagen fibres, or tendinosis, on the longer term. Microscopically, tendinosis is associated with loss of continuity of the collagen fibres; increase of mucoid ground substance, tenocyte or fibroblast hyperplasia; and increase of vascularization and cell necrosis (Khan et al. 1999; Sammarco and DiRaimondo 1989). Macroscopically, the surface of the tendon appears dull, predominantly grey and soft. If left untreated, tenosynovitis can cause fibrosis around the tendon and synovial proliferation, leading to hypertrophy and stenosis of the tendon (Wang et al. 2005). Peroneal tendinopathy can occur anywhere along the course of the tendons, but is most often found at the level where the tendons experience the most stress and angular change: around the lateral malleolus (PB), along the peroneal tubercle (PB and PL) or within the cuboid groove (PL).

35.3.2 Tears and Ruptures

Just as tendinopathies, peroneal tendon tears tend to occur in areas where the tendons experience the highest stress (Sammarco and DiRaimondo 1989); tears in the PB tendon are mostly found within the retromalleolar groove, while PL tendon tears are often located at the level of the cuboid, at the level of the os peroneum or at the level of the peroneal tubercle (Heckman et al. 2008; Sobel et al. 1991). The PB tendon is more prone to tear than the PL tendon, due to its position between the fibula and the PL tendon. In a study by Dombek et al., a PB tendon tear was found in 87.5% of patients, and a tear of the PL tendon was found in only 12.5% (Dombek et al. 2003). Redfern et al. found concomitant tearing of both tendons in 38% of patients treated operatively for peroneal tendon tears (Redfern and Myerson 2004).

35.3.3 Subluxation and Dislocation of the Tendons

Peroneal tendon dislocation has been reported in 0.3–0.5% of all traumatic ankle injuries and is most prevalent in athletes performing sports that require short-cutting movement, such as skiing (Oden 1987), soccer and gymnastics (Arrowsmith et al. 1983). Dislocation occurs when one or both tendons are displaced from the retromalleolar groove, often as a result of rupturing of the SPR. Due to its anatomical location in between the PB and the SPR, the PL is more prone to dislocate than the PB.

Predisposing factors include calcaneal fracture displacement (Wong-Chung et al. 2015) and anatomical abnormalities such as the presence of an accessory peroneal tendon (Yammine 2015), a low-lying muscle belly (Thomas et al. 2009) or a flat or convex-shaped retromalleolar groove (Kumai and Benjamin 2003; Saupe et al. 2007).

Peroneal tendon dislocation is generally classified in four grades. (Eckert and Davis 1976; Oden 1987) Grade one, approximately 51% of the cases, includes cases where the SPR is subperiosteally elevated from the fibula. In grade two, around 33%, the SPR is elevated together with the fibrocartilaginous ridge. In grade three, approximately 13%, the SPR is completely torn off the fibula together with a cortical fragment (Eckert and Davis 1976). Grade four includes cases with a ruptured posterior part of the retinaculum (Oden 1987). Later, Raikin proposed a classification of intrasheath subluxation, with the SPR remaining intact, while the peroneal tendon changes from their natural position within the retromalleolar groove (Raikin et al. 2008). In type A, the PL lies deep in relation to the PB, and in type B, the PL subluxates through a tear within the PB (Raikin et al. 2008).

35.4 Patient History and Clinical Examination

Careful patient history and clinical examination are the key to proper diagnosis of peroneal tendon injuries. Acute injuries are often reported as 'an ankle sprain that never resolved', while chronic disorders occur after a gross ankle inversion trauma in the medical history or in patients with chronic lateral ankle ligament instability. Patients typically present with lateral ankle pain or pain along the course of the peroneal tendons that worsens with activity. Other symptoms reported include swelling, tenderness, giving way and lateral ankle instability. Differentiation between a peroneal tendinopathy and a tear during physical examination is difficult. A tendon tear may appear with less pain but more weakness and swelling. In case of dislocation, the patient may report a popping or snapping sensation.

Findings during physical examination include a recognizable tenderness over the peroneal tendons, crepitus and swelling. Passive plantar flexion and inversion or active dorsiflexion and eversion often exacerbate pain, and muscle strength can sometimes be weakened when compared to the contralateral side. In tears, pain may be exacerbated on acute loosening of resistance during the provocation test (Heckman et al. 2008; Philbin et al. 2009). Possible dislocation of the tendons sometimes can be provoked during physical examination by active dorsiflexion and eversion (Safran et al. 1999).

35.5 Diagnostics

In the opinion of the authors, thorough patient history and physical examination often impart the most reliable information to pinpoint the exact diagnosis. Additional diagnostics, however, are required in most cases to rule out other pathologies and to create a treatment strategy.

To rule out acute and chronic osseous pathologies such as fractures, spurs or calcifications, weight-bearing radiographs in anteroposterior and lateral direction should be made. In case of peroneal tendon dislocation type 3, a small avulsion fracture of the lateral malleolus or 'fleck sign' may be visible on the anteroposterior view (Church 1977).

For evaluation of the peroneal tendons and surrounding structures, MRI is still used as the standard diagnostic test (Heckman et al. 2008). Park et al. reported sensitivity and specificity for peroneal pathology to be 84% and 75%, respectively (Park et al. 2010). A more recent study by Kennedy et al. documented 90% sensitivity and 72% specificity for peroneal tendinopathy (Kennedy et al. 2016). Normal peroneal tendons appear with homogenous signal intensity on T1-and T2-weighted images. Abnormalities include a C-shaped tendon, clefts, irregularity of the tendon contour and increased signal intensity due to fluid within the tendon sheath (Fig. 35.1) (Rosenberg et al. 1997; Schweitzer et al. 1997). Some of these findings such as increased signal intensity, however, are also seen in some asymptomatic patients (Wang et al. 2005). Furthermore, the so-called magic angle effect may overestimate peroneal tendon disorders (Rosenberg et al. 1998). This effect only appears on T1-weighted images, while tears display signal abnormalities on both T1- and T2-weighted images. Therefore, it is important to evaluate the tendons in both settings.

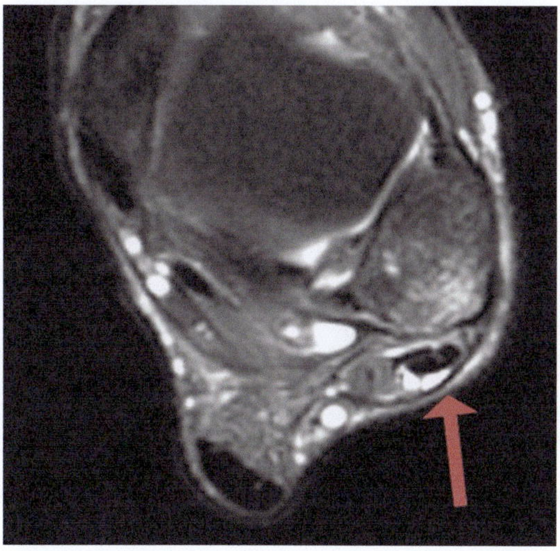

Fig. 35.1 MRI of a PB tendon tear: increased signal intensity due to fluid within the tendon sheath and a splitted tendon

Ultrasound (US) has several advantages in comparison to MRI. It is a less-expensive diagnostic method, can be employed in the outpatient clinic during physical examination and has the ability of dynamic evaluation of the tendons. This makes it easier for diagnosis of dynamic injuries such as (episodic) subluxation, dislocation and tears that are not seen on MRI. It must be noted, however, that the quality of the US is strongly correlated with the quality of the observer. Abnormalities visible on US include tendon thickening, peritendinous fluid within the tendon sheath, ruptures and luxation of the tendons over the fibular tip (Fig. 35.2).

More recent, peroneal tendoscopy is gaining popularity as a method for diagnosing peroneal tendon injuries. It is a highly sensitive and specific tool for both static and dynamic injuries and provides an easy transition to (minimally invasive) treatment (Kennedy et al. 2016; van Dijk 2014). With tendoscopy being an invasive diagnostic method for the patient, the primary indication for the procedure is important. These include posterolateral pain due to high clinical suspicion of tenosynovitis, subluxation or dislocation, partial tears or postoperative adhesion (Scholten and van Dijk 2006; van Dijk 2014). Since MRI can sometimes be inconclusive for diagnosing peroneal tendon tendinopathies, peroneal tendoscopy should be performed when clinical suspicion for a peroneal pathology is strong, with or without positive MRI findings (Kennedy et al. 2016; Marmotti et al. 2012). Not only for diagnosis but also for intervention, peroneal tendoscopy is increasingly used. Recent studies report a relatively low rate of complications with reduced costs and earlier recovery when compared with traditional open procedures (Jerosch and Aldawoudy 2007; Kennedy et al. 2016; Lui 2012; van Dijk and Kort 1998; Vega et al. n.d.).

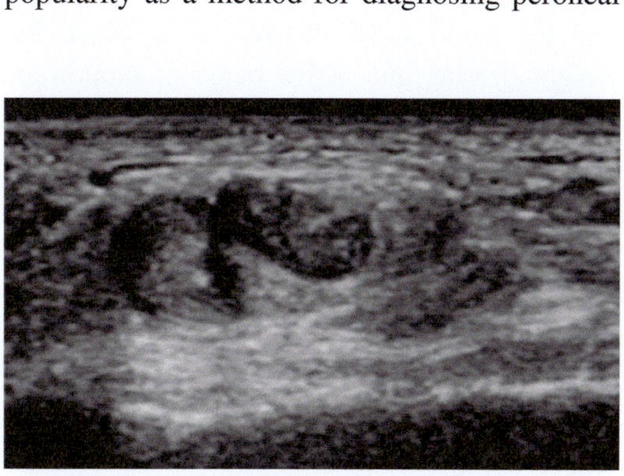

Fig. 35.2 US of the peroneal tendons

35.6 Treatment

Conservative management is the first step in treatment of peroneal tendon injuries, including a period of rest, immobilization or activity modification. Physical therapy is recommended to strengthen the peroneal tendons and surrounding muscles. In case of dislocation, patients should be immobilized in a lower leg cast for 6 weeks with the foot slightly plantar flexed and inverted, after reposing the tendons back in the retromalleolar groove (Selmani et al. 2006).

If symptoms persist, surgical treatment should be considered. Especially in tears and dislocation, surgery is often required since these pathologies rarely heal itself (Dombek et al. 2003; Redfern and Myerson 2004; Squires et al. 2007). After the release of the SPR and inspection of the tendons from the superior to interior retinacular boundaries, the tendons are debrided and decompressed (Fig. 35.3a). When a tear is found, the tendon is tubularized (Fig. 35.3b). This may not

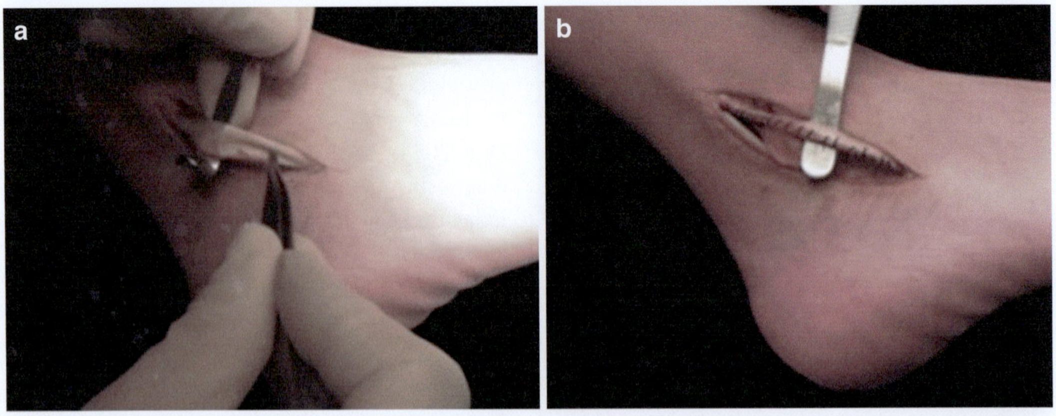

Fig. 35.3 Operative treatment of a peroneal tendon tear. (**a**) The tendon is debrided and decompressed. (**b**) Tubularization of the peroneal tendon tear

be feasible, however, when a gross part of the tendon is affected (Dombek et al. 2003). A study by Dombek et al. suggested that when more than 50% of the cross-sectional area of the tendon is involved, tenodesis to the intact peroneal tendon might be performed in case one of the tendons is still functional. If both tendons are non-functional, auto- or allograft tendon transfer should be considered (Krause and Brodsky 1998; Redfern and Myerson 2004).

For the treatment of recurrent dislocation, multiple operative techniques have been described, all with the primary purpose to restabilize the tendons back in the retromalleolar groove by restoring the anatomy of the superior peroneal tunnel. The techniques can generally be divided into four groups: (1) repair or replacement of the SPR, (2) deepening of the retromalleolar groove, (3) bone-block procedures and (4) enhancement of the SPR by rerouting of other soft tissue structures. The latter two are associated with relatively high complication rates, and therefore over the last years, attention is drawn to the first two categories. Studies looking at repair of the SPR, with or without concomitant groove deepening, show promising outcomes, high satisfaction and an 83–100% rate of return to sports (Porter et al. 2005; Raikin et al. 2008). A recent review by our group found that the combination of SPR repair and retromalleolar groove deepening provides significant higher return to sports rates as compared to SPR repair alone ($p = 0.022$) (van Dijk et al. 2015a)

During operative treatment of peroneal tendon injuries, additional predisposing factors should also be assessed (Bruce et al. 1999; Chilvers and Manoli 2008) since inadequate management of anatomical abnormalities may lead to persistent pain and dysfunction on the longer term. Therefore, additional procedures such as a lateralizing calcaneal osteotomy may be necessary in case of hindfoot varus (Molloy and Tisdel 2003)

35.7 Rehabilitation

Postoperative treatment is very important in successful managing peroneal tendon injuries and should be tailored to every individual patient (van Dijk et al. 2015b). After a tendoscopic procedure, the patient is immobilized in a compressive dressing for 2 days, with the foot in slightly inverted and the ankle at 90 degrees, after which full weight bearing and active range of motion are allowed. In case of an open procedure, including tearing down and repairing of the SPR, the ankle is best immobilized in a splint or cast up to 6 weeks. To promote early range of motion, some surgeons allow early weight bearing after 2 weeks or even shorter. Physical therapy is the key to regain strength and range of motion after a period of immobilization.

A recent review by our group recommends to tailor rehabilitation to every individual patient, for optimal functional recovery (van Dijk et al. 2015b).

Conclusion

Peroneal tendon injuries account for a significant part of posterolateral ankle complaints following acute ankle inversion trauma and can be very debilitating for patients. To prevent the tendons from chronic damage, early diagnosis and treatment are essential. MRI and US are helpful tools in diagnosing peroneal tendon injuries, but patient history and clinical examination are the key to an accurate diagnosis and choosing the optimal treatment strategy. Conservative management is still the first attempt of treatment, but surgical intervention is often necessary. In general, good to excellent results have been described after surgical intervention. To prevent treatment failure or reinjuries of the tendons, predisposing factors such as pes cavus or hindfoot varus should be addressed during initial surgery.

References

Arrowsmith SR et al (1983) Traumatic dislocations of the peroneal tendons. Am J Sports Med 11(3):142–146

Athavale SA et al (2011) Anatomy of the superior peroneal tunnel. J Bone Joint Surg Am 93(6):564–571

Bassett FH 3rd, Speer KP (1993) Longitudinal rupture of the peroneal tendons. Am J Sports Med 21(3):354–357

Borton DC et al (1998) Operative reconstruction after transverse rupture of the tendons of both peroneus longus and brevis. Surgical reconstruction by transfer of the flexor digitorum longus tendon. J Bone Joint Surg 80(5):781–784

Brandes CB, Smith RW (2000) Characterization of patients with primary peroneus longus tendinopathy: a review of twenty-two cases. Foot Ankle Int 21(6):462–468

Bruce WD et al (1999) Stenosing tenosynovitis and impingement of the peroneal tendons associated with hypertrophy of the peroneal tubercle. Foot Ankle Int 20(7):464–467

Cardone BW et al (1993) MRI of injury to the lateral collateral ligamentous complex of the ankle. J Comput Assist Tomogr 17(1):102–107

Chilvers M, Manoli A 2nd (2008) The subtle cavus foot and association with ankle instability and lateral foot overload. Foot Ankle Clin 13(2):315–324, vii. doi:10.1016/j.fcl.2008.01.003

Church CC (1977) Radiographic diagnosis of acute peroneal tendon dislocation. AJR Am J Roentgenol 129(6):1065–1068

DiGiovanni BF et al (2000) Associated injuries found in chronic lateral ankle instability. Foot Ankle Int 21(10):809–815

van Dijk CN (2006) Hindfoot endoscopy for posterior ankle pain. Instr Course Lect 55:545–554

van Dijk CN (2014) Ankle arthroscopy: techniques developed by the Amsterdam foot and ankle school. Springer, Berlin Heidelberg

van Dijk CN, Kort N (1998) Tendoscopy of the peroneal tendons. Arthroscopy 14(5):471–478

van Dijk PA et al (2015a) Return to sports and clinical outcomes in patients treated for peroneal tendon dislocation: a systematic review. Knee Surg Sports Traumatol Arthrosc. doi:10.1007/s00167-015-3833-z

van Dijk PA et al (2015b) Rehabilitation after surgical treatment of peroneal tendon tears and ruptures. Knee Surg Sports Traumatol Arthrosc 24(4):1165–1174. doi:10.1007/s00167-015-3944-6

van Dijk PA et al (2016) Peroneal tendons well vascularized: results from a cadaveric study. Knee Surg Sports Traumatol Arthrosc. doi:10.1007/s00167-015-3946-4

Dombek MF et al (2003) Peroneal tendon tears: a retrospective review. J Foot Ankle Surg 42(5):250–258

Eckert WR, Davis EA Jr (1976) Acute rupture of the peroneal retinaculum. J Bone Joint Surg Am 58(5):670–672

Edwards M (1928) The relations of the peroneal tendons to the fibula, calcaneus, and cuboideum. Am J Anat 42:213–253

Freccero DM, Berkowitz MJ (2006) The relationship between tears of the peroneus brevis tendon and the distal extent of its muscle belly: an MRI study. Foot Ankle Int 27(4):236–239

Heckman DS et al (2008) Operative treatment for peroneal tendon disorders. J Bone Joint Surg Am 90(2):404–418

Jerosch J, Aldawoudy A (2007) Tendoscopic management of peroneal tendon disorders. Knee Surg Sports Traumatol Arthrosc 15(6):806–810

Kennedy JG et al (2016) Functional outcomes after peroneal tendoscopy in the treatment of peroneal tendon disorders. Knee Surgery Sports Traumatol Arthrosc. doi:10.1007/s00167-016-4012-6

Khan KM et al (1999) Histopathology of common tendinopathies. Update and implications for clinical management. Sports Med 27(6):393–408

Krause JO, Brodsky JW (1998) Peroneus brevis tendon tears: pathophysiology, surgical reconstruction, and clinical results. Foot Ankle Int 19(5):271–279

Kumai T, Benjamin M (2003) The histological structure of the malleolar groove of the fibula in man: its direct bearing on the displacement of peroneal tendons and their surgical repair. J Anat 203(2):257–262

Lui TH (2012) Endoscopic management of recalcitrant retrofibular pain without peroneal tendon subluxation or dislocation. Arch Orthop Trauma Surg 132(3):357–361

Marmotti A et al (2012) Peroneal tendoscopy. Curr Rev Muscoskelet Med 5(2):135–144

Molloy R, Tisdel C (2003) Failed treatment of peroneal tendon injuries. Foot Ankle Clin 8(1):115–129

Mota J, Rosenberg ZS (1998) Magnetic resonance imaging of the peroneal tendons. Top Magn Reson Imaging 9(5):273–285

Oden RR (1987) Tendon injuries about the ankle resulting from skiing. Clin Orthop Relat Res 216:63–69

Park HJ et al (2010) Reliability of MRI findings of peroneal tendinopathy in patients with lateral chronic ankle instability. Clin Orthop Surg 2(4):237–243. doi:10.4055/cios.2010.2.4.237

Petersen W et al (2000) Blood supply of the peroneal tendons: injection and immunohistochemical studies of cadaver tendons. Acta Orthop Scand 71(2):168–174

Philbin TM et al (2009) Peroneal tendon injuries. J Am Acad Orthop Surg 17(5):306–317

Porter D et al (2005) Peroneal tendon subluxation in athletes: fibular groove deepening and retinacular reconstruction. Foot Ankle Int 26(6):436–441

Raikin SM et al (2008) Intrasheath subluxation of the peroneal tendons. J Bone Joint Surg Am 90(5):992–999

Redfern D, Myerson M (2004) The management of concomitant tears of the peroneus longus and brevis tendons. Foot Ankle Int 25(10):695–707

Rosenberg ZS et al (1987) Peroneal tendon injury associated with calcaneal fractures: CT findings. AJR Am J Roentgenol 149(1):125–129

Rosenberg ZS et al (1997) MR features of longitudinal tears of the peroneus brevis tendon. AJR Am J Roentgenol 168(1):141–147

Rosenberg ZS et al (1998) Normal variants and pitfalls in magnetic resonance imaging of the ankle and foot. Top Magn Reson Imaging 9(5):262–272

Safran MR et al (1999) Peroneal tendon subluxation in athletes: new exam technique, case reports, and review. Med Sci Sports Exerc 31(7 Suppl):487–492

Sammarco GJ, DiRaimondo CV (1989) Chronic peroneus brevis tendon lesions. Foot Ankle 9(4):163–170

Saupe N et al (2007) Anatomic variants associated with peroneal tendon disorders: MR imaging findings in volunteers with asymptomatic ankles. Radiology 242(2):509–517

Scholten PE, van Dijk CN (2006) Tendoscopy of the peroneal tendons. Foot Ankle Clin 11(2):415–420

Schweitzer ME et al (1997) Using MR imaging to differentiate peroneal splits from other peroneal disorders. AJR Am J Roentgenol 168(1):129–133

Selmani E et al (2006) Current concepts review: peroneal tendon disorders. Foot Ankle Int 27(3):221–228

Sobel M et al (1991) Longitudinal splitting of the peroneus brevis tendon: an anatomic and histologic study of cadaveric material. Foot Ankle 12(3):165–170

Squires N et al (2007) Surgical treatment of peroneal tendon tears. Foot Ankle Clin 12(4):675–695, vii

Strauss JE et al (2007) Chronic lateral ankle instability and associated conditions: a rationale for treatment. Foot Ankle Int 28(10):1041–1044

Thomas JL et al (2009) A preliminary report on intrasheath peroneal tendon subluxation: a prospective review of 7 patients with ultrasound verification. J Foot Ankle Surg 48(3):323–329

Truong DT et al (1995) Fracture of the os peroneum and rupture of the peroneus longus tendon as a complication of diabetic neuropathy. Skelet Radiol 24(8):626–628

Vainio K (1991) The rheumatoid foot. A clinical study with pathological and roentgenological comments. Clin Orthop Relat Res 265:4–8

Vega J, Golano P, Batista JP et al (2013) Tendoscopic procedure associated with peroneal tendons. Tech Foot & Ankle 12(1):39–48

Wang XT et al (2005) Normal variants and diseases of the peroneal tendons and superior peroneal retinaculum: MR imaging features. Radiographics 25(3): 587–602

Wong-Chung J et al (2015) Incidence and recognition of peroneal tendon dislocation associated with calcaneal fractures. Foot Ankle Surg 21(4):254–259. doi:10.1016/j.fas.2015.01.013

Wright DG, Sangeorzan BJ (1996) Calcaneal fracture with peroneal impingement and tendon dysfunction. Foot Ankle Int 17(10):650

Yammine K (2015) The accessory peroneal (fibular) muscles: peroneus quartus and peroneus digiti quinti. A systematic review and meta-analysis. Surg Radiol Anat 37(6):617–627. doi:10.1007/s00276-015-1438-3

Younger AS, Hansen ST Jr (2005) Adult cavovarus foot. J Am Acad Orthop Surg 13(5):302–315

Insertional Plantar Fasciitis

36

O. Haruki, S. Guillo, and T. Bauer

Contents

O. Haruki, M.D. • S. Guillo, M.D.
Department of Orthopaedic, Clinique du Sport, Mérignac, France

T. Bauer, M.D., Ph.D. (✉)
Department of Orthopaedic, Ambroise Paré University Hospital, West Paris University, Boulogne Billancourt, France
e-mail: thomas.bauer@aphp.fr

36.1 Introduction

Plantar Fasciitis (PF) is one of the most common causes of heel pain in adults (Abbassian et al. 2012). The population of patients suffering from PF is reported between 3 and 7% (Stephens and Walker 1997; Thomas et al. 2010), and 8% of PF patients are runners (Lysholm and Wiklander 1987; Taunton et al. 2002). The peak incidence of PF occurs between 40 and 60 years old (Furey 1975). Almost PF can be recovered without surgical intervention (Buchbinder 2004; Singh et al. 1997), PF threatens health-related quality of life (Buchbinder 2004), and it was reported that the economic burden to the US healthcare system in 2007 alone was estimated at between $192 and $376 million (Tong and Furia 2010).

36.2 Anatomy and Function

The plantar fascia consists of three bands: medial, central, and lateral. Each band is separated by an intermuscular septum that splits the intrinsic plantar muscle into their different compartments (Hicks 1954). The lateral band is superficial to

G.L. Canata et al. (eds.), *Muscle and Tendon Injuries*, DOI 10.1007/978-3-662-54184-5_36

the abductor digiti quinti minimi muscle and also attached to the lateral process of the calcaneus and the base of the fifth metatarsal. The medial band of the plantar fascia is superficial to the abductor hallucis muscle and connected to the flexor retinaculum. The flexor digitorum brevis muscle arises from the central band of the plantar fascia. The plantar fascial bands are supplied by the medial and lateral plantar nerves. The thickness of a normal plantar fascia is approximately 3 mm. In patients with plantar fasciitis, the maximum thickness is significantly increased to 7 mm (Berkowitz et al. 1991).

Hicks showed that the plantar fascia is tensioned during the latter weight bearing stage, and, as the metatarsophalangeal joints dorsiflex, this induces a tractional force at its point of insertion on the calcaneum: it's called the windlass effect (Hicks 1954). It also plays a dynamic role during the gait cycle where it elongates during the stance phase, storing potential energy during the process. It locks the midfoot during toe-off to provide a rigid structure for propulsion. The plantar fascia then passively contracts, converting the previously stored potential energy into kinetic energy and aiding acceleration.

36.3 Mechanism of Disorder

The underlying pathological changes in PF are not completely well understood. Plantar fascia can be a ligament in anatomical terms; however, deep to the superficial structure of the plantar fascia is the flexor digitorum brevis muscle with a tendon enthesis attachment to the calcaneus proximally. Therefore, it can be also explained that proximal tendinopathy of the flexor digitorum brevis muscle is involved in the pathology of PF. Lemont et al. reported 50 cases of PF who had surgery and couldn't find histological evidence of inflammation (Lemont et al. 2003). Histologically, the condition is a fasciosis; however, many PF are successfully treated by steroid injection or oral anti-inflammatory drugs. This can be explained that inflammation triggered by microtrauma.

36.4 Risk Factor

Numerous risk factors are implicated in its development. The evidence supporting these factors is limited, and their relative importance is unclear (Beeson 2014). Several causes have been hypothesized, with the most common being overuse due to prolonged weight-bearing, obesity, unaccustomed walking or running, limited ankle joint dorsiflexion, posterior muscle group tightness, and standing on hard surfaces (Beeson 2014; Bolivar et al. 2013; Puttaswarmaiah and Chandran 2007; Singh et al. 1997; Werner et al. 2010).

The presence of coexisting calcaneal spurs has often been reported (Karabay et al. 2007; McNally and Shetty 2010; Orchard 2012; Wainwright et al. 1995), but confusion exists as to whether it is a causal or significant association. Some suggest that calcaneal spurs may be an adaptive response to vertical compression of the heel rather than longitudinal traction at the calcaneal enthesis (Menz et al. 2008). A study examining prehistoric skeletal remains (Weiss 2012) concludes that plantar calcaneal spurs are a modern phenomenon resulting from long periods of standing and excess weight and associated with lower limb osteoarthritis. On the other hand, Wainwright et al. (Wainwright et al. 1995) reported a strong correlation with calcaneal spurs over 1 mm long and PF, and Johal and Milner (2012) found a higher prevalence of calcaneal spurs in patients with PF. Further research is necessary to assess whether it is a causal or significant association (Weiss 2012).

36.5 Diagnosis

The diagnosis of PF is mainly clinically performed. Patients usually complain of pain at the anteromedial prominence of the calcaneus. The pain is exacerbated by passive dorsiflexion of the toes. The pain is worse when first standing after rest, typically early in the morning. Once the patient starts walking, the pain tends to reduce. The pain eases but never fully resolves throughout the course of the day and is exacerbated by activities such as prolonged walking or exercise, particularly on hard surfaces (Berkowitz et al. 1991).

Plain x-ray is the most commonly requested investigation. X-ray shows a calcaneal spur in 50% of patients. As mentioned at the Risk Factor, the spur is not related to the plantar fascia and is the attachment of the quadratus plantar muscle.

Ultrasonography (US) is recently reported as a useful device to diagnose the PF (Berkowitz et al. 1991; Gibbon and Long 1999). Normal plantar fascia is hyperechoic and isoechoic with adjacent fat. In PF patients, the proximal end of the fascia is hypoechoic, which can clearly be seen when compared with the surrounding soft tissues. Plantar fascia is also significantly thicker in PF patients. Symptomatic patients were seen to have fascia measuring 4 mm or more in thickness, whereas those of asymptomatic patients measured 4 mm or less (Berkowitz et al. 1991; Gibbon and Long 1999). Jeong et al. reported that high proportion of atypical non-insertional PF would not be detected without US. The use of US in cases of recalcitrant plantar heel pain that have failed conservative treatment is recommended (Jeong et al. 2013; McMillan et al. 2009). It was concluded that US confirmed clinical diagnosis and classification characteristics as either insertional, non-insertional, or mixed of them (Jeong et al. 2013).

Technetium bone scintigraphy is positive in PF, with the maximum area of uptake at the point of maximum tenderness on the heel. It has also been shown to be an accurate guide in selecting the adequate site for injection therapy (Frater et al. 2006).

Computerized tomography (CT) scan can be performed if calcaneal stress fracture is suspected. Generally, MRI or CT would be considered only in those cases recalcitrant to treatment and for those patients with a high index of suspicion for the other causes of heel pain.

MRI is not a routine investigation in PF but can identify other soft tissue lesions such as soft tissue tumor, or the bone marrow edema associated with infection or if an occult fracture is suspected (Chimutengwende-Gordon et al. 2010) (Figs. 36.1 and 36.2).

Electromyography may be helpful if a neurogenic cause is suspected such as S1 nerve root entrapment, tarsal tunnel syndrome, or entrapment of the lateral plantar nerve.

Blood tests, such as a white cell count, human leucocyte antigen B27, antinuclear antibodies,

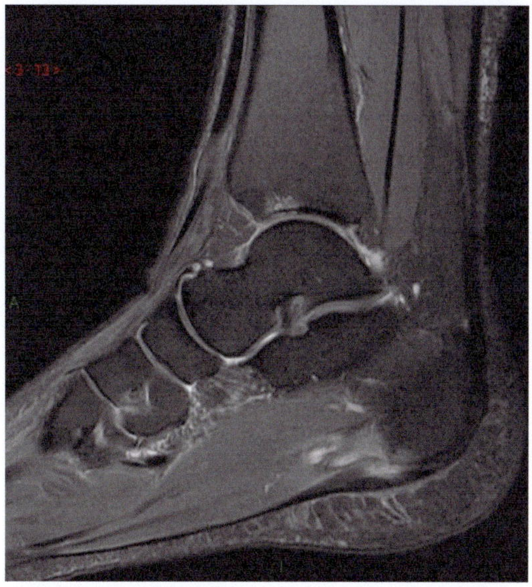

Fig. 36.1 MRI, sagittal view: partial plantar fascia rupture with bone edema

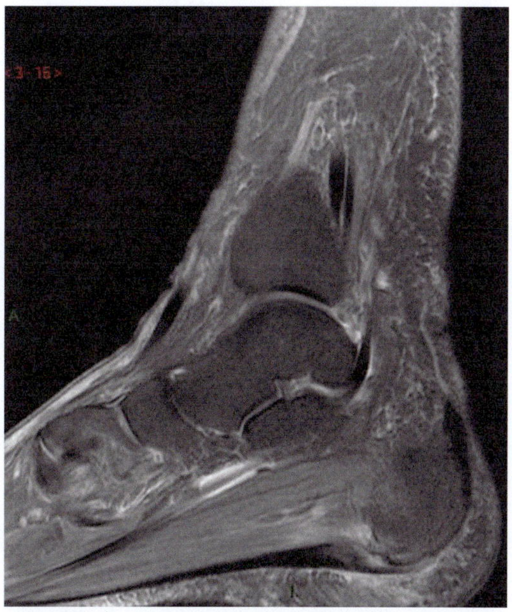

Fig. 36.2 MRI, sagittal view; plantar fasciitis with thickened fascia

and uric acid, may be needed, particularly in younger patients or with those patients who have bilateral heel pain to distinguish rheumatoid arthritis, Reiter syndrome, ankylosing spondylitis, and so on.

36.6 Conservative Treatment

36.6.1 Nonsteroidal Anti-Inflammatory Drugs (NSAIDs)

Histologically, PF is not an inflammatory disease but mainly degenerative change. However, NSAIDs are sometimes an effective treatment. In a meta-analysis study, it was found that the NSAIDs group had improved pain relief and disability compared with placebo in short to mid-term (Donley et al. 2007).

36.6.2 Stretching

Stretching is an easy treatment option. A randomized controlled trial has investigated the role of specific Achilles tendon versus plantar fascia stretching exercises in patients with established chronic plantar fasciitis. (DiGiovanni et al. 2003) This involved an eight-week program supplemented by celecoxib for the first three weeks. The short-term outcome demonstrated superior results relating to pain using the Foot Function Index in the plantar fascia-specific stretching group compared with the Achilles stretching group. The 2-year follow-up via questionnaire demonstrated 94% of respondents reported decreased pain, and 92% reported total satisfaction or satisfaction with minor reservations except late stage (DiGiovanni et al. 2006).

36.6.3 Low Dye Taping

Low dye taping is often an effective treatment modality in mild to moderate cases. The strapping uses adhesive tape to immobilize the foot and decreases the distance between the origin and insertion of the plantar fascia, thus relieving plantar strain. Tape will loosen in time, often quickly, and may prove less effective in severe cases. Relief with plantar support by strapping often gives a good indication of the efficacy of orthosis in PF patient (Yale 1974).

36.6.4 Orthotic Devices

Night splints hold the foot in a neutral position, preventing the contracture of the fascia during sleep, which helps to alleviate symptoms in the morning. However, there has been no randomized controlled trial to prove that symptoms are alleviated. Heel inserts are quite popular and can be beneficial in relieving heel pain. Wolgin et al. showed that after six months, 82% of patients had responded to time and conservative therapy (Snook and Chrisman 1972; Wolgin et al. 1994). Orthosis is very good treatment for PF, it is reported that only 1–2% of PF required surgical intervention (Furey 1975).

36.6.5 Extracorporeal Shockwave Therapy (ESWT)

ESWT in the treatment of PF has reported success rate ranging from 34 to 88% (Chen et al. 2001; Weil et al. 2002). Mechanism of ESWT is still unclear, but it is believed that the shockwaves cause micro-disruption of the thickened plantar fascia, resulting in an inflammatory response, revascularization, and recruitment of growth factors and therefore a soft tissue reparative response (Ogden et al. 2004). Before, ESWT was considered as an end-stage treatment for those patients who have failed conservative measures and are reluctant to have open surgery (Hammer et al. 2002; Wang et al. 2002). However, double-blind randomized controlled trial showed radial ESWT to be better than placebo in recalcitrant patients (Gerdesmeyer et al. 2008). Moreover meta-analysis revealed that the short-term pain relief and functional outcomes of this treatment are satisfactory (Yin et al. 2014). Radwan et al. reported that the clinical results of ESWT are comparable with those of endoscopic plantar fasciotomy for resistant PF at 3 weeks, 3 months, and 1 year postoperation (Radwan et al. 2012). Thus, ESWT can be a useful noninvasive treatment for resistant PF and leads to reduce the necessity for surgical intervention. Further studies focused on the medium-and-long term are necessary to make sure the importance of ESWT.

36.7 Injection Therapy

1. Steroid injections

Steroid injections are often effective in the short term (Crawford et al. 1999) although they have risks of fat pad atrophy and occasionally, rupture of the plantar fascia (Acevedo and Beskin 1998). One case series of six athletes with rupture of the plantar fascia noted five had previously received steroid injections (Leach et al. 1978).

2. Platelet-rich plasma (PRP)

PRP has been proposed as a potential treatment for PF. A prospective randomized study revealed that PRP was more effective and durable than steroid injection for the treatment of resistant PF (Monto 2014). PRP is also effective in long term; however, the indication must be considered with its cost-effectiveness.

3. Botulinum toxin

The effect of botulinum toxin injection for PF has shown apparently good effect; however, actually it seems not to be often used clinically (Tsikopoulos and Vasiliadis 2016).

4. Dehydrated human amniotic membrane

Konstantinos et al. reported a systematic review and network meta-analysis of 22 randomized controlled trials of injection therapy for PF (Tsikopoulos and Vasiliadis 2016). The injection therapies included as follows: corticosteroids, BTX-A, autologous whole blood, placebo, platelet-rich plasma, cryopreserved human amniotic membrane, micronized dehydrated human amniotic/chorionic membrane, dextrose prolotherapy, sham dry needling, and polydeoxyribonucleotide. This report concluded that the dehydrated amniotic membrane injection was the highest probability of being superior to placebo injection over 8 weeks and that for pain relief. Hall et al. reported the efficiency to inject guided by echography because the accuracy of US guidance is greater than that of palpation guidance; therefore, injection therapy may have more effective possibility (Hall 2013).

36.8 Surgical Treatment

When conservative management fails, which occurs in approximately 1–10% of patients, surgical options should be considered. Symptoms should be present for more than 6 months before surgery should be discussed. It is still unclear that which procedures should be selected, because there are many reports about surgical intervention for PF, but there is no evidence from randomized control trials to support surgery.

36.9 Open Plantar Fasciotomy

Open plantar fasciotomy allows for release of the tight plantar fascial bands. Open surgery has risks; approximately 25% of patients will still experience heel pain after the surgery (Buchbinder 2004). Over-release of the plantar fascia may lead to flatfoot complications. Nerve entrapments can occur, as well as pain along the scar. Contompasis (1974) performed a 3 year retrospective study of 126 surgeries for PF. Plantar fascial release provided 36% satisfactory relief (Contompasis 1974). A combination of fascial release and spur resection allowed 44.3% to have complete resolution of pain and 45.2% to have improvement in pain, whereas 10.5% had no relief.

36.10 Endoscopic Plantar Fasciotomy

The first report about endoscopic plantar fasciotomy (EPF) is by Barrett SL et al. (Barrett and Day 1991), and after that, EPF has become more popular because of its minimally invasive nature and visualization of the fascia. Basically it minimizes complications and recovery time compared with open procedures.

There are two approaches of EPF, superficial and deep fascia approach. The first method Barret et al. reported was superficial fascia approach; after that, Blanco et al. reported deep-fascia approach which has comparative results with superficial approach (Blanco et al. 2001). Komastu et al. reported that deep-fascia approach had advantages to visualize calcaneal spurs and resection of them (Komatsu et al. 2011). Whichever taking the approach, the superficial and deep layers of the medial band of the plantar fascia are released, and the width of resection is approximately halfway across the fascia (Hogan et al. 2004). Satisfaction in relief of heel pain and clinical results are superior to open procedures.

36.11 Echo-Guided Plantar Fasciotomy

Cadaveric preliminary studies proved that plantar fasciotomy can be efficiently and safely performed under US control. The portal has to be medial at the end of the plantar skin on the alignment of the sonograph. The US control has the advantage to be based on the soft tissue (to the opposite of the fluoroscan) and allow also to see structures that are not dissected like the nerve and the artery (to the opposite of the endoscopic technique) (Figs. 36.3, 36.4, and 36.5).

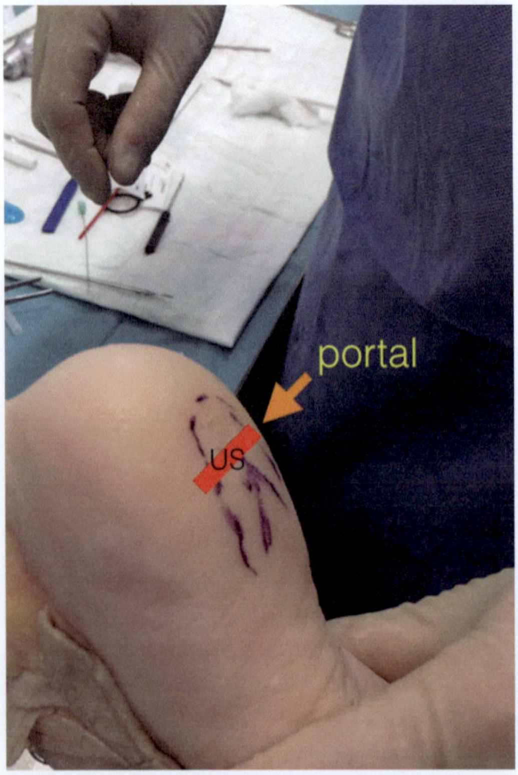

Fig. 36.3 Landmarks and portals for plantar fasciotomy under ultrasonographic control

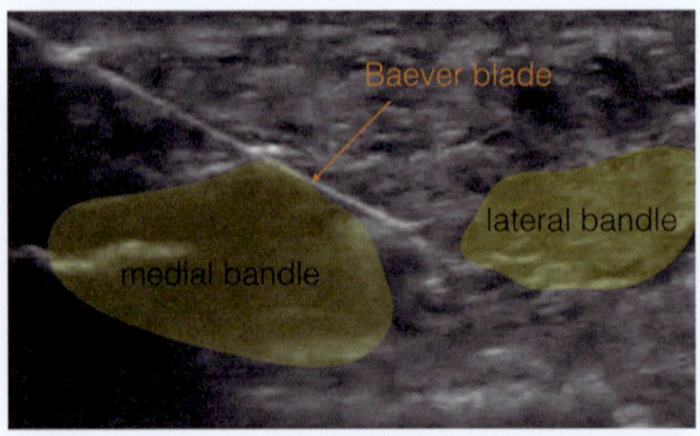

Fig. 36.4 Ultrasonographic plantar fascia visualization and fasciotomy

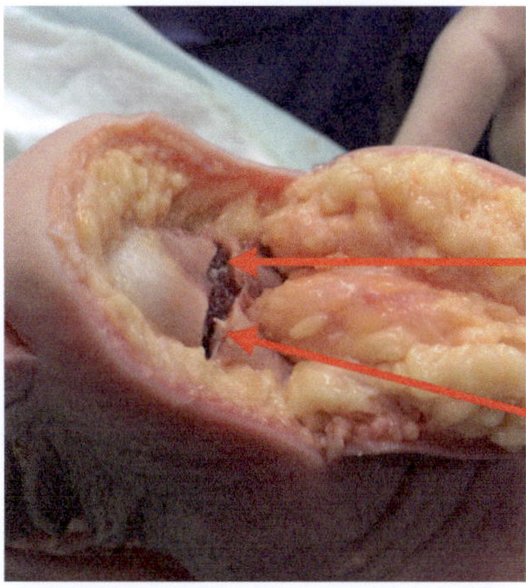

Fig. 36.5 Control of the quality of plantar fasciotomy under US control

36.12 Gastrocnemius Resection

Isolated gastrocnemius tightness has been associated with failure of conservative treatments (Patel and DiGiovanni 2011). Plantar fascia tension was directly proportional to Achilles tendon tension on cadavers in dynamic gait stimulator (Erdimir et al. 2004). Carlson et al. found that increasing tension within Achilles tendon caused increase in plantar fascia tension at four different angles of MPJ dorsiflexion (Erdimir et al. 2004). Biomechanics is believed to contribute to the onset of increasing plantar fascia tension through a decreased ankle joint range of motion. Reduced dorsiflexion of the ankle is the most important risk factor for the development of recalcitrant PF (Riddle et al. 2003). In a prospective study, the gastrocnemius resection has shown excellent results in the treatment of recalcitrant PF. Abbassian et al. reported that 17/21 patients diagnosed with PF experienced significant or total pain relief (Abbassian et al. 2012). Monteagudo et al. reported that the mean VAS pain score for a cohort of patients with PF that underwent proximal medial gastrocnemius release improved from 8.2 to 0.9. AOFAS scores improved and from 46 to 90 in this cohort as well. Moreover, open plantar fasciotomy compares poorly to PMGR about patient satisfaction (Monteagudo et al. 2013).

36.13 Radiofrequency Microtenotomy

As radiofrequency microtenotomy leads good results for Achilles tendinosis and other fasciitis, it has been proposed as a minimally invasive treatment modality for chronic PF (Akhtar et al. 2009; Shibuya et al. 2012). Radiofrequency microtenotomy induces epidermal destruction with minimal thermal damage, resulting in improved healing through controlled inflammation and focal angiogenesis (Shibuya et al. 2012). Radiofrequency microtenotomy was as effective at relieving pain, improving function, achieving patient satisfaction, and meeting patient expectations as plantar fasciotomy at 1 year follow-up (Chou et al. 2016).

36.14 Percutaneous Cryosurgery

Percutaneous cryosurgery uses subfreezing temperatures to produce analgesic effects. In a study by Cavazos et al., 77.4% of the patients were considered to have successful results after surgery. This procedure is still being studied for the effects on nerve and soft tissue after the freeze-thaw cycles (Cavazos et al. 2009).

Conclusion

PF is a common and recalcitrant disease in some cases. It is difficult to distinguish between those patients who have recovered spontaneously and those who have responded to formal treatment, because the mechanism of disorder is not fully understood and diagnosis is mostly performed clinically. Surgical MIS interventions and new treatments such as injection therapy,

Fig. 36.6 Algorithm for plantar fascia treatment

1st stage conservative treatment	Orthosis (low-dye-taping) Anti-inflammatory drugs
2nd stage treatment	ESWT Injection therapy (steroids, BTX-A, PRP, dehydrated amniotic membrane)
3rd stage surgical treatment	Endoscopic plantar fasciotomy microtenotomy

microtenotomy, and ESWT are effective for the patients who do not respond to conservative treatments; however, there are few evidence of randomized trial study (Fig. 36.6).

References

Abbassian A, Kohls-Gatzoulis J, Solan MC (2012) Proximal medial gastrocnemius release in the treatment of recalcitrant plantar fasciitis. Foot Ankle Int 33:14–19

Acevedo JI, Beskin JL (1998) Complications of plantar fascia rupture associated with corticosteroid injection. Foot Ankle Int 19:91–97

Akhtar M, Montgomery H, Shenolikar A (2009) Achilles tendon rupture following coblation for insertional Achilles tendinosis. Foot 19:55–57

Barrett SL, Day SV (1991) Endoscopic plantar fasciotomy for chronic plantar fasciitis/heel spur syndrome: surgical technique--early clinical results. J Foot Surg 30:568–570

Beeson P (2014) Plantar fasciopathy: revisiting the risk factors. Foot Ankle Surg 20:160–165

Berkowitz JF, Kier R, Rudicel S (1991) Plantar fasciitis: MR imaging. Radiology 179:665–667

Blanco CE, Leon HO, Guthrie TB (2001) Endoscopic treatment of calcaneal spur syndrome: a comprehensive technique. Arthroscopy 17:517–522

Bolivar YA, Munuera PV, Padillo JP (2013) Relationship between tightness of the posterior muscles of the lower limb and plantar fasciitis. Foot Ankle Int 34:42–48

Buchbinder R (2004) Clinical practice. Plantar fasciitis. N Engl J Med 350:2159–2166

Cavazos J, Khan KH, D'Antoni AV et al (2009) Cryosurgery for the treatment of heel pain. Foot Ankle Int 53:500–505

Chen HH, Chen LM, Huang TW (2001) Treatment of painful heel syndrome with shock waves. Clinc Orthop Relat Res 387:41–46

Chimutengwende-Gordon M, O'Donnell P, Singh D (2010) Magnetic resonance imaging in plantar heel pain. Foot Ankle Int 31:865–870

Chou AC, Ng SY, Su DH (2016) Radiofrequency microtenotomy is as effective as plantar fasciotomy in the treatment of recalcitrant plantar fasciitis. Foot Ankle Surg 22:270–273

Contompasis JP (1974) Surgical treatment of calcaneal spurs: a three-year postsurgical study. J Am Podiatr Med Assoc 64:987–999

Crawford F, Atkins D, Young P, Edwards J (1999) Steroid injection for heel pain: evidence of short-term effectiveness. A randomized controlled trial. Rheumatology 38:974–977

DiGiovanni BF, Nawoczenski DA, Lintal ME et al (2003) Tissue-specific plantar fascia stretching exercise enhances outcomes in patients with chronic heel pain. A prospective, randomized study. J Bone Joint Surg Am 85:1270–1277

DiGiovanni BF, Nawoczenski DA, Malay DP et al (2006) Plantar fascia-specific stretching exercise improves outcomes in patients with chronic plantar fasciitis. A prospective clinical trial with two-year follow-up. J Bone Joint Surg Am 88:1775–1778

Donley BG, Moore T, Sferra J et al (2007) The efficacy of oral nonsteroidal anti-inflammatory medication (NSAID) in the treatment of plantar fasciitis: a randomized, prospective, placebo-controlled study. Foot Ankle Int 28:20–23

Erdimir A, Hamel AJ, Fauth AR, Piazza SJ (2004) Sharkey NA dynamic loading of the plantar aponeurosis in walking. JBJS 86(A):546–552

Frater C, Vu D, Van der Wall H (2006) Bone scintigraphy predicts outcome of steroid injection for plantar fasciitis. J Nucl Med 47:1577–1580

Furey JG (1975) Plantar fasciitis. The painful heel syndrome. J Bone Joint Surg Am 57:672–673

Gerdesmeyer L, Frey C, Vester J et al (2008) Radial extracorporeal shock wave therapy is safe and effective in the treatment of chronic recalcitrant plantar fasciitis: results of a confirmatory randomized placebo-controlled multicenter study. Am J Sports Med 36:2100–2109

Gibbon WW, Long G (1999) Ultrasound of the plantar aponeurosis (fascia). Skeletal Radiol 28:21–26

Hall MM (2013) The accuracy and efficacy of palpation versus image-guided peripheral injections in sports medicine. Curr Sports Med Rep 12:296–303
Hammer DS, Rupp S, Kreutz A et al (2002) Extracorporeal shockwave therapy (ESWT) in patients with chronic proximal plantar fasciitis. Foot Ankle Int 23:309–313
Hicks JH (1954) The mechanics of the foot. II. The plantar aponeurosis and the arch. J Anat 88:25–30
Hogan KA, Webb D, Shereff M (2004) Endoscopic plantar fascia release. Foot Ankle Int 25(12):875–881
Jeong E, Afolayam J, Carne A, Solan M (2013) Ultrasound scanning for recalcitrant plantar faciopathy: basis of a new classification. Skeletal Radiol 42:393–398
Johal KS, Milner SA (2012) Plantar fasciitis and the calcaneal spur: fact or fiction? J Foot Ankle Surg 18(1):39–41
Karabay N, Toros T, Hurel C (2007) Ultrasonographic evaluation in plantar fasciitis. J Foot Ankle Surg 46:442–446
Komatsu F, Takao M, Innami K (2011) Endoscopic surgery for plantar fasciitis: application of a deep-fascial approach. Arthroscopy 27:1105–1109
Leach R, Jones R, Silva T (1978) Rupture of the plantar fascia in athletes. Bone Joint Surg Am 60:537–539
Lemont H, Ammirati KM, Usen N (2003) Plantar fasciitis: a degenerative process (fasciosis) without inflammation. J Am Podiatr Med Assoc 93:234–237
Lysholm J, Wiklander J (1987) Injuries in runners. Am J Sports Med 15:168–171
McMillan AM, Landorf KB, Barrett JT, Menz HB, Bird AR (2009) Diagnostic imaging for chronic plantar heel pain: a systematic review and meta-analysis. J Foot Ankle Res 2:32
McNally EG, Shetty S (2010) Plantar fascia: imaging diagnosis and guided treatment. Semin Musculoskelet Radiol 14:334–343
Menz HB, Zammit GV, Landorf KB, Munteanu SE (2008) Plantar calcaneal spurs in older people: longitudinal traction or vertical compression? J Foot Ankle Res 1:7
Monteagudo M, Maceira E, Garcia-Virto V (2013) Chronic plantar fasciitis: plantar fasciotomy versus gastrocnemius recession. Int Orthop 37(9): 1845–1850
Monto RR (2014) Platelet-rich plasma efficacy versus corticosteroid injection treatment for chronic severe plantar fasciitis. Foot Ankle Int 35:313–318
Ogden JA, Alvarez RG, Levitt RL et al (2004) Electrohydraulic high-energy shockwave treatment for chronic plantar fasciitis. J Bone Joint Surg Am 86:2216–2228
Orchard J (2012) Plantar fasciitis—clinical review. Br Med J 345:35–40
Patel A, DiGiovanni B (2011) Association between plantar fasciitisand isolated contracture of the gastrocnemius. Foot Ankle Int 32:5–8
Puttaswarmaiah R, Chandran P (2007) Degenerative plantar fasciitis: a review ofcurrent concepts. Foot 17(1):3–9
Radwan YA, Mansour AM, Badawy WS (2012) Resistant plantar fasciopathy: shock wave versus endoscopic plantar fascial release. Int Orthop 36:2147–2156
Riddle DL, Pulisic M, Pidcoe P, Johnson RE (2003) Risk factors for plantar fasciitis: a match controlled study. J Bone Joint Surg 85A:872–877
Shibuya N, Thorud JC, Humphers JM, Devall JM, Jupiter DC (2012) Is percutaneous radiofrequency coblation for treatment of Achilles tendinosis safe and effective. J Foot Ankle Surg 51:767–771
Singh D, Angel J, Bentley G et al (1997) Fortnightly review. Plantar fasciitis. BMJ 315:172–175
Snook GA, Chrisman OD (1972) The management of subcalcaneal pain. Clin Orthop Relat Res 82:163–168
Stephens MM, Walker G (1997) Heel pain: an overview of its aetiology and management. J Foot Ankle Surg 3:51–60
Taunton JE, Ryan MB, Clement DB et al (2002) A retrospective case-control analysis of 2002 running injuries. Br J Sports Med 36:95–101
Thomas JL, Christensen JC, Kravitz SR, Mendicino RW, Schuberth JM, Vanore JV et al (2010) The diagnosis and treatment of heel pain: a clinical practice guideline-revision 2010. J Foot Ankle Surg 49:S1–S9
Tong KB, Furia J (2010) Economic burden of plantar fasciitis in the United States. Am J Orthop 39:227–231
Tsikopoulos K, Vasiliadis HS (2016) Mavridis D injection therapies for plantar fasciopathy ('plantar fasciitis'): a systematic review and network meta-analysis of 22 randomised controlled trials. Br J Sports Med 50:1367–1375
Wainwright AM, Kelly AJ, Winson IG (1995) Calcaneal spurs and plantar fasciitis. Foot 5(3):123–126
Wang CJ, Chen HS, Huang TW (2002) Shockwave therapy for patients with plantar fasciitis: a one-year follow-up study. Foot Ankle Int 23:204–207
Weil LS Jr, Roukis TS, Weil LS, Borrelli AH (2002) Extracorporeal shock wave therapy for the treatment of chronic plantar fasciitis: indications, protocol, intermediate results, and a comparison of results to fasciotomy. J Foot Ankle Surg 41(3):166–172
Weiss E (2012) Calcaneal spurs: examining etiology using prehistoric skeletal remains to understand present day heel pain. Foot 22(3):125–129
Werner RA, Gell N, Hartigan A, Wiggerman N, Keyserling WM (2010) Risk factors for plantar fasciitis among assembly plant workers. Phys Med Rehabil 2:110–116
Wolgin M, Cook C, Graham C, Mauldin D (1994) Conservative treatment of plantar heel pain: long-term follow-up. Foot Ankle Int 15:97–102
Yale I (1974) Podiatric medicine. Williams and Wilkins, Baltimore, pp 219–220
Yin MC, Ye J, Yao M (2014) Is extracorporeal shock wave therapy clinical efficacy for relief of chronic, recalcitrant plantar fasciitis? A systematic review and meta-analysis of randomized placebo or active-treatment controlled trials. Arch Phys Med Rehabil 95:1585–1593

Posterior Impingement in the Ankle: "Can There Also Be a Muscular or Tendinous Entity?"

37

Pieter d'Hooghe

Contents

P. d'Hooghe
Department of Orthopaedic Surgery, ASPETAR Orthopaedic and Sportsmedicine Hospital, Aspire Zone, Sportscity Street 1, PO Box 29222, Doha, Qatar
e-mail: pieter.dhooghe@aspetar.com

37.1 Terminology

The posterior process of the talus articulates with the tibia superiorly and contributes significantly to the subtalar articulation inferiorly at the posterior facet. It consists of a more prominent lateral (Stieda's process) and a medial tubercle with the flexor hallucis longus (FHL) tendon running in the sulcus between them. Fractures of either tubercle or the complete posterior process, although rare, have been described and have been associated with sports injuries, including football. It has been common to misdiagnose these as ankle sprains initially, while the normal accessory os trigonum just posterior to the lateral tubercle can be erroneously thought to be a fracture. In individuals that have an accessory os trigonum, a fracture of the latter, or more commonly injury to its synchondrosis with the lateral tubercle, can occur after injury that can lead to subsequent "os trigonum syndrome" (Golano et al. 2002; van Dijk et al. 2000). Frequently this syndrome is closely related to inflammatory processes over the FHL in the posterior ankle area of the abovementioned sulcus. Therefore, when describing the pathogenesis and clinical features of the posterior ankle impingement syndrome, the closely related musculotendinous entities (especially FHL) need to be considered.

G.L. Canata et al. (eds.), *Muscle and Tendon Injuries*, DOI 10.1007/978-3-662-54184-5_37

37.2 Introduction

In the early 1930s—and mainly because of its anatomic features—the ankle joint was found unsuitable for arthroscopy (Burman 1931). Forty years later, in 1970, Tagaki and later Watanabe made considerable contributions to the arthroscopic surgery of the ankle, and the latter published a series of 28 ankle arthroscopies in 1972 (Watanabe M Selfoc-Arthroscope (Watanabe no. 24 arthroscope) 1972). Since then, numerous publications have followed.

Over the last three decades, arthroscopy of the ankle joint has become a standardized and important procedure, with numerous indications for both anterior and posterior intra-articular pathology, as well as for its tendinous problems around the ankle.

The advantages of arthroscopy of the ankle are the direct visualization of the structures, improved assessment of the articular cartilage, faster rehabilitation, and earlier resumption toward sports.

There is nowadays enough evidence that there is a limited value in performing a diagnostic arthroscopy because of the increased imaging modalities in ankle pathology. However, because of the lack of direct access, the nature, and deep location of its hindfoot structures, posterior ankle problems still pose a diagnostic and therapeutic challenge nowadays.

Historically, the hindfoot was approached by a three-portal technique, i.e., the anteromedial, anterolateral, and posterolateral portals, with the patient in the supine position. It is known that the traditional posteromedial portal is associated with potential damage to the tibial nerve, the posterior tibial artery, and its surrounding tendons locally. Therefore, a two-portal endoscopic technique was introduced in 2000, and since then, this technique has shown to give excellent access to the posterior ankle compartment, the subtalar joint, and the surrounding extra-articular posterior ankle structures (van Dijk et al. 2000).

Special attention to posterior ankle arthroscopy has shown the need for specific anatomical knowledge, has modified classic arthroscopic tools and skills, and has introduced a broad spectrum of new indications in posterior ankle pathology.

37.3 Functional Anatomy

The anatomical knowledge is particularly important in the arthroscopy of the ankle because of the significant risk of associated complications which can be prevented or decreased only by profound familiarity with the anatomy of the region. Adequate knowledge of the anatomy of the joint to be treated should cover not only the most common anatomic configurations (extra-articular and intra-articular) in statistical terms but also the possible anatomic variations to avoid confusion and serious technical errors (van Dijk et al. 2000; Fig. 37.1).

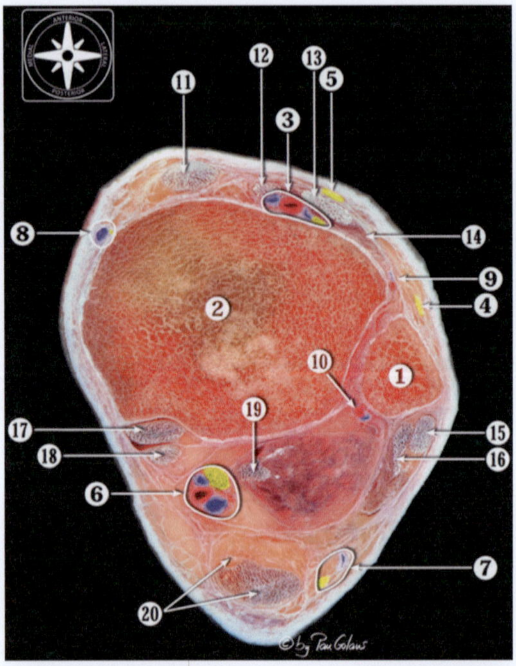

Fig. 37.1 **(Courtesy Pau Golano)** Transverse section at the level of the tibiofibular syndesmosis showing important structures susceptible to injury during ankle arthroscopy. 1 Lateral malleolus; 2 tibia; 3 anterior neurovascular bundle (deep peroneal nerve and anterior tibial artery and veins); 4 intermediate dorsal cutaneous nerve (lateral branch of the superficial peroneal nerve); 5 medial dorsal cutaneous nerve (medial branch of the superficial peroneal nerve); 6 posterior neurovascular bundle (posterior tibial nerve and posterior tibial artery and veins); 7 sural nerve and small saphenous vein; 8 saphenous nerve and great saphenous vein; 9 anterior peroneal artery; 10 posterior peroneal artery; 11 tibialis anterior tendon; 12 extensor hallucis longus tendon; 13 extensor digitorum longus tendon; 14 peroneus tertius muscle belly; 15 peroneus brevis longus; 16 peroneus brevis tendon; 17 tibialis posterior tendon; 18 flexor digitorum longus tendon; 19 flexor hallucis tendon (musculotendinous); 20 calcaneal and plantaris tendons

The main anatomical structure for the orientation and to determine the safe working area is the flexor hallucis longus tendon (FHL). Just medial to this tendon runs the posterior neurovascular bundle (tibial nerve and posterior tibial artery and veins). The posterior ankle arthroscopy should therefore routinely be performed lateral to the FHL tendon.

Proper positioning of the ankle and the hallux results in better visualization of the tendinous portion of the FHL muscle and avoids unnecessary resection of some of the muscle fibers that reach the lateral tendinous border in a semipenniform morphology. Plantar flexion of the ankle or hallux flexion facilitates visualization of the FHL tendon proximal to the lateral talar process.

The posterior ankle ligaments are also important for the orientation during the posterior ankle arthroscopy. These ligaments include the posterior talofibular ligament; the posterior intermalleolar ligament, also called the tibial slip in the arthroscopic literature; and the posterior tibiofibular ligament which is composed of a superficial and deep component or transverse ligament.

When the posterior ankle compartment is visualized arthroscopically, at first the location of the FHL tendon should be determined. Then the detailed anatomy of the posterior ankle can be identified more carefully.

The posterior talofibular ligament, component of the lateral collateral ligament, originates from the malleolar fossa, located on the medial surface of the lateral malleolus, coursing almost horizontally to insert in the posterolateral surface of the talus. This ligament is also an important reference in posterior ankle arthroscopy. Its location is important to know the site of the different working areas: subtalar and talocrural. The posterior subtalar recess is plantar to this ligament, and the talocrural joint is located dorsally (Burman 1931; Ogut et al. 2011; Golanó et al. 2006; van Dijk 2006; van Dijk et al. 2009; Ferkel and Scranton 1993).

37.4 Etiology

Posterior ankle impingement syndrome is a clinical pain syndrome that reflects the most common cause of posterior ankle pain, and it can be provoked by a forced hyperplantarflexion movement of the ankle (Andrews et al. 1985; Scholten et al. 2008; D'Hooghe and Kerkhoffs 2014). In the event of a soft tissue or bony posterior impingement of the ankle, plantar flexion induces a conflict between the posterior malleolus of the distal tibia on to the posterosuperior calcaneal bone. A bony prominent posterior processus of the ankle occurs in almost 7% of the sports population and can present itself as a hypertrophic posterior talar process or as an os trigonum. Although apparent posterior bony prominences caused by acute or repetitive overload (micro-) trauma can induce posterior ankle pain, it is not necessarily associated with the posterior ankle impingement syndrome.

Soft tissue impingement in the posterior ankle region can also occur and is frequently disregarded. It mainly is triggered by due hypertrophic FHL musculotendinous tissue, additional tendinous or doubled tendon structures, and posttraumatic scarification (van Dijk et al. 2009).

Since an acute forced hyperplantarflexion movement on the ankle or a repetitive overload induces the bony or soft-tissue conflict in the posteriorly located components of the ankle joint, we mainly see these lesions in a sports-specific population. The classical example of repetitive overload is seen in ballet dancers, where the forced plantar flexion during "en pointe" and "demi pointe" positioning induces repetitive impingement on the posteriorly located soft tissue components. Other types of sports related to the posterior ankle impingement syndrome include football, swimming, cycling, and any other sports in which the mechanism of injury is a repetitive forced plantar flexion or an acute setting (e.g., during a blocked kicking action in football). If the lesion occurs due to compression of the os trigonum between the distal tibia and calcaneal bone, it can lead to displacement of this os trigonum, disabling soft tissue inflammatory processes or even fractures of the processus posterior tali or distal tibia (van Dijk et al. 2009; Fig. 37.2).

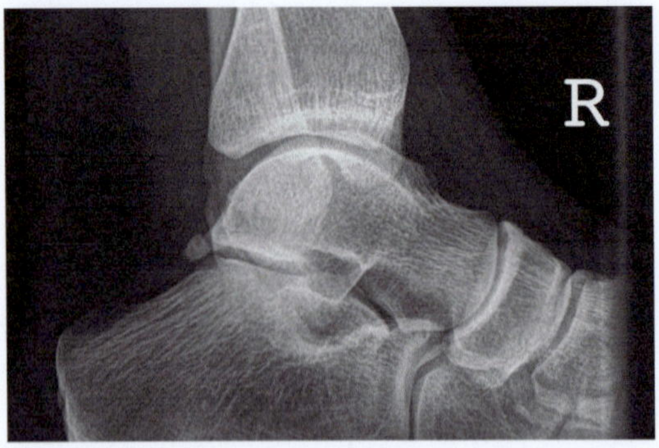

Fig. 37.2 Posterior ankle impingement due to an "os trigonum syndrome" in a right ankle

37.5 Clinical and Diagnostic Features

Clinically, posterior impingement can be much more difficult to detect and diagnose when compared to other types of ankle impingement because the affected structures lie much deeper and can be mimicked by or coexist with other disease processes such as peroneal tendinopathy, retrocalcaneal bursitis, osteochondral lesions of the posterior talar dome, Achilles tendinopathy, flexor halluces longus tendinopathy or tenosynovitis, posterior tibial osteochondral injuries, tarsal tunnel compression, tarsal coalition, and Haglund's deformity. Patients will complain of chronic deep posterior ankle pain that is worsened with push-off activities such as jumping. Physical examination includes palpation over the posterolateral process and the crunch test. Patients that suffer from posterior ankle impingement present with a posteriorly localized ankle pain during a (forced) plantar flexion movement.

The posterior ankle impingement test is a pathognomonic test to identify the clinical diagnosis of posterior ankle impingement. To have a positive test, the ankle is passively and quickly forced from neutral to hyperplantarflexion position, and during this movement, the patients encounter suddenly recognizable posteriorly located ankle pain. To increase compression on the posterolateral structures of the ankle, plantar flexion, external rotation, and eversion movements are considered during clinical testing.

Since the neurovascular structures and tendons are localized in the posteromedial region of the ankle, this area is not always easily palpated when compared to the clinical examination of the posterolateral part of the ankle (Golanó et al. 2006).

Diagnosis can be confirmed with abatement of pain following injection of an anesthetic into the posterolateral capsule of the tibiotalar joint. MRI is useful for more accurately identifying the anatomic site of abnormality, as well as revealing coexisting pathologies. Fortunately, rest is often adequate therapy regardless of whether the symptoms are acute or chronic. When nonoperative measures have failed, open or arthroscopic removal of the os can quickly return the footballer to play. Recent data has demonstrated the effectiveness of posterior ankle arthroscopy in the treatment of PAIS in the elite footballer, with return to training expected at an average of 5 weeks (D'Hooghe and Kerkhoffs 2014).

37.6 Accessory Muscles that Can Impinge on the Surrounding Musculotendinous Structures Around the Posterior Ankle

Multiple accessory, supernumerary, and anomalous muscles have been described in the radiologic, surgical, and anatomic literature. Accessory muscles of the ankle are typically asymptomatic, but can cause pain, compressive neuropathy, compartment syndrome, or rigid hindfoot deformities and can also mimic soft tissue tumors.

Magnetic resonance imaging (MRI) is the modality of choice in diagnosing accessory muscles, delineating their relationship to adjacent structures (e.g., impingement), and differentiating them from soft tissue tumors. Accessory muscles are isointense to skeletal muscle on all pulse sequences and can insert by fleshy muscular or tendinous insertions. Accessory muscles around the ankle include the flexor digitorum accessorius longus, the peroneocalcaneus internus, the accessory soleus, and the accessory peroneal muscles.

1. Peroneus quartus muscle

While a few studies have associated various symptoms with the presence of a peroneus quartus muscle in the peroneal compartment of the leg, little is known of the clinical relevance of this muscle. Originally, several accessory muscles were distinguished in the peroneal compartment:

- Peroneus quartus (PQ) (Otto)
- Peroneus-calcaneus externum (Hecker)
- Peroneus accessorius (White)
- Peroneus digiti quinti (Testut)

This terminology has been simplified by summarizing all peroneal compartment variants under the definition of a *peroneus quartus muscle* as a muscle arising from the lower leg and inserting onto the lateral hind and midfoot. This also explains the variable insertion sites of the PQ muscle:

- The retrotrochlear eminence of the calcaneus
- The metatarsal bone of the fifth toe
- The peroneal tendons
- The lateral retinaculum of the ankle
- The cuboid bone

The origin of the PQ muscle is the distal lateral portion of the fibula. It typically descends medial and posterior to the peroneal tendons. The PQ muscle is usually asymptomatic. Occasionally, it may lead to crowding in the retromalleolar groove, predisposing to peroneus brevis tendon attrition and tear. The PQ has a male predominance, is unique to humans, and is often bilateral. Classically, the peroneocalcaneal variant of peroneus quartus is the most common, originating from the peroneus brevis and inserting on the retrotrochlear eminence of the calcaneus.

2. Flexor digitorum accessorius longus muscle

The flexor digitorum accessorius longus (FDAL) is an anomalous muscle with a reported prevalence of 2–8% in cadaveric studies. The FDAL can originate from many posterior compartment structures, including the flexor retinaculum, the tibia, the fibula, the flexor hallucis longus, and the soleus. The FDAL courses through the tarsal tunnel, where it remains muscular until just prior to exiting. It lies deep to the deep aponeurosis and flexor retinaculum, differentiating it from the accessory soleus muscle.

The FDAL is intimately related to the neurovascular bundle and may abut, compress, or impinge upon the posterior tibial and/or lateral plantar nerves. Because of its close relationship to the flexor hallucis longus tendon, the FDAL has also been associated with flexor hallucis longus tenosynovitis. The FDAL either inserts onto the flexor digitorum longus (FDL) tendon prior to the FDL splitting into its four tendon slips or onto the quadratus plantae muscle. The FDAL is isointense to normal skeletal muscle on all pulse sequences. Functionally, the FDAL is thought to assist in toe flexion.

3. Accessory soleus

The accessory soleus muscle was originally described by Cruveilhier in 1843, and it is thought to represent a splitting of the soleus anlage early in its development. The accessory soleus has a reported prevalence of 0.7–5.5% in cadaveric studies. It commonly presents in the second or third decades of life and has a 2:1 male-to-female ratio.

- The accessory soleus originates from the anterior surface of the soleus muscle or from the tibia and fibula and is invested in its own fascia, distinguishing it from the normal soleus. It descends anterior or anteromedial to the Achilles tendon and superficial to the flexor retinaculum. There are five types of insertions:
- A tendinous insertion onto the upper calcaneus
- A muscular insertion onto the Achilles tendon
- A muscular insertion upon the upper surface of the calcaneus
- A tendinous insertion upon the superior calcaneus
- A tendinous insertion upon the medial calcaneus

The accessory soleus is supplied by the posterior tibial artery and innervated by the posterior tibial nerve.

Presenting signs and symptoms have included painless mass, painful mass, localized compartment syndrome, and hindfoot and clubfoot deformities. It has been suggested that pain may be related to increased intrafascial pressure, exercise-induced claudication secondary to inadequate blood supply, or compression of the posterior tibial nerve. Although the accessory soleus resides outside the tarsal tunnel, it has been implicated in tarsal tunnel syndrome, likely related to extrinsic compression. Successful surgical treatments for the symptomatic accessory soleus have included fasciotomy, muscle debulking, tendon release, and accessory muscle excision.

4. Peroneocalcaneus internus

The peroneocalcaneus internus (PCI) muscle is a rare muscle located deep to the flexor retinaculum in the posterior compartment of the lower leg. It was originally described in 1872 by Macalister. It has a prevalence of 1%. The PCI muscle originates along the inner part of the lower third of the fibula. It is bordered medially by the flexor hallucis longus muscle and tendon, where there is muscular interdigitation. The PCI is bordered anteriorly by the tibia, interosseous ligament, and tibiotalar joint. Posteriorly, the PCI is bordered by the soleus and laterally by the fascia separating the PCI from the peroneal muscles. The PCI tendon passes inferior to the sustentaculum tali, along with the flexor hallucis longus tendon, and the PCI tendon inserts onto a small tubercle on the medial calcaneus below the sustentaculum tali.

The PCI is typically asymptomatic, but it can displace the flexor hallucis longus muscle medially, indirectly compressing the neurovascular bundle. The tendons of the PCI and flexor hallucis longus course alongside of one another and can cause mechanical attrition or tenosynovitis. Symptomatic relief has been reported with steroid injection and surgical excision.

37.7 Surgical Procedure

Hindfoot endoscopy enables the surgeon to more easily assess the posterior ankle compartment. From the beginning of the description of the technique, the main indications to perform a posterior ankle arthroscopy are the treatment of an os trigonum and FHL pathology (Ogut et al. 2011; van Dijk 2006; van Dijk et al. 2009; Ferkel and Scranton 1993; Andrews et al. 1985). Nowadays, however, numerous ankle pathologies in our athletes can be treated through this minimal-invasive technique, and still indications are added.

The patient is positioned in the prone position with a tourniquet above the knee at the affected side, which should be carefully marked preoperatively. The affected ankle is positioned just over the edge of the operation table and is supported to allow free ankle movement.

The anatomical landmarks for portal placement are the sole of the foot, the lateral malleolus, and the medial and lateral borders of the Achilles tendon. With the ankle in the neutral position (90 degrees), a straight line, parallel to the sole of the foot, is drawn from the tip of the lateral malleolus to the Achilles tendon and is extended over the Achilles tendon to the medial side. The posterolateral portal is located just proximal to—and 5 mm anterior to—the intersection of the straight line with the lateral border of the Achilles tendon.

The posteromedial portal is located at the same level as the posterolateral portal, but on the medial side of the Achilles tendon.

Before addressing any pathology, the FHL tendon should be localized since just medially to where the posterior neurovascular bundle is located (Golanó et al. 2006*). The FHL tendon determines the working area, basically only lateral to this tendon (Figs. 37.3 and 37.4)***.** Once this working area is determined, the whole spectrum of posterior pathology can be treated supero-inferiorly from the tibiotalar over the subtalar joint toward the Achilles tendon insertion and mediolaterally from tarsal tunnel release toward the peroneal tendons.

Now the pathology can be addressed, ranging from debridement of soft tissue to the removal of an os trigonum or the release of the FHL tendon from its adjacent structures (Figs. 37.5 and 37.6). Also—more specifically—performing a groove deepening in case of recurrent peroneal tendon dislocation, an endoscopic tarsal tunnel release, addressing a Cedell fracture or prominent posteromedial talar tubercle, and treating a posteromedial

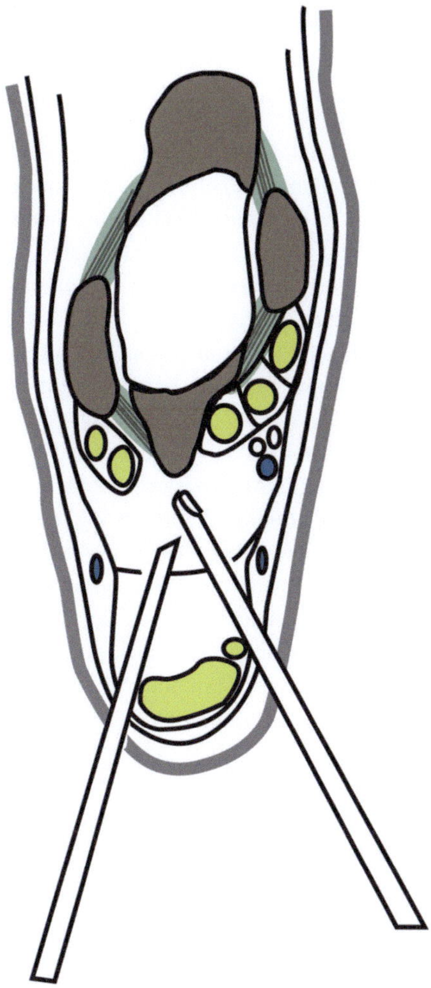

Fig. 37.3 Determining the working area for arthroscopy in posterior ankle pathology. During insertion, the arthroscope is aiming toward the first foot webspace. This enables the surgeon to determine a safe working area

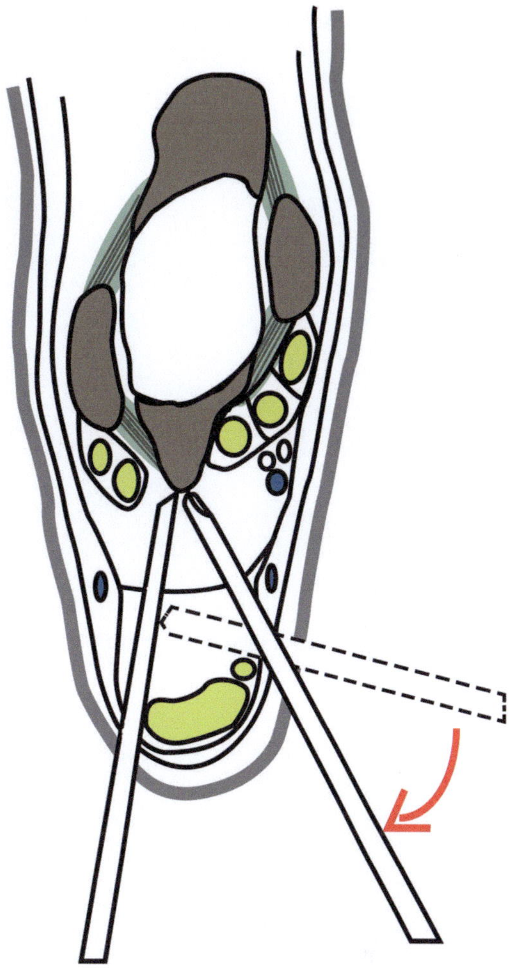

Fig. 37.4 Determining the working area for arthroscopy in posterior ankle pathology. After insertion, the arthroscope is turned in a horizontal fashion to broaden the working area after identification of the FHL

talar dome lesion are nowadays within the scope of this treatment.

Hindfoot endoscopy can be also used for the treatment of talar body fractures, intraosseous talar cysts (that are localized posteriorly in the ankle), and pigmented villonodular synovitis (PVNS). This is a condition that can be localized in the posterior ankle compartment, and it can invade the whole posterior part of the talus, extending proximally up to the FHL tendon sheath (van Dijk et al. 2009). Furthermore, Achilles tendinopathy/denervation and Haglund's syndrome pathology in the ankle can nowadays also successfully be addressed by the posterior minimal-invasive two-portal endoscopic technique in the sports population. This condition requires although a more distally aimed two-incision technique that covers the pathology all the way up to the Achilles tendon insertion.

Significant advantages of these abovementioned methods include lower morbidity, shorter postoperative hospitalization time, and quicker return to full sports. Hindfoot endoscopy is a safe and effective method for treating posterior talar cystic lesions and is an attractive alternative to

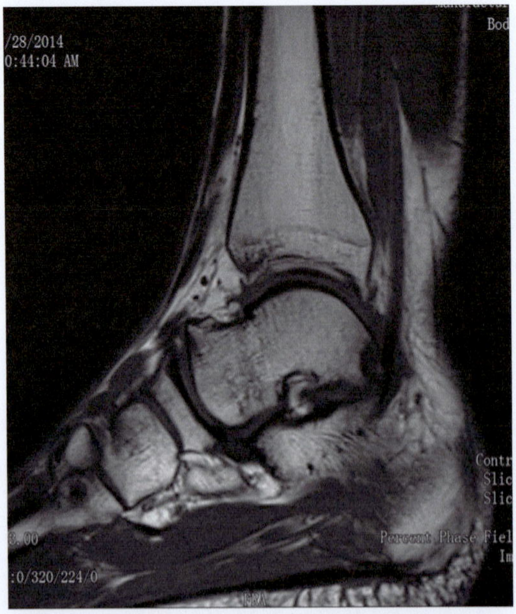

Fig. 37.5 Sagittal MRI image of a normal FHL muscle belly

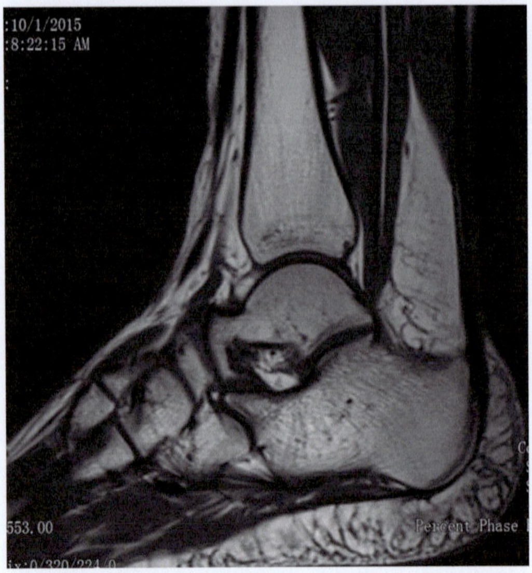

Fig. 37.6 Sagittal MRI image of a "low-lying" FHL muscle belly

open surgery for experienced arthroscopic surgeons.

Nevertheless, the most influential indication to perform posterior ankle arthroscopy remains the treatment of os trigonum and FHL release (Fig. 37.7a–d).

Conclusion

Posterior ankle arthroscopy is a challenging, but safe, reliable, and effective technique in the treatment of posterior ankle impingement.

Due to the improved functional outcome after surgery and quicker rehabilitation time, athletes can hugely benefit from this technique. The initial indications include flexor hallucis longus and os trigonum pathology. Nowadays however the technique is used—with or without an additional portal—for an increasing amount of posterior ankle pathologies. Further studies are now being performed to value the abovementioned new indications, and they show that the arthroscopic posterior technique in posterior ankle pathology has not yet reached its limits. Frequently it is wrongly thought to address only bony problems in the ankle. Many soft tissue problems (especially FHL and accessory muscles) arise in clinical posterior impingement problems over the ankle. They are a common trigger to this pathology and should always be considered and addressed.

How to diagnose posterior impingement of the ankle:

- Ask for sports-specific repetitive ankle movements.
- Perform a hyperplantarflexion movement of the ankle.
- Look for palpatory pain along the course of the flexor hallucis longus.

How to treat posterior impingement of the ankle:

- Perform a diagnostic injection.
- Start with the standardized two-portal technique after initial cadaveric training.
- Search for the flexor hallucis longus tendon and the posterior talofibular ligament as primary anatomical landmarks.

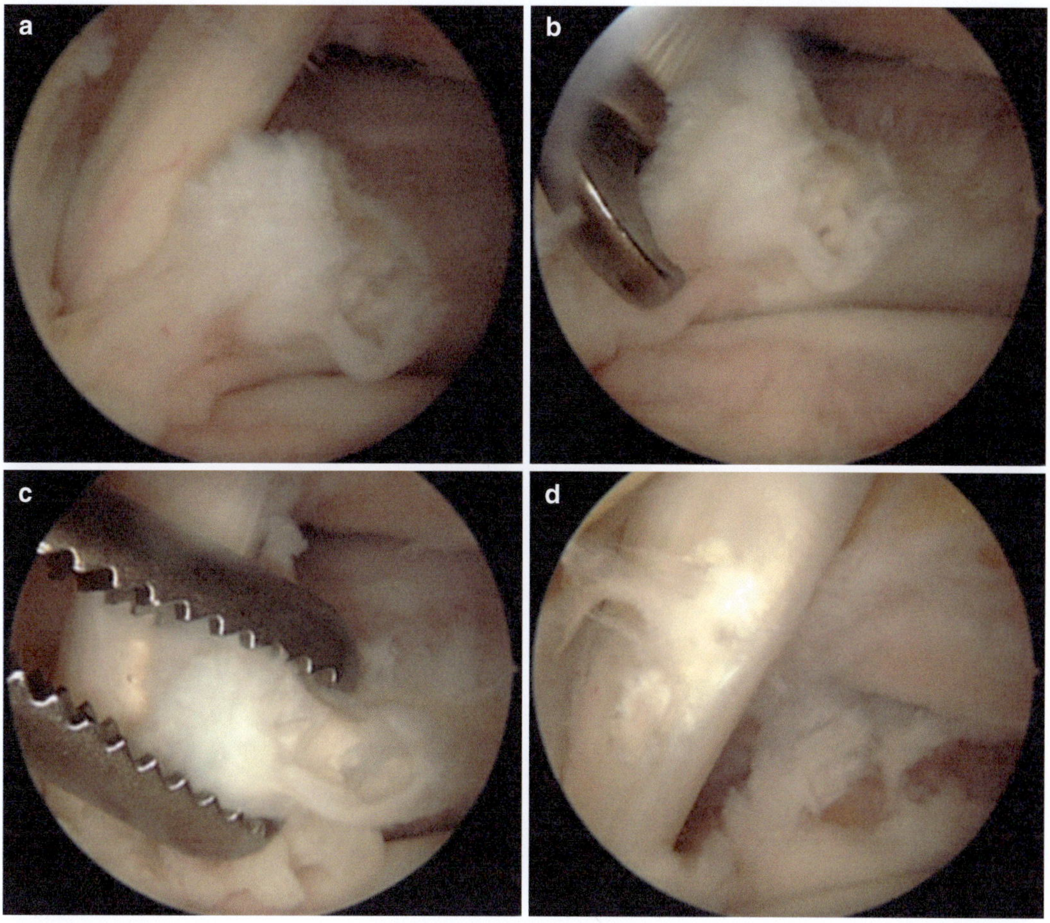

Fig. 37.7 (**a–d**) Posterior ankle arthroscopy: a four-step decompression of the FHL from an os trigonum. Mark the impingement signs on the FHL after os trigonum decompression

References

Andrews JR, Previte WJ, Carson WG (1985) Arthroscopy of the ankle: technique and normal anatomy. Foot Ankle 6:29–33

Burman MS (1931) Arthroscopy of direct visualization of joints. An experimental cadaver study. J Bone Joint Surg 13:669–695

D'Hooghe P, Kerkhoffs G (eds) (2014) The ankle in football (Springer book 2014). Chapter 15: ankle fractures, including avulsion fractures, pp 159–186

van Dijk CN (2006) Hindfoot endoscopy. Foot Ankle Clin 11:391–414

van Dijk CN, de Leeuw PA, Scholten PE (2009) Hindfoot endoscopy for posterior ankle impingement. Surgical technique. J Bone Joint Surg Am 91(Suppl 2):287–298

van Dijk CN, Scholten PE, Krips R (2000) A 2-portal endoscopic approach for diagnosis and treatment of posterior ankle pathology. Arthroscopy 16:871–876

Eirale C, Hamilton B, Bisciotti G, Grantham J, Chalabi H (2012) Injury epidemiology in a national football team of the Middle East. Scand J Med Sci Sports 22(3):323–329

Ferkel RD, Scranton PE Jr (1993) Arthroscopy of the ankle and foot. J Bone Joint Surg Am 75:1233–1242

Golano P, Mariani PP, Rodrıguez-Niedenfuhr M et al (2002) Arthroscopic anatomy of the posterior ankle ligaments. Arthroscopy 18:353–358

Golanó P, Vega J, Pérez-Carro L, Götzens V (2006) Ankle anatomy for the arthroscopist. Part I: the portals. Foot Ankle Clin N Am 11:253–273

Junge A et al (2015) Location, type and mechanism of injury in FIFA world cups. Br J Sports Med 49:599–602

Ogut T, Ayhan E, Irgit K, Sarikaya AI (2011) Endoscopic treatment of posterior ankle pain. Knee Surg Sports Traumatol Arthrosc 19:1355–1361

Scholten PE, Sierevelt IN, van Dijk CN (2008) Hindfoot endoscopy for posterior ankle impingement. J Bone Joint Surg Am 90:2665–2672

Watanabe M Selfoc-Arthroscope (Watanabe no. 24 arthroscope) (1972) Monograph. Teishin Hospital, Tokyo

Compartment Syndromes

38

Giuliano Cerulli, Matteo M. Tei, Gianpiero Cazzato, Giacomo Placella, and Marco Chillemi

Contents

G. Cerulli, M.D. (✉) • M.M. Tei • G. Cazzato
G. Placella • M. Chillemi
Institute of Orthopedics and Traumatology, Sacred Heart Catholic University—Gemelli Hospital, Rome, Italy
e-mail: giulianocerulli@gmail.com

Compartment syndromes (CS) represent an emergency involving both muscles and tendons, and their clinical diagnosis is not always easy. CS occurs when interstitial pressure increases in a fascial space, resulting in the impairment of microcirculation, causing tissue ischemia. If it is not recognized and treated early, it can lead to muscle necrosis, rhabdomyolysis, and systemic disease in severe cases. The most common causes are:

- Fractures caused by high-energy trauma
- Crush injuries
- Severe bruising
- Snakebites
- Dressings that are too tight
- Plaster casts

Pain is the earliest and most sensitive symptom, and it appears out of proportion compared to the severity of the injury. Circulatory stasis around the nerves may cause paresthesia which may lead to progressive muscle paralysis and death. When intracompartmental pressure exceeds the blood pressure, the limb is pale and it is impossible to feel peripheral pulses. For its diagnosis, there is the "5-P" rule as reported in English literature:

- Pain
- Paresthesias
- Pallor
- Paralysis
- Pulselessness

G.L. Canata et al. (eds.), *Muscle and Tendon Injuries*, DOI 10.1007/978-3-662-54184-5_38

The patient complains of severe and increasing pain that requires frequent doses of analgesic drugs. The pain increases during passive stretching of the limb; moreover, patients report tingling along the nerve distribution that passes through the affected compartment. A key point is that CS is a progressively developing condition. Maximum swelling occurs at about 30–36 h after the traumatic event; therefore, it is essential to pay careful attention to high-risk limbs during the early period post trauma. In patients with altered sensitivity, clinical signs and symptoms are less useful. These patients must be closely monitored; if there is a suspicion of compartment syndrome, it is necessary to measure intracompartmental pressure. The measurements must be taken in all compartments using specific instruments, and it should be measured as close as possible to the fracture, because in this anatomical area, the pressure is highest.

Normal intracompartmental pressure is about 5–8 mmHg. When intercompartmental pressure reaches 20 mmHg, tissue perfusion can decrease. Tissue perfusion is based on the local perfusion pressure (diastolic pressure-compartmental pressure), and if the difference between these pressures, or delta p, is less than 30 mmHg, fasciotomy is indicated. Early treatment of CS should include the removal of circumferential dressings, loosening tight bandages, and raising the limb above chest level which decreases the perfusion pressure on the muscle. If these procedures reduce symptoms, the patient should then be carefully monitored and reevaluated frequently. If these precautions are not beneficial, the patient should be taken to the operating room for fasciotomy.

38.1 Compartment Syndrome of the Upper Limbs

Compartment syndrome (CS) may occur following the inflammatory response to injury, when there is an increase in intercompartmental pressure. This increase leads to a reduction of venous outflow and increased tissue pressure with widespread tissue damage until the interruption of arterial blood flow. As a result, the tissues with a high oxygen requirement, such as skeletal muscle, become ischemic and eventually necrotic. The peripheral nervous structures that cross the compartment are also susceptible to damage due to disruptions in blood flow and increased intracompartmental pressure. This results in a limb with partial and, sometimes, complete loss of function.

Upper limb compartment syndrome may develop as a result of:

- Fractures of the distal radius
- Forearm shaft fractures
- Crush injuries of soft tissues

Several less common causes include:

- Snakebite
- Gunshot wounds
- Toxic shock syndrome
- Leukemic infiltration
- Viral myositis
- Arthroscopic infusion fluid
- Nephrotic syndrome

An open fracture does not eliminate the risk of CS. In patients with CS, early diagnosis is crucial. A delay in diagnosis can lead to serious complications, including the permanent loss of motor and sensory function of the limb.

For the clinical diagnosis of upper limb CS, the most reliable indicator is pain (McDonald and Bearcroft 2010). Patients classically experience constant and oppressive pain. For low-energy injuries, the pain may seem out of proportion. Nerve dysfunction in the compartment involved can lead to paresthesia: burning, numbness, and tingling. In patients with fractures, the pain persists and worsens despite reduction and immobilization. In CS of the forearm, patients experience excruciating pain during flexion and extension of the fingers. The patient suffers from a state of discomfort secondary to muscle compartment tension. In addition there is a reduction of sensitivity in the distribution of the peripheral nerves and widespread edema. Later there is numbness, loss of peripheral pulses, and pallor of the limb. Even if the pain is the best clinical indicator of CS, some patients are unable to report it. If the patient is a child or he has received a large amount of analgesics, is unconscious, inhibited, or sedated, he may not be able to refer clearly about the pain.

In these situations it is recommended to measure the intracompartmental pressure. Elliott and Johnstone (Elliott and Johnstone 2003) reported that 23% of forearm compartmental syndrome is caused by soft tissue injuries without fractures and 18% is caused by fractures. In our experience, there is a limited amount of available evidence regarding causes, treatment, suture wound methods, functional result, and complications of forearm CS. It has been associated with various etiologies; however, fracture of the distal radius is reported as the most common cause of forearm CS. This is contrary to what was reported in the past by Grottkau (Grottkau et al. 2005); he suggested that supracondylar fractures were the predominant cause of forearm CS in children. In a study by the National Pediatric Trauma Registry that evaluated 131 cases of pediatric CS, it was found that 74% of the cases of upper limb CS were caused by forearm fractures, and only 15% were secondary to supracondylar fractures. Bea et al. (Bae et al. 2001), studying 33 consecutive pediatric patients with 36 cases of acute compartmental syndrome, suggested that a possible reason for this decrease in CS after supracondylar fracture could be due to changes in fracture management, such as percutaneous pin osteosynthesis.

Patients under 35 years of age involved in high-energy trauma and polytrauma have an increased risk of developing forearm CS. Hwang (Hwang et al. 2009) noted that patients with distal radius fractures and ipsilateral elbow injury developed a CS in 15% of the cases, much higher than the risk (0.25%) to develop CS after an isolated fracture of the distal radius. Upper limb CS is generally diagnosed with a careful clinical examination. The removal of any tight dressings is a critical step to enable an accurate assessment of the limb. Regarding intracompartmental pressure measuring, there is almost an equal distribution between the number of patients diagnosed by clinical examination as those diagnosed by intracompartmental pressure measure.

Many authors consider the measurement of intracompartmental pressure unnecessary for diagnostic purposes; others recommend its use only in inhibited patients or in patients whose clinical findings have an ambiguous interpretation. In regard to the treatment of forearm CS, different skin incisions have been proposed. The typical ventral incision begins 1 cm proximal and 2 cm laterally and then obliquely across the antecubital fossa on the volar forearm. In the medial direction, the incision reaches the middle line at the average distal third of the forearm. Here the incision is continued only to the ulnar side of the long handheld tendon to avoid palmar skin cord of the median nerve. The incision then passes through the wrist and extends into the medial portion of the palm for the concurrent release of the carpal tunnel (Fig. 38.1). The overall rate of complications of forearm CS is about 42%. Many studies report neurological deficits as the most common complication. Acute forearm CS has more etiologies affecting patients of all ages. Without treatment it results in contractures and neurological deficits up to the complete loss of function in the forearm and hand. Emergency treatment is necessary to prevent serious consequences.

Patients under 35 years old with a forearm fracture and polytrauma are at high risk of developing CS; therefore they require careful monitoring. In inhibited patients and in those with ambiguous clinical examination results, objective diagnostic measurements are necessary (Ronel et al. 2004).

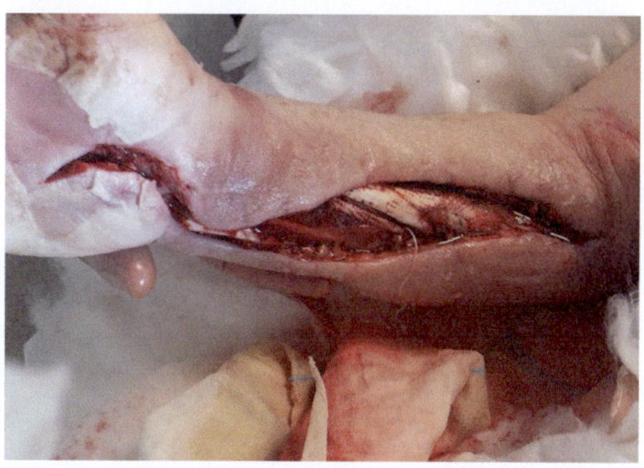

Fig. 38.1 Typical ventral incision across the volar forearm for the tretment of acute CS

38.2 Compartment Syndrome of the Lower Limbs

Acute compartment syndrome of the lower limb is a complication of fractures, soft tissue trauma, and reperfusion after acute arterial occlusion (McQueen et al. 2000). It can be caused by bleeding or swelling in a muscle compartment surrounded by fascia and bone tissue (Olson and Glasgow 2005). The long-term consequences of CS have already been described by Richard von Volkmann in the late nineteenth century as a result of a too tight plaster cast, but only after a few years was a connection made with high intracompartmental pressure. The incidence of foot CS is about 6% in patients with foot injuries caused by motorcycle accidents, while the incidence of leg CS seems lower (1.2% after closed diaphyseal fractures of the tibia). The lower limb compartment syndrome and its treatment were described in 1958, whereas until a few years ago, compartment syndrome of the foot was largely unknown and was described only in some case reports. Myerson first described this clinical entity in 1988 and presented surgical decompression as a therapeutic intervention (Myerson and Manoli 1993). The leg is composed of four compartments: anterior, lateral, surface, and deep posterior. On the contrary, there is no consensus in regard to the number of anatomical compartments of the foot. At the end of 1920, three compartments were described and later confirmed by Kamel and Sakla in 1961. After which Myerson identified four compartments (Myerson and Manoli 1993) while more recently in a cadaveric study, nine compartments were identified. However, there are only three compartments (medial, lateral, superficial) for the entire length of the foot. In a cadaveric study performed in 2008, the authors could not identify any distinct forefoot myofascial compartments, and so they concluded that a fasciotomy of the hindfoot compartments through a modified medial incision would be sufficient to decompress the whole foot (Ling and Kumar 2008). However, studies on cadavers cannot simulate physiological conditions so the conclusions of these studies should be interpreted with caution. The typical clinical presentation of leg and foot CS is no different from other regions of the body. In a systematic review of the literature, the pain has been identified as the earliest and most sensitive clinical sign of CS (Ojike et al. 2009). In a retrospective study, however, the foot pain was present in all patients with foot CS (Myerson 1990). It must be remembered that the indiscriminate use of analgesics in patients with severe pain may potentially mask the key symptom. Sensory deficits are also common in patients with CS (Ulmer 2002). Decreased discrimination between two points seems more reliable than the decreased feeling of a pinprick alone (Myerson and Manoli 1993).

When acute compartment syndrome is suspected, a careful examination is needed. Medical recommendations based on evidence (EBM) cannot, unfortunately, be made; serial laboratory tests should be performed at least hourly as it is widely recognized that muscle necrosis usually occurs within the first 3 h (Vaillancourt et al. 2004). However, contrary to what was thought in the past, muscle strength is not a good parameter to be considered, since it is difficult to determine whether the loss of strength is due to the pain or muscle necrosis. Even the examination of peripheral pulses is not reliable for the diagnosis of lower limb CS, because there may be false negatives if the intracompartmental pressure reaches the systolic blood pressure. On the other hand, invasive measurement of intracompartmental pressure is a rapid and safe procedure to reach a definite diagnosis. However, it should be emphasized that in a cohort study with more than 200 patients with diaphyseal fractures of the tibia, the continuous monitoring of intracompartmental pressure showed no differences in outcomes or possible delays in performing fasciotomy compared to the simple clinical examination of the patient (Al-Dadah et al. 2008). Another study showed that the rate of late complications was similar in patients whether they had undergone or not continuous monitoring of the intracompartmental pressure (Harris et al. 2006). Since nine compartments in the foot have been identified, it is not feasible to monitor the pressure for patients at high risk of developing CS in this anatomical area. It is also important to remember that intracompartmental pressure must be correlated with the diastolic pressure. The fasciotomy threshold is still under debate. While some authors suggest that for intracompartmental pressure the threshold for fasciotomy should be an absolute value of 30 mmHg (Willy et al. 2001), others indicate 20 mmHg less than the diastolic pressure as a threshold (Olson and Glasgow 2005). However today, the indication for fasciotomy should be based on clinical findings (neurological deficits) or on a difference between intracompartmental pressure and diastolic pressure lower than 30 mmHg (Olson and Glasgow 2005). Although most of these recommendations derive from studies of other anatomic regions, there is no reason to assume a different pathophysiological background for foot CS. Finally, it is important to remember that clinical results should be compared over time. In short, a history of trauma and the presence of serious injuries should make the physician consider the possibility of CS. Furthermore, the presence of open wounds does not implicitly decompress the compartment, for example, in the foot all nine compartments would rarely be involved. Although the management of CS consists of immediate surgical treatment, bandages and casts should be completely open in patients with severe postoperative pain. In the case of impending CS, the limb should not be raised because it reduces the blood supply that is already compromised. McQueen demonstrated that in patients with tibial fractures, the time between the onset of compartment syndrome and fasciotomy influences the outcome, rather than the time between trauma and osteosynthesis (McQueen et al. 1990). Generally, the existing literature is lacking in regard to the optimal management of tibial fractures in the presence of CS. On the other hand, multiple approaches have been used to decompress the compartments of the foot (Fulkerson et al. 2003). Although the etiology, pathophysiology, and treatment of CS are well described, little has been published about the long-term results. CS of the leg and foot has a low incidence rate (1.2% after closed tibial fractures, 6% after open tibial fractures); studies on a greater number of patients are, however, not available. A long follow-up with different surgeons and different surgical techniques does not allow a direct comparison of published results. One study has examined the quality of life after CS using the "EQ-5D score" (Giannoudis et al. 2002). Even if surgical decompression is an emergency procedure that is indicated in order to prevent further damage and long-term functional loss, several serious long-term sequelae after fasciotomy have been reported: aesthetic problems, altered sensorium, and dry and flaky skin.

In a study of 30 cases, patients with leg compartment syndrome had lower EQ-5D scores than the control group at 12 months after treatment, although their health status was not statistically different (Giannoudis et al. 2002). In addition, the authors reported that patients with faster wound closure times were healthier than those with longer wound closure times (Giannoudis et al. 2002). In another study about the results of follow-up in 26 patients with traumatic leg CS, 15.4% complained of pain at rest, and 26.9% reported pain under stress at 1–7 years after the trauma (Frink et al. 2007). In this population, more than 50% of the patients had reduced joint ROM and reported a reduction in sensitivity. Infections due to fasciotomy were described in up to 38% of the patients. Patients who had undergone a surgical flap with skin grafting for wound closure presented a lower incidence of infections. In another study, the presence of associated lesions seemed not to affect the long-term outcome after traumatic CS of the leg in regard to the joint Rom, sensory dysfunction, and loss of muscle strength. There is no information available about returning to work. Most of the studies about outcomes of foot compartment syndrome are only case reports.

In a series of 14 patients, Myerson (Myerson 1991) described the return to the previous working activity after trauma in four patients; six patients had only occasional symptoms that had developed during some daily activities, whereas three patients developed contractures with clawed fingers. No patients however needed amputation (Myerson 1991). However paresthesia and numbness of scars distal to the compartments involved were common long-term sequelae in eight patients. Complications of lower limb CS are serious and require immediate treatment. If CS is not promptly recognized, the damage caused to the affected region may be irreversible. Our experience shows that the literature available is quite limited in this specific field of orthopedics and traumatology. We found only one study using validated outcome measures to analyze the results of treatment of leg CS (Giannoudis et al. 2002). Therefore we believe that further studies are needed to describe long-term results. Although the pathophysiology of CS is well described, it is not yet clear when there is irreversible damage. A 1991 study suggested an ischemic time of 5–6 h, while other more recent studies in animal models reported muscle necrosis after less than 3 h (Verleisdonk et al. 2004). Moreover the information available in literature is inconsistent, and we believe further studies are necessary in this regard. Although clinical signs are well described (Verleisdonk et al. 2004), we believe that the most important factor in the CS diagnosis is the key figure of the doctor, who must put the patient at the center of his attention and base treatment on a "holistic-like approach."

Moreover the physician should be aware that the pain, defined as a clinical sign of CS, could be masked in patients with a reduced state of consciousness or if previously treated with analgesics. Although literature lacks recommendations about the intervals at which serial examinations should be performed in patients at risk, we believe they should be performed at least every hour, as irreversible damage has been reported to occur within the first 3 h (Verleisdonk et al. 2004). In patients with uncertain signs, the intracompartmental pressure should be measured. Literature describes various approaches for leg fasciotomy through lateral or anterolateral and posterior combined incisions. However we were unable to find a study that compared both methods; therefore, literature lacks recommendations based on EBM criteria. Recommendations for surgical treatment of foot CS are most controversial; in fact, although many approaches have been described, literature lacks comparative studies. In conclusion, lower limb CS is a rare but serious complication of which the surgeon must be aware. Although immediate fasciotomy is the indisputed treatment for patients with CS, literature lacks guidelines for high-risk patients.

38.3 Chronic Exertional Compartment Syndrome

A separate paragraph should be dedicated to the treatment of chronic exertional compartment syndrome (CECS). Considering that the first report on this syndrome was written only 30 years ago, there is still uncertainty about the development of the syndrome in the majority of affected patients.

CECS is not commonly considered as a cause of muscle pain. Typically, there is a delay of 22 months in the diagnosis of the disease. Studies on the etiology of chronic pain in the anterior leg indicate that CECS is the causal factor in 27% of the cases (Blackman 2000).

The delay in diagnosis, combined with the relative frequency, underlines the attention that physicians, not only specialists in orthopedics and traumatology, should pay toward CECS as a possible diagnosis, which can also affect the patient's performance of sports and work activities. In a list of 11 athletes with CECS, all returned to the same level of sports activities as before injury having undergone an average of 2 years of follow-up. The pathophysiology of CECS is connected to an increase in compartmental pressure occurring during exercise due to the increase in muscle volume. The prevailing theory is that during the activities, the muscle suffers a gradual increase of intracompartmental pressure with the consequent impairment of muscle tissue perfusion (Goldfarb and Kaeding 1997).

The incidence in the general population is unclear because of the difficulty to diagnose it and the delay in seeking medical care. CECS should be suspected in any athlete who presents chronic anterior leg pain that worsens with physical activity, but it is resolved upon cessation of activity. Ninety-five per cent of the cases of CECS occur in the anterior and lateral compartments of the leg (Martens et al. 1984). CECS is more frequent in young adult amateur runners and military recruits, but it is not uncommon in athletes participating in contact sports. There are no demonstrated differences in incidence between men and women (Detmer et al. 1985). The average age of onset is 20 years (Kutz et al. 1985).

The risk factors for the development of CECS include anabolic steroids and the use of creatinine which increase the muscle volume. Aberrant biomechanical factors in a runner, like the wrong foot support or over-pronation, can lead to an increased risk of compartment syndrome secondary to differences between weight and load and to high pressure on individual muscle groups in the lower leg. Acquiring a thorough history for compartment syndrome is very important because the physical examination is often irrelevant. Classically, there is the development of pain described as burning or pressure, in a compartment of the leg at the same time, at the same distance or at the same intensity (Shah et al. 2004). The pain increases in intensity as the patient continues to exercise. Symptoms occurred bilaterally in 70% of 80 cases (Mouhsine et al. 2006). Other symptoms include numbness and tingling in the dermatomal distribution of the nerve conduction through the compartment involved or weakness of the affected muscle. A classic presentation of CECS is a runner that experiences burning in the leg and numbness on the back foot after about 15 min of running continuously, with absolutely no symptoms within 30 min of stopping.

The physical examination can be used to differentiate CECS from other causes of chronic pain in leg stress. The athlete should be examined after he has completed the exercise that provokes the pain. An important diagnostic procedure could be biomechanical functional assessments, which allow stabilometric, electromyographic, and isokinetic parameters to be studied. Functional imaging studies can also give precise information about the joint kinematics and the ability to perform simple or complex gestures. Biomechanical evaluations offer a possibility for orthopedic specialists to express a precise opinion on the functional state of the musculoskeletal system and its various components through simple and more sophisticated and expensive instruments such as force plates, 16-channel EMG telemetry, instruments for isokinetic evaluation, and 3D systems to study movement. Biomechanical laboratories for the musculoskeletal system (Fig. 38.2) offer

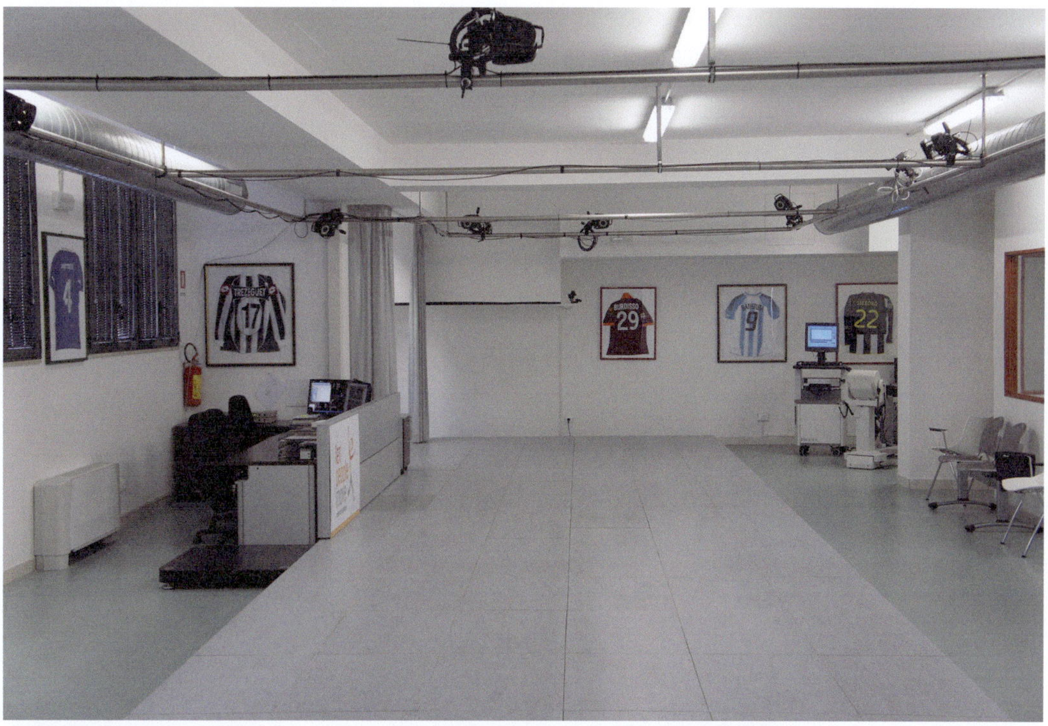

Fig. 38.2 "Let people move" biomechanical laboratory for the musculoskeletal system analysis. Arezzo-Italy

accurate and reproducible data regarding some locomotor parameters, such as reaction to the ground, proprioception, the peak of flexor and extensors of the knee muscle strength, electrical activity of various muscles of the thigh and leg evaluable in dynamic conditions, and finally the functional capacity during the most simple or the more complex gestures (Fig. 38.3).

As is well known, man, and especially athletes, should be assessed in dynamic conditions rather than in static conditions, i.e., while moving, walking, and performing specific sports gestures; in fact, the mechanical components of the "human machine" are designated to movement and spatial translocation of body units. The gold standard for the diagnosis of CECS is, however, the measurement of intracompartmental pressure. The only certain treatment of CECS is fasciotomy (Kutz et al. 1985). Nonetheless, conservative treatment has also been described, such as avoiding activities that can generate symptoms or decreasing the workout intensity. Athletes may also be advised to rest and then to slowly increase their athletic training, or especially designed orthopedic insoles might be prescribed which give plantar arch support and correct pronation while running. Other

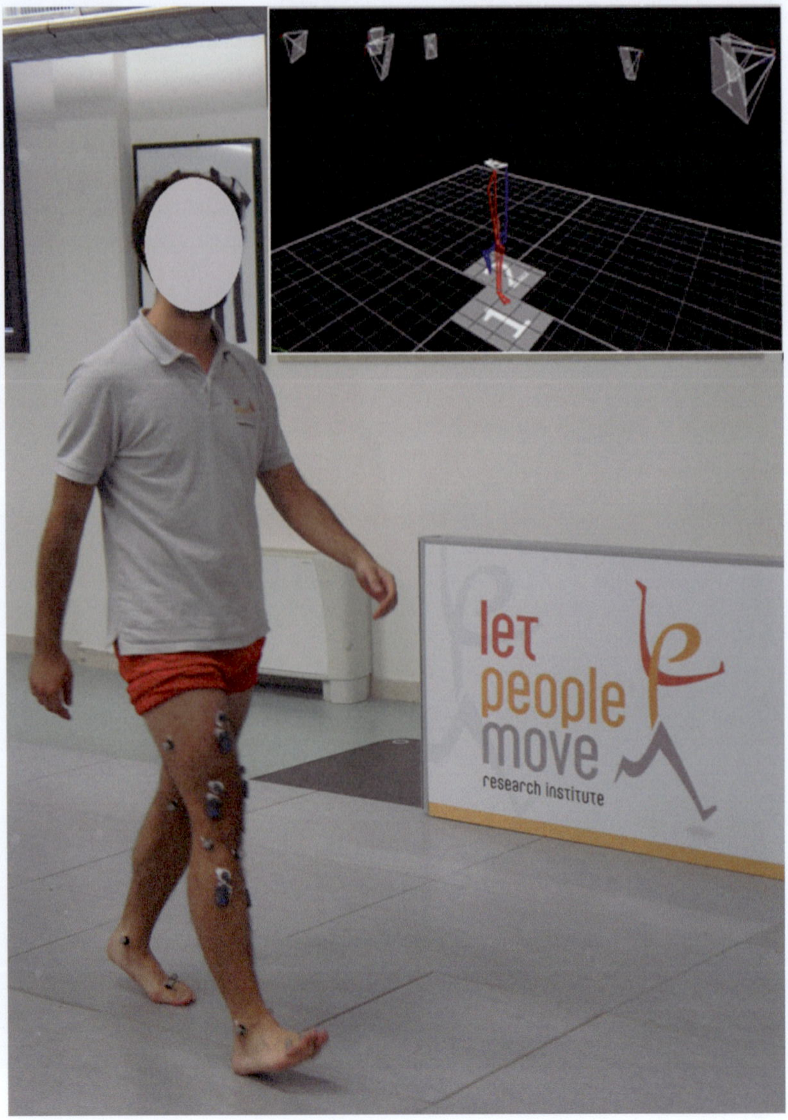

Fig. 38.3 Gait Analysis with 16-channel EMG telemetry and 3D systems

conservative treatment methods include the following: avoid running on hard surfaces, wear appropriate footwear, and try to change the sport-specific gestures on the basis of an objective biomechanical assessment. Massage therapy of the involved muscle tissue, ultrasound, and stretching before exercise are all treatment strategies that may prolong the time before symptoms appear. If athletes do not get any relief from conservative measures and they do wish to continue practicing sport at the same level and intensity, fasciotomy is the treatment of choice. According to the literature, fasciotomy of the anterior and lateral compartment gives the best results with a higher success rate of over 80%. On the contrary, deep posterior fasciotomies have a lower success rate of up to 50%.

This lower percentage is attributed to the posterior compartment's complex anatomy. Several types of fasciotomies have been described: open and subcutaneous are the most common. The advantage of fasciotomy in open is the full view of the compartment. Some types of open fasciotomy include the removal of band flaps to reduce the formation of aberrant scars and relapses.

On the other hand, subcutaneous fasciotomy involves 1–2 small incisions. Several case reports of endoscopically assisted fasciotomies have been described, but an increase in frequency of complications and relapses was reported. A compressive dressing is applied postoperatively for 2–3 days. Patients are requested to perform different types of rehabilitation exercises after surgery in order to prevent the formation of tissue adhesions. Patients can swim as soon as surgical wounds are completely healed, whereas physical therapy is usually begun 1–2 weeks after surgery. The athlete can return to full sports activity within 6–8 weeks if he/she is asymptomatic and has recovered full muscle strength and elasticity (McDermott et al. 1982), according to a postoperative biomechanical evaluation. The underlying cause of the CECS continues to be a source of debate. The initial theory about the cause of pain from CECS was thought to be ischemia. However, some medical scans such as SPECT scanning have suggested that ischemia may not be the underlying cause. The evolution of alternative diagnostic instruments will lead to a more complete understanding of the physiopathology of this syndrome. The conservative management approach may be effective at onset or in the early stages of the disease; however, there is often a delay in finding the most effective treatment as well as establishing a definite diagnosis. Nevertheless, literature is unanimous in indicating fasciotomy as the only treatment. In conclusion, a better knowledge of the physiopathology of CECS, combined with a greater awareness of the disease by both the physician and the athlete, is desirable to improve, on one hand, the success of conservative therapy and, on the other, to prescribe surgery for the patient as early as possible if necessary.

References

Al-Dadah OQ et al (2008) Continuous compartment pressure monitoring vs. clinical monitoring in tibial diaphyseal fractures. Injury 39(10):1204–1209

Bae DS, Kadiyala RK, Waters PM (2001) Acute compartment syndrome in children: contemporary diagnosis, treatment, and outcome. J Pediatr Orthop 21(5):680–688

Blackman PG (2000) A review of chronic exertional compartment syndrome in the lower leg. Med Sci Sports Exerc 32(3 Suppl):S4–10

Detmer DE et al (1985) Chronic compartment syndrome: diagnosis, management, and outcomes. Am J Sports Med 13(3):162–170

Elliott KG, Johnstone AJ (2003) Diagnosing acute compartment syndrome. J Bone Joint Surg Br 85(5):625–632

Frink M et al (2007) Long term results of compartment syndrome of the lower limb in polytraumatised patients. Injury 38(5):607–613

Fulkerson E, Razi A, Tejwani N (2003) Review: acute compartment syndrome of the foot. Foot Ankle Int 24(2):180–187

Giannoudis PV et al (2002) The impact of lower leg compartment syndrome on health related quality of life. Injury 33(2):117–121

Goldfarb SJ, Kaeding CC (1997) Bilateral acute-on-chronic exertional lateral compartment syndrome of the leg: a case report and review of the literature. Clin J Sport Med 7(1):59–61. discussion 62

Grottkau BE, Epps HR, Di Scala C (2005) Compartment syndrome in children and adolescents. J Pediatr Surg 40(4):678–682

Harris IA, Kadir A, Donald G (2006) Continuous compartment pressure monitoring for tibia fractures: does it influence outcome? J Trauma 60(6):1330–1335. discussion 1335

Hwang RW, de Witte PB, Ring D (2009) Compartment syndrome associated with distal radial fracture and ipsilateral elbow injury. J Bone Joint Surg Am 91(3):642–645

Kutz JE, Singer R, Lindsay M (1985) Chronic exertional compartment syndrome of the forearm: a case report. J Hand Surg Am 10(2):302–304

Ling ZX, Kumar VP (2008) The myofascial compartments of the foot: a cadaver study. J Bone Joint Surg Br 90(8):1114–1118

Martens MA et al (1984) Chronic leg pain in athletes due to a recurrent compartment syndrome. Am J Sports Med 12(2):148–151

McDermott AG et al (1982) Monitoring dynamic anterior compartment pressures during exercise. A new technique using the STIC catheter. Am J Sports Med 10(2):83–89

McDonald S, Bearcroft P (2010) Compartment syndromes. Semin Musculoskelet Radiol 14(2):236–244

McQueen MM, Christie J, Court-Brown CM (1990) Compartment pressures after intramedullary nailing of the tibia. J Bone Joint Surg Br 72(3):395–397

McQueen MM, Gaston P, Court-Brown CM (2000) Acute compartment syndrome. Who is at risk? J Bone Joint Surg Br 82(2):200–203

Mouhsine E et al (2006) Two minimal incision fasciotomy for chronic exertional compartment syndrome of the lower leg. Knee Surg Sports Traumatol Arthrosc 14(2):193–197

Myerson M (1990) Diagnosis and treatment of compartment syndrome of the foot. Orthopedics 13(7):711–717

Myerson MS (1991) Management of compartment syndromes of the foot. Clin Orthop Relat Res 271:239–248

Myerson M, Manoli A (1993) Compartment syndromes of the foot after calcaneal fractures. Clin Orthop Relat Res 290:142–150

Ojike NI, Roberts CS, Giannoudis PV (2009) Foot compartment syndrome: a systematic review of the literature. Acta Orthop Belg 75(5):573–580

Olson SA, Glasgow RR (2005) Acute compartment syndrome in lower extremity musculoskeletal trauma. J Am Acad Orthop Surg 13(7):436–444

Ronel DN, Mtui E, Nolan WB 3rd (2004) Forearm compartment syndrome: anatomical analysis of surgical approaches to the deep space. Plast Reconstr Surg 114(3):697–705

Shah SN, Miller BS, Kuhn JE (2004) Chronic exertional compartment syndrome. Am J Orthop 33(7):335–341

Ulmer T (2002) The clinical diagnosis of compartment syndrome of the lower leg: are clinical findings predictive of the disorder? J Orthop Trauma 16(8):572–577

Vaillancourt C et al (2004) Acute compartment syndrome: how long before muscle necrosis occurs? CJEM 6(3):147–154

Verleisdonk EJ, Schmitz RF, van der Werken C (2004) Long-term results of fasciotomy of the anterior compartment in patients with exercise-induced pain in the lower leg. Int J Sports Med 25(3):224–229

Willy C et al (2001) Acute compartment syndrome. Results of a clinico-experimental study of pressure and time limits for emergency fasciotomy. Unfallchirurg 104(5):381–391

Gold-Induced Autologous Cytokine Treatment in Achilles Tendinopathy

39

Ulrich Schneider, Reinhard Wallich, Gernot Felmet, and William D. Murrell

Contents

U. Schneider (✉)
Center for Regenerative Medicine, Wiesseer Str. 103, 83707 Ringsee, Germany
e-mail: info@prof-schneider.eu

R. Wallich
Institute for Immunology University, Heidelberg, Germany

G. Felmet
ARTICO Sportklinik, Villingen-Schwenningen, Germany

W.D. Murrell
Orthopaedic Sports Medicine, Emirates Hospitals Group, Dubai Sports Medicine, Sapphire Surgery Center, Al Razi Bldg 64, Block F, 1st Floor, PO Box 505067, Dubai Healthcare City, Dubai, UAE

Orthopaedics, Rehabilitation, and Podiatry, Ft. Belvoir Community Hospital, Ft. Belvoir, VA, USA

39.1 Introduction

In the last two decades, there has been a huge amount of clinical and scientific interest in the application of regenerative-based therapies to improve treatments for acute and chronic tendon lesions. The rationale has been to improve the quality of repair in injured tendons more towards actual tendon tissue regeneration and away from scar tissue repair that theoretically leads to a superior outcome and decreased chance of reinjury. Such therapies have had a rapid rise in clinical popularity, and while having an excellent scientific rationale, clinical evidence supporting their use has frequently been inadequate (Zhou and Wang 2016).

Most described techniques have used either cell therapy (Adams et al. 2014; Bruder et al. 1994; Chong et al. 2007, 34) and/or the administration of regenerative growth factors, sourced endogenously or exogenously (Aspenberg 2007; Cummings et al. 2012; Daher et al. 2011; Jonge et al. 2011; Gholami et al. 2016). A variety of cellular products have been created, sourced most commonly from the peripheral blood, bone marrow, and/or adipose tissue. Additionally, embryonic stem cells and induced pluripotent stem cell (iPS) products have also been described for possible clinical use (Beattie et al. 2009; Prockop 1997; Tetta et al. 2012).

In 2014, the first clinical results of a new procedure using specially designed gold particles to stimulate the expansion, a myriad of protective and regenerative proteins found naturally in a

G.L. Canata et al. (eds.), *Muscle and Tendon Injuries*, DOI 10.1007/978-3-662-54184-5_39

patient's own blood (GOLDIC®) was published. In this article, the underlying research and the effects of tendon healing will be demonstrated.

39.2 GOLDIC® Procedure

The GOLDIC® procedure was developed to enhance the therapeutic effects of gold on the cellular level in combination with the advantages of an autologous blood therapy. Extensive basic science investigation was completed to establish the most effective cultivation protocol, the best substantial gold composition, and the most promising application modality for this procedure. The primary aim of this approach was to decrease the risk of side effects.

39.3 Biological Effects of GOLDIC® Procedure on the Cellular Level

In vitro testing was initially carried out to validate the effectiveness of this novel platform. Human venous blood was incubated in GOLDIC containers for 24 hours at 37 °C. Initial analyzed serum and the control serum (incubation in non-gold-enriched containers) were analyzed by a new spectroscopic method (AquaSpec).

AquaSpec™ Technology is a unique and full-automated method for the measurement of the proteomic pattern in biological fluids like serum, plasma, urine, or synovial fluid. The methodology is based on mid-infrared spectroscopy (spectral range from 4000 to 400 cm^{-1}) that is sensitive to all chemical bonds and functional groups in molecules. This technique is suitable to print a physiological snapshot of all ingredients that reflects the composition in biological fluids. Compared to many other techniques in proteomic pattern diagnostics (e.g., MALDI-TOF), the native state of the biofluid can be accurately investigated and detects the unique proteomic pattern similar to a "fingerprint." Differences in biological samples can be considered in total, and chemometric models allow for the classification and identification of compounds present. Moreover, since the spectroscopic absorbance is linear to the concentration of a compound, the kinetics and the decay of the substrate can be quantified (Fig. 39.1).

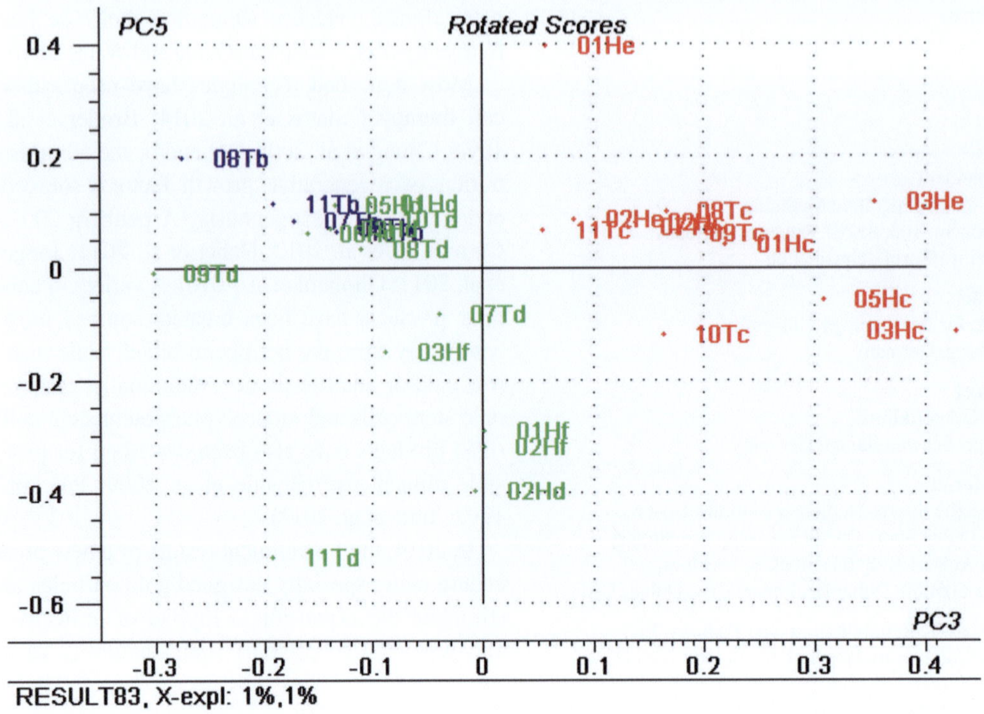

Fig. 39.1 Aqua spec analysis of 11 donors after GOLDIC® incubation: *blue*, T0; *green*, T24 GOLDIC; *red*, T24 control

Based on Aquaspec analysis, the GOLDIC® procedure leads to a significant change of protein quantities and overall composition and highlights individual differences between the different blood samples/patients.

39.4 Protein Analyses of GOLDIC®-Treated Human Serum

Using Elisa and Bioplex assays, protein levels were measured of several important cytokines/chemokines before and 24 h after treatment with the GOLDIC® procedure.

The major effect of the GOLDIC process is indicated by the significant increase of the gelsolin concentration in human serum. Gelsolin is a highly conserved, multifunctional actin-binding protein with an extracellular isoform, plasma gelsolin, for which there is not yet a clearly defined function. The secreted form of gelsolin has been implicated in a number of processes such as the extracellular actin scavenging system and the presentation of lysophosphatidic acid and other inflammatory mediators to their receptors. Additionally, gelsolin functions as a substrate for extracellular matrix-mediating enzymes (Wen et al. 1996; Spinardi and Witke 2007; Li et al. 2012) (Fig. 39.2).

Upon GOLDIC® treatment, the highest increase could be found in the following proteins, p-Gelsolin and granulocyte colony-stimulating factor (G-CSF); the following proteins were upregulated also: IL-8, macrophage chemotactic protein (MCP-3), stromal-derived protein (SDF-alpha), tumor necrosis factor-alpha (TNF-alpha), leukemia inhibitory factor (LIF), IL-10, macrophage inflammatory protein (MIP-1alpha), and MIP-1ß. Macrophage colony-stimulating factor (M-CSF), IL-15, IL-17, granulocyte-macrophage colony-stimulating factor (GM-CFS), hepatocyte growth factor (HGF), IL-2Ra, IL-12p40, chemokine (C-C motif) ligand 11 (Eotaxin/CCL11), fibroblast growth factor-basic (bFGF), and interferon-gamma (IFN-g)

GOLDIC treatment failed to induce differential expression of IL-2, IL-3, IL-4, IL-5, IL-7, IL-9, IL-13, IL-18, C-C chemokine receptor type 10 (CCR10), and interferon alpha 2 (IFN-a2).

39.5 First Clinical Results After GOLDIC® Treatment

39.5.1 Clinical Studies in Horses

The aim of the first clinical study was to determine the effectiveness of GOLDIC injections in horses with different lameness-associated diseases. In a

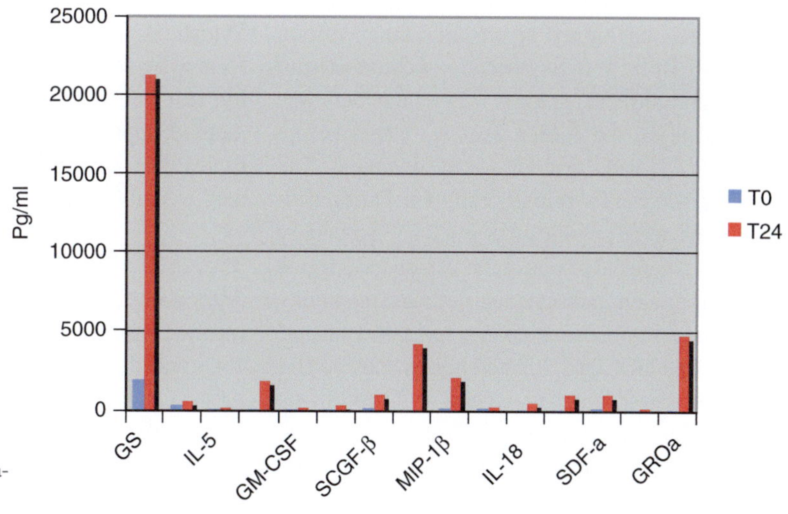

Fig. 39.2 Protein quantification in GOLDIC® serum

case series study, 36 horses (37 cases) with the clinical sign of lameness were included in this study. The causes for lameness was chondromalacia ($n = 19$) or soft tissue disorders ($n = 18$). The horses were treated by four injections of gold-induced, autologous-conditioned serum. The conditioning process included the incubation of the autologous serum with solid gold particles over 24 hours (GOLDIC procedure). Twenty-eight subjects had previously undergone therapeutic interventions, whereas nine had not. Horses were assessed for lameness using the AAEP (American Association of Equine Practitioners) grading scale (0 = no lameness, 5 = severe lameness). Swelling and/or effusion were evaluated in an equal scale between 0 and 5 (0 = no swelling/effusion, 5 = severe swelling/effusion). Scores were collected at pretreatment, and after 1, 2, and 3 weeks, and 3 and 6 months posttreatment. AAEP grading scale score was defined as the primary parameter. A *P*-value of less than 0.05 was considered statistically significant. In all 37 cases, a significant reduction of lameness, effusion (joint group), and swelling (soft tissue disorders group) within 3 weeks after treatment ($p < 0.05$) was found. Up to 3 and 6 months after treatment, all horses were free of symptoms. There were no major side effects noted throughout the study (Schneider and Veith 2013).

In a prospective randomized controlled, two-center clinical trial, 30 horses with arthrogenic lameness were enrolled in this study. The horses were treated by four injections of gold-induced, autologous-conditioned serum GOLDIC® (group B, $n = 16$) or by a single injection of corticosteroid and hyaluronic acid (group A = 14). Lameness was assessed using the AAEP grading system before and 3, 6, 12, and 36 months after treatment. The AAEP grade was the primary endpoint. Differences were considered significant at $p < 0.05$. Secondary endpoints were the results of the flexion test, degree of joint-effusion, radiographic findings, the ability to return to original performance level, and adverse effects. The GOLDIC®-treated horses showed significantly lower lameness grades at all follow-up examinations compared with the value before treatment ($p < 0.01$). In horses of group A (control HA + steroid), there was no significant decrease in lameness grade during the follow-up period. Horses of group B had significantly lower lameness grades than horses of group A at all follow-up examinations. Severe adverse events did not occur in either group.

The authors concluded that the treatment of arthrogenic lameness in horses using the gold-induced, autologous-conditioned serum (GOLDIC®) method is superior to the conventional treatment with corticosteroids and hyaluronic acid (Widmer et al. 2017).

39.5.2 Clinical Studies in Humans

In a prospective case series study, patients with chronic Achilles tendinopathy were treated with GOLDIC®. All patients received four peritendinous Achilles injections. Pain score ((VAS) visual analog scale) was evaluated at 4, 12, 24, and 52 months follow-up. MRI follow-up could be performed in five patients before and after 1 year. Adverse events were documented using MedDRA version 12.1.

39.5.2.1 Material and Methods

Nineteen patients (10 male, 9 female) were included in this study. The mean age was 44.5 years (range, 32–80). In 12 cases, the right side was affected and in 7 cases, the left side, respectively.

39.5.2.2 Statistical Analysis

Statistical analysis (Sigma Stat 3.5) was performed by an independent statistician. As normality test failed, data were analyzed by Dunn method, reporting p values with a level of >0.05 indicating significance. Data are expressed as medians and interquartile ranges.

39.5.2.3 Results

After a single four injection GOLDIC® series, the median baseline level was at 6.84 points in the VAS and dropped after 4 months down to 4.16. After 12 months, we found a further improvement in the VAS score down to 2.63. After 2 and 5 years, the VAS score further improved to 1.47

(24 months) and 1.17 (52 months), respectively. In all patient groups, a statistically significant improvement could be demonstrated at all time points compared to baseline (Figs. 39.3).

All MRIs showed fatty degeneration on the side of the tendinopathy with various sizes. One year after the treatment, all patients showed a complete regeneration of the tendon tissue. This regeneration capacity was not size or age dependent. No severe side effects could be detected (Figs. 39.4 and 39.5).

These results indicate that the treatment with GOLDIC® injections is safe and has the potential to reduce pain and increase quality of live in patients suffering under chronic Achilles tendinopathy. An impressive regenerative capacity could be demonstrated using MRI even in old patients

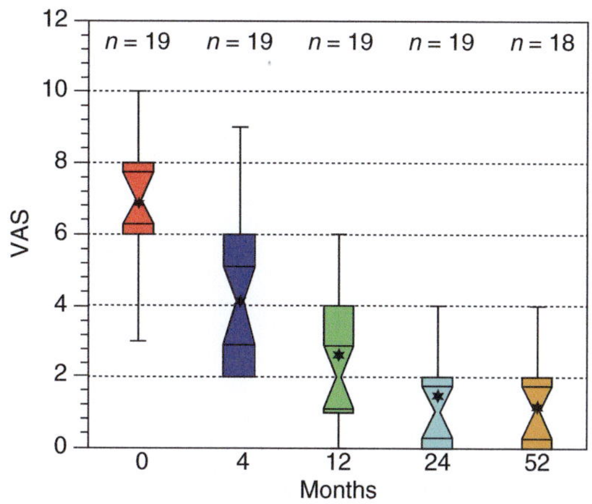

Fig. 39.3 Demonstration of the VAS score after GOLDIC® treatment. A statistically significant improvement ($p < 0.05$) compared to baseline could be demonstrated in all patient groups at all time points

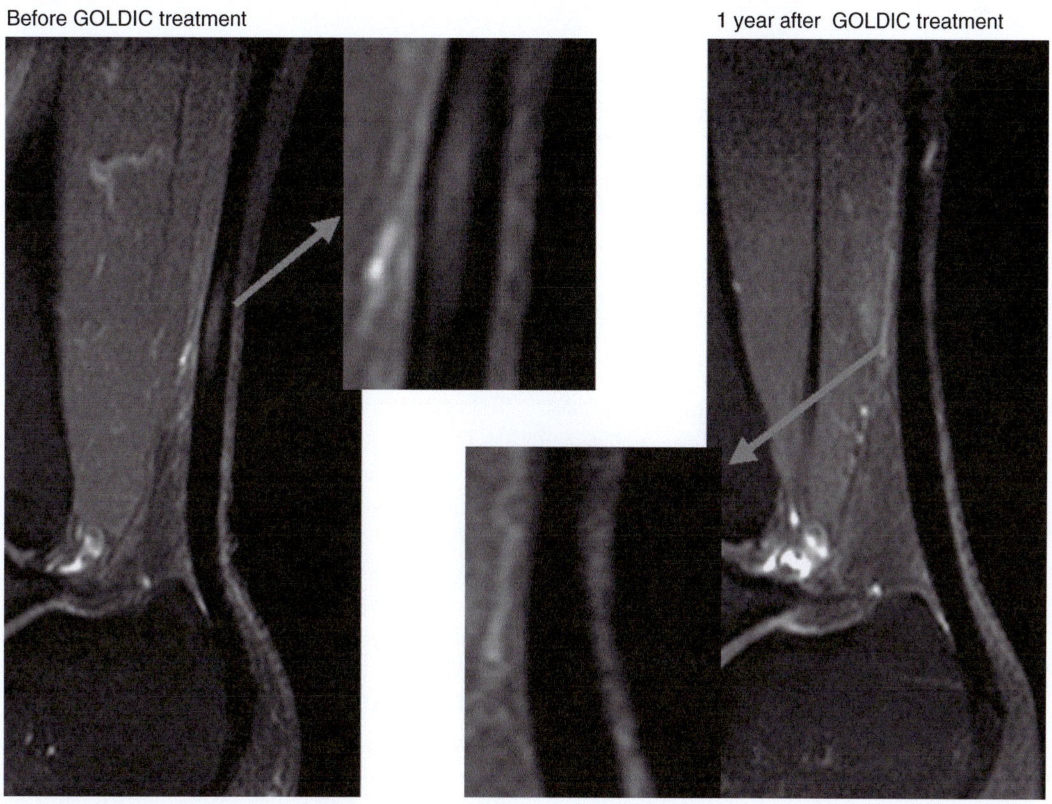

Fig. 39.4 MRI documentation of a 43-year-old female patient with chronic tendinosis of the Achilles tendon before and 1 year after GOLDIC® treatment. The necrotic tissue inside the tendon was replaced completely by original tendon tissue

Before GOLDIC treatment

1 year after GOLDIC treatment

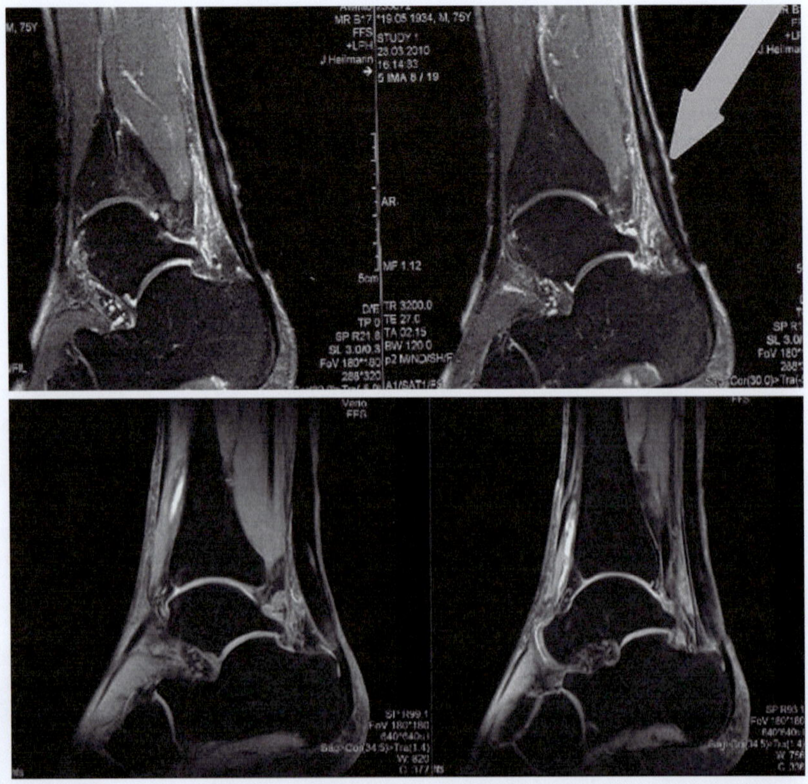

Fig. 39.5 MRI documentation of an 80-year-old male patient with chronic tendinosis and a fatty degeneration of the whole middle part of the Achilles tendon before and 1 year after GOLDIC® treatment

39.6 Discussion

While over the last two decades there has been considerable advances in the treatment of tendon disorders, new developments using cell-based and cell-free approaches are under debate. The use of these potential regenerative-acting procedures is still not fully understood, and the results are not consistent. One major problem is the inconsistency of the preparation and processing methods in the cell-based procedures like PRP. This has translated to great variability in clinical outcome of PRPs demonstrated in the literature (Gholami et al. 2016; Mlynarek et al. 2016; Zhou and Wang 2016; Filardo et al. 2016).

Currently the use of mesenchymal stromal cells (MSC) provides an exceptional alternative to conventional methods of tendinopathy treatment. Based on their proliferative potential and immunosuppressive properties, MSC are increasingly used in veterinarian and human medicine; however, the perfect conditions for an effective induction of tendon healing has not been found (Prockop 1997; Tetta et al. 2012; Huang et al. 2013).

The use of growth factors such as HGF, rhPDGF-BB, IL-6, and TGF-β in Achilles tendon repair has shown promising results (Andersen et al. 2011; Aspenberg 2007; Cui et al. 2011; Hou et al. 2009; Kashiwagi et al. 2004; Kessler et al. 2014; Kim et al. 2007; Shah et al. 2013). Bone morphogenetic proteins such as BMP-12, BMP-2, BMP-7, and BMP-14 have also shown positive results for the biological augmentation of Achilles tendon repair (Bolt et al. 2007; Dines et al. 2007; Jelinsky et al. 2011; Keller et al. 2011; Majewski et al. 2008; Rickert et al. 2005). The further investigation of these techniques in a clinical setting is warranted. Another area of great interest is the use of various scaffold material in augmentation of Achilles rupture and repair; however, these materials alone are not enough to achieve a sufficient tendon healing. Scaffolds in combination with biologic material may prove useful in order to optimize the benefits (Adams et al. 2014; Barber et al. 2008; Chen et al. 2010; Cummings et al. 2012; Farnebo et al. 2014; Gilbert et al. 2007; Lee 2007; Lee 2008; Lohan et al. 2013; Majewski et al. 2012; Ning et al. 2012; Nirmalanandhan et al. 2008; Pietschmann et al. 2013; Tang et al. 2014; Webb et al. 2013; Wisbeck et al. 2012; Yao et al. 2011; Yin et al. 2013; Zantop et al. 2006).

The GOLDIC® procedure is a completely new approach that is based on the upregulation of several important new proteins that can directly influence the body's own regenerative processes. One of the most important proteins of the GOLDIC procedure is plasma-Gelsolin (p-GSN). p-GSN is the longest known member of a family of actin-binding proteins. p-GSN regulates the integrity of the actin cytoskeletal structure and, therefore, influences on cell migration and proliferation and even ensures cell survival. Extensive research has been done, and more than 2000 papers are available to understand the various functions of this protein in all types of injuries, inflammatory conditions, or degenerative processes. Plasma-GSN is an important protective protein, and it prevents the toxic reaction, which occurs during cell death. Moreover, p-GSN is an important factor initiating healing process. The plasma concentration of GSN decreases during acute injury and inflammation, whereas application of recombinant gelsolin to animals improves recovery after sepsis or burn injuries (Zhang et al. 2011; Li et al. 2012). Osborn et al. showed that low serum levels of GSN correlate with the presence of gelsolin-actin complexes in synovial fluids, suggesting on local consumption of GSN in the inflamed joint. Therefore, one may assume that injection of GSN in the site of injury may improve the healing process, due to stabilization of cellular proliferative activity, and maintain the structural integrity of cells.

A study using fat-derived stem cells cultured with gelsolin and gelsolin combined with nucleotides showed its influence on cell morphology and growth pattern (Marycz et al. 2014). The lack of alteration in actin and vimentin expression after treatment with gelsolin may be a very desirable feature, as these proteins play essential role in governing the solid-like viscoelastic behavior of cells, whereas instability of cytoskeleton structure could be associated with cell disintegration. Translational research is currently addressing whether replenishment of plasma gelsolin could provide an efficacious and well-tolerated therapeutic intervention in several medical conditions.

Another important protein that is upregulated during the GOLDIC procedure is granulocyte colony-stimulating factor (G-CSF). G-CSF, also known as colony-stimulating factor 3 (CSF-3), is a glycoprotein that stimulates the bone marrow to produce granulocytes and stem cells and release them into the bloodstream. Functionally, it is a cytokine and hormone, a type of colony-stimulating factor, and is produced by a number of different tissues. The pharmaceutical analogs of naturally occurring G-CSF are called filgrastim and lenograstim. These pharmaceuticals are used to produce and mobilize stem cells for treatment after chemotherapy. Philpott et al. (1997) showed a significant reduction in the proportion of apoptotic cells in the CD34 + population mobilized by G-CSF compared to CD34 + cells in unstimulated PB (peripheral blood), consistent with the theory that G-CSF is acting, at least in part, by suppressing apoptosis. They also found that G-CSF-mobilized CD34 + cells are less apoptotic than CD34 + cells of unstimulated normal bone marrow, indicating that G-CSF is significantly altering the survival capacity of the mobilized cells. This protein is not detectable under normal conditions in the blood and serum. During the incubation process with gold particles, we found a significant increase in the activated serum. Therefore, G-CSF can be seen as an inductor for an endogenous stem cell treatment. In conjunction with other proteins like p-GSN, this might explain the enormous regenerative capacity of the GOLDIC® procedure.

This first clinical study in humans on tendon healing showed promising clinical results. In comparison with other modern approaches like PRP and MSC transplantation, GOLDIC® is the only procedure that can upregulate p-GSN and G-CSF. These two proteins can play an important role to achieve the highest grade of regeneration. The healing capacity that could be found in the follow-up MRIs is impressive. To our knowledge, there is no other procedure on the market that shows comparable long-lasting clinical results and a similar regenerative effect. Future comparative clinical studies have to be performed to investigate the potential of this new approach in comparison to other regenerative therapies.

References

Adams SB Jr et al (2014) Stem cell-bearing suture improves Achilles tendon healing in a rat model. Foot Ankle Int 35(3):293–299

Andersen MB et al (2011) Interleukin-6: a growth factor stimulating collagen synthesis in human tendon. J Appl Physiol 1985 110(6):1549–1554

Aspenberg P (2007) Stimulation of tendon repair: mechanical loading, GDFs and platelets. A mini-review. Int Orthop 31(6):783–789

Barber FA et al (2008) A biomechanical study of Achilles tendon repair augmentation using GraftJacket matrix. Foot Ankle Int 29(3):329–333

Beattie AJ et al (2009) Chemoattraction of progenitor cells by remodeling extracellular matrix scaffolds. Tissue Eng Part A 15(5):1119–1125

Bolt P et al (2007) BMP-14 gene therapy increases tendon tensile strength in a rat model of Achilles tendon injury. J Bone Joint Surg Am 89(6):1315–1320

Bruder SP, Fink DJ, Caplan AI (1994) Mesenchymal stem cells in bone development, bone repair, and skeletal regeneration therapy. J Cell Biochem 56: 283–294

Chen JL et al (2010) Efficacy of hESC-MSCs in knitted silk-collagen scaffold for tendon tissue engineering and their roles. Biomaterials 31(36):9438–9451

Chong AK et al (2007) Bone marrow-derived mesenchymal stem cells influence early tendon-healing in a rabbit Achilles tendon model. J Bone Joint Surg Am 89(1):74–81

Cui Q et al (2011) HGF inhibits TGF-beta1-induced myofibroblast differentiation and ECM deposition via MMP-2 in Achilles tendon in rat. Eur J Appl Physiol 111(7):1457–1463

Cummings SH et al (2012) Effect of recombinant human platelet-derived growth factor-BB-coated sutures on Achilles tendon healing in a rat model: a histological and biomechanical study. J Tissue Eng 3(1):2041731412453577

Daher RJ et al (2011) Tendon repair augmented with a novel circulating stem cell population. Int J Clin Exp Med 4(3):214–219

Dines JS et al (2007) The effect of growth differentiation factor-5-coated sutures on tendon repair in a rat model. J Shoulder Elbow Surg 16(5 Suppl):S215–S221

Farnebo S et al (2014) Decellularized tendon-bone composite grafts for extremity reconstruction: an experimental study. Plast Reconstr Surg 133(1):79–89

Filardo G et al (2016) Platelet-rich plasma in tendon-related disorders: results and indications. Knee Surg Sports Traumatol Arthrosc

Gholami M et al (2016) A systematic review and meta-analysis of the application of platelet rich plasma in sports medicine. Electron Physician 8(5):2325–2332

Gilbert TW et al (2007) Degradation and remodeling of small intestinal submucosa in canine Achilles tendon repair. J Bone Joint Surg Am 89(3):621–630

Hou Y et al (2009) Effects of transforming growth factor-beta1 and vascular endothelial growth factor 165 gene transfer on Achilles tendon healing. Matrix Biol 28(6):324–335

Huang TF et al (2013) Mesenchymal stem cells from a hypoxic culture improve and engraft Achilles tendon repair. Am J Sports Med 41(5):1117–1125

Jelinsky SA et al (2011) Treatment with rhBMP12 or rhBMP13 increase the rate and the quality of rat Achilles tendon repair. J Orthop Res 29(10):1604–1612

de Jonge S et al (2011) One-year follow-up of platelet-rich plasma treatment in chronic Achilles tendinopathy: a double-blind randomized placebo-controlled trial. Am J Sports Med 39(8):1623–1629

Kashiwagi K et al (2004) Effects of transforming growth factor-beta 1 on the early stages of healing of the Achilles tendon in a rat model. Scand J Plast Reconstr Surg Hand Surg 38(4):193–197

Keller TC et al (2011) Growth/differentiation factor-5 modulates the synthesis and expression of extracellular matrix and cell-adhesion related molecules of rat Achilles tendon fibroblasts. Connect Tissue Res 52(4):353–364

Kessler MW et al (2014) Enhancement of Achilles tendon repair mediated by matrix metalloproteinase inhibition via systemic administration of doxycycline. J Orthop Res 32(4):500–506

Kim HJ et al (2007) The role of transforming growth factor-beta and bone morphogenetic protein with fibrin glue in healing of bone-tendon junction injury. Connect Tissue Res 48(6):309–315

Lee DK (2007) Achilles tendon repair with acellular tissue graft augmentation in neglected ruptures. J Foot Ankle Surg 46(6):451–455

Lee DK (2008) A preliminary study on the effects of acellular tissue graft augmentation in acute Achilles tendon ruptures. J Foot Ankle Surg 47(1):8–12

Li GH et al (2012) Multifunctional roles of gelsolin in health and diseases. Med Res Rev 32:999–1025

Lohan A et al (2013) Human hamstring tenocytes survive when seeded into a decellularized porcine Achilles tendon extracellular matrix. Connect Tissue Res 54(4–5):305–312

Majewski M et al (2008) Ex vivo adenoviral transfer of bone morphogenetic protein 12 (BMP-12) cDNA improves Achilles tendon healing in a rat model. Gene Ther 15(16):1139–1146

Majewski M et al (2012) Improvement of tendon repair using muscle graft transduced with TGF-beta1 cDNA. Eur Cell Mater 23:94–101. discussion 101–102
Marycz K et al (2014) The autologous gelsolin combined with exogenous nucleotides enhance chondrogenic differentiation in equine adipose derived mesenchymal stromal cells—an in vitro research. J Cell Sci Ther 5:174
Mlynarek RA et al (2016) Platelet-Rich Plasma (PRP) in orthopedic sports medicine. Am J Orthop (Belle Mead NJ) 45(5):290–326
Ning LJ et al (2012) Preparation and characterization of decellularized tendon slices for tendon tissue engineering. J Biomed Mater Res A 100(6):1448–1456
Nirmalanandhan VS et al (2008) Effect of scaffold material, construct length and mechanical stimulation on the in vitro stiffness of the engineered tendon construct. J Biomech 41(4):822–828
Philpott NJ et al (1997) G-CSF-mobilized CD34 peripheral blood stem cells are significantly less apoptotic than unstimulated peripheral blood CD34 cells: role of G-CSF as survival factor. Br J Haematol 97(1):146–152
Pietschmann MF et al (2013) Comparison of tenocytes and mesenchymal stem cells seeded on biodegradable scaffolds in a full-size tendon defect model. J Mater Sci Mater Med 24(1):211–220
Prockop DJ (1997) Marrow stromal cells as stem cells for nonhematopoietic tissues. Science 276:71–74
Rickert M et al (2005) Adenovirus-mediated gene transfer of growth and differentiation factor-5 into tenocytes and the healing rat Achilles tendon. Connect Tissue Res 46(4–5):175–183
Schneider U, Veith G (2013) First results on the outcome of gold induced, autologous-conditioned serum (GOLDIC) in the treatment of different lameness-associated equine diseases. J Cell Sci Ther 5:151
Shah V et al (2013) Dose-response effect of an intra-tendon application of recombinant human platelet-derived growth factor-BB (rhPDGFBB) in a rat Achilles tendinopathy model. J Orthop Res 31(3):413–420
Spinardi L, Witke W (2007) Gelsolin and diseases. Subcell Biochem 45:55–69
Tang SW et al (2014) Stringent requirement for spatial arrangement of extracellular matrix in supporting cell morphogenesis and differentiation. BMC Cell Biol 15:10
Tetta C et al (2012) The role of microvesicles derived from mesenchymal stem cells in tissue regeneration; a dream for tendon repair? Muscles Ligaments Tendons J 2:212–221
Webb WR et al (2013) The application of poly(3-hydroxybutyrate-co-3-hydroxyhexanoate) scaffolds for tendon repair in the rat model. Biomaterials 34(28):6683–6694
Wen D et al (1996) The plasma and cytoplasmic forms of human gelsolin differ in disulfide structure. Biochemistry 35:9700–9709
Widmer A et al (2017) A prospective comparison of the Goldic® technique and corticosteroid plus hyaluronic acid injections for arthrogenic lamness in horses. Vet Comp Orthop Traumatol in review
Wisbeck JM et al (2012) Xenograft scaffold full-wrap reinforcement of Krackow Achilles tendon repair. Orthopedics 35(3):e331–e334
Yao J et al (2011) Viability and proliferation of pluripotential cells delivered to tendon repair sites using bioactive sutures-an in vitro study. J Hand Surg Am 36(2):252–258
Yin Z et al (2013) The effect of decellularized matrices on human tendon stem/progenitor cell differentiation and tendon repair. Acta Biomater 9(12):9317–9329
Zantop T et al (2006) Extracellular matrix scaffolds are repopulated by bone marrow-derived cells in a mouse model of Achilles tendon reconstruction. J Orthop Res 24(6):1299–1309
Zhang QH et al (2011) Treatment with gelsolin reduces brain inflammation and apoptotic signaling in mice following thermal injury. J Neuroinflammation 8:118
Zhou Y, Wang JH (2016) PRP treatment efficacy for tendinopathy: a review of basic science studies. Biomed Res Int 2016:9103792

Shock Wave Therapy for Tendinopathies

40

Maria Cristina d'Agostino, Elisabetta Tibalt, Kenneth Vincent Craig, and Stefano Respizzi

Contents

M.C. d'Agostino (✉) • E. Tibalt • S. Respizzi
Shock Wave Therapy & Research Unit, Humanitas Clinical and Research Hospital, Milan, Italy
e-mail: cristina.d'agostino@humanitas.it; elisabetta.tibalt@humanitas.it

K.C. Vincent
Kompass Health Associates, Auckland, New Zealand

Shockwave & Isokinetic Centre, Melbourne, VIC, Australia

Extracorporeal shock wave therapy (ESWT) originally introduced in medicine as lithotripsy (extracorporeal shock wave lithotripsy or ESWL) for the treatment of urolithiasis, in the 1980s has expanded its scope of application into the field of orthopedics and musculoskeletal medicine, mainly for the treatment of tendon and bone pathologies (Notarnicola and Moretti, Muscles Ligaments Tendons J 33–37, 2012; Wang, J Orthop Surg Res 11, 2012; Romeo et al., Med Princ Pract 7–13, 2014; d'Agostino et al., Int J Surg 147–153, 2015, J Biol Regul Homeost Agents 323–332, 2016). ESWT in orthopedic applications, unlike originally introduced to urology, is not utilized as a destructive force to disintegrate calcific deposits but conversely to induce tissue-specific beneficial effects and *regeneration*, via a constellation of biocellular response modulation (d'Agostino et al. 2015, 2016). More recently, due to its regenerative and angiogenetic properties, ESWT has been successfully applied across medical disciplines including dermatology, vulnology (i.e., complex non-healing wounds, ulcers, and painful scars) (Saggini et al. 2008; Arno' et al. 2010; Qureshi et al. 2011; Fioramonti et al. 2012; Mittermayr et al. 2012), and andrology (Chung and Cartmill 2015; Bechara et al. 2015; Abu-Ghanem et al. 2014; Lei et al. 2013; Gruenwald et al. 2013). In orthopedics, ESWT is considered where tendinopathies prove resistant and indocile to conventional management and where high risks of surgical complications are present or in the instance where surgery has failed (Haupt 1997). In certain instances, ESWT conducted in combination with

G.L. Canata et al. (eds.), *Muscle and Tendon Injuries*, DOI 10.1007/978-3-662-54184-5_40

conventional management of tendinopathies is seen to yield better therapeutic outcomes over purely conventional management alone (Rompe et al. 2009; Al-Abbad and Simon 2013). ESWT offers a revolutionary clinical treatment option for unresponsive tendinopathies that are indocile to conventional interventions, given its known biocellular responses (i.e., inflammatory modulation), and tissue regenerative properties (Notarnicola and Moretti 2012; Romeo et al. 2014; Wang 2012; Wang 2003; d'Agostino et al. 2015, 2016).

The biocellular responses that are attributed to ESWT are seen to occur based on the principle of *mechanosensory* and *mechanotransductive feedback*, where the introduction and the ensuing transduction of the shock waves (SW) stimulus derive a myriad of positive biological responses, aimed to influence and encourage homeostatic return (Huang et al. 2013; d'Agostino et al. 2015, 2016).

When applied by an experienced and trained *SW operator*, ESWT offers a strategic, efficacious, safe, noninvasive, and systemically neutral therapeutic intervention that is easily complied with and tolerated by patients for the management of tendinopathies (Notarnicola and Moretti 2012; Romeo et al. 2014; Wang 2012; Ioppolo et al. 2014; Notarnicola et al. 2012).

ESWT could revolutionize the nature and standard of tendinopathy management, elevating it from being *palliative* toward a more *curative* approach.

40.1 Brief History

SW are supersonic acoustic energy waves, considered to be the most efficient method for energy dispensation. They are ubiquitous in nature, like thunder following lightning during a storm, or man-made like the supersonic jet burst from an aircraft (d'Agostino et al. 2016). Early recognized as a physical entity in the beginning of the nineteenth century, only after the *Second World War* did scientists begin to consider the possible useful application of SW in medicine, and in 1974 a research grant titled "Application of Extracorporeal Shock Wave Lithotripsy" was approved. The first patient with kidney stone would later be treated with SW in Munich (Germany) in 1980, making it the world's first minimally invasive surgical procedure that would become the *gold standard* for the treatment of urolithiasis and solidify the utility of the ESWL procedure up to the present day (Herr 2008; Thiel 2001).

Valchanou and Michailov in 1991 would soon observe and publish their findings, noting that the action of SW was not purely disruptive in nature, nor only limited to kidney stone disintegration but could be potentially utilized in a regenerative manner, as SW were seen to modulate bone healing (Valchanou and Michailov 1991). This landmark discovery heralded the interest and further investigation of SW application for bone pathology and shifted the paradigm of SW application from the singular *mechanical destructive* type application, associated with ESWL toward becoming a potential intervention for regenerative application in orthopedics. The expansion of SW from urology (ESWL) into orthopedics (ESWT) yielded positive results on several pathologies, including pseudarthrosis, stress fractures, and some degenerative bone conditions, further demonstrating ESWT clinical safety and efficacy (Schaden et al. 2001; Schaden et al. 2015; Cacchio et al. 2009; Furia et al. 2010a; Furia et al. 2010b; Alves et al. 2009; d'Agostino et al. 2011; Vulpiani et al. 2012; Leal et al. 2015a).

Since the late 1999s, ESWT has demonstrated similar clinical efficacy for the treatment of a variety of tendinopathic conditions with admirable positive treatment outcomes and survival curve (Notarnicola et al. 2011, 2012; Notarnicola and Moretti 2012; Leal et al. 2015b; Thiele et al. 2015; Gerdesmeyer et al. 2015; Agil et al. 2013; Moya et al. 2015, 2016).

Yet despite the plethora of scientific publications over the past decade, that continuously report on the safety, efficacy, and regenerative nature of ESWT, there remains some reluctance toward its wider application in orthopedics and musculoskeletal medicine. This could be due to several factors, including the ambiguity associated with device choice and treatment parameters, as well as the results of some earlier studies reporting of the ineffectiveness of SW in clinical practice (Buchbinder et al. 2002a, b; Haake et al. 2002). The reports of these earlier well-designed trials concluded that ESWT was ineffective for both plantar fasciitis (Buchbinder et al. 2002b) and lateral epicondylitis (Buchbinder et al. 2002a; Haake et al. 2002), and this may have significantly contributed some of the reluctance toward the wider use of ESWT. However, on a positive note, these trials highlighted the pertinence for adequate training and protocol selection when applying ESWT, as well as designed trials (Buchbinder et al. 2002; Haake et al. 2002) and appropriate treatment protocols (Ogden 2004). Nowadays, after a relevant number of clinical investigations have been carried out, there is greater appreciation and clarity when selecting ESWT protocols. Furthermore, a great majority of the investigators report highly successful results when utilizing ESWT for plantar heel pain syndromes and elbow epicondylitis and some other tendinopathic conditions as well (Notarnicola et al. 2011, 2012; Notarnicola and Moretti 2012; Leal et al. 2015b; Thiele et al. 2015; Gerdesmeyer et al. 2015; Agil et al. 2013; Moya et al. 2016).

The International Society for Medical Shockwave Treatment (ISMST) is the international society that is leading the way encouraging continuous scientific research, education, and collaboration with regard to ESWT. With two decades of scientific background and expertise in this field, the ISMST and all its affiliate national societies continue to organize congresses and ESWT instructional courses, attended by many from all over the globe. The ISMST develops and updates safe treatment recommendations while encouraging scientific research for the safe and effective use of this therapy (ISMST web-site: www.shockwavetherapy.org).

As with any medical breakthrough and intervention, there will always be proponents and opponents, and ESWT is no exemption to this. However, we must consider and acknowledge the fact that, in this modern era, every technology is extremely susceptible to redundancy, but after over four decades since its maiden investigatory application (1974) in medicine (lithotripsy), the utility and investigation in *SW* continue to expand across medical disciplines, which may be classified as a phenomenon in its own right. In this chapter, the authors will highlight the current understanding associated with ESWT and its clinical application for the management of tendinopathies. Given the safety profile, systemic neutrality, noninvasiveness, and regenerative capacity associated with this modality, it is plausible that ESWT could revolutionize the standard of tendinopathy management, elevating it from being mainly palliative toward a more curative approach (d'Agostino et al. 2015).

40.2 General Characteristics of Shock Waves (SW)

Most pertinently, a shock wave differs from an ultrasound wave in that SW are biphasic supersonic waves, which transmit in a non-sinusoidal motion pattern, achieving peak pressure amplitudes approximately 1000 times greater than that produced by an ultrasound wave (Coombs et al. 2000; Delius et al. 1997; Coleman and Saunders 1993; Ogden and Toth-Kischkat 2001). The physical characteristics and clinical applications of SW were established by an *International Consensus Conference* in 1997, and according to the parameters outlined and recognized by national and international scientific societies, a shock wave displays and possesses the characteristics as described in Fig. 40.1.

There are three methods for generating SW: electrohydraulic source (EH), electromagnetic (EM), and piezoelectric (PE) ones. All of them have in common that the waves are generated in water (inside the applicator), as the impedance of water and biologic tissue are similar and comparable; as a result, reflection is limited and waves are better transferred into the body (van der Worp et al. 2013).

The shock wave created by each of these three sources is primarily generated by a controlled high-voltage discharge within a three-dimensional (3D) fluid-filled chamber, causing a transient high-pressure disturbance; each discharge propagates a biphasic sonic impulse within the chamber. This sudden rise from ambi-

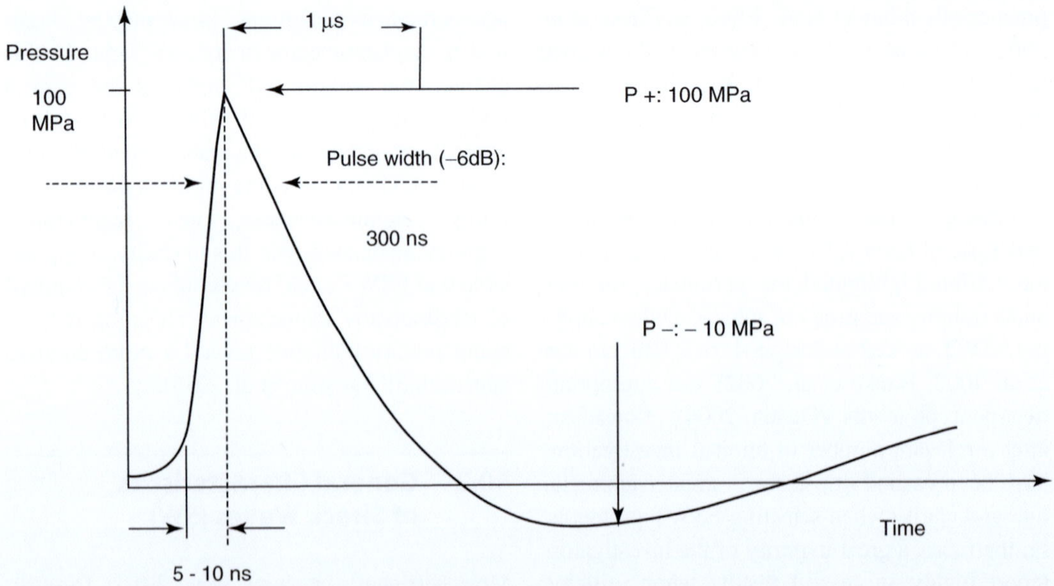

Fig. 40.1 Characteristics of a shock wave: **Phase 1**: High pressure wave rise time from basic ambient value to a pressure value of approximately 100 MPa within <10 nanoseconds (ns). **Phase 2**: Wave implosion to a negative pressure value of approx. −10 MPa of within microseconds (Ueberle 1997; Wess et al. 1997; Speed 2014; Gerdesmeyer et al. 2002, 2006; Ogden and Toth-Kischkat 2001; Coombs et al. 2000; Delius et al. 1997; Coleman and Saunders 1993) (www.shockwavetherapy.org)

ent pressure within the chamber creates an extremely short duration broad frequency spectrum (16–20 MHz) SW, that within nanoseconds (ns) of the SW life cycle, creates an initial peak pressure known to rise above 100 MPa (500 bar), which negatively implodes to approximately −10 MPa within microseconds (Fig. 40.1) (Coombs et al. 2000; Delius et al. 1997; Coleman and Saunders 1993; Ogden and Toth-Kischkat 2001). For all of them, SW are produced as a consequence of a rapid increase in pressure (like a "micro-explosion") into the water, and sooner, for medical purposes, they are concentrated or "focused" on the anatomical "target"; thanks to a parabolic lens, which directs SW, as soon as they are produced from the source (Ogden and Toth-Kischkat 2001; Gerdesmeyer et al. 2002, 2006; Speed 2014). Based on these specific technical characteristics, SW are defined also as "focused" SW (fSW), implying different treatment protocols, for the different types of sources, relatively to the number of shots and the recommended energy levels (expressed as Energy Flux Density in mJ/mm^2) to be applied for the different kinds of treatments (Speed 2014).

The rapid sequence of alternating positive and negative phases, during SW propagation, is responsible of the "mechanical" effects (most probably as *shear stresses*) on the interfaces between different tissues, with their own specific and different densities (acoustic impedance). At higher energies, the negative (or tensile) phase of the SW curve can produce cavitation at the tissue interfaces: gas bubbles are formed and subsequently implode at higher speed, thus generating a second front of SW or *microjets* of fluid. Overall, these physical phenomena can be responsible, as final result, of the direct (physical) and indirect (biological) effects of SW on the treated tissues (Ueberle 1997; Gerdesmeyer et al. 2002, 2006; Ogden and Toth-Kischkat 2001).

Based on the type of tissue we have to treat ("soft tissues" or bone), it is appropriate to use one specific SW generator (lithotripter), as the energy levels requested for obtaining a certain biological effect are different: briefly, for tendinopathies, low–medium energy levels are adequate, while medium–high ones are requested for bone (Notarnicola and Moretti 2012; Notarnicola et al. 2012; Romeo et al. 2014; Haupt 1997).

Regarding the different modalities of applying SW, national and international recommendations established all essential requirements for a correct treatment (*ISMST Consensus Conference*, www.shockwavetherapy.org).

40.3 Radial or Pressure Waves (Radial Pulse Therapy or RPT)

In the early 2000s, some other devices featuring "ballistic" or "radial" pressure waves were introduced into the field of ESWT clinical practice. That new technology produced "pressure waves" and not properly fSW, but the term "radial shock waves" was used since that time (Lohrer et al. 2016).

Radial waves (RW also named as Radial Pulse Therapy or RPT) can be considered as "ordinary sound waves" differently generated: in fact, the source (or applicator) is consisting of a barrel handpiece, where, by the action of compressed air or by the influence of a magnetic field, a metallic bullet is accelerated at a very high speed. This high kinetic energy makes it to impact against the tip of the applicator itself, directly applied on the skin; energy is accumulated during run and transmitted directly to the body surface in the target area. Moreover, RW continue to propagate into the body as spherical or ball-shaped waves that are in a radial way, thus deriving the suggestive definition of *radial waves* (RW). The energy produced by these *pressure waves* is highest at the level of skin surface but diverges and weakens as it penetrates deeper. Based on the particular mechanism of generation, in Radial Pulse Therapy, the "focal point" is not targeted on the anatomical area (as occurs in fSW) but rather on the tip of the applicator; moreover, RW are not focused in depth but, due to the radial transmission, are restricted to the more superficial layers of the body to be treated. From the physical point of view, although both fSW and RW are *acoustic waves*, they differ in shape and, although sharing some clinical indications, nevertheless diverge for some other ones (Ogden and Toth-Kischkat 2001; Gerdesmeyer et al. 2002, 2006; Speed 2014; d'Agostino et al. 2015; Lohrer et al. 2016).

As some authors confirmed, the equipments that produce RW, in comparison with those generating fSW, are relatively smaller, cheaper, and easier to handle. Moreover, the maximum energy for RW is delivered at the applicator to skin interface, and fSW peak pressure is about 100 times higher, while the pulse duration is 1000 times shorter (Novak 2015). In any case, the clinical efficacy of RW could be demonstrated for some specific diseases, and nowadays, it is a widely accepted method in clinical practice, with comparable results, although specifically for superficial musculoskeletal disorders (Lohrer et al. 2016; Novak 2015; Foldager et al. 2012; Speed 2014).

Classically, the main differences between fSW (focused SW) and RPT (Radial Pulse Therapy) can be listed as follows (Novak 2015; Lohrer et al. 2016):

- Principle of generation = pneumatic for RPT versus electrohydraulic, piezoelectric, or electromagnetic for fSW
- Wavelength = 0.15 to 1.5 m (RPT) versus 1.5 mm (fSW)
- Maximum pressure = 1 (RPT) versus 10–100 (fSW) MPa
- Penetration depth = 2–5 cm (RPT) versus 5–20 cm (fSW)

According to what was described by Alkhamaali ZK et al., it is not correct to characterize RW as low-energy shock wave treatment and fSW as high-energy shock wave treatment. Furthermore, RPT, due to the possibility to generate cavitation, must be differentiated from vibrating devices. The capacity to create a cavitation effect has been demonstrated in new-generation RW devices and sharply separates them from certain vibrating devices that do not generate a cavitational effect (Alkhamaali et al. 2016) (Fig. 40.2).

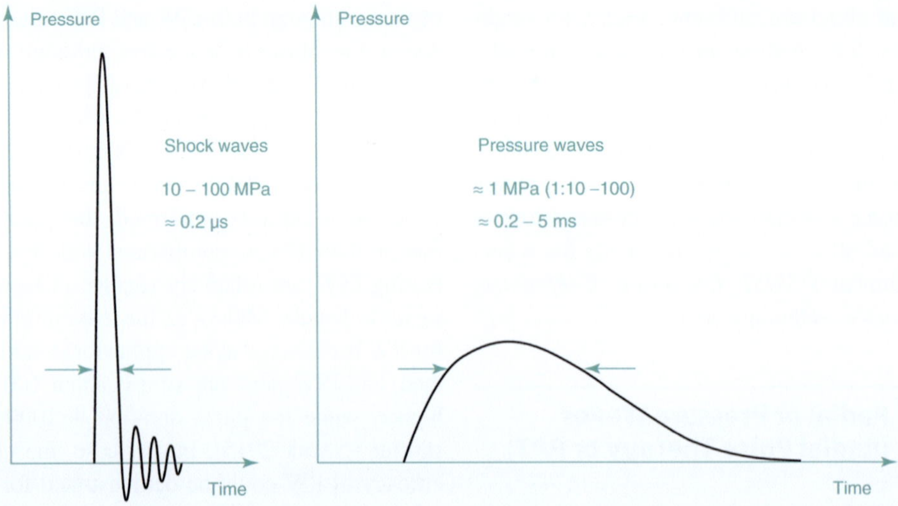

Fig. 40.2 Divergence between a shock wave (fSW) (on the *left*) and a radial (pressure or pulse) wave (RPT) (on the *right*)

40.4 SW Mechanisms of Action: Biocellular Action and Responses

The exact mechanism of action of many clinical interventions remains incompletely elucidated, and ESWT is not excluded from being in the same category. However, advances have been made in recent years to help provide greater illumination of the actions of SW and the biocellular responses derived from this treatment over several indications, including tendinopathies (d'Agostino et al. 2015, 2016).

The science of *mechanobiology* helps elucidate the actions and responses of ESWT on human tissue, as it assists researchers to analyze and appreciate the effects of SW after it disperses its physical acoustic energy onto tissues and cells, in a process termed *mechanotransduction* (d'Agostino et al. 2015; Chiquet et al. 2009; Jaalouk and Lammerding 2009; Kolahi and Mofrad 2010). Mechanotransduction describes the processing of an extracellular stimulus (SW), where the force from the stimulus is processed and converted, resulting in a myriad of biochemical responses that influences cellular function (proliferation, migration, apoptosis, and differentiation) (d'Agostino et al. 2015; Chiquet et al. 2009; Jaalouk and Lammerding 2009; Kolahi and Mofrad 2010).

ESWT transmits a SW stimulus that has been known to induce positive biological effects on the cells and tissues, including tendons, thus restoring tissue *homeostasis* and ultimately function (Notarnicola and Moretti 2012; Romeo et al. 2014; Haupt 1997). This suggests that the homeostatic influence of ESWT on tissue may be considered an indirect, rather than a direct action, yet none the less, an ameliorating intervention (d'Agostino et al. 2015).

The influences of ESWT on the cellular, biochemical, and tissue levels are seen to be multiple and complex. From a cellular level, ESWT is seen to action its influence on pattern recognition Toll-like receptors (TLRs) and macrophages (Holfeld et al. 2014b, 2016; Tepekoylu et al. 2015; Davis et al. 2009; Mariotto et al. 2009; Kuo et al. 2009; Shao et al. 2010; Sukubo et al. 2015), influencing inflammation, angiogenesis, tissue perfusion, and progenitor cell expression, among other factors (Holfeld et al. 2014a; Huang et al. 2013; Tara et al. 2014; Tepekoylu et al. 2013; Visco et al. 2014; Sansone et al. 2012; Ciampa et al. 2005; Gotte et al. 2002; Davis et al. 2009). Its biochemical influences are known to act on neurotransmitters (i.e., substance P or SP and calcitonin gene-related peptide or CGRP), thus assisting in analgesic action and pain modulation even in chronic conditions (Richardson and Vasko 2002; Saggini et al. 2015). ESWT regenerative influences are known to stimulate the progenitor cells of tenocyte, fibroblasts, osteoblast, and endothelial cells, as well as inducing TGF-ß1 production (d'Agostino et al. 2015; Tara et al. 2014; Visco et al. 2014; Sansone et al. 2012; Suhr et al. 2013; Raabe et al. 2013; Kearney et al. 2012; Tamma et al. 2009; Hausdorf et al. 2011; Wang et al. 2002a, b; Tepekoylu et al. 2013), while downregulating pro-fibrotic proteins (i.e., MMP2), reducing fibrous capsule formation, and increasing fibrotic tissue resorption and remodeling (Fischer et al. 2015). These are some of the reasons why ESWT for the management of tendinopathies is gaining more consideration and acceptance.

40.5 ESWT for Tendinopathies?

Tendons, the tough connective tissue of various forms that commonly connects muscles to bone, is primarily comprised of tenoblasts (immature cells), tenocytes (mature cells), collagen, elastin and ground substances. Tendinopathies are a clinical commonality, yet the exact intrinsic pathomechanics of this condition still remains partly unclear. Tendinopathies often present with pain, degeneration, with or without swelling, and with varying levels of debilitations (Sharma and Maffulli 2005; Abate et al. 2009; Scott and Danielson 2009; Cook and Purdam 2009). The disruptions to the tendon's regenerative process (including aberrances of resident tenocytes proliferation, collagen matrix syntheses), which combined with the ensuing hypoxia, are considered to be some of the primary causes for tendinopathies and further disease progression (Sharma and Maffulli 2005; Abate et al. 2009; Scott and Danielson 2009; Cook and Purdam 2009). Although the presence of overt inflammation has been questioned and in most cases rejected as a primary contributor (Sharma and Maffulli 2005; Abate et al. 2009; Scott and Danielson 2009; Cook and Purdam 2009), yet the presence of covet inflammation, as well as the aberrant immune activity (Agil et al. 2013; Sharma and Maffulli 2005; Rees et al. 2009; Wang et al. 2003; Tsuzaki et al. 2003a, b; Archambault et al. 2002), its role in the maintenance of tendon pathology, and its contributions toward disease progression requires greater elucidation.

The general consensus, to date, is that ESWT may be considered for tendinopathies that are resistant and indocile to conservative management. ESWT is at times recommended in combination with loading exercise routines. At the present time, there is uncertainty in some quarters as to whether ESWT (fSW) or Radial Pulse Therapy (RPT) is more suitable for the management of tendinopathies (Lohrer et al. 2016), and this therapeutic choice remains at the clinician's individual discretion and expertise.

From the clinical point of view, the most important thing to be underlined is that the maximum energy in RPT is transmitted at the interface between the applicator head of the device and the skin and diminishes its energy inside the treated tissue by the square of the penetration depth (Lohrer et al. 2016). As a consequence, since the beginning, RPT was applied to tendon pathologies, primarily by their immediately subcutaneous localization and by a large area of injured tissue. Midportion Achilles tendinopathy and patellar tendinopathy seem, for example, to fulfill these criteria, and some of the authors demonstrated those can be an indication for RPT (Lohrer et al. 2016).

Based on current evidence, some of the authors in the literature stated to be unable to prefer ESWT or RPT for musculoskeletal soft tissue injuries. Conflicting evidence exists from the results of two studies that directly compared fSW to radial waves in patients affected by plantar fasciitis and patellar tendinopathy (Lohrer et al. 2016). As a whole, in clinical practice, RPT has been proven to be as effective and safe noninvasive treatment option for tendon pathologies in several randomized controlled trials. Currently there is no scientific evidence in favor of either RPT or ESWT (fSW), with respect to the treatment outcome (Speed 2014; Schmitz et al. 2015).

According to the ISMST *Consensus Statement (2014)*, fSW should be applied by a trained physician, while radial waves can be applied, after medical prescription, by physiotherapists or *allied health professionals* as well, limited to superficial tendinopathies and muscle pathologies (ISMST-website: www.shockwavetherapy.org).

Regarding local anesthesia, nowadays, while still considered as helpful for bone treatments (Schaden et al. 2015; Lohrer et al. 2016), it is not indicated for soft tissue SW applications, including tendinopathies (Schmitz et al. 2015; Lohrer et al. 2016) (as stated also in the *ISMST Recommendations*), due to the risk of diminishing its therapeutic efficacy. Some experimental researches, in fact, seem to point out that "pain perception" induced by SW application is responsible for releasing neuropeptides (as substance P), thus determining both central and local trophic effects to increase metabolism in bradytrophic tissues (Schmitz et al. 2015; Klonschinski et al. 2011; Lohrer et al. 2016). In an experimental setting, it was demonstrated in fact that "...ESWT dose-dependently activates and sensitizes primary afferent nociceptive C-fibers, and that both activation and sensitization were prevented if local anesthesia was applied" (Klonschinski et al. 2011; Lohrer et al. 2016).

Regardless of the SW equipments, if the treatment is carried out in respect of the rules of "*Good Clinical Practice*" and ISMST Recommendations, by an expert operator, from a general point of view, this therapy can be considered a very safe and effective treatment (Pettrone and McCall 2005; Wang et al. 2000; Furia 2005); furthermore, no device-related problems nor systemic and/or local complications are reported (Ko et al. 2001).

40.6 ESWT for Tendinopathies: Basic Science

The safe and effective application of ESWT over a decade ago onto the plantar fascia prompted the further exploration of ESWT application in tendinopathies (Notarnicola and Moretti 2012). Seil and colleagues, in 2006, noted the success rates of tendinopathy management with ESWT ranged from 60 to 80% (Seil et al. 2006). What was noted by investigators as to the action of ESWT, when applied on tendinopathies in vivo and in vitro experimental studies, were typical changes in tendon structures in the form of transient dose-dependent inflammatory response; proliferation at tendon-bone complex, along with the release of pro-angiogenic regulatory factors (nitric oxide and vascular endothelial growth factor); and proliferating growth factors (PCNA, TGF-ß1), all assisting in tendon regeneration and functional restoration (Wang et al. 2003; Chen et al. 2004; Bosch et al. 2007, 2009; Berta et al. 2009; Frairia and Berta 2011; Chao et al. 2008; Hans et al. 2009; Vetrano et al. 2011; Leone et al. 2016; Zhang et al. 2011; De Girolamo et al. 2014). Histological examinations in animal models noted that ESWT, on pathological tendons, reduced edema, swelling, and inflammatory cell infiltration. Moreover, after ESWT exposure, the lesion site undergoes intensive progenitor tenocyte proliferation and progressive tendon tissue regeneration, together with increased expression levels in mRNA for TGF-beta1, IGF-1 expression, and collagen type I while suppressing synthesis of matrix metalloproteinase (MMPs), thus suggesting that ESWT may increase mitogenic tendon proliferative responses (Chen et al. 2004; Bosch et al. 2007, 2009; Berta et al. 2009; Frairia and Berta 2011; Chao et al. 2008; Hans et al. 2009; Vetrano et al. 2011; Leone et al. 2016; Zhang et al. 2011; De Girolamo et al. 2014; Notarnicola and Moretti 2012). Lubricin expressions were similarly increased, thus indicating modulation against tendon erosion and adhesions, while providing pain relief as well (Zhang et al. 2011).

Very interestingly, in 2015, in humans, by using microdialysis, Waugh CM and coauthors examined the real-time biological response of healthy and pathological tendons to SW exposure, reporting no statistical differences between the biological tissue response to SW in healthy and pathological tendons. In addition, the biological response to this treatment could be differentiated between *possible responders* and *nonresponders* based on a minimum fivefold increase in any inflammatory marker or MMP from pre- to post-ESWT. Based on their research, they suggested that the mechanical stimulus provided by ESWT might aid tendon remodeling in tendinopathy, by promoting the inflammatory and catabolic processes that are associated with removing damaged matrix constituents. The failed response of some individuals may help to explain why ESWT does not improve symptoms in all patients and provides a potential focus for future research (Waugh et al. 2015).

Again, more recently, Leone et al. showed that ESWT is able in vitro to accelerate the differentiation of human primary-cultured tendon stem/progenitor cells, describing how cultures of tenocytes, derived from ruptured tendons, were more susceptible to SW mediated activation, thus suggesting a possible recruitment of undifferentiated progenitors at the site of injury. They were able to demonstrate that SW induce cell proliferation, although in different stages of differentiation and presenting a heterogeneous natural differentiation potential, probably initiated by tendon injuries. Therefore, the authors concluded that aligned with some other reports, the clinical benefits of ESWT can be attributed to the mechanical stress, promoting the in vivo regenerative capacity of the tissue. Moreover, they showed for the first time that ESWT significantly enhances hTSPCs-induced differentiation, as indicated by cytochemical and molecular findings. Taken together, previous reports and the present observations seem to corroborate the long-held idea that ESWT may enhance recruitment, proliferation, and differentiation of tissue-derived stem cells. Leone et al. propose that such treatment, applied on injured tendons, is able to accelerate stem cell differentiation—probably through the release of different cytokines and growth factors—mainly toward tenocytic lineage, contributing to tendon repair. Further investigations will certainly help to better clarify that ESWT clinical benefits are amenable to mechanisms triggering tendon healing promoted by resident stem cells recruitment (Leone et al. 2016).

In addition to all these tissue-specific *trophic* actions of SW, it is interesting to remember that from a general point of view, ESWT may influence the regulation and modulation of both overt and covert inflammatory markers, including TLRs, macrophages, cytokines, and tumor necrosis factor-alpha (TNFα), thus helping to restore *homeostatic* return of tendon turnover (Holfeld et al. 2014b, 2016; Tepekoylu et al. 2013, 2015; Davis et al. 2009; Mariotto et al. 2009; Kuo et al. 2009; Shao et al. 2010; Sukubo et al. 2015; Lowbenwein et al. 2015).

40.7 Brief Overview of ESWT in Tendinopathies

Plantar heel pain syndrome. Ogden et al. (2002) conducted a meta-analysis of 20 studies ranging from 1990 to 2000, with a sample size totaling 1655 patients (Ogden et al. 2002). Briefly, one study utilized ballistic RPT, and the others utilized fSW. 18 studies reported success rate ranging from 61 to 88%, all with minimal to no adverse effects. Always Ogden and coauthors, in 2004, published a double-phased double-blind placebo-randomized controlled trial, with a total of 285 patients, where n = 144 were allocated ESWT, (n = 141) and placebo at follow-up (3 months), 67% (ESWT) recorded complete healing compared to 42% some improvement (control). No adverse effects were noted (Ogden 2004; Ogden et al. 2004). Since that time until recent years, many articles were published in the literature on this topic; some of them reporting controversial results about the efficacy of SW in clinical practice. Finally, in 2015, Gollwitzer and coauthors published a randomized, controlled, multicenter study whose objective was to test whether focused extracorporeal shock wave therapy is effective in relieving chronic heel pain diagnosed as plantar fasciitis. The results provided proof of the clinically relevant effect size of focused extracorporeal shock wave therapy without local anesthesia in the treatment of recalcitrant plantar fasciitis, with success rate between 50 and 65% (Gollwitzer et al. 2015).

Achilles tendinopathy (AT). Gerdesmeyer et al. (2015), published a review of six separate studies on chronic Achilles tendinopathy (AT) carried out between 2005 and 2008. Four studies utilized fSW, and two other ones utilized RPT. The authors concluded that both of them were effective for the treatment of AT. There were two reports of mild adverse effect out of a total sample size of 347 across all six studies. There was a consensus that treatments should be carried out without local anesthesia in order to obtain optimal results (Gerdesmeyer et al. 2015).

Patellar tendinopathy. Leal et al. recently reviewed 15 studies from 2000 to 2015, where both fSW and radial waves were utilized for the treatment of chronic patellar tendinopathy (CPT). The author's conclusions were that ESWT provided good results for the treatment of CPT, where pathological pain scores reduced with functional improvement. They found that there were insufficient grounds to recommend RPT for treating CPT. The authors recommended that ESWT was unsuitable in acute cases of patellar tendinopathy. No significant adverse effects were reported (Leal et al. 2015b).

Lateral epicondylitis. Thiele et al. (2015) reviewed two set of studies allocated into two groups: Group 1 negative results reporting and Group 2 positive results reporting. The studies that described negative results were seven in total, with a total sample size of 700 patients, with a date ranging from 2002 to 2008. The studies that reported positive outcomes were ten in total, with a total sample size of 758 patients, with a date ranging from 1996 to 2012. The authors' comments were as follows: where negative or inconclusive reporting was the conclusion of each of the study, it was noted that recommended treatment guidelines and protocols of the ISMST were not followed. Some of the flaws noted in these instances were the use of incorrect SW energy levels, inclusion of acute conditions, and control groups receiving ESWT. This highlights the necessity for clinicians to obtain adequate training for the use of ESWT. The overall conclusion was that there was adequate evidence to support the use of ESWT for chronic later epicondylitis. The note to clinicians assessing clinical evidence is to ensure that recommended treatment parameters were being correctly utilized and not to just focus on the general study design. ESWT is effective for lateral epicondylitis where recommended guidelines are applied (Thiele et al. 2015).

Shoulder tendinopathies. Moya et al. (2015) reviewed 17 studies ranging from 1999 to 2013, assessing both calcific (n = 11) and noncalcific shoulder (n = 6) pathologies utilizing both fSW (n = 15) and radial waves (n = 2) (Moya et al. 2015). Some studies compared ESWT to surgical intervention, where investigators found no difference in the outcome between surgical intervention and ESWT. In the studies investigating efficacy of SW for calcific shoulder pathology, all investigators (n = 10) reported significant improvement of pathology after ESWT. The one investigator utilizing rWT similarly reported positive outcomes as well. In the studies investigating efficacy of SW on noncalcific shoulder pathology, one investigator found some short-term benefit, while all other investigators reported no significant change to report. From a general point of view, the authors concluded that (Moya et al. 2015):

- SW can be considered an efficacious and efficient alternative to surgery for calcific rotator cuff (RC) tendinopathy, thus a treatment of choice for this pathology, as well as an effective treatment modality when other conservative methods have failed.
- Clinical efficacy of SW in noncalcific shoulder tendinopathy is still controversial but with promising perspectives.
- Although the available evidence does not allow conclusions of the effectiveness in *frozen shoulder*, preliminary studies encourage to continue with larger series of patients.
- Promising results on other shoulder diseases have been reported, but it lacks solid evidence.
- Although the persistence of calcification may be associated with good clinical outcome, complete resorption has better results than partial disappearance or persistence.
- Both high- and low-energy SW result effective, although more sessions in the second case are required.

- RPT would seem to be effective in calcium deposit resolution as well.
- The absence of dense calcification rim around the RC is a good predictor of treatment outcome with SW.
- The mechanism of calcium absorption has not yet been elucidated, although some authors proposed *neo-lymphangiogenesis* as a possible biological substrate (Moya et al. 2015).

Moreover, in calcium deposit dissolution after SW exposure, a possible beneficial interference with some inflammatory pathways could not be excluded and would imply further investigations. This is particularly evident, when considering the influence of SW in the mechanism of innate immunity and self-healing processes, that regulate pro-resolving and pro-regenerative reactions to pathogens and some other *noxae* (d'Agostino et al. 2015; Holfeld et al. 2014b; Sukubo et al. 2015). In fact, as it has been recently demonstrated for the first time in human histological samples, in calcific tendinitis lesions of the shoulder, there seems to be a significant increase in neovascularization and neoinnervation, along with an eightfold increase in mast cells and macrophages. The findings are consistent with the hypothesis that in calcific tendinitis, the calcific material is inducing a vigorous inflammatory response within the tendon with formation of new blood vessels and nerves (Hackett et al. 2016), and these data surely provide a glimpse on future therapeutic perspectives in calcific tendinopathies.

40.8 Comparison of ESWT with Some Other Therapies

When comparing some alternative therapeutic procedures with ESWT, the greater efficacy of the *bio-mechanotransductive* properties of ESWT is clearly more evident. Ozturan et al. (2010) compared the short-, medium-, and long-term effects of corticosteroid injection, autologous blood injection, and ESWT in epicondylitis for example. Corticosteroid (CS) injection showed a higher success rate in the short term, while autologous blood injection and ESWT were more efficacious over the long term; there was a higher percentage of recurrence after CS injection. These authors reported a success rate of 50% relative to CS therapy, 83.3% to autologous blood injection, and 89.9% to ESWT (Ozturan et al. 2010). It is pertinent to mention that in another study for the treatment of tendinopathies, ESWT proved to be an effective and noninvasive therapeutic intervention that reduced the need for surgery (Radwan et al. 2008); it was shown to be similarly a treatment of choice for patients where local steroid injections are ineffective or contraindicated (Lee et al. 2012). Rebuzzi and coauthors reported, in a retrospective study comparing arthroscopy and ESWT after a 2 year follow-up, that ESWT was the better treatment option for calcifying tendonitis of the shoulder (Rebuzzi et al. 2008). We found in more recent scientific literature for various tendinopathies that certain agents such as hyaluronic acid injection have been already compared to SW efficacy rates for Achilles tendinopathy (Lynen et al. 2016) and painful noncalcific rotator cuff tendinopathy (Frizziero et al. 2016). Moreover, according to some of the authors, the use of ultrasound-guided percutaneous lavage (UGPL) for calcific shoulder tendinopathies would seem similarly less effective than previously considered (Arirachakaran et al. 2016).

From a general point of view, it is quite plausible to suggest that, where ESWT is noted to be ineffective or less effective, the common reason is due more to incorrect methodology and pathology selection, rather than its real inefficacy (Rompe and Maffulli 2007; Thiele et al. 2015; Moya et al. 2016). In other words, it seems that the reason of controversial results in the literature, regarding the success of ESWT in tendinopathies could be not a "biological" matter, but rather a "methodological" criticism (Rompe and Maffulli 2007).

In clinical practice, as well as in designing clinical studies and comparing methodologies, always according to the ISMST Recommendations, it is important to consider that the clinical results can be strongly affected by the following factors (ISMST-website, www.shockwavetherapy.org):

- Degree of experience of the SW operator (physician or physiotherapist or other allied health professionals)
- Type of equipment utilized for applying SW
- Adequate therapeutic approach, in the context of a so-called integrated personalized program, where SW are combined, for example, with therapeutic exercise (especially in tendinopathies). Nevertheless, we must consider that ESWT efficacy can be negatively influenced in clinical practice by the following factors:
  - If inclusion/exclusion criteria for SW application have not been met or when there is no consensus on them
  - When the disease we are going to treat with SW is the secondary manifestation of a general or primary disease
  - When some concurrent not orthopedics diseases are present
- Based on the level of chronicity. In the specific field of tendinopathies, it has been described that effectiveness of ESWT may depend also on the stage of tendinopathy. A recent model of tendinopathy differentiates between a reactive tendinopathy/early tendon disrepair phase and a late tendon disrepair/degeneration phase. ESWT would seem most appropriate in the latter, when the tendinopathy is mostly degenerative and when conservative treatment has no effect (Rees et al. 2009).This is also supported by some studies that showed no effect of ESWT in the early stage of tendinopathy (Rompe et al. 2010; Zwerver et al. 2011). Until now, studies have not differentiated between subjects in the study based on these different stages; therefore, different studies may have used populations that are not comparable (van der Worp et al. 2013). Again, if we consider the different treatment parameters, as van der Worp et al. described, many instrumental settings that can be varied during ESWT must be taken into account. The precise relationship between these settings and the effectiveness of the treatment are often unclear, although for some settings there is some indication as to how they may influence effectiveness (van der Worp et al. 2013). For example, according to some authors, energy flux densities above 0.50 mJ/mm^2 should be avoided (Maier et al. 2002; Rompe et al. 1998), while Bosch et al. in an animal study demonstrated that EH-generated shock waves already have a major impact on healthy tendon tissue at an intensity of 0.14 mJ/mm^2 (Bosch et al. 2009).

Furthermore, some of the authors provide some suggestions for the use of ESWT in clinical practice. When SW are applied for treating tendinopathies, it seems best to apply it in a later stage (van der Worp et al. 2013), in combination with tendon load management (Kountouris and Cook 2007), after other conservative options have been tried and before more radical options like surgery are considered (van der Worp et al. 2013).

40.9 SW and Sports Activities

Nowadays, ESWT turns out to be a valid tool also for improving recovery and healing in tendinopathies also related to sports activities. It is well recognized that treating and relieving this kind of tendinopathies can represent a great challenge, both due to biomechanical overload and almost always for the inability to stay away from training and racing, which could affect the biological pathways of recovery, independently of the kind of treatment applied. It derives that while applying ESWT for these specific cases, its effectiveness could be invalidated (or reduced)—as a biological therapeutic tool—by the same factors abovementioned, as well as the final results, if below expectations. About it, the *TOPGAME Study* (randomized controlled trial, level of evidence, 1) was designed by Zwerver et al. for determining the effectiveness of ESWT on pain, symptoms, and function in athletes with early symptomatic patellar tendinopathy, who are still in training and competition. Patellar tendinopathy is a common overuse injury among jumping athletes, for which no evidence-based treatment guidelines exist. ESWT appears to be a promising treatment but its effectiveness had to be studied in athletes with patellar tendinopathy, having symptoms for 3–12 months and who are still playing. In this study, the authors were able to demonstrate that ESWT, as a unique treatment during the competitive season, does not show benefit over a placebo treatment, in the management of actively competing jumping athletes with patellar tendinopathy, who have symptoms for less than 12 months (Zwerver et al. 2011). Obviously, this study does not affect the validity of ESWT as a good choice of treatment for tendinopathies (patellar one and so on) from a general point of view, also in sports. Rather it shifts attention on the necessity to a "proper" application, not only in terms of a correct diagnosis and practical technique (adequate device and professional competence of the operator) but also of a "strategic" timing of intervention and expectation of results, especially while considering that biological reactions induced by SW mechanotransduction take time to appear and act (from a few weeks up to 2–3 months) (d'Agostino et al. 2015).

Conclusions

From a general point of view, after its original introduction in medicine for urological applications, ESWT, already surpassed the relatively long *pioneristic phase*, progressively has now gained a recognized therapeutic dignity in orthopedics and rehabilitation, thus representing a valid, noninvasive therapeutic tool for tendinopathies, especially for all those conditions where other therapies (included surgery) have failed. Moreover, it presents, at the same time, the characteristics of safety and effectiveness, together with the advantage of repeatability and compatibility, if indicated to combine SW with some other conservative treatments (physical, biophysical, or medical ones) (d'Agostino et al. 2016).

As Zwerver et al. correctly wrote, SW are commonly applied in the management of tendon injuries, and, nowadays, pain relief and mechanotransduction-induced tissue regeneration and remodeling of the tendons, together with dissolution of calcifications, are considered to be the most important working mechanisms. The heterogeneity of the systems (fSW and radial waves), treatment protocols, and study populations and the fact that there seem to be a heterogeneity in the population ("responders" and "nonresponders") continue to make it difficult, at the moment, to give firm recommendations with regard to the most optimal ESWT approach. Moreover, specific knowledge with regard to the effects of SW in patients affected by tendinopathies related to metabolic disorders is not yet available. Further fundamental and clinical researches are required to determine the value of ESWT in the management of tendinopathies (Zwerver et al. 2016) and its therapeutic dignity, not only in "standard" conditions but also in all more complicated situations, where SW could act as a real biological tool in restoring physiological tendon tissue tropism and metabolism, as "biosurgery" (or "noninvasive surgery") (d'Agostino et al. 2015, 2016).

As Lohrer et al. pointed out, an increasing number of excellent SW studies for musculoskeletal diseases were published in the literature, and perhaps, without being exaggerated, ESWT can be considered the best analyzed treatment modality in orthopedics. Almost all systematic musculoskeletal ESWT reviews regarding this argument conclude that high-level studies are requested; nevertheless, Lohrer underlines that "the question to be answered in future is not if ESWT works, but rather which treatment protocol and parameters are the best for specific and well described conditions." Research finally has to follow clinical practice, where treatment protocols have to be individualized (Lohrer et al. 2016), especially in orthopedics and rehabilitation.

Until now, always in agreement with Lohrer, main or exclusive goal of clinical SW research seems to be detecting the success of ESWT applied, following a standardized protocol. The question, however, if ESWT is likewise effective in each stage of a given musculoskeletal indication, is still completely unanswered at the moment (Lohrer et al. 2016).

Moreover, as a "tendon pathology continuum model" has been described (Cook and

Purdam 2009) and tendinopathy is "no longer a 'one size fits all' diagnosis" (Cook 2011), it is reasonable to expect that different stages of a given pathology may respond differently to SW, especially in consideration of the fact that SW acts as a biological tool on the tendon homeostasis. Again, also considering that "monotherapies" are rarely used in clinical practice, especially for tendinopathies, it would be desirable that future randomized controlled work should focus on assessing and comparing more realistic treatment protocols (Lohrer et al. 2016).

In 1997, Haupt wrote "…in patients in whom conservative treatment has failed, surgery used to be the only choice, but its success rate barely exceeds that of SW therapy, and surgery can still be done if SW therapy fails. Extracorporeal Shock Waves will have an impact on orthopedics comparable to its effect in urology. Scientific evaluations, professional certifications, quality assurance and reimbursement issues present great challenges…" (Haupt 1997; d'Agostino et al. 2015, 2016).

Much progress has been made since SW were initially applied in urology and soon after in the musculoskeletal field: nowadays, based on *SW Science* and clinical evidences, it seems that the "prophetic" thought of Haupt became reality, and perhaps we have exceeded also expectations. We can declare the "SW pioneering phase" as closed while opening the innovative and revolutionary era of the "biophysical" stimulation and tissue regeneration in musculoskeletal diseases, with important clinical and therapeutic implications also in the field of that one we can define as "regenerative rehabilitation" (d'Agostino et al. 2015, 2016).

References

Abate M, Silbernagel KG, Siljeholm C, Di Iorio A, De Amicis D, Salini V, Werner S, Paganelli R (2009) Pathogenesis of tendinopathies: inflammation or degeneration? Arthritis Res Ther 11(3):235

Abu-Ghanem Y, Kitrey ND, Gruenwald I, Appel B, Vardi Y (2014) Penile low-intensity shock wave therapy: a promising novel modality for erectile dysfunction. Korean J Urol 55(5):295–299

Agil A, Siddiqui MR, Solan M, Redfern DJ, Gullati V, Cobb JP (2013) Extracorporeal shock wave therapy is effective in treating chronic plantar fasciitis: a meta-analysis of RCTs. Clin Orthp Relat Res 471(11):3645–3652

Al-Abbad H, Simon JV (2013) The effectiveness of extracorporeal shock wave therapy on chronic Achilles tendinopathy: a systematic review. Foot Ankle Int 34(1):33–41

Alkhamaali ZK, Crocombe AD, Solan MC, Cirovic S (2016) Finite element modelling of radial shock wave therapy for chronic plantar fasciitis. Comput Methods Biomech Biomed Engin 19(10):1069–1078

Alves EM, Angrisani AT, Santiago MB (2009) The use of extracorporeal shock waves in the treatment of osteonecrosis of the femoral head: a systematic review. Clin Rheumatol 28(11):1247–1251

Archambault J, Tsuzaki M, Herzog W, Banes AJ (2002) Stretch and interleukin-1beta induce matrix metalloproteinases in rabbit tendon cells in vitro. J Orthop Res 20:36–39

Arirachakaran A, Boonard M, Yamaphai S, Prommahachai A, Kesprayura S, Kongtharvonskul J (2016) Extracorporeal shock wave therapy, ultrasound-guided percutaneous lavage, corticosteroid injection and combined treatment for the treatment of rotator cuff calcific tendinopathy: a network meta-analysis of RCTs. Eur J Orthop Surg Traumatol Aug 23

Arnó A, García O, Hernán I, Sancho J, Acosta A, Barret JP (2010) Extracorporeal shock waves, a new non-surgical method to treat severe burns. Burns 36(6):844–849

Bechara A, Casabé A, De Bonis W, Nazar J (2015) Effectiveness of low-intensity extracorporeal shock wave therapy on patients with Erectile Dysfunction (ED) who have failed to respond to PDE5i therapy. A pilot study. Arch Esp Urol 68(2):152–160

Berta L, Fazzari A, Ficco AM, Enrica PM, Catalano MG, Frairia R (2009) Extracorporeal shock waves enhance normal fibroblast proliferation in vitro and activate mRNA expression for TGF-beta1 and for collagen types I and III. Acta Orthop 80(5):612–617

Bosch G, de Mos M, van Binsbergen R, van Schie HT, van de Lest CH, van Weeren PR (2009) The effect of focused extracorporeal shock wave therapy on collagen matrix and gene expression in normal tendons and ligaments. Equine Vet J 41(4):335–341

Bosch G, Lin YL, van Schie HT, van De Lest CH, Barneveld A, van Weeren PR (2007) Effect of extracorporeal shock wave therapy on the biochemical composition and metabolic activity of tenocytes in normal tendinous structures in ponies. Equine Vet J 39(3):226–231

Buchbinder R, Green S, White M, Barnsley L, Smidt N, Assendelft WJ (2002a) Shock wave therapy for lateral elbow pain. Cochrane Database Syst Rev 1:CD003524

Buchbinder R, Ptasznik R, Gordon J, Buchanan J, Prabaharan V, Forbes A (2002b) Ultrasound-guided

extracorporeal shock wave therapy for plantar fasciitis: a randomized controlled trial. JAMA 288(11):1346–1372
Cacchio A, Giordano L, Colafarina O, Rompe JD, Tavernese E, Ioppolo F, Flamini S, Spacca G, Santilli V (2009) Extracorporeal shock-wave therapy compared with surgery for hypertrophic long-bone nonunions. J Bone Joint Surg Am 91(11):2589–2597
Chao YH, Tsuang YH, Sun JS, Chen LT, Chiang YF, Wang CC, Chen MH (2008) Effects of shock waves on tenocyte proliferation and extracellular matrix metabolism. Ultrasound Med Biol 34(5):841–852
Chen YJ, Wang CJ, Yang KD, Kuo YR, Huang HC, Huang YT, Sun YC, Wang FS (2004) Extracorporeal shock waves promote healing of collagenase-induced Achilles tendinitis and increase TGF-beta1 and IGF-I expression. J Orthop Res 22(4):854–861
Chiquet M, Gelman L, Lutz R, Maier S (2009) From mechanotransduction to extracellular matrix gene expression in fibroblasts. Biochem Biophys Acta 1793(5):911–920
Chung E, Cartmill R (2015) Evaluation of clinical efficacy, safety and patient satisfaction rate after low-intensity extracorporeal shockwave therapy for the treatment of male erectile dysfunction: an Australian first open-label single-arm prospective clinical trial. BJU Int 115(Suppl 5):46–49
Ciampa AR, de Prati AC, Amelio E, Cavalieri E, Persichini T, Colasanti M, Musci G, Marlinghaus E, Suzuki H, Mariotto S (2005) Nitric oxide mediates anti-inflammatory action of extracorporeal shock waves. FEBS Lett 579(30):6839–6845
Coleman AJ, Saunders JE (1993) A review of the physical properties and biological effects of the high amplitude acoustic field used in extracorporeal lithotripsy. Ultrasonics 31:75–89
Cook J (2011) Tendinopathy: no longer a 'one size fits all' diagnosis. Br J Sports Med 45(5):385
Cook JL, Purdam CR (2009) Is tendon pathology a continuum? A pathology model to explain the clinical presentation of load-induced tendinopathy. Br J Sports Med 43(6):409–416. doi:10.1136/bjsm.2008.051193
Coombs R, Schaden W, Zhou SSH (2000) Musculoskeletal shockwave therapy. Greenwich Medical Media, London
d'Agostino MC, Craig K, Tibalt E, Respizzi S (2015) Shock wave as biological therapeutic tool: from mechanical stimulation to recovery and healing, through mechanotransduction. Int J Surg 24(Pt B):147–153
d'Agostino MC, Frairia R, Romeo P, Amelio E, Berta L, Bosco V, Gigliotti S, Guerra C, Messina S, Messuri L, Moretti B, Notarnicola A, Maccagnano G, Russo S, Saggini R, Vulpiani MC, Buselli P (2016) Extracorporeal shockwaves as regenerative therapy in orthopedic traumatology: a narrative review from basic research to clinical practice. J Biol Regul Homeost Agents 30(2):323–332
d'Agostino C, Romeo P, Amelio E, Sansone V (2011) Effectiveness of ESWT in the treatment of Kienböck's disease. Ultrasound Med Biol 37(9):1452–1456
Davis TA, Stojadinovic A, Anam K, Amare M, Naik S, Peoples GE, Tadaki D, Elster EA (2009) Extracorporeal shock wave therapy suppresses the early proinflammatory immune response to a severe cutaneous burn injury. Int Wound J 6(1):11–21
de Girolamo L, Stanco D, Galliera E, Viganò M, Lovati AB, Marazzi MG, Romeo P, Sansone V (2014) Soft-focused extracorporeal shock waves increase the expression of tendon-specific markers and the release. Ultrasound Med Biol 40(6):1204–1215
Delius M, Draenert K, Draenert Y et al (1997) Effects of extracorporeal shock waves on bone: a review of shock wave experiments and the mechanism of shock wave action. In: Siebert W, Buch M (eds) Extracorporeal shock waves in orthopaedics. Springer Verlag Berlin, pp 91–107
Fioramonti P, Cigna E, Onesti MG, Fino P, Fallico N, Scuderi N (2012) Extracorporeal shock wave therapy for the management of burn scars. Dermatol Surg 38(5):778–782
Fischer S, Mueller W, Schulte M, Kiefer J, Hirche C, Heimer S, Köllensperger E, Germann G, Reichenberger MA (2015) Multiple extracorporeal shock wave therapy degrades capsular fibrosis after insertion of silicone implants. Ultrasound Med Biol 41(3):781–789. doi:10.1016/j.ultrasmedbio.2014.10.018
Foldager CB, Kearney C, Spector M (2012) Clinical application of extracorporeal shock wave therapy in orthopedics: focused versus unfocused shock waves. Ultrasound Med Biol 38(10):1673–1680
Frairia R, Berta L (2011) Biological effects of extracorporeal shock waves on fibroblasts. A review. Muscles Ligaments Tendons J 1(4):137–146
Frizziero A, Vittadini F, Barazzuol M, Gasparre G, Finotti P, Meneghini A, Maffulli N, Masiero S (2016) Extracorporeal shockwaves therapy versus hyaluronic acid injection for the treatment of painful non-calcific rotator cuff tendinopathies: preliminary results. J Sports Med Phys Fitness Apr 12
Furia JP (2005) Safety and efficacy of extracorporeal shock wave therapy for chronic lateral epicondylitis. Am J Orthop (Belle Mead NJ) 34(1):13–9; discussion 19
Furia JP, Juliano PJ, Wade AM, Schaden W, Mittermayr R (2010a) Shock wave therapy compared with intramedullary screw fixation for nonunion of proximal fifth metatarsal metaphyseal-diaphyseal fractures. J Bone Joint Surg Am 92(4):846–854
Furia JP, Rompe JD, Cacchio A, Maffulli N (2010b) Shock wave therapy as a treatment of nonunions, avascular necrosis, and delayed healing of stress fractures. Foot Ankle Clin 15(4):651–662
Gerdesmeyer L, Henne M, Gobel M, Diehl P (2006) Physical principles and generation of shock waves in: extracorporeal shock wave therapy: clinical results, technologies, basics. Data Trace Publishing Company, Towson, pp 11–20
Gerdesmeyer L, Maier M, Haake M, Schmitz C (2002) Physical-technical principles of extracorporeal shockwave therapy (ESWT). Orthopade 31:610–617

Gerdesmeyer L, Mittermayr R, Fuerst M, Al Muderis M, Thiele R, Saxena A, Gollwitzer H (2015) Current evidence of extracorporeal shock wave therapy in chronic Achilles tendinopathy. Int J Surg 24(Pt B):154–159

Gollwitzer H, Saxena A, DiDomenico LA, Galli L, Bouché RT, Caminear DS, Fullem B, Vester JC, Horn C, Banke IJ, Burgkart R, Gerdesmeyer L (2015) Clinically relevant effectiveness of focused extracorporeal shock wave therapy in the treatment of chronic plantar fasciitis: a randomized, controlled multicenter study. J Bone Joint Surg Am 97(9):701–708. doi:10.2106/JBJS.M.01331

Gotte G, Amelio E, Russo S, Marlinghaus E, Musci G, Suzuki H (2002) Short-time non-enzymatic nitric oxide synthesis from L-arginine and hydrogen peroxide induced by shock waves treatment. FEBS Lett 520(1–3):153–155

Gruenwald I, Appel B, Kitrey ND, Vardi Y (2013) Shockwave treatment of erectile dysfunction. Ther Adv Urol 5(2):95–99

Haake M, Konig IR, Decker T, Riedel C, Buch M, Muller HH (2002) Extracorporeal shock wave therapy in the treatment of lateral epicondylitis: a randomized multicenter trial. J Bone Joint Surg Am 84-A(11):1982–1991

Hackett L, Millar NL, Lam P, Murrell GA (2016) Are the symptoms of calcific tendinitis due neoinnervation and/or neovascularization? J Bone Joint Surg Am 98(3):186–192

Han SH, Lee JW, Guyton GP, Parks BG, Courneya JP, Schon LC (2009) J.Leonard Goldner award 2008. Effect of extracorporeal shock wave therapy on cultured tenocytes. Foot Ankle Int 30(2):93–98

Haupt G (1997) [Shock waves in orthopedics]. [Article in German]. Urologe A 36(3):233–238

Hausdorf J, Sievers B, Schmitt-Sody M, Jansson V, Maier M, Mayer-Wagner S (2011) Stimulation of bone growth factor synthesis in human osteoblasts and fibroblasts after extracorporeal shock wave application. Arch Orthop Trauma Surg 131(3):303–309

Herr HW (2008) 'Crushing the stone': a brief history of lithotripsy, the first minimally invasive surgery. BJU Int 102(4):432–435

Holfeld J, Tepeköylü C, Blunder S, Lobenwein D, Kirchmair E, Dietl M, Kozaryn R, Lener D, Theurl M, Paulus P, Kirchmair R, Grimm M (2014a) Low energy shock wave therapy induces angiogenesis in acute hind-limb ischemia via VEGF receptor 2 phosphorylation. PLoS One 9(8):e103982

Holfeld J, Tepeköylü C, Kozaryn R, Urbschat A, Zacharowski K, Grimm M, Paulus P (2014b) Shockwave therapy differentially stimulates endothelial cells: implications on the control of inflammation via toll-like receptor 3. Inflammation 37(1):65–70

Holfeld J, Tepekoylu C, Reissig C, Lobenwein D, Scheller B, Kirchmair E, Kozaryn R, Albrecht-Schgoer K, Krapt C, Zins K, Urbschat A, Zacharowski K, Grimm M, Kirchmir R, Paulus P (2016) Toll-like receptor 3 signaling mediates angiogenic response upon shockwave treatment of ischemic muscle. Cardiovasc Res 109(2):331–343

Huang C, Holfeld J, Schaden W, Orgill D, Ogawa R (2013) Mechanotherapy: revisiting physical therapy and recruiting mechanobiology for a new era in medicine. Trends Mol Med 19(9):555–564

Ioppolo F, Rompe JD, Furia JP, Cacchio A (2014) Clinical application of SWT in musculoskeletal disorders. Eur J Phys Rehab Med 50:217–230

Jaalouk DE, Lammerding J (2009) Mechanotransduction gone awry. Nat Rev Mol Cell Biol 10(1):63–73

Kearney CJ, Hsu HP, Spector M (2012) The use of extracorporeal shock wave-stimulated periosteal cells for orthotopic bone generation. Tissue Eng Part A 18(13–14):1500–1508

Klonschinski T, Ament SJ, Schlereth T, Rompe JD, Birklein F (2011) Application of local anesthesia inhibits effects of low-energy extracorporeal shockwave treatment (ESWT) on nociceptors. Pain Med 12(10):1532–1537

Ko JY, Chen HS, Chen LM (2001) Treatment of lateral epicondylitis of the elbow with shock waves. Clin Orthop Relat Res 387:60–67

Kolahi KS, Mofrad MR (2010) Mechanotransduction: a major regulator of homeostasis and development. Wiley Interdiscip Rev Syst Biol Med 2(6):625–639

Kountouris A, Cook J (2007) Rehabilitation of Achilles and patellar tendinopathies. Best Pract Res Clin Rheumatol 21:295–316

Kuo YR, Wang CT, Wang FS, Yang KD, Chiang YC, Wang CJ (2009) Extracorporeal shock wave treatment modulates skin fibroblast recruitment and leukocyte infiltration for enhancing extended skin-flap survival. Wound Repair Regen 17(1):80–87

Leal C, d'Agostino C, Garcia SG, Fernandez A (2015a) Current concepts of shockwave therapy in stress fractures. Int J Surg 24(Pt B):195–200

Leal C, Ramon S, Furia J, Fernandez A, Rumero L, Hernandez-Sierra L (2015b) Current concepts of shockwave therapy in chronic patella tendinopathy. Int J Surg 24(Pt B):160–164

Lee SS, Kang S, Park NK, Lee CW, Song HS, Sohn MK, Cho KH, Kim JH (2012) Effectiveness of initial extracorporeal shock wave therapy on the newly diagnosed lateral or medial epicondylitis. Ann Rehabil Med 36(5):681–687

Lei H, Liu J, Li H, Wang L, Xu Y, Tian W, Lin G, Xin Z (2013) Low-intensity shock wave therapy and its application to erectile dysfunction. World J Mens Health 31(3):208–214

Leone L, Raffa S, Vetrano M, Ranieri D, Malisan F, Scrofani C, Vulpiani MC, Ferretti A, Torrisi MR, Visco V (2016) Extracorporeal Shock Wave Treatment (ESWT) enhances the in vitro-induced differentiation of human tendon-derived stem/progenitor cells (hTSPCs). Oncotarget 7(6):6410–6423

Lohrer H, Nauck T, Korakakis V, Malliaropoulos N (2016) Historical ESWT paradigms are overcome: a narrative review. Biomed Res Int 2016:3850461. doi:10.1155/2016/3850461. Review

Lowbenwein D, Tepekoylu C, Kozaryn R, Pechriggl EJ, Bitchse M, Graber M, Fritsch H, Samsroth S, Stefanova N, Paulus P, Czerny M, Grimm M, Holfeld J (2015) Shock wave treatment protects neuronal degeneration via a toll-like receptor 3 dependent mechanism: implications of a first-ever causal treatment for ischemic spinal cord injury. J Am Heart Assoc 4(10):e002440

Lynen N, De Vroey T, Spiegel I, Van Ongeval F, Hendrickx NJ, Stassijns G (2016) Comparison of peritendinous hyaluronan injections versus extracorporeal shock wave therapy in the treatment of painful Achilles' tendinopathy: a randomized clinical efficacy and safety study. Arch Phys Med Rehabil. doi:10.1016/j.apmr.2016.08.470

Maier M, Tischer T, Milz S, Weiler C, Nerlich A, Pellengahr C, Schmitz C, Refior HJ (2002) Dose-related effects of extracorporeal shock waves on rabbit quadriceps tendon integrity. Arch Orthop Trauma Surg 122(8):436–441

Mariotto S, de Prati AC, Cavalieri E, Amelio E, Marlinghaus E, Suzuki H (2009) Extracorporeal shock wave therapy in inflammatory diseases: molecular mechanism that triggers anti-inflammatory action. Curr Med Chem 16(19):2366–2372

Mittermayr R, Antonic V, Hartinger J, Kaufmann H, Redl H, Téot L, Stojadinovic A, Schaden W (2012) Extracorporeal shock wave therapy (ESWT) for wound healing: technology, mechanisms, and clinical efficacy. Wound Repair Regen 20(4):456–465

Moya D, Ramón S, d'Agostino MC, Leal C, Aranzabal JR, Eid J, Schaden W (2016) Incorrect methodology may favor ultrasound-guided needling over shock wave treatment in calcific tendinopathy of the shoulder. J Shoulder Elbow Surg 25(8):e241–e243

Moya D, Ramón S, Guiloff L, Gerdesmeyer L (2015) Current knowledge on evidence-based shockwave treatments for shoulder pathology. Int J Surg 24(Pt B):171–178

Notarnicola A, Moretti B (2012) The biological effects of extracorporeal shock wave therapy (ESWT) on tendon tissue. Muscles Ligaments Tendons J 2(1):33–37

Notarnicola A, Moretti L, Tafuri S, Forcignanò M, Pesce V, Moretti B (2011) Reduced local perfusion after shock wave treatment of rotator cuff tendinopathy. Ultrasound Med Biol 37(3):417–425

Notarnicola A, Pesce V, Vicenti G, Tafuri S, Forcignanò M, Moretti B (2012) SWAAT study: extracorporeal shock wave therapy and arginine supplementation and other nutraceuticals for insertional Achilles tendinopathy. Adv Ther 29(9):799–814

Novak P (2015) Physics: F-SW and R-SW. Basic information on focused and radial shock wave physics. In: Lohrer H, Gerdesmeyer L (eds) Multidisciplinary medical applications. Level 10 Buchverlag Daniela Bamberg, Heilbronn, pp 28–49

Ogden JA (2004) Extracorporeal shock wave therapy for plantar fasciitis: randomised controlled multicentre trial. Br J Sports Med 38(4):382

Ogden J, Alverez RG, Levitt RL, Johnson JE, Marlow ME (2004) Electrohydraulic high-energy shock-wave treatment for chronic plantar fasciitis. J Bone Joint Surg 86(10):2216–2228

Ogden JA, Alvarez RG, Marlow M (2002) Shockwave therapy for chronic proximal plantar fasciitis: a meta-analysis. Foot Ankle Int 23(4):301–308

Ogden JA, Toth-Kischkat A (2001) Schultheiss reiner. Principles of shock wave therapy. Clin Orthop 387:8–17

Ozturan KE, Yucel I, Cakici H, Guven M, Sungur I (2010) Autologous blood and corticosteroid injection and extracorporeal shock wave therapy in the treatment of lateral epicondylitis. Orthopedics 33(2):84–91

Pettrone FA, McCall BR (2005) Extracorporeal shock wave therapy without local anesthesia for chronic lateral epicondylitis. J Bone Joint Surg Am 87(6):1297–1304

Qureshi AA, Ross KM, Ogawa R, Orgill DP (2011) Shock wave therapy in wound healing. Plast Reconstr Surg 128(6):721e–727e

Raabe O, Shell K, Goessl A, Crispens C, Delhasse Y, Eva A, Scheiner-Bobis G, Wenisch S, Arnhold S (2013) Effect of extracorporeal shock wave on proliferation and differentiation of equine adipose tissue-derived mesenchymal stem cells in vitro. Am J Stem Cells 2(1):62–73. Print 2013

Radwan YA, ElSobhi G, Badawy WS, Reda A, Khalid S (2008) Resistant tennis elbow: shock-wave therapy versus percutaneous tenotomy. Int Orthop 32(5):671–677

Rebuzzi E, Coletti N, Schiavetti S, Giusto F (2008) Arthroscopy surgery versus shock wave therapy for chronic calcifying tendinitis of the shoulder. J Orthop Traumatol 9(4):179–185

Rees JD, Maffulli N, Cook J (2009) Management of tendinopathy. Am J Sports Med 37:1855–1867

Richardson JD, Vasko MR (2002) Cellular mechanisms of neurogenic inflammation. J Pharmacol Exp Ther 302(3):839–845

Romeo P, Lavanga V, Pagani D, Sansone V (2014) Extracorporeal shock wave therapy in musculoskeletal disorders: a review. Med Princ Pract 23(1):7–13

Rompe JD, Cacchio A, Haist J, Reiners V, Furia JP, Schmitz C, Weil L, Maffulli N (2010) Plantar fascia-specific stretching versus radial shock-wave therapy as initial treatment of plantar fasciopathy. J Bone J Surg Am 92:2514–2522

Rompe JD, Furia J, Maffulli N (2009) Eccentric loading versus eccentric loading plus shock-wave treatment for midportion achilles tendinopathy: a randomized controlled trial. Am J Sports Med 37(3):463–470

Rompe JD, Kirkpatrick CJ, Küllmer K, Schwitalle M, Krischek O (1998) Dose-related effects of shock waves on rabbit tendo Achillis. A sonographic and histological study. J Bone Joint Surg Br 80(3):546–552

Rompe JD, Maffulli N (2007) Repetitive shock wave therapy for lateral elbow tendinopathy (tennis elbow): a systematic and qualitative analysis. Br Med Bull 83:355–378

Saggini R, Di Stefano A, Saggini A, Bellomo RG (2015) Clinical application of shock wave therapy in musculoskeletal disorders: part II related to myofascial and nerve apparatus. J Biol Regul Homeost Agents 29(4):771–785

Saggini R, Figus A, Troccola A, Cocco V, Saggini A, Scuderi N (2008) Extracorporeal shock wave therapy for management of chronic ulcers in the lower extremities. Ultrasound Med Biol 34(8):1261–1271

Sansone V, MC D'A, Bonora C, Sizzano F, De Girolamo L, Romeo P (2012) Early angiogenic response to shock waves in a three-dimensional model of human microvascular endothelial cell culture (HMEC-1). J Biol Regul Homeost Agents 26(1):29–37

Schaden W, Fischer A, Sailler A (2001) Extracorporeal shock wave therapy of nonunion or delayed osseous union. Clin Orthop Relat Res 387:90–94

Schaden W, Mittermayr R, Haffner N, Smolen D, Gerdesmeyer L, Wang CJ (2015) Extracorporeal shock wave therapy (ESWT)—first choice treatment of fracture non-unions? Int J Surg 24:179–183

Schmitz C, Császár NB, Milz S, Schieker M, Maffulli N, Rompe JD, Furia JP (2015) Efficacy and safety of extracorporeal shock wave therapy for orthopedic conditions: a systematic review on studies listed in the PEDro database. Br Med Bull 116:115–138

Scott A, Danielson P (2009) An emerging role for angiogenesis in tendinopathy. Eur Musculoskelet Rev 4(1):75–76

Seil R, Wilmes P, Nührenbörger C (2006) Extracorporeal shock wave therapy for tendinopathies. Expert Rev Med Devices 3(4):463–470

Shao PL, Chiu CC, Yuen CM, Chua S, Chang LT, Sheu JJ, Sun CK, Wu CJ, Wang CJ, Yip HK (2010) Shock wave therapy effectively attenuates inflammation in rat carotid artery following endothelial denudation by balloon catheter. Cardiology 115(2):130–144. doi:10.1159/000262331

Sharma P, Maffulli N (2005) Tendon injury and tendinopathy: healing and repair. J Bone Join Surg AM 87A(1):187–202

Speed C (2014) A systematic review of shockwave therapies in soft tissue conditions: focusing on the evidence. Br J Sports Med 48(21):1538–1542

Suhr F, Delhasse Y, Bungartz G, Schmidt A, Pfannkuche K, Bloch W (2013) Cell biological effects of mechanical stimulations generated by focused extracorporeal shock wave applications on cultured human bone marrow stromal cells. Stem Cell Res 11(2):951–964

Sukubo NG, Tibalt E, Respizzi S, Locati M, d'Agostino MC (2015) Effect of shock waves on macrophages: a possible role in tissue regeneration and remodeling. Int J Surg 24(Pt B):124–130

Tamma R, dell'Endice S, Notarnicola A, Moretti L, Patella S, Patella V, Zallone A, Moretti B (2009) Extracorporeal shock waves stimulate osteoblast activities. Ultrasound Med Biol 35(12):2093–2100

Tara S, Miyamoto M, Takagi G, Kirinoki-Ichikawa S, Tezuka A, Hada T, Takagi I (2014) Low-energy extracorporeal shock wave therapy improves microcirculation blood flow of ischemic limbs in patients with peripheral arterial disease: pilot study. J Nippon Med Sch 81(1):19–27

Tepeköylü C, Lobenwein D, Blunder S, Kozaryn R, Dietl M, Ritschl P, Pechriggl EJ, Blumer MJ, Bitsche M, Schistek R, Kotsch K, Fritsch H, Grimm M, Holfeld J (2015) Alteration of inflammatory response by shock wave therapy leads to reduced calcification of decellularized aortic xenografts in mice. Eur J Cardiothorac Surg 47(3):e80–e90

Tepekoylu C, Wang FS, Kozaryn R, Albrecht-Schgoer K, Theurl M, Schaden W, Ke HJ, Yang Y, Kircmair R, Grimm M, Wand CJ, Holfeld J (2013) Shock wave treatment induces angiogenesis and mobilizes endogenous CD31/CD34-positive endothelial cells in a hindlimb ischemic model: implications for angiogenesis and vasculogenesis. J Thorac Cardiovasc Surg 146(4):971–978

Thiel M (2001) Application of shock waves in medicine. Clin Orthop Relat Res 387:18–21

Thiele S, Thiele R, Gerdesmeyer L (2015) Lateral epicondylitis: this is still a main indication for extracorporeal shock wave therapy. Int J Surg 24(Pt B):165–170

Tsuzaki M, Bynum D, Almekinders L, Yang X, Faber J, Banes AJ (2003a) ATP modulates load-inducible IL-1beta, COX 2, and MMP-3 gene expression in human tendon cells. J Cell Biochem 89:556–562

Tsuzaki M, Guyton G, Garrett W, Archambault JM, Herzog W, Almekinders L, Bynum D, Yang X, Banes AJ (2003b) IL-1 beta induces COX2, MMP-1, -3 and -13, ADAMTS- 4, IL-1 beta and IL-6 in human tendon cells. J Orthop Res 21:256–264

Ueberle F (1997) Shock wave technology. In: Siebert W, Buch M (eds) Extracorporeal shock waves in orthopaedics. Springer, Berlin, pp 59–87

Valchanou VD, Michailov P (1991) High energy shock waves in the treatment of delayed and nonunion of fractures. Int Orthop 15(3):181–184

Vetrano M, d'Alessandro F, Torrisi MR, Ferretti A, Vulpiani MC, Visco V (2011) Extracorporeal shock wave therapy promotes cell proliferation and collagen synthesis of primary cultured human tenocytes. Knee Surg Sports Traumatol Arthrosc 19(12):2159–2168

Visco V, Vulpiani MC, Torrisi MR, Ferretti A, Pavan A, Vetrano M (2014) Experimental studies on the biological effects of extracorporeal shock wave therapy on tendon models. A review of the literature. Muscles Ligaments Tendons J 4(3):357–361

Vulpiani MC, Vetrano M, Trischitta D, Scarcello L, Chizzi F, Argento G, Saraceni VM, Maffulli N, Ferretti A (2012) Extracorporeal shock wave therapy in early osteonecrosis of the femoral head: prospective clinical study with long-term follow-up. Arch Orthop Trauma Surg 132(4):499–508

Wang CJ (2003) An overview of shock wave therapy in musculoskeletal disorders. Chang Gung Med J 26(4):220–232

Wang CJ (2012) Extracorporeal shockwave therapy in musculoskeletal disorders. J Orthop Surg Res 7:11. doi:10.1186/1749-799X-7-11

Wang CJ, Chen HS, Chen WS, Chen LM (2000) Treatment of painful heels using extracorporeal shock wave. J Formos Med Assoc 99(7):580–583

Wang CJ, Wang FS, Yang KD, Huang CS, Hsu CC, Yang LC (2003) Shock wave therapy induced neovascularization at the tendon–bone junction. A study in rabbits. J Orthop Res 21:984–989

Wang FS, Wang CJ, Sheen-Chen SM, Kuo YR, Chen RF, Yang KD (2002a) Superoxide mediates shock wave induction of ERK-dependent osteogenic transcription factor (CBFA1) and mesenchymal cell differentiation toward osteoprogenitors. J Biol Chem 277(13):10931–10937

Wang FS, Yang KD, Chen RF, Wang CJ, Sheen-Chen SM (2002b) Extracorporeal shock wave promotes growth and differentiation of bone-marrow stromal cells towards osteoprogenitors associated with induction of TGF-beta1. J Bone Joint Surg Br 84(3):457–461

Waugh CM, Morrissey D, Jones E, Riley GP, Langberg H, Screen HR (2015) In vivo biological response to extracorporeal shockwave therapy in human tendinopathy. Eur Cell Mater 29:268–80; discussion 280

Wess O, Ueberle F, Duhrsen RN et al (1997) Working group technical developments—consensus report. In: Chaussy C, Eisenberger F, Jocham D, Wilbert D (eds) High energy shock waves in medicine. Thieme, Stuttgart, pp 59–71

van der Worp H, van den Akker-Scheek I, van Schie H, Zwerver J (2013) ESWT for tendinopathy: technology and clinical implications. Knee Surg Sports Traumatol Arthrosc 21(6):1451–1458

Zhang D, Kearney CJ, Cheriyan T, Schmid TM, Spector M (2011) Extracorporeal shockwave-induced expression of lubricin in tendons and septa. Cell Tissue Res 346(2):255–262

Zwerver J, Hartgens F, Verhagen E, van der Worp H, van den Akker-Scheek I, Diercks RL (2011) No effect of extracorporeal shockwave therapy on patellar tendinopathy in jumping athletes during the competitive season: a randomized clinical trial. Am J Sports Med 39:1191–1199

Zwerver J, Waugh C, van der Worp H, Scott A (2016) Can shockwave therapy improve tendon metabolism? Adv Exp Med Biol 920:275–281

Index

G.L. Canata et al. (eds.), *Muscle and Tendon Injuries*, DOI 10.1007/978-3-662-54184-5

MIX
Papier aus verantwortungsvollen Quellen
Paper from responsible sources
FSC® C105338

If you have any concerns about our products,
you can contact us on
ProductSafety@springernature.com

In case Publisher is established outside the EU,
the EU authorized representative is:
Springer Nature Customer Service Center GmbH
Europaplatz 3, 69115 Heidelberg, Germany

Printed by Libri Plureos GmbH
in Hamburg, Germany